Molecular Endocrinology

SECOND EDITION

Molecular Endocrinology

SECOND EDITION

Franklyn F. Bolander

Department of Biology
University of South Carolina
Columbia, South Carolina

Academic Press

San Diego   New York   Boston
London   Sydney   Tokyo   Toronto

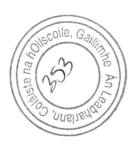

This book is printed on acid-free paper. ∞

Academic Press, Inc.
A Division of Harcourt Brace & Company
525 B Street, Suite 1900, San Diego, California 92101-4495

United Kingdom Edition published by
Academic Press Limited
24-28 Oval Road, London NW1 7DX

Library of Congress Cataloging-in-Publication Data

Bolander, Franklyn F.
    Molecular endocrinology / by Franklyn F. Bolander. -- 2nd ed.
        p.   cm.
    Includes bibliographical references and index.
    ISBN 0-12-111231-4
    1. Molecular endocrinology.   I. Title.
    QP187.3.M64M62   1994
    599'.0142--dc20   94-10458
                                                                    CIP

PRINTED IN THE UNITED STATES OF AMERICA
94   95   96   97   98   99   MM   9   8   7   6   5   4   3   2   1

Dedicated to all of my teachers.
May I return their favors to the
next generation.

Contents

Part 4
Gene Regulation by Hormones 387

Part 5
Special Topics 491

Preface to the Second Edition

The publication of one's first book is a cause for both celebration and consternation. Obviously, one is proud of the accomplishment, but one is also acutely aware of its shortcomings: inadvertent errors, topics omitted or poorly covered, and so on. The second edition is my chance to correct these oversights, incorporate changes suggested by colleagues, and update the material. A summary of the major changes is described here.

The biggest explosion in information over the past few years has been in the areas of growth factors and hematopoietic-immune factors; both of these areas are highly relevant to cancer and transplantation research. To accommodate this new information, Part 1 of the second edition adds a third chapter that presents nonclassical hormones, including parahormones, growth factors, hematopoietic-immune factors, and nonvertebrate and plant hormones. The last two lay the foundation for the chapter on evolution later in the book.

The material on receptors (Part 2) has also been expanded and updated. Since publication of the first edition, the structure–function relationships of many hormone receptors have been studied in great depth; furthermore, the DNA-binding domain of several nuclear receptors and the extracellular domain of some membrane receptors have had their three-dimensional structures solved. In addition to this general information, several entirely new groups of receptors, which did not even exist at the time of the first edition, have been added: guanylate cyclase, serine kinase, and the cytokine and RXR receptors. Finally, several new subfamilies of the serpentine receptors are also covered.

Part 3 (Transduction) contains several new topics, including small G proteins, pH, and the protein tyrosine phosphatases. The chapter on phosphorylation has been completely rewritten. In particular, the number of kinases discussed has increased and their hierarchy and interrelationships are explored.

The chapter on transcriptional regulation has also been completely revised. Since the first edition, many transcription factors have been sequenced and their regulation, especially by phosphorylation, has been characterized. These data form the new core of the chapter, which emphasizes how hormones regulate them and how they regulate transcription.

The chapters in Part 5 (Special Topics) have been expanded. The number of clinical syndromes attributed to molecular defects in the endocrine pathway has grown and now includes defects in transcription factors, receptors, G proteins, kinases, and phospholipases. This chapter also now includes somatic mutations in tumors, for example, estrogen receptor mutations in breast cancer and androgen receptor mutations in prostate cancer. The chapter on oncogenes has been enlarged to include both the entire range of host–pathogen interactions as they pertain to the endocrine system and a new section on antioncogenes.

Throughout all of these revisions, I have tried not to change the original intent and style of the first edition: the text should be self-contained, focused, and easily readable, and it should emphasize perspective and interrelationships. I believe that I have succeeded.

Finally, I thank Clint Cook for the computer graphics, Kimberly Loman and Elizabeth Knapp for artwork, and many colleagues for helpful suggestions. I also acknowledge Grant CA-42009 from the National Institutes of Health for supporting some of the research discussed herein.

Preface to the First Edition

For several years I have taught a graduate level course in molecular endocrinology. The recent, explosive growth of this field is both exciting and awesome. Unfortunately, it has also made the teaching of my course extremely difficult: there is more and more information to cover in less and less time, and the reading lists have become unreasonably long. I searched in vain for a textbook that would give my students a solid background in the basics of molecular endocrinology so that I could use class time more effectively. It was from that futile search that this text was conceived. It is hoped that professionals in related fields will also find this book to be a helpful summary and general reference source.

This book has several objectives: (1) to present a succinct summary of molecular endocrinology, (2) to offer a perspective and synthesis of this information, and (3) to introduce certain useful techniques to the reader. Although this text attempts to cover, in one place, all of the major facets of this field, it is not meant to be an all-inclusive compendium. Rather, it covers basic principles using selected examples. This allows for a streamlined text, where major concepts are preeminent. However, the information should be easily transferable to other systems that may be of more interest to the reader.

Perspective is achieved in two ways. First, by having all of the aspects of molecular endocrinology in a single book, interrelationships become more apparent. Second, selected controversial topics are discussed in depth in order to give the reader a better feel for the current attitudes in these areas.

Finally, certain useful techniques are presented, both because of their importance to particular topics and to alert students that such methodology exists and may be of use to them in their research. The text does not go into "recipe" details but rather tries to concentrate on advantages, disadvantages, and applicability of each technique.

The book begins with a brief summary of general endocrinology. I have found that my students have diverse backgrounds and many have never had a course in endocrinology. Therefore, this section was added to provide a basic introduction; for those readers with a better background, it may serve as a brief review and reference source. The remainder of the text discusses the molecular aspects of hormone action in chronological order: hormone–

receptor interactions, second messenger generation, gene induction, and post-transcriptional control. At the end, certain special topics are covered.

I would like to thank the staff of Academic Press for their patience and editorial assistance, the anonymous reviewers for their many helpful comments and corrections, Melanie Trimble for most of the art work, and Debra Williams for her secretarial assistance. I would also like to acknowledge Grants HD-16283 and CA-42009 from the National Institutes of Health for supporting some of the research discussed herein.

PART *1*

Introduction and General Endocrinology

CHAPTER **1**

Introduction

CHAPTER OUTLINE

I. Definitions

Endocrinology is the study of hormones; but what are hormones? The question is far more difficult to answer today than it was a few decades ago. The classic definition is that hormones are chemical substances produced by specialized tissues and secreted into blood, in which they are carried to target organs (1). However, this definition was constructed when most of the available knowledge of endocrinology was restricted to vertebrate systems. As the field of endocrinology has expanded, new hormones and new systems that would not be included under this definition have been discovered. It is useful to describe these discrepancies so that a more functional definition can be developed:

1. Specialized tissues for hormone synthesis. Discrete endocrine glands exist only in arthropods, mollusks, and vertebrates, although chemical substances that have hormonal activity have been identified throughout the animal, plant, and fungal kingdoms. Even in vertebrates, a class of hormones, the *parahormones*, exists that is designed to act locally. Since these compounds are made wherever they are needed, they tend to have a nearly ubiquitous distribution. Finally, many vertebrate growth factors are synthesized in multiple locations.

2. Blood for hormone distribution. First, blood is unique to vertebrates. The addition of hemolymph to the definition would permit arthropod hormones to be included, but hormones of plants and lower animals would still be omitted. Second, even in vertebrates the parahormones diffuse through the extracellular fluid to reach their local targets. Other hormones are released by neurons and also have local effects. Finally, the classic definition would exclude *ectohormones*, hormones that traverse air or water to act between or among individuals. These hormones are particularly well developed in certain insect species and include *pheromones* (sexual attractants), *gamones* (inducers of sexual development), and *allomones* and *kairomones* (interspecies attractants).

3. A separate target organ. Some parahormones, once secreted, not only diffuse to surrounding cells but also stimulate the cells originally synthesizing them. This positive feedback is referred to as *autocrine* function, and results in the synthesizing cell becoming its own target organ. Furthermore, bacteria make several regulatory molecules for internal use. These signal molecules, called *alarmones*, are usually modified nucleotides and are produced in response to a particular stress such as starvation or a vitamin deficiency.

Because of these limitations, this book will use a broader definition: A *hormone* is a chemical, nonnutrient, intercellular messenger that is effective at micromolar concentrations or less. In other words, hormones are chemical substances that carry information between two or more cells. This definition would include all the preceding examples except the alarmones. That exclusion is clearly the bias of the author, but the essence of *endocrinology* is the chemical coordination of bodily functions and alarmones are used exclusively in single cells. The restriction of hormones to chemical substances seems initially to be a logical one, although species such as fireflies can use light to induce behavioral patterns in others. However, now that the visual pigment rhodopsin and the catecholamine receptor have been shown to be homologous, one must begin to wonder whether this exclusion is also arbitrary. Finally, metabolic pathways can be induced or repressed by substrate levels; indeed, substrate flow is an important regulator in many systems. Therefore, nutrients are also excluded. The inclusion of the concentration clause is used to eliminate other miscellaneous inducers; the one thing that sets hormones apart from other chemical regulators is their effectiveness at extremely low concentrations, usually in the nanomolar range or below. Plant hormones are unusual because they are often required in larger amounts; for this reason the micromolar limit was used.

Having established working definitions for endocrinology and hormones, it is now appropriate to consider one for molecular endocrinology: *molecular endocrinology* is the study of hormone action at the cellular and molecular level. In particular, this book will concentrate on the molecular mechanisms of hormone action and interaction. However, the topic of hormonal synergism and antagonism at the molecular level is better understood against a background knowledge of hormone action in the whole organism; for example, the progesterone inhibition of prolactin receptors and second messengers in the mammary gland is merely an isolated fact unless one knows the general function of these hormones in the reproductive cycle. Therefore, the function of this part of the book is to provide the reader in general, and the novice in particular, with sufficient background information to appreciate the molecular interrelationships that will be developed in later parts. Obviously a complete presentation of general endocrinology cannot be accomplished in only three chapters: the coverage is specifically oriented and only sufficient to prepare the reader for the remainder of the book. However, it is hoped that the reader will become interested enough to consult any of the excellent, and far more comprehensive, texts listed in the general references at the end of this chapter.

The rest of this chapter is concerned with identifying the basic characteristics of hormones and their regulation and concludes with an illustrative example — the hormonal control of calcium metabolism. Chapter 2 then examines the other classical endocrine systems. Finally, Chapter 3 briefly covers nonclassical and nonvertebrate hormones such as growth factors, parahormones, and the hormones of plants and insects.

II. Hormone – Target Relationships

As noted earlier, the classical endocrine system involves a hormone being made in one part of the body and reaching its target in another part of the body via the bloodstream (Fig. 1-1A). However, many other types of interactions can occur. In a paracrine system, the hormone remains in the tissue, where it reaches nearby cells by diffusion (Fig. 1-1B). The hormone may even influence the cell that originally secreted it; this is often part of a negative or positive feedback loop (Fig, 1-1C). This system is called an autocrine system. All these systems are open, that is, there are no diffusion barriers and selectivity of target cells is determined by the presence or absence of receptors to that hormone. In contrast, a *cryptocrine* system involves the secretion of a hormone into a closed environment. This system obviously requires a very special intimacy between cells, as occurs between Sertoli cells and spermatids or thymic nurse cells and T lymphocytes (Fig. 1-1D). Another example of this phenomenon is the transfer of second messengers, such as

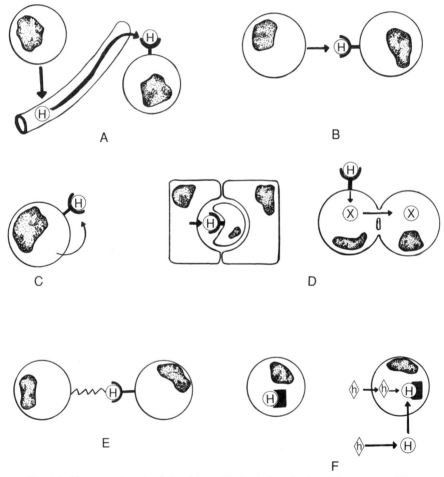

Fig. 1-1. Hormone–target relationships: (A) classical endocrine, (B) paracrine, (C) autocrine, (D) cryptocrine, (E) juxtacrine, (F) intracrine. H, Hormone; encircled H, active hormone; h within a diamond, prohormone; X, second messenger.

cyclic nucleotides or inositol trisphosphate, through gap junctions between adjacent cells.

The *juxtacrine* system represents another mechanism for limiting the diffusion of hormones. In this case, the hormone is synthesized as a membrane-bound precusor. Although this precursor is usually cleaved to yield a soluble peptide, it may also remain attached to the plasma membrane, where it retains its biological activity. Therefore, its effects are limited to the length of its tether (Fig. 1-1E). Hormones that may act in this fashion include the epidermal growth factor, transforming growth factor-α, tumor necrosis factor-α, colony stimulating factor-1, and the kit ligand (see Chapter 3).

Finally, the *intracrine* system is one in which hormone synthesis and receptor binding occur intracellularly; a possible example is the *Ah* (*a*romatic *h*ydrocarbon) receptor (Fig. 1-1F). This receptor was originally identified as the dioxin-binding protein and is responsible for mediating the induction of enzymes that metabolize aromatic hydrocarbons. Researchers believe that its natural ligand is some hydrophobic metabolite or nutrient within the cell. Normally, this system would not be considered a hormone system in this text, but several variations of the definition would qualify. For example, intracrine systems would also include the endogenous generation of hormones from precursors synthesized elsewhere. The thyroid gland secretes predominantly thyroxine; this compound is converted to the active form, triiodothyronine, by peripheral enzymes. The sex steroids represent another example; 40% of all androgens in males and 75–100% of estrogens in postmenopausal females are generated in target tissues from adrenal precursors (2). This generation can be both positively and negatively regulated: aromatase and 5α-reductase can synthesize the active steroid, whereas sulfotransferases can inactivate these compounds. These enzymes allow the tissue to adjust the hormone levels to local conditions. Another mechanism by which this can be accomplished is through the production of hormone-binding proteins that can either inhibit hormone action by sequestration or enhance activity by maintaining a high local concentration, depending on the particular binding protein and other conditions (see Chapter 2).

III. Chemical Nature

Structurally, hormones are extremely diverse (Fig. 1-2). The most abundant and most versatile of these are the peptide and protein hormones, which range in size from a simple tripeptide (thyrotropin-releasing hormone) to 198 amino acids (prolactin). Some protein hormones, such as human chorionic gonadotropin, are even larger because of multiple subunits and glycosylation. In addition to full proteins, individual amino acids have been modified to yield hormones; the most common amino acid precursors are tyrosine (the catecholamines and thyroid hormones), histidine (histamine), and tryptophan (serotonin and indoleacetic acid).

The lipids constitute another rich source of hormones. The steroids form

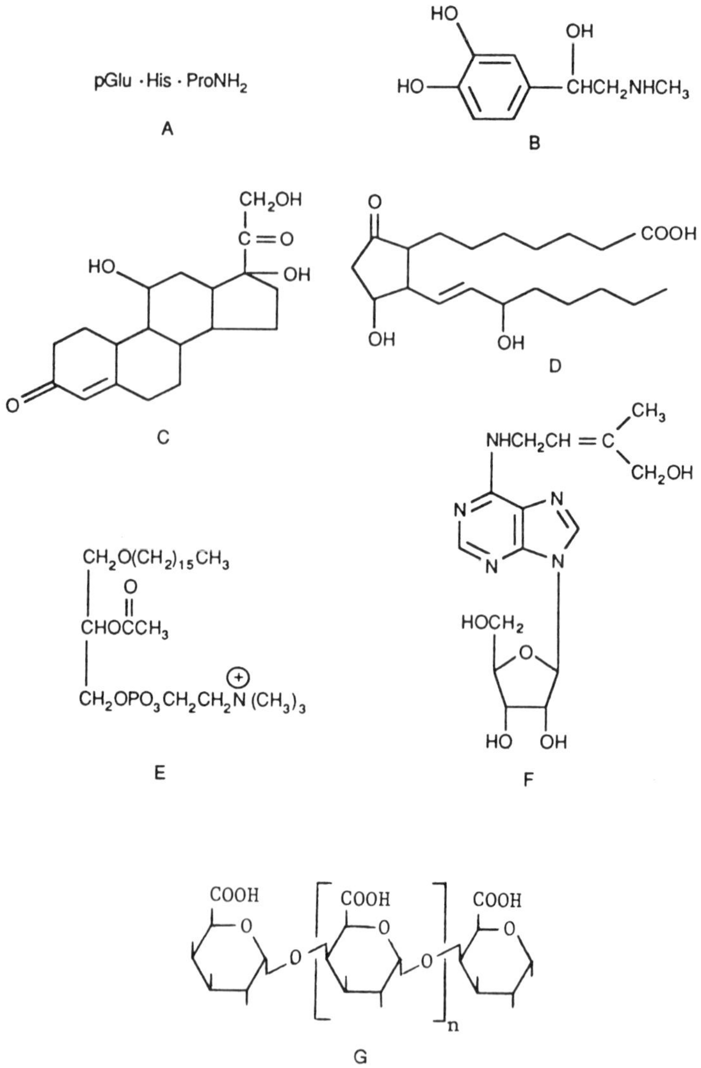

Fig. 1-2. Structural diversity of hormones. (A) thyrotropin-releasing hormone, (B) epinephrine, (C) cortisol, (D) prostaglandin, (E) platelet-activating factor, (F) zeatin (a cytokinin), (G) α-1,4-oligogalacturonide (an elicitor).

an entire group by themselves. Fatty acid derivatives include the prostaglandins and related compounds; some insect pheromones are also synthesized from fatty acids. Finally, the structure of platelet-activating factor is similar to that of phosphatidylcholine (3).

The nucleotides would seem to be an unusual source, but they too are well represented: some pheromones, the cytokinins (plant hormones), 1-methyladenine (a starfish hormone), cyclic AMP (in slime molds), and, if the reader lacks the bias of the author, many alarmones are nucleotide derivatives.

Oligosaccharides form the most recently identified group of hormones. They were first characterized in plants, in which they are produced from the breakdown of the plant cell wall in response to certain plant infections. These *elicitors* then trigger a defense response within the plant cell (4). Carbohydrate hormones have now been postulated to occur in animals: the *aggregation factor* of sponges is a glycan (5), one of the mediators of insulin action appears to be an oligosaccharide (see Chapter 10), and β-glucan and pectin can act as secretagogues (secretion stimulators) in vertebrates (6). In the latter case, the physiological relevance is still uncertain.

Although the structural diversity of hormones is great, one property is particularly important: water solubility (Table 1-1). Hydrophobic hormones are difficult to store because they pass through membranes so easily; as a result, they are synthesized as they are needed. The thyroid hormones are an exception and will be discussed further later. Hydrophobic hormones do not dissolve readily in water; therefore, they require serum transport proteins with hydrophobic pockets. Because they are partially hidden in these pockets, these proteins are protected and their half-lives are long. Finally, their hydrophobicity allows them to cross the plasma membrane, bind to cytoplasmic or nuclear receptors, and elicit direct cellular effects.

Hydrophilic hormones, however, can be contained within membrane vesicles so they can be stored. Although a few of the smaller peptides are known to bind to serum proteins, most of the water-soluble hormones are transported free in the serum, however, as a result they are rapidly eliminated from the circulation. Because they cannot cross the plasmalemma, they must interact with their receptors at the cell surface and generate a second signal to affect cellular processes, that is, their mechanism of action is indirect.

IV. Biological Activity

What are the functions of hormones? Hormones coordinate nearly all the biological activities within an organism; these activities are primarily metabolism, growth, and reproduction (Table 1-2). *Metabolism* is the sum of all

Table 1-1
A Comparison of Hydrophobic and Hydrophilic Hormones

Characteristic	Hydrophobic	Hydrophilic
Examples	Steroids and thyronines	Peptides and catecholamines
Storage after synthesis	Minimal except for thyronines	Yes
Binding proteins	Always	Sometimes, especially smaller peptides
Half-life	Long (hours or days)	Short (minutes)
Receptors	Cytoplasmic or nuclear	Plasma membrane
Mechanism of action	Direct	Indirect (second messenger)

Table 1-2

Some Major Vertebrate Hormones and Their Characteristics

Hormone	Structure	Mechanism[a]	Source	Target	Action
Calcium metabolism					
Parathormone (PTH)	Peptide	cAMP, calcium	Parathyroid gland	Bone, kidney	Bone resorption; renal calcium resorption
PTH-related protein	Peptide	cAMP	Mammary gland and uterus	Mammary gland, placenta	Local calcium transport
Calcitonin (CT)	Peptide	cAMP, calcium	C cells (thyroid gland)	Bone	Inhibits bone resorption
1,25-Dihydroxycholecalciferol (1,25-DHCC)	Steroid derivative	DNA binding	Skin, liver kidney	Intestine, kidney	Intestinal calcium absorption; renal resorption
Tropic hormones					
Adrenocorticotropic hormone (ACTH)	Protein	cAMP	Adenohypophysis	Adrenal cortex	Stimulates glucocorticoid synthesis and secretion
Luteinizing hormone (LH)/human chorionic gonadotropin (hCG)	Protein	cAMP	Adenohypophysis/placenta	Gonads	Stimulates progesterone (♀) and testosterone (♂) synthesis and secretion
Follicle-stimulating hormone (FSH)	Protein	cAMP	Adenohypophysis	Gonads	Stimulates estrogen synthesis and secretion (♀) and gamete development
Thyroid-stimulating hormone (TSH)	Protein	cAMP	Adenohypophysis	Thyroid	Stimulates thyroid hormone synthesis and secretion
Melanocyte-stimulating hormone (MSH)	Peptide	cAMP	Hypophysis	Melanocyte	Skin darkening
Sodium and water metabolism/blood pressure					
Antidiuretic hormone (ADH)/vasopressin (VP)	Peptide	cAMP, calcium	Neurohypophysis	Kidney, liver	Renal water resorption and glycogenolysis
Angiotensin II (AT)	Peptide	Calcium	Liver	Adrenal cortex, vasculature	Stimulates aldosterone synthesis and secretion; vasoconstriction
Aldosterone	Steroid	DNA binding	Adrenal cortex	Kidney	Renal sodium and water resorption

Hormone	Chemical class	Second messenger	Source	Target	Action
Atrial natriuretic factor (ANF)	Peptide	cGMP	Atria	Kidney, vasculature	Sodium diuresis; angiotensin II antagonist
Endothelins (ETs)	Peptide	Calcium	Endothelium	Vasculature	Vasoconstriction and smooth muscle growth
Nitric oxide (NO)	NO	cGMP	Endothelium and other tissues	Vasculature	Vasodilates and decreases platelet adhesion
Reproductive hormones					
Estrogens	Steroids	DNA binding	Ovary, placenta	Reproductive tract, etc.	Sexual characteristics
Androgens	Steroids	DNA binding	Testis, adrenal cortex	Reproductive tract, etc.	Sexual characteristics; spermatogenesis
Progesterone	Steroid	DNA binding	Ovary, placenta	Reproductive tract, etc.	Pregnancy maintenance
Relaxin	Peptide	cAMP	Ovary	Public symphysis	Parturition
Prolactin (PRL)	Peptide	Unknown	Adenohypophysis	Mammary gland	Lactation
Oxytocin (OT)	Peptide	Calcium	Neurohypophysis	Mammary gland, uterus	Milk ejection, parturition
Inhibin/activin	Peptides	Serine kinase	Gonads	Hypothalamopituitary axis, gametes	Inhibition of FSH (inhibin); gametogenesis
Energy metabolism					
Growth hormone (GH)/somatotropin	Peptide	Unknown	Adenohypophysis	Multiple	Lipolysis; glucose sparing; general body growth
Glucocorticoids	Steroids	DNA binding	Adrenal cortex	Muscle, liver	Gluconeogenesis
Triiodothyronine (T$_3$)	Tyrosine derivative	DNA binding	Thyroid gland	Multiple	Lipolysis; glycogenolysis
Glucagon	Peptide	cAMP	α Cells (pancreas)	Liver	Glycogenolysis; gluconeogenesis
Epinephrine (E)	Tyrosine derivative	cAMP, calcium	Adrenal medulla	Fat, muscle	Lipolysis; glycogenolysis
Insulin	Peptide	Tyrosine kinase, oligosaccharides	β Cells (pancreas)	Multiple	Lipid, protein, and glycogen synthesis
Neurotransmitters					
Norepinephrine (NE)	Tyrosine derivative	cAMP, calcium	Central and sympathetic nervous system	Multiple	"Fight-or-flight" response

continues

continued

Hormone	Structure	Mechanism[a]	Source	Target	Action
Dopamine	Tyrosine derivative	cAMP, calcium	Hypothalamus, etc.	Adenohypophysis, etc.	Inhibition of PRL secretion
Acetylcholine (ACh)	Amino alcohol derivative	Sodium	Central and parasympathetic nervous system	Muscles, etc.	Maintenance of involuntary activity and muscle contraction
Glutamate (Glu)	Amino acid	Calcium	Central nervous system	Central nervous system	Stimulatory transmitter
γ-Aminobutyric acid (GABA)	Glutamate derivative	Chloride	Central nervous system	Central nervous system	Inhibitory transmitter
Glycine (Gly)	Amino acid	Chloride	Spinal cord	Spinal cord	Inhibitory transmitter

Release and inhibiting factors: see Table 2-1
Local gastrointestinal hormones: see Table 2-5
Growth and growth-inhibiting factors: see Table 3-1
Immuno-inflammatory hormones: see Table 3-2
Parahormones: see Table 3-3

[a] The mediators listed are the primary or best characterized ones; the list is not meant to be all-inclusive. The given mediators may be either positively or negatively affected, depending on the particular hormone.

processes that handle or alter materials within living organisms and can be divided into (i) mineral and water metabolism and (ii) energy metabolism. Hormones involved in the former regulate the absorption, storage, and secretion of electrolytes and water; their function is to maintain a constant ionic environment inside the body. Hormones involved in energy metabolism regulate the flow of organic substrates through chemical pathways to maintain appropriate ATP levels within the cell. Insulin is a hormone of energy storage because it shunts substrates into macromolecular reservoirs: glucose into glycogen, amino acids into protein, and fatty acids into triacylglycerides. Most of the other hormones regulating energy metabolism are involved in energy expenditure, that is, they break down these reservoirs and shunt the liberated substrates into chemical pathways that generate ATP.

Growth is the enlargement of a cell, tissue, or organism by the net accumulation of material and/or an increase in cell number. This is a very complex process requiring the coordination of both mitosis and metabolism, which must supply the necessary materials and energy. Not surprisingly, some of these hormones, such as growth hormone, are involved in regulating both growth and metabolism. In addition to generalized growth, hormones can selectively affect certain tissues, such as epidermal or neural tissues.

Reproduction is the process by which an organism generates and (sometimes) nourishes a new member of the species. It too is a very complex process: sex steroids and gonadotropins promote gametogenesis; relaxin and oxytocin stimulate lactation and suckling.

In addition to these broad functions, many more specialized functions are served by hormones. Both the tropic hormones and the releasing and inhibiting factors participate in a regulatory hierarchy and merely stimulate or block the synthesis and secretion of hormones from other glands. The parahormones are made and act locally; for example, most of the eicosanoids are involved in inflammation, blood clotting, or smooth muscle contraction. Finally, the gastrointestinal tract contains many hormones that act regionally to facilitate the digestion and absorption of ingested material.

One other group of hormones listed in Table 1-2 is the neurotransmitters. At first, the group may seem somewhat out of place, since the endocrine and nervous systems have classically been considered distinct entities. However, neurotransmitters satisfy the definition of a hormone developed in Section I. In addition, many molecules can function as hormones or as neurotransmitters, for example, the catecholamines and the gastrointestinal hormones. Consequently, the two systems have become partially fused into a neuroendocrine system, which may be considered appropriate subject matter for an endocrinology text.

V. Control

In the following sections, many different hormones will be discussed. Although their actions may vary considerably, their regulation will conform to a limited number of mechanisms. The simplest is *negative feedback*: rising levels of a hormone shut off its production so that a constant or desired concentration can be maintained. Because many glands in the body are under hierarchical control, this negative feedback can occur at several levels (Fig. 1-3A). For example, the hypothalamus produces releasing factors that stimulate the secretion of hormones from the anterior pituitary; most of these hormones will, in turn, stimulate other glands in the body (see Chapter 2, Section II). The hormones from these peripheral glands may have a feedback effect primarily on the anterior pituitary or on the hypothalamus.

Positive feedback, in which rising hormone levels stimulate further hormone production, is less common because it can produce a vicious cycle.

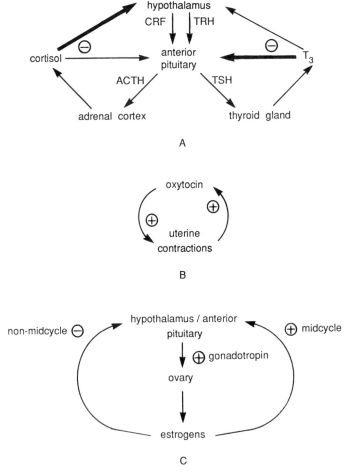

Fig. 1-3. Feedback regulation of hormone secretion. (A) negative feedback, (B) positive feedback, (C) cycle-dependent feedback. ACTH, Adrenocorticotropic hormone; CRF, corticotropin-releasing factor; T_3, triiodothyronine; TRH, thyrotropin-releasing hormone; TSH, thyroid-stimulating hormone (thyrotropin).

However, if there is a clear termination point in the cycle, such positive feedback can greatly augment the initial stimulus without going out of control. An example is the stimulus control of oxytocin, a hormone secreted by the posterior pituitary (Fig. 1-3B). As parturition nears, uterine contractions begin and stimulate the release of oxytocin, a potent inducer of smooth muscle contraction. As a result, the uterus contracts harder and further stimulates oxytocin secretion. When the fetus is finally expelled, the cycle is broken.

Finally, the type of feedback may be dependent on other physiological parameters. For example, estrogen normally has a negative feedback effect on the hypothalamic–pituitary axis (Fig. 1-3C). However, at midcycle, the axis suddenly becomes stimulated by estrogen, a positive feedback is established, and estrogen levels rise until they trigger a surge of luteinizing hormone, which leads to ovulation.

VI. Hormonal Control of Calcium Metabolism

A. Introduction

The hormonal regulation of calcium homeostasis represents an ideal introduction to endocrinology because it is a relatively simple, closed system involving three hormones (parathormone, calcitonin, and the active form of vitamin D) and three organs (bone, kidney, and the gastrointestinal tract). The function of these hormones is to maintain a constant calcium concentration in the blood, because this ion is critically involved in the activity of excitable tissues such as nerves and muscles. Elevated calcium levels depress electrical activity, whereas low calcium levels enhance such activity. For example, patients with hypercalcemia exhibit muscular weakness, bradycardia (slow heartbeat), lethargy, and confusion and, in severe cases, may become comatose. Patients with hypocalcemia, however, may demonstrate muscular spasms (tetany), irritability, psychosis, and even seizures. Another problem requiring tight regulation of calcium levels is its poor solubility; if the concentration of calcium in biological fluids becomes too high, it can precipitate out of solution anywhere. This phenomenon is called *ectopic calcification*. Therefore, it is readily understandable why the body controls calcium levels so rigidly.

The concentration of calcium in the blood is kept between 2.2 and 2.55 mM and exists in three forms: bound, complexed, and free. About 30% of the calcium is bound to protein, primarily serum albumin; another 10% is complexed to various chelators such as citrate; the remaining 60% is free or ionized. Only the latter form is important in biological activities; therefore, free calcium is the fraction that is tightly regulated. For example, in certain liver diseases the synthesis of serum albumin levels declines, so total calcium declines also. However, the patient shows no evidence of hypocalcemia, because the free calcium is still normal.

Although the blood level of calcium is regulated, blood and the extracellular fluid make up the smallest calcium reservoir in the body (0.1%). Some calcium is stored intracellularly (1%) but most resides in bone and teeth (99%). Therefore, an understanding of bone composition, structure, and metabolism is essential to any discussion of calcium metabolism.

B. Bone

Bone is composed of osteoid, calcium salts, and cells. *Osteoid* is the organic matrix into which the calcium salts are deposited. The osteoid gives the bone resilience, whereas the minerals impart rigidity. This is best seen in cadaveric long bones treated with either alkali, which digests the osteoid, or acid, which removes the calcium: the alkali-treated bone is rigid but crumbles easily, whereas the acid-treated bone is so flexible that it can be tied into a knot.

The primary component of the osteoid is *collagen* (90%), a fibrous protein composed of three chains. Each mature chain contains about 1000 amino acids, and all three chains tightly twist around each other to form a long rod, 1.5 nm × 300 nm (Fig. 1-4). This triple helix is possible because the individual chains possess a large number of small amino acids, that eliminate steric

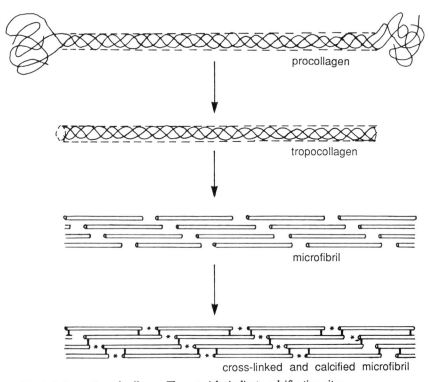

procollagen

tropocollagen

microfibril

cross-linked and calcified microfibril

Fig. 1-4. Formation of collagen. The asterisks indicate calcification sites.

interference: approximately one-third is glycine and another third is proline or hydroxyproline. Collagen is initially synthesized as a precursor, *procollagen*, by the bone cells or *osteoblasts*. After secretion, the ends of the procollagen are proteolytically removed to form *tropocollagen*, which then polymerizes by lining up in a quarter-staggered array with other tropocollagen rods. Initially the polymerization is noncovalent, but subsequently covalent crosslinks are established. The remainder of the osteoid is composed of miscellaneous glycoproteins, mucopolysaccharides, and osteocalcin. Osteocalcin, a 49-amino-acid globular peptide, contains an unusual amino acid — γ-carboxyglutamic acid — which is synthesized from glutamic acid via a vitamin K-dependent reaction. This amino acid is an excellent calcium chelator. It is thought that osteocalcin may sequester calcium to allow for a more gradual and more controlled precipitation of bone mineral.

The major calcium salt is *hydroxyapatite*, which has the following formula: $3Ca_3(PO_4)_2 \cdot Ca(OH)_2$. The salt is deposited in the gaps between the collagen molecules and within the fibrils (Fig. 1-4); the crystals have their long axes aligned with that of the collagen.

Both the synthesis of the osteoid and its calcification are performed by the third component, the cells. The *osteoblast* arises from the osteoprogenitor cell, a fibroblast-like cell located on the bone surface. In addition to synthesizing collagen, this cell also secretes calcium into the extracellular fluid until the salt concentration exceeds its solubility. This supersaturation is possible because various pyrophosphates are also secreted; these compounds act as crystal growth inhibitors by absorbing onto and stabilizing the hydroxyapatite crystal embryos. According to one hypothesis, calcium precipitation is initiated when these pyrophosphates are hydrolyzed by alkaline phosphatase, an enzyme very abundant in osteoblasts. As calcification proceeds, some osteoblasts become entrapped and are relegated to the maintenance of the bone in their immediate vicinity; these are the *osteocytes*. Finally, since bone acts, in part, as a calcium reserve for the body, there must be a mechanism to reclaim these salts during calcium deprivation or loss. This bony dissolution is accomplished by large multinucleated cells with ruffled borders. These *osteoclasts*, as they are called, are very rich in lysosomal and mitochondrial enzymes.

C. Hormones

Parathormone (PTH) is an 84-amino-acid peptide, although only the first 34 amino acids are required for full biological activity. The parathyroid glands, which synthesize and secrete PTH, are derived from the third and fourth pharyngeal pouches and migrate caudally until they become embedded in the posterior wall of the thyroid gland (Fig. 1-5), one each in the superior and inferior pole of each lateral lobe. A single gland measures only 6 x 4 x 2 mm and histologically contains two cell types. The *chief cells* synthesize PTH whereas the *oxyphil* cells, which do not appear until after puberty, have no known function. A homologous peptide, *parathyroid hormone-related protein*

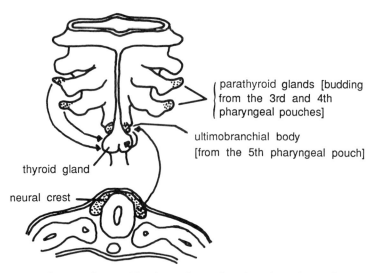

parathyroid glands [budding from the 3rd and 4th pharyngeal pouches]

ultimobranchial body [from the 5th pharyngeal pouch]

thyroid gland

neural crest

Fig. 1-5. Embryonic pharynx. The skin and mesoderm have been dissected away to show the outside of the pharyngeal lining with its pouches and the thyroid diverticulum. Future glandular tissue is stippled. Adapted and reproduced by permission from J. R. McClintic, *Human Anatomy*. Copyright © 1983 The C. V. Mosby Company.

(PTHrP), was first identified in tumors associated with hypercalcemia, but has now been found in many normal tissues such as the mammary gland, bladder and uterus (7). PTHrP may act as a parahormone for local calcium transport and/or smooth muscle relaxation.

Calcitonin (CT) is a 32-amino-acid peptide with an amino-terminal disulfide loop and an amidated carboxy terminus. The cells that synthesize CT originate from the neural crest and initially migrate to the ultimobranchial body of the fifth pharyngeal pouch. From there they invade the thyroid gland, which is descending the neck after having invaginated from the floor of the primitive mouth (Fig. 1-5). Histologically, the cells are located between, or partially embedded in, the thyroid follicles; for this reason, they are called parafollicular cells. Since they secrete CT, they are also known as C cells.

The active form of *vitamin D* is 1,25-dihydroxycholecalciferol (1,25-DHCC) and is synthesized by a fascinating pathway involving three different tissues and a nonenzymatic step (Fig. 1-6). The precursor is either 7-dehydrocholesterol from animals or ergosterol from plants; these molecules differ only in their side chains. Although 7-dehydrocholesterol can be synthesized in some human tissues, the amounts may be inadequate to meet the needs of the body, especially during rapid growth. Consequently, either 7-dehydrocholesterol or ergosterol is required in the diet, generating their designation as vitamins. After absorption from the digestive tract, the sterol travels to the skin where ultraviolet light aromatizes the B ring, causing it to rupture. After

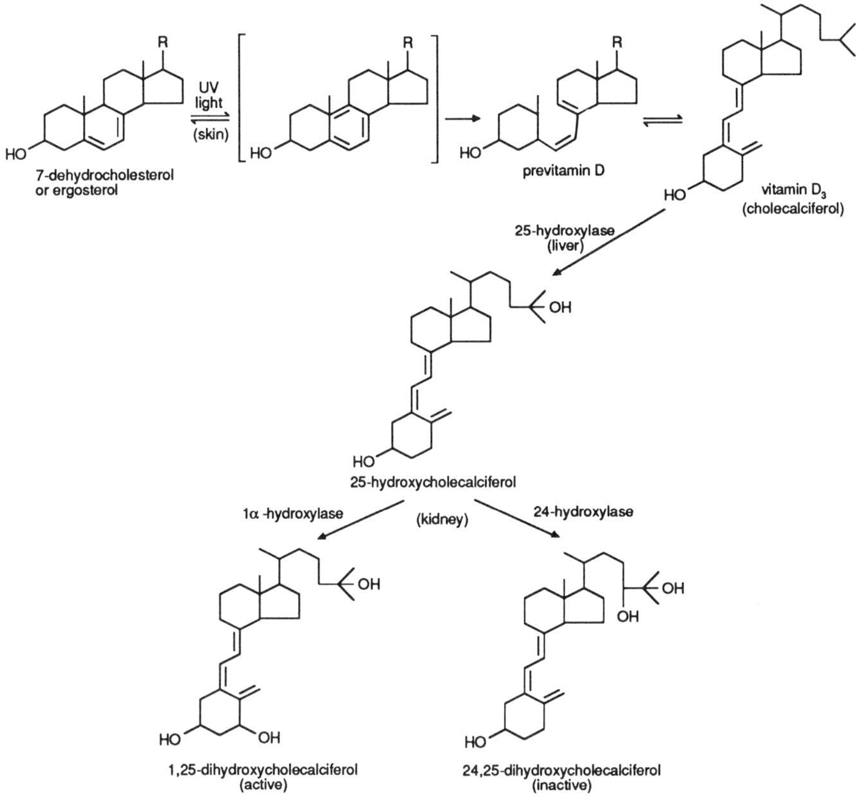

Fig. 1-6. Synthetic pathway for vitamin D and its active metabolites.

rearrangement of the double bonds, vitamin D goes to the liver, where it is 25-hydroxylated. Finally, the compound is carried to the kidney, where it is hydroxylated on either the 1 or the 24 position. 1,25-DHCC is the form active in elevating serum calcium whereas 24,25-DHCC was merely thought to be an inactive metabolite. However, it is now known that 24,25-DHCC actively opposes the effects of 1,25-DHCC. First, 24,25-DHCC stimulates the metabolism of 1,25-DHCC, thereby lowering the serum levels of the latter. Second, in chondrocytes, 24,25-DHCC inhibits a transduction signal activated by 1,25-DHCC. Therefore, the choice between the 1 and 24 positions has dramatically different effects and is highly regulated (see subsequent discussion). The importance of this sterol is reflected in the increased incidence of rickets in children during the Industrial Revolution. Inadequate exposure to the sun as a result of the children spending all day working in factories impaired the synthesis of 1,25-DHCC at the first step. Without 1,25-DHCC, the body absorbs calcium very poorly and rapidly growing bones become soft because of inadequate calcification.

D. Hormonal Regulation

Parathormone elevates calcium levels by dissolving the salts in bone and preventing their renal excretion. In bone, PTH activates the osteoclasts and induces their lysosomal enzymes. In the kidney, PTH stimulates calcium resorption while promoting phosphate and bicarbonate excretion. The hormone acts, in part, through cyclic AMP (cAMP) and protein kinase C (PKC), second messengers discussed in Chapters 8 and 9.

Calcitonin was once believed to stimulate bone synthesis, but more recent data show that it only blocks the action of PTH, that is, it is only a PTH antagonist. Calcitonin also stimulates cAMP and PKC. This paradox of agonist and antagonist acting through the same second messengers was initially explained by proposing that the two hormones affected different cell types. However, it is now known that both hormones act on the same cell, the osteoclast. It is likely that these, and possibly other, second messengers are differentially activated by hormone concentration, temporal exposure, or other factors (see Chapter 8 for a more detailed discussion). Another unresolved problem is the apparent insignificance of CT in calcium metabolism: total thyroidectomy without CT replacement does not result in any abnormality of calcium regulation. For this reason, some authorities consider CT to be an evolutionary vestige, however, if this were true, the gene for this hormone should have been inactivated or lost through random mutation, since enough time has elapsed for these changes to occur. The answer may lie in its gene, which actually encodes two peptides: CT and a homologous peptide called *calcitonin gene-related peptide* (CGRP). In the parafollicular cells, the mRNA is processed and translated to give CT but in certain parts of the nervous system, such as the trigeminal ganglion, the mRNA is processed and translated to yield CGRP (8). This peptide induces analgesia, inhibits gastric acid secretion, and is associated with other activities of the autonomic nervous system. These functions, as well as other yet undiscovered activities, may be sufficiently important to the organism to cause selection for the entire gene. Seemingly useless DNA that is maintained in the genome because of its close association with vital DNA has been termed *selfish DNA*, and CT may be an example of this phenomenon.

1,25-Dihydroxycholecalciferol has at least two target organs: the gastrointestinal tract and bone. In the digestive tract, 1,25-DHCC induces a calcium-binding peptide that is required for calcium absorption. This peptide is a member of the calmodulin family (see Chapter 9). In bone, pharmacological doses of 1,25-DHCC mimic the effects of PTH; at physiological concentrations, it synergizes with PTH. Previously, no effects for 1,25-DHCC could be documented in the kidney. However, in vitamin D-deficient animals, this sterol stimulates calcium resorption in the distal renal tubule. Although this effect resembles the action of PTH, the hormones use different mechanisms: PTH activates the (Na^+, Ca^{2+}) exchanger, whereas the resorption stimulated by 1,25-DHCC is ATP dependent.

These hormones also affect phosphate metabolism. Calcitonin facilitates the transport of phosphate into cells and 1,25-DHCC promotes the absorption of phosphate from the intestines. Finally, PTH induces the excretion of phosphate in the kidneys. This effect was originally thought to facilitate the solubilization of calcium from bone, but it is now known that PTH can still resorb bone without increasing phosphate excretion. Another possible explanation for this effect is that it enables PTH to elevate calcium concentrations without risking ectopic calcification, which would be more likely to occur if both calcium and phosphate were elevated.

E. Summary

These actions can now be integrated into a general scheme (Fig. 1-7). Low serum calcium levels stimulate PTH and inhibit CT secretion; these two hormones are always reciprocally regulated, since their effects antagonize one another (Fig 1-8A). Parathormone releases calcium from bone and reduces its excretion from the kidney. Both hypocalcemia and PTH induce the 1α-hydroxylase; hypophosphatemia, which frequently accompanies low serum calcium levels, further augments this induction while inhibiting the 24-hydroxylase. The final result is a shift in vitamin D from the inactive 24,25-DHCC form to the active 1,25-DHCC form (Fig. 1-8B). The latter stimulates calcium uptake from the digestive tract and resorption from the

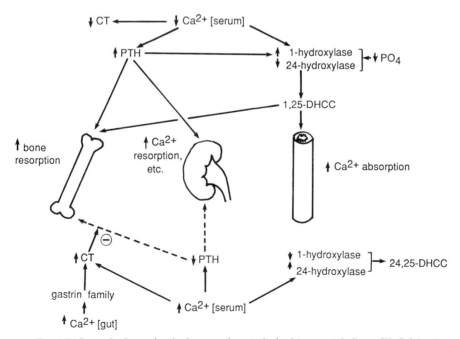

Fig. 1-7. General scheme for the hormonal control of calcium metabolism. CT, Calcitonin; DHCC, dihydroxycholecalciferol; PTH, parathormone.

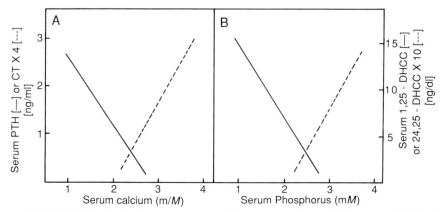

Fig. 1-8. (A) Relationship between serum calcium concentrations and the levels of PTH and CT. (B) Relationship between serum phosphorus concentrations and the levels of 1,25-DHCC and 24,25-DHCC.

kidney while synergizing with PTH in releasing calcium from bone. Therefore, hypocalcemia is corrected by recruiting calcium from the bone and digestive tract while restricting its loss through the kidney. If calcium levels are high, the reverse occurs. Parathormone secretion is inhibited and CT is stimulated to antagonize what little PTH may still be circulating. Furthermore, the 24-hydroxylase is induced while the 1α-hydroxylase is inhibited, resulting in a shift to 24,25-DHCC. This metabolite induces the degradation of 1,25-DHCC and blocks the activity of any residual 1,25-DHCC. Finally, an interesting anticipatory signal is generated by the gastrointestinal tract; one of the functions of the digestive tract is to identify the contents of a meal and relay this information to the body to prepare it metabolically for these substrates (see Chapter 2, Section VI). In this case, calcium in the digestive tract stimulates the release of members of the gastrin family of hormones; these in turn stimulate the secretion of CT. After all, if calcium is about to be absorbed from the intestines, it does not have to be resorbed from bone.

References

General References

DeGroot, L. J. (ed.) (1989). "Endocrinology," 2d Ed. Saunders, Philadelphia.
Gorbman, A., Dickhoff, W. W., Vigna, S. R., Clark, N.B., and Ralph, C. L. (1983). "Comparative Endocrinology." Wiley, New York.
Hadley, M. E. (1992). "Endocrinology." Prentice Hall, Englewood Cliffs, New Jersey.
Martin, C. R. (1985). "Endocrine Physiology." Oxford University Press, London.
Norman, A. W., and Litwack, G. (1987). "Hormones." Academic Press, Orlando, Florida.
Wilson, J. D., and Foster, D. W. (eds.) (1992). "Textbook of Endocrinology." 8th Ed. Saunders, Philadelphia.

Cited References

1. Bern, H. A. (1990). The "new" endocrinology: Its scope and its impact. *Am. Zool.* **30,** 877–885.
2. Labrie, F. (1991). Intracrinology. *Mol. Cell. Endocrinol.* **78,** C113–C118.
3. Prescott, S. M., Zimmerman, G. A., and McIntyre, T. M. (1990). Platelet-activating factor. *J. Biol. Chem.* **265,** 17381–17384.
4. Darvill, A., Augur, C., Bergmann, C., Carlson, R. W., Cheong, J. J., Eberhard, S., Hahn, M. G., Ló, V. M., Marfà, V., Meyer, B., Mohnen, D., O'Neill, M. A., Spiro, M. D., van Halbeek, H., and Albersheim, P. (1992). Oligosaccharins-oligosaccharides that regulate growth, development and defence responses in plants. *Glycobiology* **2,** 181–198.
5. Misevic, G. N., and Burger, M. M. (1990). The species-specific cell-binding site of the aggregation factor from the sponge *Microciona prolifera* is a highly repetitive novel glycan containing glucuronic acid, fucose, and mannose. *J. Biol. Chem.* **265,** 20577–20584.
6. Sepehri, H., Renard, C., and Houdebine, L. M. (1990). α-Glucan and pectin derivatives stimulate prolactin secretion from hypophysis *in vitro. Proc. Soc. Exp. Biol. Med.* **194,** 193–197.
7. Martin, T. J., Moseley, J. M., and Gillespie, M. T. (1991). Parathyroid hormone-related protein: Biochemistry and molecular biology. *Crit. Rev. Biochem. Mol. Biol.* **26,** 377–395.
8. Breimer, L. H., MacIntyre, I., and Zaidi, M. (1988). Peptides from the calcitonin genes: Molecular genetics, structure and function. *Biochem. J.* **255,** 377–390.

CHAPTER 2

Classical Endocrinology

CHAPTER OUTLINE

I. Introduction

In Chapter 1, the basic characteristics of hormones and their regulation were reviewed and illustrated with an example. In this chapter, the other classical hormones are discussed (Table 1-2). The chapter begins with the most centralized endocrine system: the hypothalamic–pituitary axis whose output controls the adrenal glands, the thyroid gland, and the gonads. After this axis and its dependent glands are discussed, the hormones involved in energy metabolism are examined. These hormones are closely associated with the gastrointestinal tract and include insulin and glucagon, among others.

II. Hypothalamus and Pituitary Gland

A. Introduction

The pituitary, or hypophysis, is really two glands fused together; each gland has a different embryonic origin, secretes a different class of hormones, and is regulated differently. The posterior pituitary, or neurohypophysis, is an outgrowth of the floor of the third ventricle and is still connected to the ventricle via the infundibulum (Fig. 2-1). In most species, the anterior pituitary, or adenohypophysis, arises as an ectodermal invagination (Rathke's pouch) from the primitive mouth, the stomodeum. However, there are exceptions: it arises from the endoderm in the hagfish and from the ectoderm of the face in the lamprey. The intermediate lobe of the pituitary is really just

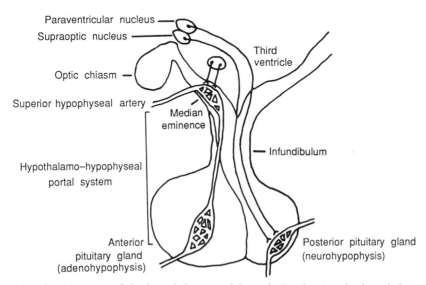

Fig. 2-1. Anatomy of the hypothalamus and hypophysis, showing the hypothalamo–hypophyseal portal system to the adenohypophysis and the neural pathways to the neurohypophysis.

a subdivision of the adenohypophysis; in birds and some mammals, it is completely absent.

B. Posterior Pituitary

The neurohypophysis secretes two nonapeptides, vasopressin and oxytocin, each of which contains a carboxy-terminal amide and a disulfide loop between residues 1 and 6. However, the two peptides are actually synthesized in the peptidergic neurons of the supraoptic and paraventricular nuclei of the hypothalamus. The sequences of these peptides are encoded within a larger protein that also contains the sequences of other biologically active peptides; such a molecule is known as a *polyprotein*. The polyprotein precursor for the neurohypophyseal hormones is cleaved into three pieces: the nonapeptide is the amino terminus, a neurophysin occupies the central region, and a 40-amino-acid glycoprotein forms the carboxy terminus. The neurophysin is a 10-kDa protein that binds the peptide hormone and protects it from rapid degradation. Larger proteins can form enough internal bonds to form a stable, tight globular structure with no exposed amino or carboxy termini. Such a structure is relatively resistant to proteolysis. The neurohypophyseal hormones overcome the handicap of their small size by binding to a larger carrier protein. Further protection is afforded by the primary structure of the hormones themselves: each has its amino and carboxy termini blocked, as noted earlier. The third product of the polyprotein, the carboxy-terminal glycoprotein, has no known function but may be involved in the processing of the precursor. After synthesis and cleavage of the polyprotein, the hormone and its neurophysin are packaged into vesicles, travel down the axons through the infundibulum, and are stored in the nerve endings in the posterior pituitary until they are released.

Vasopressin (VP), or *antidiuretic hormone* (ADH), is involved in water conservation. The most important stimulus for its secretion is an elevated blood osmolarity. Secretion can also be elicited by a 10–25% decrease in blood volume or by stress and nausea. The major effects of this hormone include the stimulation of water resorption in the kidneys and glycogenolysis in the liver. The former would obviously dilute the blood concentration and the latter may be part of the "fight-or-flight" response to stress (see Section III). ADH may also cause vasoconstriction, but this effect requires pharmacological concentrations of the hormone. Clinically, ADH deficiency results in diabetes insipidus and the inability to concentrate urine. As a result, patients can excrete as much as 15 liters of urine daily and must consume equal amounts of liquids to prevent dehydration.

The other peptide hormone is *oxytocin*, which stimulates smooth muscle contraction; it functions in both parturition and suckling. Uterine contractions at the time of parturition stimulate oxytocin release via a positive feedback loop that is broken when the fetus is finally expelled. Suckling triggers another neural reflex leading to oxytocin secretion, which stimulates the contraction of the myoepithelial cells around the alveoli and ducts of the mammary gland. This contraction forces milk toward the nipple, resulting in the milk "letdown," and facilitates suckling. This is another example of positive feedback; the loop is interrupted when the infant is sated and stops nursing. Maternal deficiency of oxytocin does not impair delivery but it is likely that fetal oxytocin crosses into the maternal circulation.

C. Hypothalamus

The hypothalamus also controls the anterior pituitary, although there are no neural pathways connecting the two structures. Instead, the control is exerted by hormones, which are carried from the hypothalamus to the adenohypophysis via a special circulatory system: the hypothalamo–hypophyseal portal system (Fig. 2-1). The superior hypophyseal artery supplies both the pituitary stalk and the median eminence; the latter forms part of the floor of the third ventricle. The primary capillary plexus is drained by the hypophyseal portal vessel, which opens into a second capillary bed in the anterior pituitary. The neurons in the hypothalamic–hypophysiotropic nuclei send their axons to the median eminence, where they secrete releasing and inhibiting factors into the primary plexus. These factors are then delivered directly to the anterior pituitary, where they regulate the secretion of hormones synthesized in the adenohypophysis.

The structures for several of these factors are known (Table 2-1). Most

Table 2-1

Releasing and Inhibiting Factors Synthesized by the Hypothalamus

Hormone	Action	Structure	Precursor
Thyrotropin-releasing hormone (TRH)	↑ TSH, PRL	Blocked tripeptide (pGlu–His–Pro–NH$_2$)	29-kDa precursor containing five copies of TRH
Gonadotropin-releasing hormone (GnRH, LHRH)	↑ LH, FSH	Blocked decapeptide (pGlu . . . Gly–NH$_2$)	Amino terminus of 90-amino-acid precursor; carboxy-terminal 56 amino acids may be a PRL-inhibiting factor
Somatotropin (GH) release-inhibiting factor (SRIF, somatostatin)	↓ GH	14-Amino-acid peptide with disulfide bond between residue 3 and 14	Carboxy terminus of 92-amino-acid precursor
Corticotrophin-releasing factor (CRF)	↑ ACTH	41-Amino-acid peptide with amidated carboxy terminus	Carboxy terminus of 190-amino-acid precursor
Growth hormone-releasing factor (GHRF)	↑ GH	44-Amino-acid peptide with amidated carboxy terminus	Residues 32–75 from 107-amino-acid precursor
Pituitary adenylate cyclase-activating polypeptide (PACAP)	↑ LH, PRL, GH, ACTH	27- or 38-Amino-acid peptide with amidated carboxy terminus	Residues 132–169 from 176-amino-acid precursor
Dopamine	↓ PRL, ↑ GH	Catechol	

are small peptides that are synthesized as a larger precursor. In the case of the thyrotropin–releasing hormone (TRH), the precursor contains five copies of the sequence Gln–His–Pro–Gly flanked by pairs of basic amino acids. Couplets of basic residues indicate cleavage sites, a carboxy-terminal glycine is a signal for amidation, and the amino-terminal glutamine forms an intra-amino acid peptide bond between the α amino group and the γ carboxy group to produce pyroglutamic acid (pGlu). Amino-terminal pyroglutamic acids and amidated carboxy termini protect the free ends of these peptides from degradation by exopeptidases. This is important for the releasing and inhibiting factors, because their small size precludes any significant secondary or tertiary structure into which loose ends could be tucked. In the case of the gonadotropin-releasing hormone (GnRH) precursor, two factors may be produced: the GnRH forms the amino terminus while a GnRH-associated peptide forms the carboxy terminus. This latter peptide has prolactin (PRL)-inhibiting activity, but its physiological significance has not been determined. The pituitary adenylate cyclase-activating polypeptide (PACAP) is unique in its wide distribution and broad specificity. This peptide is a member of the vasoactive intestinal peptide family (see Section VI,B) and can stimulate the release of several pituitary hormones from the adenohypophysis, as well as epinephrine from the adrenal medulla and insulin from the pancreas.

D. Anterior Pituitary

The cells of the anterior pituitary can be histologically classified by the stains they take up. The *chromophobes* do not stain at all and have no known function. The *acidophils* stain with acid dyes and synthesize members of the growth hormone–prolactin family. The cells may be specialized: somatotrophs secrete only GH, whereas mammotrophs or lactotrophs secrete PRL. However, a few cells may secrete both hormones. In female mice, the somatotrophs and mammotrophs are nearly equal in abundance, but in male mice the somatotrophs outnumber the mammotrophs 6:1; this ratio may explain the larger size of the male in most species. The basophils stain with basic dyes and secrete the tropic hormones; a *tropic hormone* is one that regulates another gland. The thyrotrophs synthesize thyroid-stimulating hormone (TSH); gonadotrophs make luteinizing hormone (LH) and follicle-stimulating hormone (FSH); and cortico-lipotrophs produce adrenocorticotropic hormone (ACTH) and related peptides.

1. Growth Hormone–Prolactin Family

GH and PRL are homologous hormones that arose by gene duplication. Each contains nearly 200 amino acids and has a large central disulfide loop and a small carboxy-terminal one. In addition, PRL has another small loop at the amino terminus. GH has both direct and indirect actions. Many of its metabolic effects are direct and include the stimulation of lipolysis, amino acid uptake, and protein synthesis; the latter two effects are especially pronounced in muscle. GH also induces peripheral resistance to insulin so glucose cannot be utilized and blood glucose levels rise; this is known as the *diabetogenic effect*. GH also stimulates linear growth of the skeleton; originally, this action was thought to be indirect: GH stimulated the secretion of *insulin-like growth factor-I* (IGF-I), previously called somatomedin C, from the liver. The IGF-I, in turn, stimulated both chrondrocyte mitosis and sulfate incorporation into the cartilage matrix; the growth of long bones occurs at the cartilaginous growth plates. Although the role of IGF-I in chrondrocyte proliferation is clearly established, it is now known that GH plays an equally important and direct role in chrondrocyte differentiation (1). Finally, IGF-I promotes the uptake of amino acids and glucose into muscle. Many other hormones also stimulate IGF-I secretion, but in these cases IGF-I acts as a parahormone. For example, parathormone stimulates the production of IGF-I in bone and ACTH does the same in adrenal cortex. In summary, GH has two major actions: (i) direct metabolic effects that facilitate muscle growth and glucose sparing and (ii) skeletal growth effects that are partially direct (differentiative) and partially mediated by IGF-I (proliferative).

PRL is an ancient hormone with multiple functions within the vertebrate lineage; these will be discussed more fully in Chapter 15. In mammals, PRL has three major activities: lactogenic, gonadotropic, and immunologic. In all mammals, PRL is essential for the development of the mammary glands in preparation for milk production. In rodents, it is also gonadotropic and is essential for the maintenance of pregnancy. Except for lactation, PRL is not required for human reproduction; nonetheless, the human ovary still has abundant receptors for PRL, and pathologically elevated levels of this hormone can cause amenorrhea. Hyperprolactinemia can also produce impotence in men, but at physiological concentrations PRL is not thought to play a role in male reproduction. The newest activities of PRL to receive attention are its immunological effects (2). PRL is synthesized and secreted by several parts of the immune system in which it may act as a parahormone, it is mitogenic for some immune cells, and its receptor is homologous to those of the cytokine family of immune and hematopoietic hormones (see Chapter 3).

Prolactin is the only adenohypophyseal hormone that is under tonic inhibitory control, that is, the mammotrophs are programmed to secrete PRL unless otherwise inhibited. This is dramatically demonstrated when the hypothalamo–hypophyseal portal system is disrupted. In the absence of any releasing or inhibiting factors, serum levels of all the adenohypophyseal hormones except PRL fall; PRL serum levels, however, rise. PRL secretion is also stimulated by suckling via a neural reflex; this is essential for the continuation of lactation. Indeed, if a woman does not wish to nurse her infant, she is given postpartum a dopamine agonist that suppresses PRL secretion and prevents lactation (Table 2-1). The secretion of both GH and PRL occurs as short pulses that are most abundant during sleep. For GH, this pattern is necessary for its biological activity. For example, clinically, certain patients have short stature but normal basal and stimulated serum GH levels (3). However, the spiking pattern is absent. These patients will grow if exogenous GH is administered intermittently. However, other biological activities may require chronically elevated levels. For example, in experimental animals, the continuous administration of GH induces PRL receptors but inhibits a major urinary protein whereas a pulsatile administration induces the protein but inhibits the receptors (4).

2. Glycoprotein Hormones

These hormones from the basophilic cells form another family: all are dimers sharing a common 89-amino-acid α subunit. The β subunit, containing 112–115 amino acids, is different and imparts specificity to the biological actions of each hormone, but it is inactive alone. All these hormones are glycosylated to generate a final molecular mass of 32 kDa and all stimulate their target organs via cAMP. Thyrotropin stimulates the synthesis and release of thyroxine (T_4) from the thyroid gland; FSH promotes gametogenesis in both sexes and estradiol secretion in the female, and LH stimulates progesterone production in the corpus luteum of the ovary and testosterone production in the Leydig cells of the testis.

3. Proopiomelanocortin

The final tropic hormone, ACTH, is synthesized as part of a 31-kDa polyprotein containing 265 amino acids. This polyprotein is called *proopiomelanocortin* (POMC) and contains three melanocyte-stimulating hormones (α-, β-, and γ-MSH), three endorphins (α-, β-, and γ-endorphin), and ACTH (Fig. 2-2). Many of these sequences are overlapping, so only a certain subset of hormones can be produced from a single precursor. Therefore, post-translational processing regulates the expression of these hormones.

MSH is generated in the cells of the intermediate lobe of the pituitary in fish, reptiles, and amphibians. Humans do not have this lobe, but these cells are still present, scattered in the remaining anterior and posterior lobes. In these lower vertebrate, MSH causes the pigment granules in melanocytes to disperse so the skin will darken. Because genetic factors are much more important in the skin color of mammals and birds, MSH appears to be less important, although it still transiently increases pigment synthesis in these vertebrates.

ACTH stimulates the synthesis and secretion of adrenal steroids. Primarily it promotes the uptake of cholesterol and its conversion to pregneno-

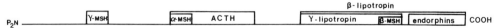

Fig. 2-2. Proopiomelanocortin and the individual hormones into which it can be cleaved. ACTH, Adrenocorticotropic hormone; MSH, melanocyte-stimulating hormone.

lone. This is the first, and rate-limiting, step in the pathway (see Section III). Like the other tropic hormones, ACTH uses cAMP as a second messenger (see Chapter 8). The endorphins will be discussed in Chapter 3.

III. Adrenal Glands

A. Anatomy

Like the pituitary, the adrenal gland is two glands in one: the outer layer, the *adrenal cortex*, synthesizes steroids and the center layer, the *adrenal medulla*, synthesizes catecholamines, primarily epinephrine. The medulla originates from the neural crest and is, in fact, a sympathetic ganglion modified to secrete its "neurotransmitter" into the circulatory system rather than into a synaptic cleft. The cortex develops from the mesothelium of the abdominal cavity and envelops the medulla during embryogenesis. Eventually, the pyramidal gland comes to rest at the superior pole of each kidney.

Each part of the adrenal gland has its own blood supply. The cortex is divided into three layers: the *zona glomerulosa* contains ball-like clusters of cells and lies just underneath the adrenal capsule; the *zona fasciculata* contains cells arranged in columns and is the middle layer; the *zona reticularis* contains cells in a netlike pattern and is the innermost layer (Fig. 2-3). The capsular arteries penetrate the capsule and form the capsular plexus in the zona glomerulosa. From there the straight capillaries carry the blood between

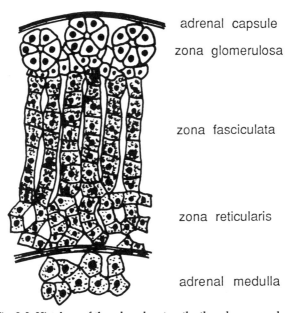

adrenal capsule

zona glomerulosa

zona fasciculata

zona reticularis

adrenal medulla

Fig. 2-3. Histology of the adrenal cortex; the three layers are shown.

the columns of the zona fasciculata to the reticular plexus of the zona reticularis. Finally, the blood is drained into the alar and emissary veins. The medulla is supplied by the medullary artery, which gives rise to the medullary capillaries; the medulla is drained by the central vein. One important connection occurs between these two circulatory systems; the reticular plexus also drains into the medullary capillaries, exposing the medulla to high concentrations of corticosteroids. These steroids are involved in regulating epinephrine synthesis (see Section III,D,2).

B. Zonae Fasciculata and Reticularis

The major products of these layers are the *glucocorticoids* (cortisol in humans and corticosterone in rodents) and the *androgens* (Fig. 2-4). The pathway is regulated by ACTH, which stimulates P450scc (*P450* cytochrome responsible for side-chain cleavage) in the first step. This is accomplished in two ways: first, ACTH induces the enzyme itself through its second messengers. cAMP and calcium. Second, ACTH also induces an endopeptidase that converts a precursor into a 34-amino-acid peptide called *diazepam-binding inhibitor* (DBI). The name comes from the ability of this peptide to displace the drug diazepam from endogeneous receptors, some of which reside on the mitochondria. Binding of this receptor activates cholesterol transport into the mitochondria, where the first step occurs. Acutely, ACTH can activate this receptor in the absence of protein synthesis, suggesting that ACTH may directly stimulate the receptor by phosphorylation as well as by induction of the processing enzyme for its ligand (5). Initially, researchers believed that each of the reactions shown in Fig. 2-4 was catalyzed by a separate enzyme; however, it is now known that the steroidogenic enzymes all belong to a family of P450 cytochromes that have multiple activities (6). For example, a desmolase cleaves carbon-carbon bonds when each carbon has an oxygen. Originally, the hydroxylation of adjacent carbons and the subsequent cleavage of the intervening bond were thought to be catalyzed by separate enzymes, but single proteins can possess both hydroxylase and desmolase activities.

ACTH is only one portion of a regulatory loop: ACTH elevates serum cortisol, which inhibits the hypothalamus from secreting corticotropin-releasing factor (CRF). Without CRF, the adenohypophysis will not release any more ACTH. Cortisol also has a feedback effect on the pituitary. Superimposed on this control is a circadian rhythm in which ACTH is secreted during sleep; hence cortisol levels are highest in the morning. Finally, stress also induces the adenohypophysis to secrete ACTH; both the circadian rhythm and the stress effect are mediated through the hypothalamus and CRF.

Glucocorticoids have one major function: gluconeogenesis (Fig. 2-5). These steroids inhibit protein synthesis and, at higher concentrations, may even stimulate protein degradation; the resulting amino acids will serve as precursors for glucose. The steroids then induce enzymes to remove and detoxify the amino acids' nitrogen so only the carbon skeleton remains.

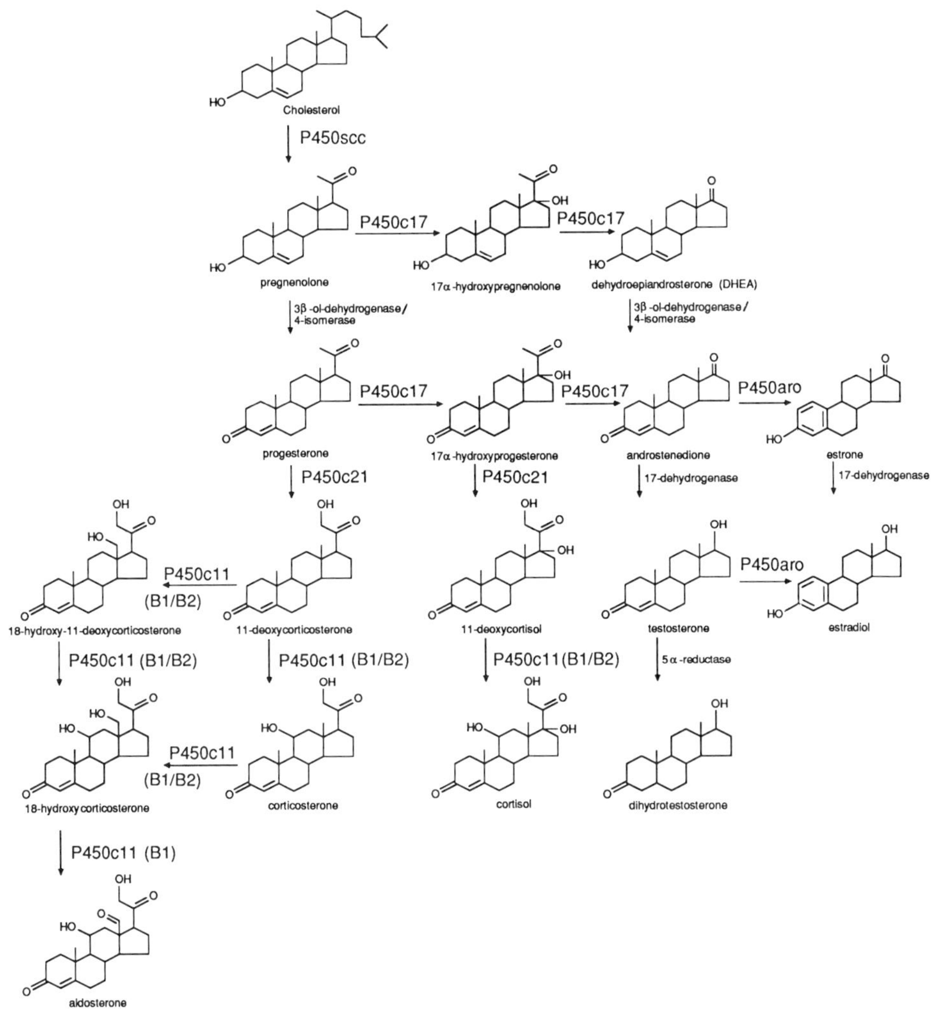

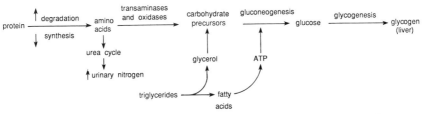

Fig. 2-4. Steroid biosynthetic pathway. This is a composite scheme; not all of these steps occur in each layer.

Fig. 2-5. The steps in gluconeogenesis stimulated by glucocorticoids.

Glucocorticoids can also promote lipolysis, which provides another carbon skeleton, glycerol, for gluconeogenesis. Finally, these steroids induce enzymes critical in reversing glycolysis (see Section VI). Therefore, these steroids are involved with every facet of gluconeogenesis. Glucocorticoids are also potent anti-inflammatory agents: they can stabilize lysosomes, inhibit leukocyte migration, lower antibody levels, and destroy lymphocytes. These actions make glucocorticoids very useful in the treatment of inflammatory diseases and certain leukemias and lymphomas. However, these effects are only manifest at pharmacological concentrations and probably have no physiological relevance. Indeed, at low concentrations, glucocorticoids have been shown to actually stimulate lymphocyte differentiation, such as antibody production.

The sex steroids are only by-products of the glucocorticoid pathway. Dehydroepiandrosterone is the major androgen secreted by the adrenal gland. It is of no importance in males, whose primary sources of androgens are the testes. In women, however, the adrenals are a major source of androgens, which are important in the development of sexual hair. Only insignificant amounts of estrogens are synthesized. Even in males, the major sources of estrogens are not the adrenals but the testicular androgens, which are aromatized in peripheral tissues.

Because steroids are so hydrophobic, they must have serum carrier proteins. Both the steroid- and thyroid hormone-binding proteins are of two types: (i) proteins specifically designed for a particular group of steroids and (ii) general carriers with hydrophobic pockets. The former usually have a single high-affinity binding site per molecule, whereas the latter have many lower affinity sites. The most important general carrier is albumin: although its affinity is only $10^3 - 10^6$/M for most steroids, its serum concentration is so high that it still binds a significant portion of these hydrophobic hormones (Table 2-2). In contrast, more specific carriers have affinities in the range of $10^7 - 10^{10}$/M. In addition to solving the solubility problem, these proteins also protect the hormones from degradation. Indeed, the half-life of these molecules is inversely related to the proportion of free hormone: 36% of aldosterone is free and its half-life is only 20–30 min, whereas only 0.02% of T_4 is free and its half-life is 6 days. Another contributing factor to the half-lives of hydrophobic hormones is their membrane permeability, which allows them to be resorbed passively from the urine. Nonetheless, the free hormone is the most important fraction because it is biologically active. For example, during pregnancy, estrogens induce many of the carrier proteins, so *total* hormone levels rise, but pregnant women have no signs or symptoms of hormone excess because the *free* fraction remains the same.

Binding proteins may also influence the biological activity of their ligands in more specific and highly regulated ways; one of the best examples is actually the binding protein for a peptide, IGF. The IGF-binding protein (IGFBP) can either enhance or inhibit the activity of IGF. When phosphorylated or solubilized, IGFBP binds IGF very tightly and sequesters it from its

Table 2-2
Steroid-Binding Proteins in Serum

Steroid-binding protein	Serum concentration (mg/dl)	Bound or free (%)					
		Cortisol	Aldos-terone	Testos-terone	Estrogen	T_3	T_4
Corticosteroid-binding globulin (CBG)	3.0–3.5	70	17	—	—	—	—
Testosterone–estrogen-binding globulin (TeBG)	0.09–0.28	—	—	30	38	—	—
Thyronine-binding globulin (TBG)	1–2	—	—	—	—	60	78
Thyronine-binding prealbumin (TBPA)	25–33	—	—	—	—	30	3
Albumin	3500–4500	22	47	68	60	10	19
Free		8	36	2	2	0.2	0.02

membrane receptor. However, when glycosylated, IGFBP binds to the membrane and increases IGF activity, presumably by concentrating the hormone near its receptor (7).

C. Zona Glomerulosa

This layer makes only *aldosterone*. This restriction was originally thought to be due to both the absence of P450c17, so it cannot synthesize the sex steroids or many glucocorticoids, and to the exclusive presence of an 18-hydroxylase, which is essential for the synthesis of aldosterone. However, with the cloning of the enzymes of steroid synthesis, it became apparent that the 11β-hydroxylase, 18-hydroxylase, and 18-ol-dehydrogenase activities all resided in a single enzyme, renamed P450c11. Since the zonae fasciculata and reticularis have 11β-hydroxylase activity, they must also have 18-ol-dehydrogenase activity because both catalytic activities occur within the same enzyme. So why is aldosterone made exclusively in the zona glomerulosa? The answer lies in the fact that there are actually two isoforms of this enzyme, CYP11B1 and CYP11B2. Although they are 93% identical, only the CYP11B2 has 18-ol-dehydrogenase activity; this isoform is unique to the zona glomerulosa. The function of this mineralocorticoid is to stimulate sodium resorption from the distal renal tubule; water is passively resorbed with the sodium. The major stimuli for aldosterone secretion are hypovolemia (low blood volume), hyponatremia (low serum sodium levels), and low renal perfusion pressure. However, none of these stimuli directly affects the zona glomerulosa; instead, they are channeled through the kidney. Why are the kidneys involved? The reason is simple: they have the most to lose if blood pressure falls too much. The kidneys remove wastes from the body, and to accomplish this they receive 25% of the cardiac output. If blood pressure falls excessively, they will not be able to perform their function. In addition, the kidneys are metabolically very active and a severe drop in blood pressure, even for a short period of time, can lead to tubular necrosis.

Therefore, the kidney has a special sensor in the juxtaglomerular complex, which is located where the distal convoluted tubule meets the afferent arteriole. These *juxtaglomerular cells* can measure sodium concentrations and the renal perfusion pressure (Fig. 2-6). They do not monitor blood volume directly, but the sympathetic nervous system does and stimulates these cells when the volume gets too low. The secretory product of the juxtaglomerular cells is a proteolytic enzyme, *renin*. Its substrate is *angiotensinogen*, an

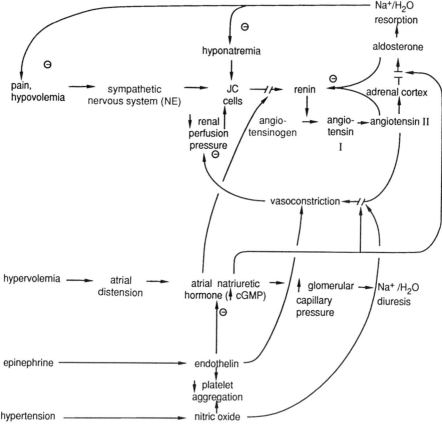

Fig. 2-6. The control of water–sodium balance and blood pressure by the renin–angiotensin–aldosterone system, atrial natriuretic hormone, endothelin, and nitric oxide. Parallel lines indicate those steps blocked by the indicated hormone. JG, Juxtaglomerular; NE, norepinephrine.

α_2-globulin made in the liver and secreted into the blood. Angiotensinogen is actually a prohormone; *prohormones* are are inactive precursors and must be modified in some way to yield the active hormone. In this case, angiotensinogen is initially cleaved in the blood by renin to form *angiotensin I*, an inert peptide. Then, in the lungs, a converting enzyme removes two more amino acids to form the active *angiotensin II*. This octapeptide is the most potent vasopressor known, and the resulting vasoconstriction helps restore the renal perfusion pressure. Angiotensin II also stimulates aldosterone synthesis by inducing the desmolase complex, and both angiotensin II and aldosterone inhibit further renin secretion via a short feedback loop. As noted earlier, aldosterone promotes sodium and water resorption, which corrects the hyponatremia and hypovolemia.

A counter-regulatory mechanism involves another hormone, *atrial natriuretic hormone* (ANF) (8–10). This peptide is synthesized as a 126-amino-acid precursor in the atria of the heart. The active hormone is cleaved from the carboxy terminus; various fragments are produced, but the most likely form *in vivo* has about 30 amino acids. This fragment is released when the atria become distended, as by hypervolemia (volume overload), and its function is to eliminate this excess volume. To produce this effect, ANF dilates the afferent arterioles and constricts the efferent arterioles of the nephron, resulting in an increased glomerular capillary pressure. This higher pressure increases filtration and induces a sodium and water diuresis (Fig. 2-6). Its other effects are related to opposing the renin–angiotensin–aldosterone system: it inhibits both renin and aldosterone secretion and antagonizes the vasoconstriction of angiotensin II. The actions of ANF appear to be mediated by cyclic GMP (cGMP) (see Chapter 8). Two other isoforms are produced in the central nervous system; their roles are less clear than those of the atrial hormone.

Nitric oxide (NO) is another hormone that opposes the renin–angiotensin–aldosterone system (11). NO is a parahormone that is synthesized in the endothelium from arginine by progressive oxidation and induces relaxation in the adjacent smooth muscle layer of the blood vessels by elevating cGMP, like ANF. It can also decrease platelet aggregation and adhesion, and its presence in macrophages and neural tissues suggests that other functions will be discovered as well (12). In endothelium, NO is stimulated by hypertension and several hormones, and its vasodilatory action would facilitate the reduction of blood pressure.

Like NO, *endothelins* are parahormones made in the endothelium (13,14). These 21-amino-acid peptides are cleaved from a larger precursor in response to several hormones such as epinephrine. This catechol is released during stress (see subsequent discussion) and elevates blood pressure, in part through endothelins, which induce vasoconstriction and smooth muscle growth, suppress ANF serum levels, and inhibit the production of cGMP by ANF (15). As such, they complement the renin–angiotensin–aldosterone system. Like NO, they also inhibit platelet aggregation.

D. Adrenal Medulla

1. Autonomic Nervous System

The adrenal medulla developed from the autonomic nervous system (ANS) and remains functionally linked to it; therefore, one cannot discuss one without the other. The ANS is concerned with regulating unconscious activities, and is divided into two opposing components. The parasympathetic nervous system is concerned with the maintenance of bodily activities under basal conditions; for example, it slows the heart rate and stimulates visceral functions such as the secretion of digestive enzymes and increased gut motility. The sympathetic nervous system is concerned with energy expenditure during times of stress; for that reason, it is frequently referred to as the "fight-or-flight" system. For example, it mobilizes substrates for conversion into energy, it dilates bronchioles to increase oxygen uptake, and it increases the perfusion of liver, brain, skeletal muscle, and heart to facilitate the delivery of these substrates and oxygen.

Most organ systems in the body are innervated by both components of the ANS; the net effect on the system is determined by a balance between the two. Each component has a two-neuron pathway from the central nervous system to the target organ. In the sympathetic nervous system, the first neuron synapses with the second in a *ganglion*; the second then travels to its target organ, where it secretes norepinephrine. The adrenal medullae are actually derived from a pair of these sympathetic ganglia, except that the second neurons empty their secretions into the blood instead of leaving the ganglia for some peripheral tissue. Another difference is that the medullae secrete epinephrine rather than norepinephrine.

2. Catecholamine Synthesis

Catecholamine synthesis in the second neuron begins with the hydroxylation of tyrosine to dihydroxyphenylalanine (DOPA) by tyrosine hydroxylase (Fig. 2-7). ACTH is required to maintain basal levels of this enzyme;

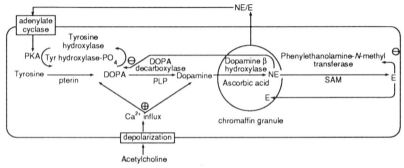

Fig. 2-7. Catecholamine biosynthetic pathway in the adrenal medulla. DOPA, Dihydroxyphenylalanine; E, epinephrine; NE, norepinephrine; PKA, cAMP-dependent protein kinase; PLP, pyridoxal phosphate; SAM, S-adenosylmethionine.

this effect is achieved via cAMP-dependent phosphorylation. After DOPA is decarboxylated, the product, dopamine, is transported into the chromaffin granule where dopamine is further hydroxylated to form norepinephrine, the distal neurotransmitter in the sympathetic nervous system. As norepinephrine accumulates, it acts through a feedback mechanism to inhibit the tyrosine hydroxylase. In the adrenal medulla, norepinephrine is converted to epinephrine in a methylation step catalyzed by phenylethanol-N-methyltransferase; S-adenosylmethionine (SAM) is the methyl donor. This reaction takes place in the cytoplasm, but the epinephrine re-enters the granule after its methylation. The methyltransferase is induced by glucocorticoids and inhibited by epinephrine. The former originate in the adrenal cortex, which drains, in part, through the medulla (see Section III,A); the latter represents product inhibition.

Synthesis and secretion is stimulated by the first neuron, whose neurotransmitter is acetylcholine (ACh). Acetylcholine stimulates both the tyrosine hydroxylase and the dopamine β-hydroxylase via a calcium-dependent mechanism. Once secreted, the catecholamines not only enter the blood but also have a feedback effect on the secretory cell, elevating cAMP levels and activating tyrosine hydroxylase. Intracellular catecholamines represent accumulated products that turn synthesis off, but extracellular catecholamines represent a depleted reserve and stimulate further synthesis.

3. Catecholamine Actions

Norepinephrine has very specific effects; it is the compound of choice for neurotransmission. Its primary effect is to increase total peripheral resistance in the circulatory system. Epinephrine has more general effects, and therefore is distributed in the blood. Its major actions can be divided into metabolic, cardiovascular, and smooth muscle effects. The metabolic effects involve the mobilization of substrates for energy expenditure: it stimulates lipolysis in adipocytes and glycogenolysis in liver and muscle. It actually plays an ancillary role in liver glycogenolysis, which is more strongly affected by glucagon. Furthermore, because muscle lacks glucose-6-phosphatase, the glucose liberated from glycogen cannot leave the cell; instead, the glucose is broken down to lactate, which is released into blood and resynthesized into glucose in the liver.

In the cardiovascular system, epinephrine stimulates the vasoconstriction of the subcutaneous, splanchnic, renal, and mucosal beds, although the skeletal muscle bed vasodilates; this shunts blood from the viscera to the skeletal muscles, which receive circulatory priority in the "fight-or-flight" response. Epinephrine also increases the heart rate and cardiac output and thus facilitates the delivery of nutrients to the skeletal muscles.

Finally, epinephrine relaxes the smooth muscles of the uterus, bladder, and bronchioles, although it constricts the sphincters. Dilated airways improve oxygenation of the blood. As for the rationale behind the sphincter and bladder effects, it it presumed that, when one's life is threatened, one cannot be bothered by the more earthy bodily functions.

IV. The Thyroid Gland

A. Introduction

The thyroid originates as an invagination from the floor of the mouth and migrates down the neck. It consists of two lateral lobes connected by an isthmus; occasionally, there is also a central pyramidal lobe. The thyroid is yet another gland containing two different secretory components: during its migration, it incorporates the C cells, which originate from the neural crest after passing through the ultimobranchial body (see Fig. 1-5). The C cells synthesize calcitonin and were discussed in Section VI, Chapter 1. Histologically, the thyroid contains follicles: epithelial cells surrounding a colloid material. The C cells are located between or attached to the follicles (Fig. 2-8).

B. Synthesis of Thyroid Hormones

Triiodothyronine (T_3) and thyroxine (T_4) are basically iodinated tyrosines with an extra phenyl ring. However, their synthesis presents a problem: both T_3 and T_4 are very hydrophobic, which makes their storage difficult. The gland could simply synthesize the hormones on demand, the way the adrenals and gonads solve the same problem with the hydrophobic steroids. Unfortunately, this solution for the thyroid hormones is not satisfactory because one of the essential ingredients, iodide, is not always readily available. Ideally, the gland should build up a reserve of T_3 and T_4 when iodide is abundant; then it could draw on this store when iodide is scarce. The solution is to synthesize T_3 and T_4 from tyrosines that are already incorporated into a

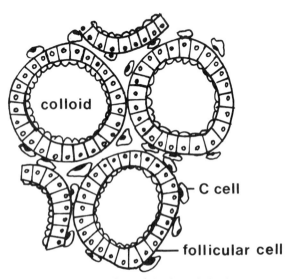

Fig. 2-8. Histology of the thyroid gland.

protein; the residues may be hydrophobic, but the entire protein is hydrophilic and can be easily compartmentalized. When thyroid hormones are needed, some of the protein is digested to liberate the T_3 and T_4. In this way, as much as a 6-month supply of thyroid hormones can be maintained.

The first step in the biosynthetic pathway is the procurement of the iodide (Fig. 2-9), which is accomplished by an iodide pump that can concentrate iodide against a 25- to 40-fold gradient. Another preliminary step is the synthesis of the iodination enzyme and substrate. The substrate is thyroglobulin, a huge protein composed of two identical 330-kDa subunits. It is a glycoprotein with a large number of cysteines. The enzyme is thyroid peroxidase and is packaged within the same vesicles as the thyroglobulin. However, it is not active until it is released into the colloid at the apical surface of the follicular cell. There, the enzyme oxidizes I^- to I^+. *In vitro*, the oxidized iodide spontaneously incorporates itself into the tyrosine ring; however, *in vivo* there is evidence that this organification is also facilitated by the peroxidase. Finally, the iodinated ring from one tyrosine is coupled to that of another (Fig. 2-10). *In vitro*, the coupling can also occur spontaneously, but the existence of a coupling enzyme has been postulated for the *in vivo* reaction. Because the sole purpose of thyroglobulin is to be a precursor for thyroid hormones, one might suppose it to be rich in tyrosines; however, this is not the case. One molecule has 140 tyrosines; about 25 of which are iodinated; only 8 iodinated tyrosines are coupled to form 4 T_3 and/or T_4 residues. Four to ten times more T_4 than T_3 is made.

When thyroid hormones need to be secreted, the iodinated thyroglobulin is taken up by the follicular cell. The endocytotic vesicle fuses with lysosomes and the protein is degraded. The T_3 and T_4 are released and diffuse into the blood. The uncoupled tyrosines, both mono- and diiodotyrosines, are deiodinated and the iodide recycled. One final activation step is the conversion of T_4 to T_3. Several data support the importance of this step:

1. In all systems studied to date, T_3 is more potent than T_4.

2. Nuclear receptors for the thyroid hormones prefer T_3 over T_4 (see Chapter 5).

3. T_3 deficiency produces hypothyroidism even in the presence of normal T_4 levels.

4. Iopanoic acid, a specific 5'-deiodinase inhibitor, blocks all the biological actions of T_4.

Therefore, it is generally assumed that T_3 is responsible for most, if not all, of the biological activities of the thyroid hormones and that T_4 is only a prohormone. This conversion of T_4 to T_3 takes place in the peripheral tissues, which contain the iodothyronine deiodinase.

The activity of the follicular cell is controlled by TSH from the pituitary gland. This tropic hormone stimulates synthesis by promoting iodide uptake

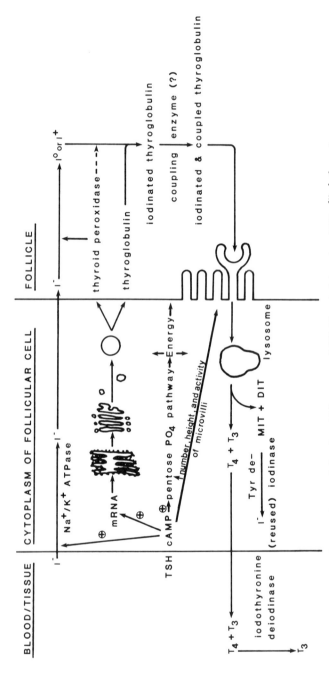

Fig. 2-9. Biosynthetic pathway of the thyroid hormones. MIT, Monoiodotyrosine; DIT, diiodothyronine.

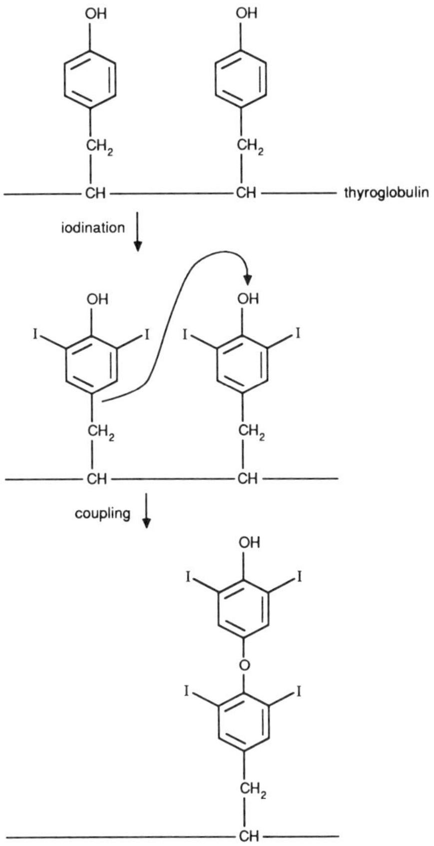

Fig. 2-10. Coupling reaction in thyroid hormone synthesis.

and inducing the genes for thyroid peroxidase and thyroglobulin. TSH stimulates secretion by increasing the number, height, and activity of the microvilli, which internalize the iodinated thyroglobulin. Finally, TSH stimulates the pentose phosphate pathway to provide the energy for all the aforementioned processes.

C. Actions of Thyroid Hormones

Thyroid hormones elicit a bewildering, and often conflicting, array of actions in vertebrates. One of the first and most prominent effects is the stimulation of calorigenesis, as evidenced by increased oxygen consumption. The muscular, gastrointestinal, and renal systems appear to be the most responsive whereas the nervous, reproductive, and immunological systems are relatively unresponsive. The molecular basis for this effect appears to be a series of futile cycles activated by T_3. For example, in carbohydrate metabolism, T_3 potentiates the effect of insulin on glucose uptake and glycogen synthesis but also potentiates the effects of the catecholamines on glycogenolysis. The latter predominates, but blood glucose levels do not rise as much as would be expected, because much of the glucose is oxidized. T_3 also stimulates both lipid synthesis and lipolysis; again, degradation predominates. These effects on lipolysis are both direct and indirect; the latter actions are a result of the potentiation of the effects of catecholamines, GH, glucocorticoids, and glucagon. In fact, T_3 potentiates the effects of so many hormones that it has frequently been called a *permissive hormone*. At least part of this potentiation is due to the T_3 induction of the receptors for these hormones; more receptors would increase the responsiveness of the tissue to these hormones. In an action also related to lipid metabolism, T_3 stimulates hydroxymethylglutaryl coenzyme A reductase, the rate-limiting enzyme in cholesterol synthesis; however, cholesterol levels actually fall because its elimination via bile acids exceeds its enhanced synthesis. It may be that T_3 does not exert any specific metabolic effects; rather, it may simply adjust the overall metabolic rate in the tissues. In addition to its metabolic and calorigenic effects, the thyroid hormone also exerts many important developmental and growth effects. At physiological concentrations, T_3 promotes protein synthesis, linear growth, and skeletal maturation. In amphibians it stimulates molting and metamorphosis. However, even in growth and development the specific role played by T_3 is unclear. For example, T_3 is known to exert a "permissive" effect on other growth-related hormones. Furthermore, some of its effects on metamorphosis can be explained by assuming that T_3 is merely triggering a preprogrammed event. For example, a T_3 pellet implanted in frog skin will cause the epidermis to thicken everywhere except the opercular window, where the forelimb will emerge; here the epidermis thins (16). This result has been interpreted to mean that each cell in the tadpole is genetically programmed to execute certain activities during metamorphosis. Although T_3 triggers this program, the response of the cell is determined by its genetic program.

V. Reproduction

A. Androgens

In males, androgens are primarily synthesized in the Leydig cells of the testes and are secreted as testosterone. In females, the adrenal cortex is the major source and secretes *dihydroepiandosterone* (DHEA); the ovary makes a minor contribution.

1. Actions

Androgens act in one of three molecular forms: dihydrotestosterone (DHT), testosterone (T), and estradiol (E_2). The peripheral tissues possess a 5α-reductase that converts testosterone to DHT. This is the active androgen in all adult tissues except muscle, that is, testosterone is usually a prohormone. Nonetheless, testosterone does have some direct effects in several embryonic structures and in adult muscles. Finally, testosterone can be converted to E_2 by an aromatase in peripheral tissues; this is the form in which testosterone acts on certain parts of the brain.

Although the sex chromosomes determine whether the gonad will become a testis or an ovary, the development of the other genital structures results from the interaction between the genetic elements and the sex steroids. Genetically, all embryos are programmed to develop a female phenotype. As a consequence, female embryos do not require the presence of estrogen or any other sex steroid to generate a female genital pattern; indeed, castration of female embryos does not interfere with the development of this pattern. However, in male embryos, androgens will stimulate the growth of the genital tubercle into a penis, induce the fusion of the labioscrotal swellings to form the scrotum, and promote the descent of the testes into this sac. If a male embryo is castrated, the genital tubercle forms a clitoris, the swellings never fuse and become the labia majora, and the gonads remain in the abdomen, that is, a female phenotype prevails. In male embryos, androgen secretion by the Leydig cells is initiated by a placental gonadotropin, *human chorionic gonadotropin* (hCG), but hCG is only elevated during the first trimester. The embryonic pituitary gland must take over or the genitalia will be incompletely masculinized, that is, the penis will be small, the testes undescended, and so on. The Leydig cells secrete testosterone, which stimulates the external genitalia, including the penis and scrotum. DHT is responsible for the development of the internal genitalia, including the epididymis, vas deferens, seminal vesicles, and prostrate gland. In nonprimates, androgens may have two other important targets: the mammary gland and the hypothalamus. In the mammary gland, DHT destroys all or part of the epithelium and thwarts nipple formation. In the hypothalamus, testosterone, after conversion to E_2, changes the secretory pattern of the gonadotropins from the cyclic female pattern to the tonic male pattern. In females, serum E_2 is sequestered in α-fetoprotein so the cyclic pattern persists. If female animals are given enough estrogen to exceed the binding capacity of this protein, the hypothalamus will become masculinized, that is, gonadotropins will be secreted tonically. In human fetuses, serum gonadotropin and testosterone levels return to basal levels by 28 weeks of gestation and the testes will remain quiescent until puberty.

In adolescence, androgens have important developmental, psychological, and sexual effects. Androgens stimulate both linear growth and skeletal maturity, that is, although the longitudinal growth of bones is accelerated, the growth plate shrinks and eventually becomes obliterated when the epiphyses and diaphyses fuse. This fusion marks the permanent termination of linear growth. Growth is also facilitated by the anabolic actions of androgens, especially by increased protein synthesis, which is most marked in muscles. Behaviorally, androgens induce aggression and libido. Finally, androgens promote the development of both primary and secondary male sexual characteristics.

Secondary sexual characteristics are those not required for reproduction per se, although they may facilitate the attraction of mating partners. They include sexual hair and a deep voice. Primary male sexual characteristics are those essential for successful intromission and insemination. They include the penis, testes, and accessory sexual structures.

2. Control

The testes are composed of *seminiferous tubules* and *Leydig cells*. The tubules are responsible for spermatogenesis and contain both the *spermatogonia* and the *Sertoli cells*. The latter nurture the sperm as they progress through their developmental stages. Spermatogenesis requires both FSH and very high levels of testosterone. The testosterone is supplied by the surrounding Leydig cells and is concentrated in the tubules by a special androgen-binding protein induced by FSH. LH stimulates testosterone synthesis by inducing P450scc in the Leydig cells. As for ACTH, this induction is accompanied by the stimulation of cholesterol transport into the mitochondria (Section III,B). Note that all steroid-synthesizing tissues are regulated at the initial P450scc step: both LH in the testis and ovary and ACTH in the zonae fasciculata and reticularis work through cAMP, whereas the effects of angiotensin II in the glomerulosa are mediated by calcium. The differences in the type of steroids secreted are determined by the other enzymes present in the tissues.

The regulation of testosterone secretion is relatively simple (Fig. 2-11; 17): low steroid levels release the hypothalamus and pituitary from feedback inhibition. The resulting GnRH secretion stimulates LH release which, in turn, activates steroid synthesis in the Leydig cells. When steroid levels have been restored, feedback inhibition is re-established. Control of spermatogenesis is more problematic: the product of the pathway is not a hormone that can exert feedback effects on the brain but a cell that remains in the tubule. It appears that the Sertoli cells monitor spermatogenesis and, whenever appropriate, release a hormone, *inhibin*, that specifically inhibits FSH secretion (18). It has, however, been discovered that this molecule has a dual function. Inhibin is a heterodimer containing a disulfide-linked 18-kDa α subunit and a 14-kDa β subunit; homodimers of the β subunit have also been discovered *in vivo*. Because the β-subunit homodimer selectively stimulated FSH secretion *in vitro*, it was called *activin*. Subsequently, this activity could not be demonstrated *in vivo*; rather, activin receptors have been found on spermatogonia, so this peptide is now thought to be a parahormone growth factor for these cells (19).

B. Estrogens and Progestins

The major sources of estrogens in women are the ovaries; in men, estrogens are formed from the peripheral conversion of androgens. The adrenal glands do not synthesize estrogens in any significant amounts. As in male embryos, hCG and the embryonic pituitary gonadotropins stimulate sex steroid pro-

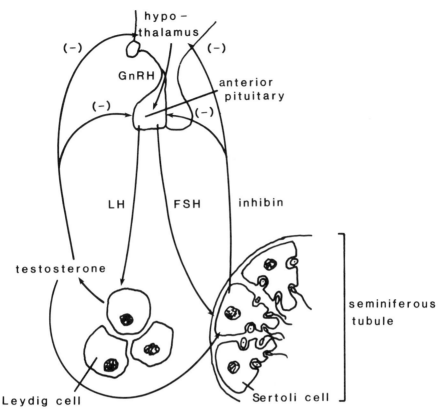

Fig. 2-11. Hormonal regulation of steroidogenesis and spermatogenesis in the testis. Adapted and reprinted by permission from Ref. 17. Copyright © 1979 McGraw-Hill Book Company.

duction from the gonads. However, there is no known role for estrogens in embryogenesis, since the basic phenotype is already female. For example, females with metabolic defects that prevent estrogen synthesis are morphologically normal at birth.

During puberty, estrogens have actions very similar to those of androgens. They stimulate linear growth and skeletal maturation, but are much less active in inducing muscle protein synthesis. They cause behavioral changes and promote the development of both primary and secondary female sexual characteristics. Primary female sexual characteristics include the internal and external genitalia; secondary sexual characteristics include breast development and the female pattern of fat deposition.

1. Oogenesis

In male humans, spermatogenesis requires 10 weeks to progress from spermatogonia to spermatozoa. However, the entire testis is not synchronized, although short stretches of the seminiferous tubule are; therefore, because the development of the male gametes is distributed throughout the gonad, there is a continuous supply of spermatozoa. Furthermore, because of attrition during storage and, eventually, during their trek in the female reproductive tract, the spermatozoa are made in large numbers.

Female animals, however, exemplify a different reproductive strategy. Because a female will carry the fetuses to term within her body, they have an excellent chance for survival; therefore, females need to produce only a few mature ova. In humans, a female usually produces only one ovum per reproductive cycle. Furthermore, because the female retains the fetuses, the development of her reproductive tract must be coordinated with oogenesis, intromission, and implantation. All these events require a synchronized series of hormonal and anatomical events called the *estrous* or *menstrual cycle*, depending on whether or not the mammal sheds blood during the cycle.

In humans, oogenesis begins *in utero*. The oogonia divide to produce between 6 and 7 million cells by 5 months of gestation. Then all of them become *primary oocytes* and enter prophase of meiosis I, at which stage they will remain until puberty. In males, spermatogonia are always reproducing themselves and thus maintain a reserve population; this allows spermatogenesis to continue well into old age. However, because there is no such reserve of oogonia, no further oocytes can be produced. In fact, almost immediately, oocytes begin to undergo atresia so that only 2 million are present at birth and only 300,000 remain by the time puberty approaches. Further atresia takes place during each menstrual cycle (see below), so women generally deplete their supply of oocytes when they are about 50 years of age.

During puberty in humans, the menstrual cycle begins. It consists of four phases: the follicular phase, ovulation, the luteal phase, and the menstrual phase. The *follicular* phase is also known as the *estrogenic* or *proliferative* phase and lasts 10–14 days. It begins when FSH recruits 10–20 primordial follicles to develop into primary follicles; this development involves proliferation of the granulosa cells surrounding the primary oocyte (Fig. 2-12; 20). The follicles also become invested with stroma: the outer layer, or *theca externa*, is merely a connective tissue capsule but the inner layer, or *theca interna*, is steroidogenic. LH, aided by inhibin, stimulates P450scc in the theca interna but, because these cells lack aromatase activity, the major products are androstenedione and testosterone. However, this androgen production is partially checked by activin. These steroids are then transported to the adjacent granulosa cells, which convert them to E_2 by a FSH-induced aromatase. E_2 further stimulates LH secretion but inhibits FSH secretion. The FSH concentrations decline and the follicles compete with one another for the available hormone. At this stage the follicles begin to develop a fluid-filled cavity, the *antrum*, and are now called secondary follicles. As FSH concentration becomes a limiting factor, the less successful follicles degenerate and, in humans, only one usually survives. When the antrum is

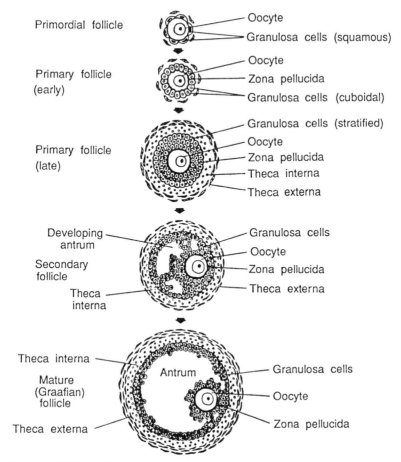

Primordial follicle — Oocyte — Granulosa cells (squamous)

Primary follicle (early) — Oocyte — Zona pellucida — Granulosa cells (cuboidal)

Primary follicle (late) — Granulosa cells (stratified) — Oocyte — Zona pellucida — Theca interna — Theca externa

Secondary follicle — Developing antrum — Theca interna — Granulosa cells — Oocyte — Zona pellucida — Theca externa

Mature (Graafian) follicle — Theca interna — Antrum — Theca externa — Granulosa cells — Oocyte — Zona pellucida

Fig. 2-12. Follicular development in the ovary. Reprinted by permission from Ref. 20. Copyright © 1979 Roberta Dilk Bruck.

complete, the entire structure is called a *mature* or *Graafian follicle*. In the meantime, the primary oocyte completes meiosis I to form the *secondary oocyte* and the first polar body, which usually degenerates. The secondary oocyte then enters meiosis II but becomes arrested in metaphase, in which state it will remain until fertilization. The rising levels of E_2 (Fig. 2-13) thicken the vagina and stimulate mucus production in preparation for intromission by the male copulatory organ. E_2 also stimulates hypertrophy (increase in cell size) and hyperplasia (increase in cell number) of the myometrium and endometrium, which are the muscle and inner lining of the uterus, respectively. Finally, E_2 promotes myometrial contractility, which may facilitate the transfer of the sperm from the vagina to the oviducts.

The positive feedback by E_2 results in a dramatic rise in LH levels at midcycle (Fig. 2-13). LH alters the integrity of the follicle, which ruptures and releases the oocyte and its surrounding granulosa cells. This is ovulation.

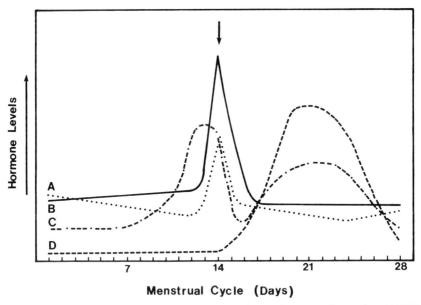

Fig. 2-13. Hormone levels during the menstrual cycle. The hormones depicted are (A) FSH, (B) LH, (C) estradiol, and (D) progesterone.

The *luteal* phase is also known as the *progestational* or *secretory* phase and lasts another 10–14 days. After ovulation, the follicle collapses and a new protein, *follistatin*, becomes elevated. This molecule binds activin, thereby neutralizing its inhibition of the androgen production needed for sex steroid synthesis (18). LH, now unhampered by activin, stimulates the collapsed follicle to produce large amounts of progesterone. In fact, it is so rich in cholesterol and steroids that it has a yellow color, which gives the structure its name: *corpus luteum* (yellow body). *Progesterone* stimulates the proliferation of the uterine glands, the secretion of glycogen, and the development of the spiral arterioles, all of which prepare the uterus for implantation and nourishment of the embryo. It also suppresses uterine contractions, which might otherwise endanger implantation. Finally, it inhibits both the synthesis and the secretion of LH but only the secretion of FSH, that is, although the levels of both gonadotropins decline, the pituitary content of FSH increases because synthesis continues. However, the pituitary LH content is totally depleted. Since LH is required for progesterone synthesis by the corpus luteum, the synthesis of this steroid likewise declines.

Another hormone secreted by the corpus lutem is *relaxin*. It has two major functions: first of all, it induces collagenases that soften the uterine cervix and loosen the public symphysis. Both effects facilitate delivery of the infant at parturition. These enzymes also weaken the follicular cell wall prior to its rupture during ovulation. The second function is to inhibit myometrial activity, but this effect is not seen in all species. Relaxin can also be synthesized by the mammary and prostate glands, although its functions in these tissues are unknown (21).

The superficial layer of the endometrium, the *stratum functionalis*, is totally dependent on progesterone for its maintenance. When progesterone levels fall, the stratum functionalis atrophies and is shed along with the unfertilized ovum. This is the *menstrual phase*. The decline of progesterone levels also releases the pituitary from inhibition. FSH is immediately secreted because intracellular stores are filled, and it recruits more primordial follicles for the next cycle. LH secretion is delayed, since it must first be synthesized. If LH were to be secreted too quickly, the LH-induced E_2 production would inhibit FSH secretion and follicular development.

2. Pregnancy

If fertilization takes place, the secondary oocyte will complete meiosis II and the female and male pronuclei will fuse to form a *zygote*. Fertilization occurs in the upper third of the oviducts and cleavage begins promptly; by the time the embryo reaches the uterus, it is a *blastocyst*. The blastocyst is divided into two components: the *inner cell mass* will become the embryo proper and the *trophoblast* will become the fetal placenta. The human trophoblast invades the endometrium during implantation and secretes hCG (Fig. 2-14), which is a placental homolog of LH. Therefore, when the pituitary LH level falls, LH is replaced by a placental gonadotropin, which continues to stimulate the corpus luteum to produce progesterone. This prevents menstruation and maintains the pregnancy. Eventually, the fetoplacental unit will take over all steroid synthesis. In fact, if the mother is ovariectomized

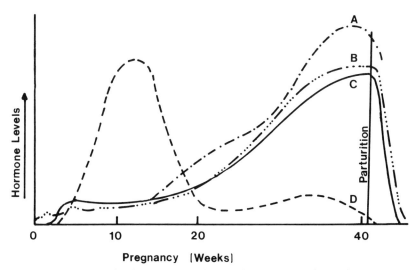

Fig. 2-14. Hormone levels during pregnancy. The hormones depicted are (A) human placental lactogen, (B) estrogen, (C) progesterone, and (D) hCG.

after 30 days of gestation or hypophysectomized after 12 weeks, the pregnancy still continues normally.

The major sources of steroids during pregnancy are the placenta, the maternal adrenal cortex, and the fetal adrenal cortex and liver. The fetal adrenal cortex is located between the adult cortex and the medulla; it makes up a large portion of the fetal adrenal gland but disappears by 1 year postpartum. The interrelationships among these sources are depicted in Fig. 2-15.

Although the placenta is the immediate source of the sex steroids during pregnancy, it lacks certain enzymes and relies heavily on other tissues for appropriate precursors. For example, it lacks hydroxymethylglutaryl coenzyme A reductase, the rate-limiting enzyme in cholesterol synthesis. The placental cholesterol comes from the mother, who also supplies at least 50% of the cholesterol for the fetal adrenal gland. From cholesterol, the placenta can synthesize progesterone but, lacking 17α-hydroxylase, it cannot go beyond this step. This second enzyme deficiency is bypassed if both the fetal and the maternal adrenal gland supply the placenta with DHEA. The placenta, which has very high aromatase activity, converts DHEA to estrone and E_2. The fetal adrenal gland also sulfates the DHEA; the resulting steroid is hydroxylated in the fetal liver and aromatized in the placenta to form estriol.

The function of progesterone is to prevent abortion by maintaining the endometrium. However, the functions of the other hormones, especially at the high concentrations found in the serum, are unknown. Indeed, humans are among the very few species that have high estrogen levels during pregnancy. The placenta also secretes large amounts of human placental lactogen (hPL), a member of the GH–PRL family, but its role is likewise unclear, since

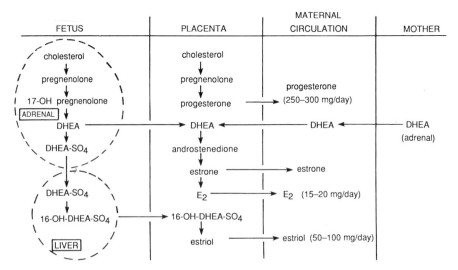

Fig. 2-15. Interrelationships among the placenta, fetus, and mother with respect to steroidogenesis during pregnancy. DHEA, Dihydroepiandrosterone; E_2, estradiol.

patients with hPL gene deletions and no serum hPL levels can still have normal pregnancies (see Chapter 17).

VI. Gastrointestinal Hormones

The function of the gastrointestinal (GI) tract is to digest and absorb ingested nutrients. This act requires the close coordination of the entire GI system, much of which is provided by hormones. Furthermore, since eating is intermittent, the body must be prepared to handle periodic surges of nutrients from the GI tract; again, hormones are the major regulators. Finally, it is only appropriate that some of these hormones also control metabolism during times of fasting. This section is divided into two parts: the first deals with the major hormones of the pancreas and the metabolic shifts that they induce throughout the body; the second part focuses on the GI tract itself and examines the local endocrine control of digestion.

A. Pancreas

The pancreas is both an endocrine and an exocrine gland. This chapter is concerned only with the endocrine function, which resides in nests of cells between the acini. These islets of Langerhans are histologically composed of several cell types, each occupying a specific position in the islet and each secreting a different hormone (Table 2-3).

1. Insulin

Although insulin consists of two peptides linked by disulfide bonds, it is originally synthesized as an 81-amino-acid precursor, proinsulin. The entire molecule is required to approximate the appropriate cysteines, and the disulfide bridges form while the prohormone is in the rough endoplasmic reticulum. Once this linkage occurs, the intervening piece, or C peptide, must be

Table 2-3
Histochemical Characteristics of Some Pancreatic Hormones

Hormone	Location	Structure
Glucagon	A (α) cells: Outermost rim of islets	29-Amino-acid linear poly-peptide
Insulin	B (β) cells: Core of islet	Two chains (21 and 30 amino acids) connected by disulfide bonds
SRIF	D (δ) cells: Inner rim of islets	14-Amino-acid cyclic peptide (via disulfide bond)
Pancreatic polypeptide	F cells	36-Amino acid linear poly-peptide

removed since proinsulin is only about 10% as active as insulin. Cleavage is accomplished by a trypsin-like protease attracted to two pairs of basic amino acids (Fig. 2-16). Cleavage begins when the molecule is in the Golgi apparatus and continues in the secretory granules, although it is never complete: about 6% of insulin is secreted as proinsulin. Finally, zinc is transported into the granules and triggers the crystallization of insulin as dimers and hexamers.

To understand the control of insulin secretion, it is necessary to discuss its actions briefly. Insulin is an anabolic hormone, that is, it is involved with energy storage. Primarily, this action is manifested as an increase in glucose and amino acid transport into cells and as the stimulation of conversion of these precursors into storage forms such as glycogen, protein, and triglycerides. Therefore, elevated blood levels of glucose, fatty acids, or amino acids will stimulate insulin release. However, this would result in the secretion are insulin after the substrate levels had already risen in the blood; to regulate these blood concentrations more smoothly, several anticipatory signals have been developed. For example, GI tract motility and secretion are stimulated by the parasympathetic nervous system (see Section III,D), whose activity means that the GI tract is actively digesting food and that nutrients will soon be absorbed into the bloodstream. As a result, ACh, the distal neurotransmitter of the parasympathetic nervous system, stimulates insulin secretion. Finally, the presence of carbohydrate in the intestines results in the release of gastric inhibitory peptide, which is also an insulin secretagogue.

Mechanistically, the actions of insulin are quite complex. Some of the effects merely involve blocking or reversing the actions of other hormones. For example, several of the cAMP-dependent hormones stimulate glycogenolysis and lipolysis by phosphorylating critical enzymes in these pathways (see Chapter 11). However, insulin promotes the storage of glucose and fatty acids and inhibits the breakdown of glycogen and triglycerides. It does so by activating specific phosphatases that remove the phosphate from enzymes,

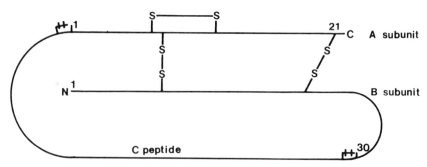

Fig. 2-16. Schematic diagram of the proinsulin molecule showing the A, B, and C peptides, as well as the pairs of basic residues that are attacked by proteases during the conversion of proinsulin to insulin.

that is, it reverses the phosphorylation induced by the cAMP-dependent protein kinase.

Insulin can also affect metabolism by altering substrate flow. For example, insulin stimulates the uptake of glucose within cells; the resulting high levels of glucose 6-phosphate allosterically activate glycogen synthase (Fig. 2-17). In another example, insulin stimulates glycolysis but eventually the cell becomes sated with ATP, which shuts down the tricarboxylic acid cycle by allosterically inhibiting several important enzymes, including isocitrate dehydrogenase. As a result, citrate begins to accumulate and will allosterically activate the committed step in fatty acid synthesis.

Insulin can also have more direct effects. For example, the immediate stimulation of metabolite transport and certain enzymes is mediated by still-unknown second messengers. Finally, the delayed activation of other enzymes occurs via gene induction.

2. Glucagon

Glucagon is considerably simpler to discuss. It is a 29-amino-acid linear peptide whose major action is to elevate blood glucose levels; therefore, it is catabolic and antagonizes the actions of insulin. More specifically, it stimulates liver glycogenolysis and inhibits glycolysis; it is aided by epinephrine, which triggers glycogenolysis in muscle and lipolysis in adipose tissue. Both hormones act via a cAMP-dependent protein kinase, which phosphorylates critical enzymes in these pathways (see Chapter 11). Cortisol also plays a complementary role by stimulating gluconeogenesis in the liver and providing this organ with amino acid metabolites. At low concentrations, cortisol inhibits protein synthesis; at higher concentrations, it promotes protein breakdown. The resulting amino acids are deaminated and the ammonia is detoxified in the urea cycle. Except for its effects on protein synthesis, all these processes are accomplished by enzyme induction via steroid receptors. The effects of all these hormones are listed in Table 2-4 and schematically depicted in Fig. 2-18. Note that Table 2-4 only summarizes the major actions of each hormone to emphasize the complementary nature of these hormones. In truth, each hormone has a wide variety of overlapping activities; for example, epinephrine can stimulate hepatic glycogenolysis, although not to the same extent as glucagon. Similarly, glucocorticoids can induce lipolysis and glucagon can promote hepatic proteolysis.

B. Local Gastrointestinal Hormones

Several hormones are secreted by the GI tract in response to nutrients or acidity. Their major functions appear to involve the coordination of digestive secretions, GI tract motility, and visceral blood flow (Table 2-5).

For example, amino acids stimulate gastrin release, which in turn elevates gastric acid secretion to facilitate further proteolysis. If hydrogen ion concentrations become too high, gastrin secretion is inhibited. In another example, *cholecystokinin* (CCK), formerly called pancreozymin, is concerned

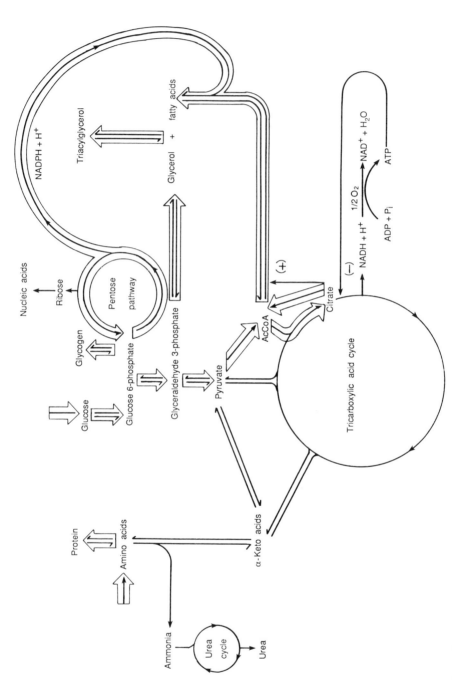

Fig. 2-17. Schematic representation of the biochemical actions of insulin. The arrow overlays indicate substrate flow during insulin stimulation.

Table 2-4
Biochemical Effects of Some Catabolic Hormones

Hormone	Carbohydrate	Protein	Lipid
Glucagon	↑ Glycogenolysis (liver); ↓ Glycolysis		
Epinephrine	↑ Glycogenesis (muscle)		↑ Lipolysis
Cortisol	↑ Gluconeogenesis	↓ Protein synthesis ↑ Transaminases ↑ Urea cycle	

with the digestion of triglycerides; therefore, its secretion is stimulated by fatty acids. In turn, this hormone stimulates the secretion of pancreatic enzymes, including the pancreatic lipase. However, the effectiveness of the lipase alone is limited because triglycerides are not soluble in water. However, CCK also stimulates contraction of the gallbladder, which contains bile. Bile salts are amphipathic and thus are excellent detergents; they emulsify the fat, which then becomes more susceptible to the lipase. One final example of the regulation of digestion is provided by *secretin*. When the stomach empties its acidic contents into the duodenum, the acid stimulates the release of secretin, which promotes bicarbonate secretion in bile and pancreatic fluids. The bicarbonate is used to neutralize the acid.

Digestion involves the synthesis and secretion of enzymes, muscular activity, and active transport. To support this high metabolic rate, *vasoactive intestinal peptide* (VIP) and *substance P* dilate the mesenteric circulatory system. This increased blood flow also helps dilute the absorbed nutrients, which are present in the hepatic portal system at high concentrations. These two hormones, along with *motilin,* also regulate GI motility.

Finally, there is coordination among the hormones themselves. The role of *gastric inhibitory peptide* (GIP) in alerting the pancreas that carbohydrate is in the gut has already been mentioned. *Gastrin releasing peptide* (GRP), a member of the bombesin peptide family, is another anticipatory signal. The sight or odor of food activates the parasympathetic nervous system, which then triggers the release of GRP via the vagus nerve. Somatostatin (SRIF), which was first discovered as an inhibitor of GH release, also inhibits the release of many other hormones. It is synthesized in the D cells of the islets, where it affects the secretion of insulin and glucagon. VIP however, is a general stimulator of hormone release.

Many of these hormones are members of one of three families. All the hormones in the gastrin family have the same carboxy-terminal pentapeptide (−Gly−Trp−Met−Asp−Phe−NH$_2$). All the activity of gastrin is found in this pentapeptide, whereas the actions of CCK can be fully mimicked by its carboxy-terminal octapeptide. *Cerulein,* a decapeptide found in the skin and GI tract of amphibians, is also a member of this family. In contrast, the

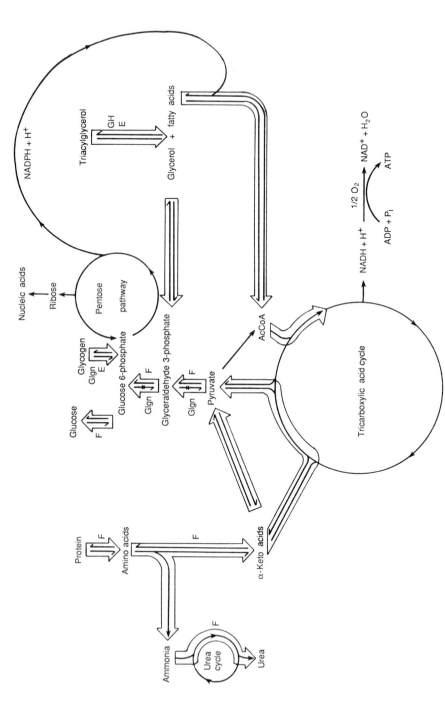

Fig. 2-18. Schematic representation of the biochemical actions of several catabolic hormones, including cortisol (F), glucagon (Glgn), epinephrine (E), and growth hormone (GH). The arrow overlays indicate substrate flow during stimulation by these hormones.

Table 2-5
Physiochemical and Physiological Characterization of Several Gastrointestinal Hormones

Hormone	Size (amino acids)	Location	Stimulators	Actions
Gastrin	17	Antrum	Amino acids (H^+, inhibitor)	Stimulates HCl secretion; stimulates mucosal and pancreatic growth
Gastrin-releasing peptide (GRP)	27	Stomach and small intestine	Vagus	Stimulates gastrin secretion and growth of GI tract
Cholecystokinin (CCK)	33	Duodenum and jejunum	Fatty acids	Stimulates gallbladder contraction and pancreatic enzyme secretion; inhibits sphincter of Oddi and gastric emptying
Secretin	27	Duodenum	Acid	Stimulates pancreatic and bile secretion of bicarbonate
Gastric inhibitory peptide (GIP)	43	Duodenum and jejunum	Carbohydrate	Stimulates insulin secretion
Vasoactive intestinal peptide (VIP)	28	Jejunum and colon	Unknown	Visceral vasodilator; inhibits smooth muscle of GI and genitourinary tract; general hormone releaser (gut, pancreas, and pituitary)
Substance P	11	Gut	Mixed meal	Vasodilator and sialogogue; stimulates GI motility
Motilin	22	Duodenum	Unknown	Stimulates GI motility in the fasting state
Somatostatin (SRIF)	14	D (δ) cells of pancreas	Unknown	General hormone release inhibitor (gut, pancreas, and pituitary)

a GI, Gastrointestinal.

members of the secretin family require the entire molecule for activity. This family includes secretin, VIP, and glucagon. The *tachykinin* family includes substance P, substance K, and neuromedin K. These molecules only have about a dozen amino acids and all end with a carboxy-terminal sequence of $-Phe-X-Gly-Leu-Met-NH_2$, where X represents any amino acid.

References

General References

DeGroot, L. J., (ed.) (1989). "Endocrinology," 2d Ed. Saunders, Philadelphia.
Hadley, M. E. (1992). "Endocrinology." Prentice Hall, Englewood Cliffs, New Jersey.
Martin, C. R. (1985). "Endocrine Physiology." Oxford University Press, London.
Norman, A. W., and Litwack, G. (1987). "Hormones." Academic Press, Orlando, Florida.
Wilson, J. D., and Foster, D. W., (eds.) (1992). "Textbook of Endocrinology," 8th Ed. Saunders, Philadelphia.
See also Refs. 1, 2, 6, 8–14, 18, and 21.

Cited References

1. Isaksson, O. G. P., Lindahl, A., Nilsson, A., and Isgaard, J. (1987). Mechanism of the stimulatory effect of growth hormone on longitudinal bone growth. *Endocr. Rev.* **8**, 426–438.
2. Gala, R. R. (1991). Prolactin and growth hormone in the regulation of the immune system. *Proc. Soc. Exp. Biol. Med.* **198**, 513–527.
3. Spiliotis, B. E., August, G. P., Hung, W., Sonis, W., Mendelson, W., and Bercu, B. B. (1984). Growth hormone neurosecretory dysfunction. A treatable cause of short stature. *JAMA J. Am. Med. Assoc.* **251**, 2223–2230.
4. Norstedt, G., and Palmiter, R. (1984). Secretory rhythm of growth hormone regulates sexual differentiation of mouse liver. *Cell* **36**, 805–812.
5. Papadopoulos, V. (1993). Peripheral-type benzodiazepine/diazepam binding inhibitor receptor: Biological role in steroidogenic cell function. *Endocr. Rev.* **14**, 222–240.
6. Miller, W. L. (1988). Molecular biology of steroid hormone synthesis. *Endocr. Rev.* **9**, 295–318.
7. Clemmons, D. R. (1992). IGF binding proteins: Regulation of cellular actions. *Growth Regul.* **2**, 80–87.
8. Inagami, T. (1989). Atrial natriuretic factor. *J. Biol. Chem.* **264**, 3043–3046.
9. Brenner, B. M., Ballermann, B. J., Gunning, M. E., and Zeidel, M. L. (1990). Diverse biological actions of atrial natriuretic peptide. *Physiol. Rev.* **70**, 665–699.
10. Ruskoaho, H. (1992). Atrial natriuretic peptide: Synthesis, release, and metabolism. *Pharmacol. Rev.* **44**, 479–602.
11. Marletta, M. A. (1989). Nitric oxide: Biosynthesis and biological significance. *Trends Biochem. Sci.* **14**, 488–492.
12. Collier, J., and Vallance, P. (1989). Second messenger role for NO widens to nervous and immune systems. *Trends Pharmacol. Sci.* **10**, 427–431.
13. Rubanyi, G. M., and Botelho, L. H. P. (1991). Endothelins. *FASEB J.* **5**, 2713–2720.
14. Simonson, M. S. (1993). Endothelins: Multifunctional renal peptides. *Physiol. Rev.* **73**, 375–411.
15. Shirakami, G., Nakao, K., Saito, Y., Magaribuchi, T., Mukoyama, M., Arai, H., Hosoda, K., Suga, S. I., Mori, K., and Imura, H. (1993). Low doses of endothelin-1 inhibit atrial natriuretic peptide secretion. *Endocrinol. (Baltimore)* **132**, 1905–1912.
16. Kaltenbach, J. C. (1953). Local action of thyroxin on amphibian metamorphosis.

III. Formation and perforation of the skin window in *Rana pipiens* larvae effected by thyroxin–cholesterol implants. *J. Exp. Zool.* **122**, 449–467.

17. Smith, E. L., Hill, R. L., Lehman, I. R., Lefkowitz, R. J., Handler, P., and White, A. (1983). "Principles of Biochemistry: Mammalian Biochemistry," 7th ed., McGraw-Hill, New York.

18. Findlay, J. K. (1993). An update on the roles of inhibin, activin, and follistatin as local regulators of folliculogenesis. *Biol. Reprod.* **48**, 15–23.

19. Kaipia, A., Parvinen, M., and Toppari, J. (1993). Localization of activin receptor (ActR-IIB2) mRNA in the rat seminiferous epithelium. *Endocrinol. (Baltimore)* **132**, 477–479.

20. Bruck-Kan, R. (1979). "Introduction to Human Anatomy," Harper & Row, New York.

21. Bryant-Greenwood, G. D., and Schwabe, C. (1994). Human relaxins: Chemistry and biology. *Endocr. Rev.* **15**, 5–26.

CHAPTER 3

Non-Classical Endocrinology

CHAPTER OUTLINE

I. Introduction

In the preceding chapters, chemicals closely fitting the classical definition of a hormone were described. In this chapter, the renegades will be discussed. These hormones are frequently synthesized at multiple sites and may act locally (1). However, their most bewildering characteristics are their extensively overlapping biological activities, their large repertoire of effects, and their occasional contradictory activities. All these properties are probably related to the fact that most of these hormones are growth factors: all hormones stimulating mitosis are going to activate a number of common pathways; therefore, some overlap in activity is inevitable. Furthermore, growth is a complex process requiring coordination with metabolism, which will supply the materials and energy for growth, and with reproduction, which will be its chief competitor for these limited nutrients. As such, these hormones will have a wide range of effects.

Finally, many of these hormones can exert opposite activities such as growth promotion and inhibition. This phenomenon can be explained if one assumes that the action of a hormone will be influenced by the history and environment of its target (2). All growth is not the same: the growth manifested during embryogenesis is very different from that seen during simple enlargement or that required to repair tissue damage. In addition, it must be remembered that hormones usually have no intrinsic activity: only two are known to be enzymes and none are transport proteins. Their effect is actually the cellular response to their presence. This response is not stereotyped: the cell integrates all the information it has received and then initiates action appropriate to the circumstances.

Invertebrate and plant hormones will also be discussed here, since many of them are somewhat atypical with respect to the classical definition of a hormone. The following discussion cannot hope to cover every growth factor or invertebrate hormone. Rather, it will concentrate on those hormones that will be encountered again later in this text.

II. Growth Factors

A. Cell Cycle

Actively dividing cells undergo a repetitive sequence of events known as the *cell cycle*. This cycle is divided into four stages (Fig. 3-1): M, G_1, S, and G_2. M and S are easy to recognize. M is mitosis, when the cell is visibly undergoing cell division. The mitotic stages, prophase through telophase, can be followed by light microscopy. S is when DNA synthesis is occurring and has no visible correlate; however, it can be detected using radiolabeled thymidine incorporation. G_1 and G_2 are the gaps between M and S and between S and M, respectively. Unfortunately, these gaps are still black boxes. Although the actions of various growth factors can be mapped within these stages, it is not clear exactly what processes are occurring.

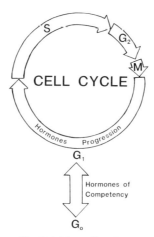

Fig. 3-1. The cell cycle.

Most growth factors act in G_1 to speed the advance of an already actively dividing cell toward S, but they often have no effect on nondividing cells. These factors are known as *hormones of progression*. Other growth factors can make nondividing cells sensitive to the hormones of progression, although they themselves cannot actually initiate cell division. These latter factors are called *hormones of competency* and their requirement has led to the speculation that nondividing cells are not simply stalled in G_1 but actually lie outside of the cell cycle, in a stage known as G_0. These cells must first be brought back into the cycle by the hormones of competency before they can be stimulated by the hormones of progression.

B. General Growth Factors

1. Epidermal Growth Factor Family

The epidermal growth factor family (EGF) consists of EGF, *transforming growth factor-α* (TGF-α), and *amphiregulin* (Table 3-1) (3-6). Both EGF and TGF-α are synthesized as membrane-bound precursors that are cleaved to yield the 6-kDa soluble hormone. However, both precursors are active and the EGF precursor appears to persist in some tissues such as the alveolar membrane in the lactating mammary gland. Therefore, EGF may have a juxtacrine, as well as an endocrine, mode of action. Both EGF and TGF-α bind to the same receptor and have very similar activity. Less is known about amphiregulin, which was purified from conditioned medium from breast cancer cells. Because it has a lower affinity for the EGF receptor and because its range of target cells is more restricted, amphiregulin is believed to have its own receptor. Both EGF and TGF-α are hormones of progression that act early in G_1 to stimulate epithelial cell proliferation. They can also stimulate anchorage-independent growth and the formation of new blood vessels to supply the expanding tissue (*neovascularization*).

Table 3-1

Some Growth and Growth Inhibiting Factors in Vertebrates

Hormone[a]	Source	Action
EGF family: Single peptide chain		
EGF	Salivary glands	Epithelial proliferation; anchorage independence; neovascularization
TGF-α	Many	Same
Amphiregulin	Unknown	Same, but less effective in some cell types (for example, renal)
TGF-β family: Identical or homologous dimers		
TGF-βs	Ubiquitous	Inhibits proliferation of epithelial and immune cells; induces mesoderm
Müllerian inhibiting substance	Mammalian testes	Regression of Müllerian ducts in males
Inhibins/activins	Gonads and hypothalamus	Inhibits FSH secretion; spermatogenesis
Bone morphogenetic protein	Bone	Osteogenesis; bone repair
PDGF family: Identical or homologous dimers		
PDGF	Platelets	Proliferation of connective tissue; tissue repair
Vascular endothelial growth factor (VEGF)	Neural tissues and vascular smooth muscle	Vascular endothelial mitogen; increases vascular permeability
Insulin family: Intact or cleaved peptide chain		
IGF-I	Liver	GH-Dependent cartilage growth
IGF-II	Many	Fetal growth
Relaxin	Ovary	Inhibits uterine contractions; elongates interpubic ligament; softens cervix
FGF family: Single peptide chain		
Acidic FGF	Neural tissues	Proliferation of vasular endothelium and certain fibroblasts; mesoderm induction (with TGF-β); chemotaxic; adipocyte and neuron differentiation
Basic FGF	Many	Same
Keratinocyte growth factor (KGF)	Stroma of epithelia	Epithelial cell mitogen
IL-1α and β	Macrophages	Stimulate helper T cells to produce IL-2
NGF family: Peptides		
NGF	Brain, heart, spleen	Neuronal survival, outgrowth, and differentiation, especially dorsal root and paravertebral ganglia
Brain-derived neurotrophic factor (BDNF)	Brain, heart	Same, especially dorsal root and nodose ganglia
Neurotrophin-3 (NT-3)	Brain, heart, kidney, liver, thymus	Same, including all three ganglia
Hematopoietic growth factors: Glycoproteins (not homologous)		
Erythropoietin	Kidney	Proliferation of RBC progenitor cell
CSFs	Endothelium, T cells, fibroblasts, macrophages	Proliferation of WBC progenitor cells

continues

continued

Hormone[a]	Source	Action
IL-3	Helper T cells	Proliferation of multilineage colonies
SCF (=KL, MGF, SLF)		Proliferation of hematopoietic cells (especially mast cells), germ cells, and melanoblasts
Retinoic acid	Diet (stored in liver)	Epithelial differentiation

[a] CSFs, Colony stimulating factors; EGF, epidermal growth factor; FGF, fibroblast growth factor; IGF, insulin-like growth factor; IL, interleukin; NGF, nerve growth factor; PDGF, platelet-derived growth factor; RBC, red blood cell; SCF, stem cell factor; TGF, transforming growth factor; WBC, white blood cell.

2. Transforming Growth Factor-β Family

Transforming growth factor-β (TGF-β) is a 25-kDa homodimer that forms the carboxy terminus of a larger precursor (6–9). After cleavage, the homodimer remains noncovalently attached to the amino-terminal halves as an inactive tetramer. TGF-β is eventually liberated by the protease *plasmin*, which is elevated during injury; this association has led to the speculation that TGF-β may play a role in wound repair.

TGF-β and the other members of this family are interesting for their ability to inhibit, as well as stimulate, growth. In addition, many members have important functions in embryogenesis. TGF-β itself inhibits the proliferation of most epithelial and immune cells by arresting them in G_1. However, it has two other effects that can reverse this inhibition: first, it can stimulate the synthesis and secretion of growth factors that, along with TGF-β, can induce mesoderm and blood vessel formation and stimulate the proliferation of keratinocytes and intestinal epithelium. Also, it can promote the production and deposition of extracellular matrix, which can further promote mitogenesis.

Müllerian inhibiting substance (MIS), also called anti-Müllerian hormone, is a 70- to 72-kDa homodimer whose carboxy terminus exhibits homology to TGF-β. In males, it is produced by the testes during embryogenesis when it thwarts the development of the Müllerian duct derivatives, including the uterus and oviducts. In persistent Müllerian duct syndrome, this hormone is absent and male pseudohermaphroditism results. Such males appear to be normally virilized with the sole exception of possessing uteri and oviducts that are usually discovered during incidental surgery.

The inhibins and activins were covered in Chapter 2 (Section V) when their role in regulating FSH secretion was discussed. However, these hormones are also active in the embryonic formation of axial and anterior structures such as the notochord, neural tube, and segmented somites.

Finally, there are several *bone morphogenetic proteins* in this family (10,11). Other than their sequences, production by bone tissue, and osteogenic activity, not much is known about them. Researchers believe that they may be involved in bone repair as well as in cartilage and bone differentiation during limb morphogenesis.

3. Platelet-Derived Growth Factor Family

Like inhibin/activin, platelet-derived growth factor (PDGF) is composed of two homologous subunits that can form either homo- or heterodimers. The A subunit is 12 kDa whereas the B subunit is 18 kDa. The B subunit has a carboxy-terminal extension that electrostatically interacts with the plasma membrane, where it remains bound. As such, it resembles the EGF precursor. This membrane-binding region is also present in the A subunit, but it is proteolytically removed during processing; as a result, PDGF A homodimers are secreted and not retained on the cell surface. The ratio of these isoforms depends on the species and the tissue being examined; for example, in human platelets, the AB isoform represents 70% of PDGF whereas the BB isoform accounts for the remainder. Note that the PDGF receptor also has two isoforms that form homo- and heterodimers and that show relative specificity for different PDGF isoforms (see Chapter 6). PDGF is involved in chemotaxis and the proliferation of connective tissue, especially in wound repair. PDGF is a hormone of competency.

Vascular endothelial growth factor (VEGF) is a dimer of apparently identical 23-kDa subunits. It is produced by a number of neural cell types as well as by vascular smooth muscle. VEGF stimulates mitogenesis in vascular endothelium and increases vascular permeability. Its site of action in the cell cycle has not yet been investigated.

4. Fibroblast Growth Factor Family

The fibroblast growth factor (FGF) family consists of *acidic FGF, basic FGF, keratinocyte growth factor* (KGF), and *interleukin-1* (IL-1) (12,13). Both acidic and basic FGF have 154 amino acids, bind to the same receptor, and have identical biological activities. FGF has both growth-promoting and differentiative effects: it stimulates the proliferation of vascular endothelium and certain fibroblasts, but also promotes adipocyte and neuronal differentiation. Finally, it is critical for the formation of the posterior and lateral mesoderm during embryogenesis. Like PDGF, it is a hormone of competency. KGF is produced by epithelial stroma and also stimulates epithelial mitosis. The function of IL-1 is described in Section II,D. Some members of this family are bound to the cell surface, presumably by their cationic carboxy termini, in a manner similar to PDGF.

5. Insulin Family

Insulin is a metabolic hormone that was covered in Chapter 2 (Section VI). However, this family has several other members that are better known for their growth-promoting activity (14,15). *Insulin-like growth factors-I* and *-II* (IGF-I and IGF-II) are both insulin homologs whose C peptide has been reduced in length and retained; they utilize different receptors. They are both found in the serum associated with binding proteins. Although IGF-I and -II are hydrophilic, the binding proteins may serve functions other than solubilization. For example, these proteins can inhibit the activity of IGF, presumably by sequestering the hormone; they may also protect these small peptide hormones from rapid degradation.

IGF-I is secreted primarily from the liver in response to growth hormone. Its major systemic effect is the stimulation of cartilage growth resulting in linear growth of the skeleton. However, IGF-I can also be produced in many tissues under the control of tropic hormones to promote local growth and/or differentiation, for example, in leukocytes and mammary gland by growth hormone; in bone by parathormone and sex steroids; in adrenocortical cells by ACTH; in testis by LH and FSH; in granulosa cells by LH, FSH, and estradiol; in uterus by estradiol and progesterone; and in fibroblasts by EGF, FGF, and PDGF. IGF-II appears to be important for fetal growth. Both factors are hormones of progression that act late in G_1. Relaxin is another member of this family and was discussed in Chapter 2 (Section V).

6. Nerve Growth Factor Family

The nerve growth factor family (NGF), consists of NGF, *brain-derived neurotrophic factor* (BDNF), and *neurotrophin-3* (NT-3). All three peptides are synthesized as precursors that are cleaved to generate an approximately 120-amino-acid hormone; the sequences of the mature peptides are about 50% identical and appear to be distantly related to the TGFβ and PDGF families. Their biological activities also significantly overlap: all three hormones are involved in the survival, outgrowth, and differentiation of neurons. Their major differences are found in their target tissues and their sites of synthesis. NGF acts on the dorsal root and paravertebral sympathetic ganglia and is made in many tissues, especially the brain, heart, and spleen. BDNF affects the dorsal root and nodose ganglia and has a more restricted distribution, being found in high levels in brain and heart with lesser concentrations in lung and muscle. NT-3 stimulates all three ganglia and, like NGF, is synthesized in most tissues. However, the levels in these tissues are much higher, often equaling or exceeding those found in brain.

A fourth neurotrophin, *ciliary neurotrophic factor* (CNTF), is functionally, but not structurally, related to the NGF family. As the name implies, it stimulates ciliary ganglion growth; it can also promote cholinergic and glial differentiation. Unlike the NGF family, it is not cleaved from a precursor and may not even be secreted: it has no signal sequence and accumulates in the cytoplasm of all transfected cells. With its 200 amino acids, it is larger than NGF. CNTF has a very restricted distribution: it is only found in abundance in the sciatic nerve, whereas the spinal cord has low levels.

C. Hematopoietic Growth Factors

All blood cells are generated from a single stem cell in the bone marrow, the *hematocytoblast* (Fig. 3-2; 16–19). This cell, in turn, gives rise to five blast cells. The proerythroblast develops into the *erythrocyte*, or red blood cell, which is important in transporting oxygen. The myeloblast produces cells with secretory granules, the *granulocytes;* they include the *neutrophil, eosinophil,* and *basophil.* The neutrophil phagocytizes bacteria and the eosinophil is involved in allergic reactions and parasitic infections. The basophil, called a *mast cell* when it is found in tissues, contains histamine and heparin and is involved in allergic responses and blood clotting. The monoblast gives rise to *monocytes,* which are elevated during viral and tuberculous infections. Monocytes can also develop into *macrophages,* which are concerned with removing debris from injuries or infections. The lymphoblast produces both *B lymphocytes,* which produce antibodies, and *T lymphocytes,* which are involved in cell-mediated immunity (see Section II,D). The megakaryoblast will eventually give rise to a cell that fragments. These cellular pieces are called *thrombocytes* or *platelets* and form a critical part of the blood clotting system.

1. Erythropoietin

Erythropoietin is a 39-kDa glycoprotein secreted by the renal peritubular cells in response to low oxygen tension (*hypoxia*); it is not clear whether the interstitial cells or the capillary endothelial cells produce erythropoietin. The kidney is a highly metabolic organ that receives 25% of the cardiac output; as such, the kidney is very susceptible to damage from hypoxia. Under these circumstances, it releases erythropoietin, which stimulates erythrocyte progenitor cell proliferation, increases the hemoglobin content per red blood cell, and promotes the early release of erythrocytes from the marrow. The absence of this hormone produces the severe anemia seen in end-stage kidney disease.

2. Colony Stimulating Factors

The colony-stimulating factors (CSFs) stimulate the proliferation of one or more leukocytic lines and are produced by a wide variety of cell types, including endothelium, fibroblasts, T lymphocytes, and macrophages, especially when these cells originate in the lungs, kidneys, spleen, or salivary glands.

The *granulocyte/macrophage CSF* (GM-CSF) is an 118- to 127-amino-acid glycoprotein with a molecular mass of 16–41 kDa, depending on the species and the degree of glycosylation. The carbohydrate portion of the molecule is not necessary for biological activity, a fact that also applies to all other CSFs. GM-CSF has the most wide-ranging effects: at low concentrations it selectively stimulates the proliferation of the monocyte–macrophage cell line, whereas at higher concentrations it affects all the granulocytes, especially the basophils and mast cells.

The *macrophage CSF* (M-CSF or CSF-1) is more selective and only stimulates the monoblast cell line. It is a homodimer of 47–70 kDa, depending on glycosylation, and is initially synthesized as a membrane-bound precursor. Both the membrane-bound and the soluble forms enhance the survival, proliferation, and differentiation of monocytes and macrophages.

The effect of the *granulocyte CSF* (G-CSF) depends on the concentration

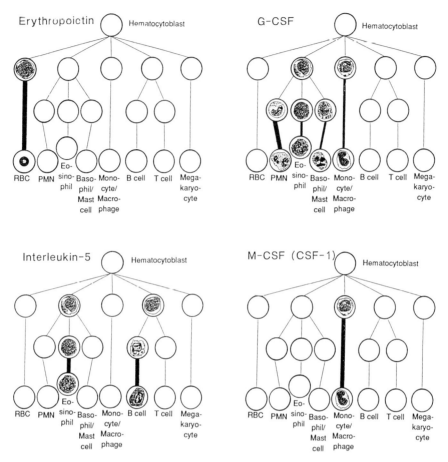

Fig. 3-2. Stem cell lines in hematopoiesis and the hormones that regulate them. Thick lines represent major effects; thin lines represent effects only observed at higher concentrations. RBC, Red blood cell; PMN, polymorphonuclear leukocyte.

of this 25- to 30-kDa glycoprotein. At low concentrations, it selectively stimulates the proliferation of the neutrophil progenitor cell; however, at higher concentrations, it can affect all the granulocytes, as well as the monoblast lineage.

The last CSF was discovered by several groups working independently; unfortunately, each group gave it a different name and, as yet, no consensus has arisen concerning the nomenclature. The synonyms are listed below with an explanation of each: *Kit ligand* (KL, its receptor is the *kit* gene product), *mast cell growth factor* (MGF), *stem cell growth factor* (SCF), and *steel factor* (SLF, it complements the *steel* mutation in mice). This factor stimulates hematopoiesis, especially the mast cell line, but, unlike others CSFs, it also promotes mitosis in other stem cells such as germ cells and melanoblasts.

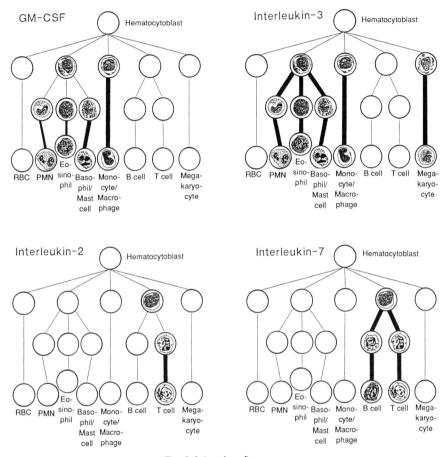

Fig. 3-2 *(continued)*

3. Interleukins

The interleukins are primarily concerned with the proliferation and differentiation of T and B lymphocytes and are, therefore, considered in Section II, D. However, two of these hormones are important for other cell types. In fact, *interleukin-3* (IL-3 or multi-CSF) does not have any effect at all on lymphocytes, although it stimulates all the other white blood cells and even the megakaryoblast cell line. *IL-5* does affect B lymphocytes, but also promotes the production of eosinophils.

D. Immuno-inflammatory Hormones

To understand the immuno-inflammatory hormones (Table 3-2), one must first understand the immuno-inflammatory reaction (20–23). In general, this reaction is two-fold: first there is the production of *antibodies*, proteins with a

Table 3-2

Some Immuno-inflammatory Hormones in Vertebrates

Hormone[a]	Source	Action
IL-1	Macrophages	Stimulates helper T cells to produce IL-2; inflammatory
IL-2	Helper T cells	Stimulates T cell proliferation
IL-3	Helper T cells	Hematopoeisis; mast cell growth factor
IL-4	Helper T cells	Activates B cells; immunoglobulin class switching
IL-5	Helper T cells	Stimulates B cell proliferation; eosinophil growth and differentiation
IL-6	Helper T cells, fibroblasts, epithelium, macrophages	Stimulates B cell maturation to antibody-secreting cells; inflammatory
IL-7	Bone marrow stromal cells	B cell precursor and T cell proliferation
IL-8	Fibroblasts, epithelium, hepatocytes, macrophages	Neutrophil chemotaxis
TNFs	Immune cells	B and T cell activation, growth, and differentiation; inflammation; cytotoxicity; proliferation of vascular epithelium and fibroblasts; catabolism
CSFs	Immune cells, fibroblasts	Hematopoiesis; inflammation
IFNs	Helper T cells	B and T cell activation, growth, and differentiation; inflammation; cytotoxicity; inhibition of protein synthesis

[a] CSFs, Colony stimulating factors; IFNs, interferons; IL, interleukins; TNFs, tumor necrosis factors.

high affinity for a foreign substance, the *antigen*. Since many antibodies are secreted into the blood, this type of response is known as *humoral immunity*. Another type of defense response is the generation of cytotoxicity, called *cell-mediated immunity*.

1. Humoral Immunity

Antibodies are modular proteins: each of the two heavy chains consists of four repeating domains and each of the two light chains has two such repeating units (Fig. 3-3). The amino termini line up and the first domain of all four chains forms two antigen binding pockets, the *immunoglobulin folds*. The carboxy termini of the heavy chains determine antibody localization or trigger other immune responses, such as complement fixation. Each of the five major classes of heavy chains has its own unique spectrum of immune activities.

There are only two genes for the light chains and one for the heavy chains. The origin of the different antibody classes and antigen specificity lies in the genomic organization of these genes (Fig. 3-4). Each light chain gene contains one exon encoding the second domain, known as C_L for constant region. However, there are several hundred exons encoding the first domain, known as V_L for variable region. There are also several small exons that encode a few amino acids located at the junction between V_L and C_L; these are the J (junctional) exons. The heavy chain gene has a similar organization

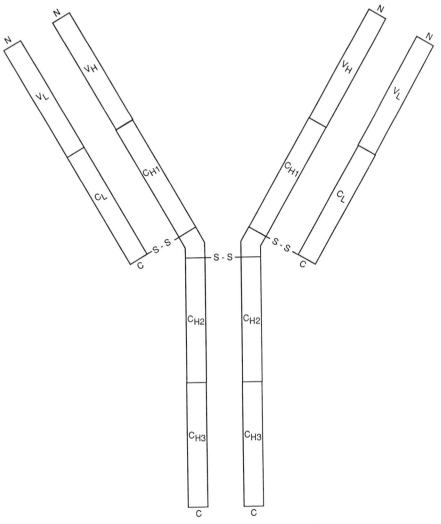

Fig. 3-3. An antibody molecule. Each heavy chain is composed of one variable domain (V_H) and three constant domains (C_H); each light chain has only one of each type of domain (V_L, C_L). N and C represent the amino termini and carboxy termini, respectively.

except that there is an additional group of small exons like the J exons and just preceding them; these are the D (diversity) exons. Another difference is generated by the exons for the constant domains, which number three in the heavy chain. Each one has its own exon (C_{H1}, C_{H2}, and C_{H3}) with a small hinge exon between C_{H1} and C_{H2}. The first set of constant exons encodes the immunoglobin M (IgM) heavy chain; this is followed by sets for the other antibody classes and their isoforms.

During embryogenesis, the B lymphocytes (B cells) differentiate. The

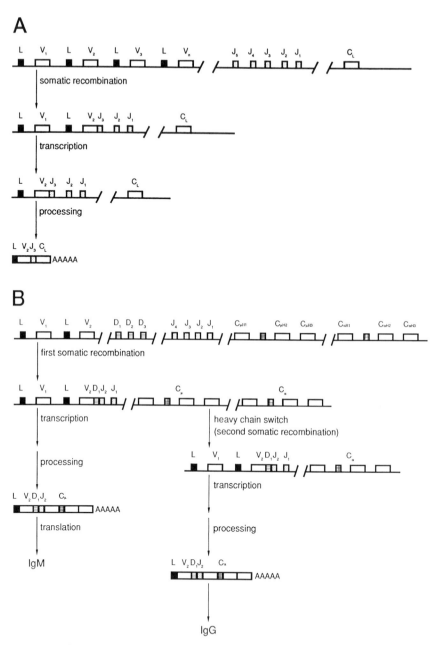

Fig. 3-4. Somatic recombination: (A) light chain recombination, (B) heavy chain recombination (see the text for description). C, Constant exon; D, diversity exon; hnRNA, heterologous nuclear RNA (mRNA precursor); Ig, immunoglobulin; J, junctional exon; L, leader sequence; V, variable exon.

heavy and light chain genes in each cell randomly couple one V_L and J exon to the C_L exon and one V_H, J, and D exon to the first C_H set. All intervening exons are spliced out and lost; this process is called *somatic recombination*. The resulting antibody will be of the IgM class and have an antigen specificity determined by the random association of multiple exons. Each B lymphocyte will produce a unique IgM and display it on its plasma membrane.

If the B lymphocyte ever encounters an antigen matching the specificity of its antibody, the antigen will bind to the IgM and be internalized, partially degraded, and finally displayed on the cell surface bound to *Class II major histocompatibility complexes* (MHCs) (Fig. 3-5). The class II MHCs are merely two light chains with hydrophobic carboxy termini that anchor the chains in the plasma membrane. At the same time, this entire process is being mimicked by antigen-presenting cells, including macrophages, dendritic cells of lymphoid organs, and Langerhans cells of the skin. This antigen processing is necessary because the T cell receptor (see subsequent discussion) only recognizes unfolded peptides.

Another group of lymphocytes, the helper T cells, also has receptors that resemble the class II MHCs and are called T cell receptors. The helper T cell with a receptor with appropriate specificity will bind to the partially degraded antigen on the macrophage cell surface; this interaction is facilitated by special adhesion proteins such as CD4. CD4 is particularly noteworthy

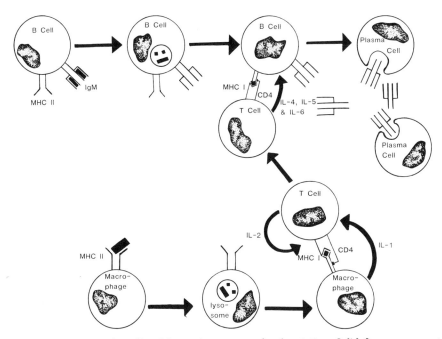

Fig. 3-5. Humoral mediated immunity; see text for description. Solid figures represent intact or processed antigens. IL, Interleukins; MHC I and II, class I and II major histocompatibility complexes.

since it is used by the human immunodeficiency virus (HIV) to gain entry into T cells, which the virus eventually destroys. As a result of its interaction with the T cell, the macrophage secretes interleukin 1 (IL-1), which mediates several infammatory responses such as fever, and also stimulates the helper T cell to produce IL-2. IL-2 acts in an autocrine manner to stimulate the proliferation of helper T cells; this is called *clonal selection*, since it amplifies only those cells producing a helper T cell receptor with specificity for the antigen in question.

The helper T cell can now bind to the same antigen on the B cell; this interaction leads to the secretion of IL-4, IL-5, and IL-6 by the helper T cell. IL-4 stimulates a second somatic recombination event in which the V_H-D-J exon complex is now randomly spliced to a constant domain set. In this way, the antigen specificity of the original IgM can be transferred to an IgG or any other antibody class; this phenomenon is known as *heavy chain switching*. IL-5 stimulates B cell proliferation, which results in the clonal selection of B cells making antibodies with specificity for this particular antigen. Finally, IL-6 matures the B cell into an antibody-producing plasma cell.

2. Cell-Mediated Immunity

Cell-mediated immunity is often used in response to viral and fungal infections. The initial response is very similar to that for humoral immunity: antigen-presenting cells phagocytizes the antigen, partially degrade it, and display it on the cell surface via class II MHCs. However, the macrophage interacts with a different T cell, the cytotoxic T cell. Nonetheless, the response is the same: the macrophage secretes IL-1, which stimulates the cytotoxic T cell to produce IL-2. The latter acts in an autocrine manner to stimulate T cell proliferation (clonal selection).

Meanwhile, cells infected with viruses or fungi are leaking foreign antigens to the cell surface where they are bound to *class I MHCs*. Class I MHC is a single light chain with a carboxy-terminal hydrophobic extension that anchors it in the plasma membrane. The immunoglobulin fold is intact because this light chain has an extra variable domain at the amino terminus. The cytotoxic T cell binds the antigen on the infected cell and injects *perforins* into the target cell membrane where they polymerize into pores; this phenomenon is very similar to the formation of C9 pores in complement fixation. The cellular contents begin to leak out and the infected cell dies.

3. Miscellaneous Immuno-inflammatory Hormones

a. Tumor Necrosis Factor Family.   This family consists of *tumor necrosis factor-α (TNF-α)* and *TNF-β* (24,25). TNF-α has 157 amino acids and is not glycosylated in humans, although this modification does occur in the murine hormone. It is synthesized as a membrane-bound precursor. TNF-β is larger because of a 17-amino-acid amino-terminal extension and the presence of glycosylation; it is not synthesized as a membrane-bound precursor. Both hormones are trimers, forming a pyramid with 3-fold symmetry. They are secreted from macrophages, natural killer cells, and some T lymphocytes.

The most remarkable biological effect of the TNFs is their ability to induce regression, and sometimes total destruction, of certain tumors by redirecting electrons in mitochondria to the formation of oxygen radicals that are primarily responsible for the damage. In normal cells, TNFs induce protective proteins, such as the manganese superoxide dismutase; but malignant cells are often deficient in this detoxifying enzyme and are very sensitive to oxygen radicals. In addition, there is some evidence that the hormone itself may insert into membranes and produce functional channels in a pH-dependent manner. Finally, TNF exerts some of its effects through other hormones. For example, it activates phospholipase A_2, which liberates arachidonic acid for the formation of eicosanoids (see subsequent discussion), and stimulates the release of IL-6, which is a major inducer of *acute phase proteins*. Acute phase proteins are associated with the acute phase response that accompanies profound systemic injury or infection. They include protease inhibitors; complement components; fibrinogen; C-reactive protein, which promotes phagocytosis; and haptoglobulin and hemopexin, both of which bind hemoglobin released during hemolysis to prevent kidney damage and to recycle the iron.

A functionally related, although structurally distinct, peptide is the *leukemia inhibitory factor (LIF)*. This is a 179-amino-acid 58-kDa glycoprotein with a unique amino acid sequence. Its biological activity is very similar to that of IL-6: it stimulates the proliferation and differentiation of various blood cells and induces the acute phase response. However, it differs from IL-6 in its inhibition of adipogenesis, sometimes leading to wasting (cachexia). In this respect, it resembles TNF. *Oncostatin M* is another member of the LIF family. It stimulates the growth of fibroblasts and HIV-infected cells, inhibits proliferation of normal endothelial and cancer cells, and increases IL-6 production by endothelium. It is produced by activated T lymphocytes and monocytes.

b. Interferon Family.   The *interferon (IFN)* family consists of the type I IFNs, IFN-α and IFN-β, and type II IFN, IFN-γ. The type I IFNs have 166 amino acids and share about 30% homology; their genes have no introns. However, IFN-α is not N-glycosylated whereas IFN-β is, leading to a slightly higher molecular weight for the latter. IL-6 appears to be a distant cousin of this family. The type II IFN, IFN-γ, is a homodimer whose glycosylated subunits have 143 amino acids each. It does not appear to be structurally related to the type II IFNs, but its activity is so similar that all three IFNs are considered functionally related.

The IFNs are best known for their antiviral activity. One major effect of these hormones is to halt protein synthesis via two routes. First they induce an eIF-2 kinase that phosphorylates and inactivates the translation initiation factor eIF-2. Second, they induce an oligo-2′,5′-adenylate synthetase that, when activated by double-stranded RNA, synthesizes oligo-2',5'-adenylates. These short polynucleotides activate an endonuclease that degrades mRNA. Furthermore, in macrophages the IFNs are potent inducers of MHC antigens and trigger a respiratory burst that generates superoxides and peroxides for phagocytosis. The latter effect is reminiscent of the activity of TNF; indeed, IFN and TNF are highly synergistic in killing tumor cells.

E. Parahormones

Parahormones are hormones that exert their effects within the tissues that synthesize them; that is, they are local hormones. There are simply too many parahormones to describe all of them in a brief synopsis. However, three groups will become important in future sections: the eicosanoids, the opiate peptides, and the purine derivatives.

1. Eicosanoids

The *eicosanoids* are derivatives of arachidonic acid and include the *prostaglandins, thromboxanes* (both from the cyclo-oxygenase pathway), *leukotrienes* (products of the 5-lipoxygenase enzyme), and *lipoxins* (from the 12-lipoxygenase pathway) (26,27). According to standardized nomenclature, the first two letters signify the particular group to which the compound belongs. For example, PG designates a prostaglandin; TX, a thromboxane; and LX, a lipoxin. The third letter denotes a series within each group. Each compound within a particular series has an identical head (ring) group, including substitutions and double bonds (Fig. 3-6). The numerical subscript indicates the number of double bonds in the side chains.

The major synthetic steps in the formation of eicosanoids are shown in Fig. 3-7. The prostaglandins are made everywhere, but the synthesis of the thromboxanes, leukotrienes, and lipoxins has a more restricted distribution. All three groups are made in platelets, neutrophils, and the lung; thromboxanes are also synthesized in the brain, and leukotrienes and lipoxins in mast cells. *Eicosatetraynoic acid* (ETYA) is an arachidonic acid analog containing

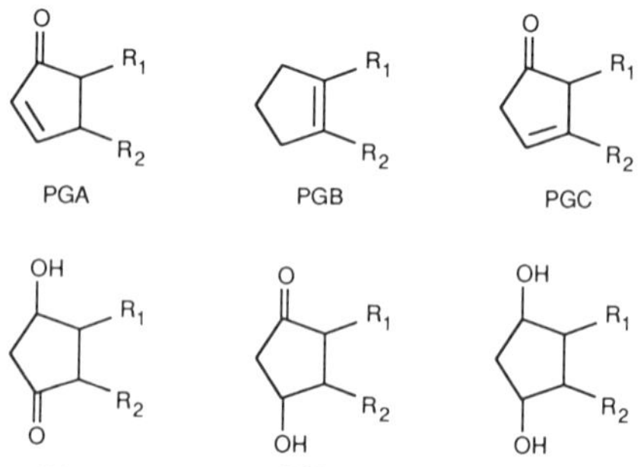

Fig. 3-6. Head (ring) groups for the different series of prostaglandins.

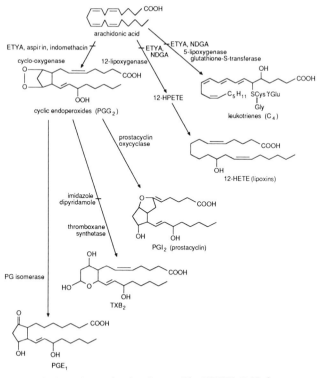

Fig. 3-7. Biosynthetic pathway for the eicosanoids. HPETE, 5-Hydroxy-peroxy-6,8,11,14-eicosatetraenoic acid; HETE, 5-hydroxy-6,8,11,14-eicosatetraenoic acid; EYTA, eicosatetraynoic acid; NDGA, nordihydroguaiaretic acid.

triple bonds in place of the double bonds, and inhibits any enzyme using this fatty acid as substrate. Although ETYA is not used clinically, several other inhibitors are useful drugs. Certainly the most common one is aspirin, which inhibits the cyclo-oxygenase involved in prostaglandin synthesis. Aspirin is an anti-inflammatory agent and many prostaglandins mediate the inflammatory response (see subsequent text). Another drug is *dipyridamole*, a coronary vasodilator. This compound inhibits the synthesis of the thromboxanes, which are vasoconstrictors. The lipoxygenase pathway can be selectively inhibited by *nordihydroguaiaretic acid* (NDGA).

Eicosanoids have one of three major actions: mediation of inflammation, prevention of blood loss, or contraction of smooth muscle. PGA, PGE, and the leukotrienes belong to the first group and elicit all the classic signs of inflammation. They dilate blood vessels to produce erythema, increase their permeability so they leak and produce edema, provoke pain and fever, stimulate lysosome release, and are chemotactic. The lipoxins appear to counteract the inflammatory activity of these other eicosanoids. As such, they may play a role in maintaining tight control over this process. Thromboxanes fall into the second group; they constrict blood vessels and promote platelet aggregation, thereby facilitating blood clotting. PGF is a member of the last group; it is a potent stimulator of virtually all smooth muscle, including that in the vasculature, bronchioles, and GI and reproductive tracts. The function of this latter group of hormones depends on the particular tissue and circumstances. For example, the prostaglandins in semen stimulate uterine contractility, which is thought to aid in the transport of sperm up the female reproductive tract.

2. Opiate Peptides

While studying the mechanism of action of narcotics, pharmacologists discovered that animals possessed receptors for these drugs. Why would animals have a specific receptor for a plant alkaloid unless these receptors were originally designed for an endogenous narcotic-like compound? Such a compound was sought and [Met^5]- and [Leu^5]enkephalin were eventually isolated. Two other groups of opiate peptides have now also been purified and characterized. All three groups have the same amino terminal pentapeptide: $H_2N-Tyr-Gly-Gly-Phe-Met-$ or $H_2N-Tyr-Gly-Gly-Phe-Leu-$. Indeed, this part of the molecule is recognized by all the different opiate receptors; the carboxy-terminal extension merely enhances the binding of each class of opiate peptides to a particular receptor (see subsequent discussion).

What do a plant alkaloid and a pentapeptide have in common? The three-dimensional conformation of the narcotics has been determined and much information on structure – function relationships has been obtained: all potent narcotics have a phenol ring, an amine, and, usually, a phenyl ring. These groups are also present in the opiate peptides (Fig. 3-8). Presumably, the three-dimensional structure of these peptides is such that these groups occupy the same relative positions as they do in the narcotics (28). However, small peptides rarely form stable three-dimensional structures and, although some structures for opiate peptides have been proposed, there is still considerable controversy over which, if any, is correct.

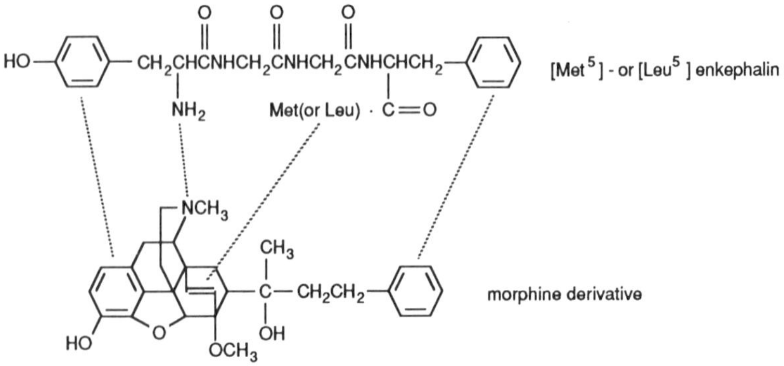

Fig. 3-8. Structural comparison of enkephalin and a morphine derivative.

The opiate peptides can be divided into three groups based on their origin. The *endorphins* are incorporated in the polyprotein proopiomelano-cortin (POMC), which can give rise to ACTH, three different MSHs, or three different endorphins, depending on how the protein is processed (see Chapter 2). There is only one copy of the endorphin sequence within POMC; the three forms are generated by proteases, which give rise to carboxy termini of different lengths. The endorphins have between 16 and 27 amino acids, depending on how much of the carboxy terminus is removed. The *enkephalins* were the first opiate peptides isolated and are only 5–7 amino acids long; they are derived from another precursor, *proenkephalin*. Finally, the *dynorphins* and *neoendorphins* are 10–17 amino acids long and are encoded within *prodynorphin*. Both proenkephalin and prodynorphin contain multiple copies of their respective opiate peptide, and all three precursors are believed to be evolutionarily related (29).

Like many parahormones, opiate peptides are made in multiple locations; the highest concentrations are found in the pituitary gland, adrenal medulla, and peptidergic neurons. There are at least three different receptors for these peptides (see Chapter 5). The δ receptor mediates analgesia, the μ receptor mediates euphoria, and the κ receptor mediates sedation, dysphoria, and anorexia. In general, the δ receptor has a higher affinity for [Leu^5]enkephalin; the μ receptor, for β-endorphin and [Met^5]enkephalin; and the κ receptor, for dynorphin. However, there is considerable overlap in receptor binding activities.

3. Purines

The metabolic role of adenine compounds is well known and the function of cyclic AMP as a second messenger is commonly appreciated. However, some of these nucleotides also act as parahormones (30–32). Adenosine is released during times of stress, such as hypoxia, and acts on the P_1 purinergic receptors. It appears to exert a protective effect on highly metabolic tissues by reducing their energy expenditures; for example, it slows the heart, relaxes smooth muscle, and raises the threshold of certain neurons (Table 3-3). For this reason, it has often been called a "retaliatory metabolite." ATP also appears to be released during stress, but its effects are not easily classified. ATP binds to P_2 purinergic receptors, where it usually induces vasodilation and platelet aggregation and affects glandular secretion and the immune system. It is secreted by certain neurons, platelets, and the adrenal medulla.

F. Miscellaneous Factors

1. Retinoic Acid

Retinoic acid (33), like 1,25-DHCC, cannot be made by the human body; its precursor, β-carotene, must be consumed in the diet. For that reason it is also known as vitamin A. It is perhaps best recognized as a component of rhodopsin, a retinal pigment necessary for light detection; however, it is also

Table 3-3
Purinergic Receptors, Agonists, Mediators, and Actions

Receptor class	Subclass	Endogenous agonists	Second messengers[a]	Actions
P$_1$	A$_1$	Adenosine	Decreases cAMP, K$^+$	Bradycardia; anticonvulsant; negative inotropism (atria); anti-adrenergic
	A$_2$	Adenosine	Increases cAMP	Sedation; vasodilation
	A$_3$	Adenosine	Calcium	Neuronal hyperpolarization (brain striatum only)
P$_2$	P$_{2X}$	ATP, ADP	Cation channels	Vasoconstriction
	P$_{2Y}$	ATP, ADP	NO, PG, K$^+$, IP$_3$– Ca^{2+}	Smooth muscle relaxant; exocrine– endocrine secretion
	P$_{2Z}$	ATP^{4-}	Unknown	Mast cell degranulation; inhibits lymphocyte cytotoxicity; increases membrane permeability (mast cells only)
	P$_{2T}$	ADP	Decreases cAMP	Platelet aggregation (platelets only)

[a] IP$_3$, Inositol trisphosphate; NO, nitric oxide; PG, prostaglandins.

important in epithelial cell differentiation. *In vivo*, vitamin A deficiency causes secretory epithelium to become highly keratinized whereas vitamin A replacement restores mucous and ciliated epithelium. *In vitro*, retinoic acid can inhibit the proliferation of some tumor cell lines by inducing terminal differentiation.

Because derivatives of vitamin A are hydrophobic, they must be carried by specialized transport proteins like those for steroids and thyroid hormones. β-Carotene is absorbed by the intestinal mucosa, oxidized to retinol, esterified, and packaged into chylomicrons. In the liver, the retinol is liberated and repackaged into a 21-kDa globulin called retinol-binding protein. Each protein has one binding site for retinol and complexes with one prealbumin molecule, a T$_3$-binding protein. Epithelial cells have high affinity binding sites for the retinol-binding protein; this cell–protein interaction releases the retinol, which is transported inside the cell where it is bound to *cellular retinol-binding protein*. It can also be oxidized to retinoic acid and be bound to another carrier, *cellular retinoic acid-binding protein*. The function of these cytoplasmic proteins is not clear, since retinoic acid exerts its biological activity by binding to nuclear receptors. Although these proteins may help transport the retinoic acid to the nucleus, steroids, which have an identical mechanism of action, do not need such help. Perhaps the proteins maintain a cytoplasmic reservoir for retinoids or aid in some nongenomic effects of these hormones.

2. Local Inflammatory Peptides

N-Formylpeptides are unusual in eukaryotic systems; they are thought to arise from the breakdown of bacterial proteins during infection and of mitochondrial proteins after tissue damage. Either case, infection or injury, represents a potentially dangerous situation that requires a prompt defensive reponse. The formyltripeptide *formylmethionylleucylphenylalanine* (fMLP) primarily affects neutrophils and macrophages; its effects include the induction of chemotaxis, phagocytosis, and degranulation, as well as the generation of superoxides, which are used to kill ingested organisms. *Interleukin-8*, a 10-kDa nonglycosylated peptide, has a similar spectrum of activities but is a member of the C–X–C chemokine family specific for neutrophils. This family has a conserved cysteine motif and can be subdivided depending on whether the first two cysteines are adjacent (the C–C chemokines) or separated by an intervening amino acid (the C–X–C chemokines). The C–X–C chemokines include IL-8 and *melanocyte growth-stimulatory activity* (MGSA); the C–C chemokines are specific for monocytes and include the *macrophage inflammatory proteins 1α* and *1β* (MIP-1α and MIP-1β).

Bradykinin is one of several small inflammatory peptides, the *kinins*, released from precursors called *kininogens*. Bradykinin is generated by the action of a serine protease, *kallikrein*, which circulates in the blood as the inactive precursor *prekallikrein*. As such, bradykinin is produced at the end of a cascade in which the blood coagulation factor XIIa converts prekallikrein to kallikrein, which then digests kininogen to release bradykinin.

Bradykinin is a local vasodilator and increases capillary permeability. It also produces pain and prostaglandins, which mediate some of the actions of bradykinin. Finally, it can affect smooth muscle contractility by inducing contractions or relaxation, depending on the source of the smooth muscle.

Thrombin is a most unlikely growth factor. It is a serine protease that is most commonly associated with the blood coagulation cascade in which it catalyzes the conversion of fibrinogen to fibrin during clot formation. However, it is a very potent activator of platelets, which it induces to aggregate, secrete serotonin, and produce prostaglandins. It is also mitogenic for fibroblasts and monocytes–macrophages, increases endothelial permeability, and is chemotaxic for monocytes–macrophages. Finally, it can induce a slow sustained contraction in smooth muscle, although it can also promote relaxation in previously contracted smooth muscle. Most, if not all, of these actions are associated with the binding of thrombin to the target cells, like a hormone, yet its biological activity also requires an intact catalytic site, like an enzyme. Its mechanism of action will be discussed further in Chapter 6.

Hepatocyte growth factor (HGF), formerly called scatter factor, is also related to a serine protease involved in blood coagulation. HGF is synthesized from a 728-amino-acid precursor having a 38% identity with plasminogen, a protease that dissolves blood clots. The precursor is cleaved to separate the four kringle domains in the original amino terminus from the pseudocatalytic domain in the carboxy terminus. The subunits remain together to form the heavy and light chains, respectively, of the mature hormone. HGF stimulates the proliferation of hepatocytes, fibroblasts, and cells of epithelial origin; in addition, it promotes the dispersion of epithelial cells.

A third hormone that appears to be related to an enzyme is *platelet-der-*

ived endothelial cell growth factor (PD-ECGF), a 45-kDa protein with homology to and the activity of thymidine phosphorylase. *In vivo*, it stimulates chemotaxis and thymidine incorporation in endothelial cells; *in vitro*, it induces angiogenesis.

Another unusual hormone is *platelet-activating factor* (PAF) (34,35), a phospholipid with a *sn*-1 ether, a *sn*-2 acetate, and a choline head group (Fig. 1-1E). Many of its actions are involved in mediating inflammation and allergic reactions. In addition to activating platelets, neutrophils, monocytes, and macrophages, PAF has major effects on the circulatory system, including increased vascular permeability and decreased cardiac output and blood pressure. It can also stimulate hepatic glycogenolysis and smooth muscle contractions in both the uterus and the bronchioles.

III. Invertebrate Hormones

A. Insects

Although most of the known hormones involved in insect endocrinology are given in Table 3-4 (36–38), only a few will be mentioned later in this text. Many of these latter hormones are related to either ecdysis (molting) or reproduction.

Table 3-4
The Major Insect Hormones

Hormones	Structure	Source	Action
Molting			
Prothoracicotropic hormone (PTTH-B)	Peptide[a]	Neurosecretory cells – corpus cardiacum (NSC – CC)	Stimulates ecdysone release (prothoracic glands)
PTTH-S (Bombyxin)	Peptide[a]	See PTTH-B	Like PTTH-B, but not believed to be the physiological PTTH
Ecdysone	Sterol[a]	Prothoracic glands, ovary	Ecdysis; vitellogenesis in some Diptera
Juvenile hormones (JH)	Sesquiterpenes[a]	Corpus allatum	Inhibits metamorphosis; stimulates vitellogenesis (fat body) and oocyte growth
Allatotropin	Peptide[a]	Brain	Stimulates JH synthesis
Allatostatin	Peptide[a]	Brain	Inhibits JH synthesis
Bursicon	Protein	NSC, thoracic ganglion	Cuticular tanning (sclerotization)
Eclosion hormone (EH)	Peptide[a]	CC	Ecdysis behavior and eclosion

continues

continued

Hormones	Structure	Source	Action
Reproduction			
Antigonadotropin	Peptide[a]	Abdominal neuro-secretory organs	Inhibits previtellogenic oocyte development
Egg development neurosecretory hormone (EDNH)	Peptide	NSC–CC complex	Oocyte maturation
Oostatic hormone	Sterol(?)	Vitellogenic oocytes	Inhibits EDNH secretion
Follicle cell tropic hormone (FCTH)	Peptide	Neurosecretory cells	Stimulates ovarian ecdysone
Diapause hormone (DH)	Peptide[a]	Subesophageal ganglion	Arrests embryonic develop-ment; glycogen synthesis
Pheromones	Terpene and aliphatic derivatives[a]	Epidermal glands	Sexual attractants
Pheromone bio-synthesis activat-ing neuropeptide (PBAN)	Peptide	Subesophageal ganglion–CC complex	Stimulates pheromone syn-thesis
Metabolism			
Trehalagon	Peptide	NSC–CC complex	Glycogenolysis (fat body)
Adipokinetic hor-mone (AKH)	Peptide[a]	NSC–CC complex	Lipolysis and glycogenolysis (fat body)
Diuretic hormone	Peptide[a]	NSC–CC or mes-othoracic gan-glion	Diuresis (Malpighian tubules)
Chloride transport-stimulating hor-mone (CTSH)	Peptide/protein	NSC–CC complex	K^+ and Cl^- resorption (rec-tum)
Myotropism			
Proctolin	Peptide[a]	CC	Stimulates cardiac and smooth muscle
Leukokinins	Peptide[a]	CC	Stimulates smooth muscle
Sulfakinins	Peptide[a]	CC	Stimulates smooth muscle
Melanotropism			
Melanization and reddish color-ation hormone (MRCH)	Peptide[a]	Subesophageal gan-glion	Melanization and red-brown pigment concentration
Pigment-dispers-ing factor (PDS)	Peptide[a]	Brain–ventral cord	Pigment dispersion

[a] The exact structure is known. DH and PBAN are from the same polyprotein precursor and have the same carboxy terminus (-F-X-P-R-L-NH$_2$).

1. Ecdysis

Ecdysis and metamorphosis are regulated by two major hormones: *ecdysone* and *juvenile hormone*. The neurosecretory cells and the *corpus cardiacum*, a transformed ganglion closely associated with the heart, produce a peptide called the *prothoracotropic hormone* (PTTH) that stimulates the prothoracic gland to produce ecdysone, a sterol hormone (Fig. 3-9). There are really two PTTHs: PTTH-B and PTTH-S. Although PTTH-B is believed to be the physiological tropin, PTTH-S is an extremely interesting peptide because of its close homology to the mammalian hormone insulin.

Ecdysone alone will produce both molting and metamorphosis. However, this is undesirable during early development: insect larvae need several molts to grow before they metamorphose. To delay metamorphosis until the last larval molt, a metamorphosis-inhibiting hormone must be produced at each ecdysis: this is juvenile hormone. It is secreted by an epithelial gland, the *corpus allatum*, in response to two tropic hormones from the brain. Only when ecdysone is produced and juvenile hormone is suppressed does metamorphosis accompany a molt.

There are also several ancillary hormones. *Bursicon* is produced by the

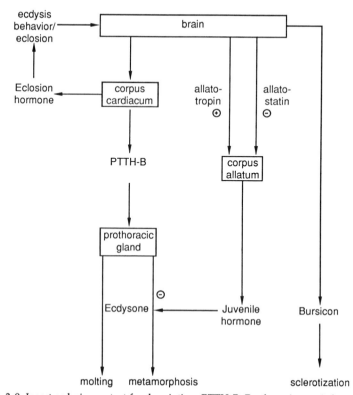

Fig. 3-9. Insect ecdysis; see text for description. PTTH-B, Prothoracicotropic hormone B.

brain and is responsible for tanning the new cuticle. *Eclosion hormone* is secreted by the corpus cardiacum and induces either molting behavior or behavior leading to the emergence of the insect from its pupa (eclosion).

2. Reproduction

Both ecdysone and juvenile hormone are also involved in reproduction. The following is a general discussion of insect oogenesis (Fig. 3-10); details in any given species may differ. Various tropic hormones from the brain stimulate the ovary to produce ecdysone and the corpus allatum to secrete juvenile hormone; another tropic hormone triggers oocyte development. Juvenile hormone stimulates progression of the oocyte to the vitellogenic stage and, along with ecdysone, promotes vitellogenin production by the fat body. The vitellogenic oocytes also provide negative feedback to both the brain and the previtellogenic oocytes.

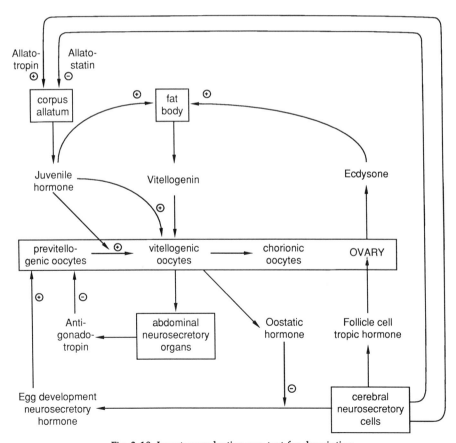

Fig. 3-10. Insect reproduction; see text for description.

Table 3-5

The Major Hormones in Crustaceans

Hormones	Structure	Source	Target	Action
Molting				
Molt inhibiting hormone (MIH)	Peptide[a]	X-organ–sinus gland	Y gland	Inhibits ecdysone synthesis
Ecdysterone	Sterol[a]	Y gland	Epidermis	Ecdysis
Reproduction				
Gonad-inhibiting hormone (GIH)	Peptide[a]	X-organ–sinus gland	Fat body, oocyte	Inhibits oocyte growth and vitellogenesis
Androgenic hormone (AH)	Peptide/ protein	Androgenic gland		♂ Secondary sexual development
Vitellogenin-stimulating ovarian hormone (VSOH)	Unknown	Ovary	Fat body, etc	Vitellogenesis and ♀ secondary sexual characteristics
Permanent ovarian hormone (POH)	Unknown	Ovary		Induction of oostegites
Juvenile hormones (JH)	Sesquiterpene[a]	Mandibular organs	Fat body, oocyte	Inhibits vitellogenesis and oocyte growth

	Type	Source	Target	Action
Pigmentation				
Red pigment-concentration hormone (RPCH)	Peptide[a]	X-organ–sinus gland, postcommissural organs	Chromatophores	Concentration of red pigment granules
Black pigment-concentration hormone (BPCH)	Peptide	Same	Chromatophores	Concentration of black pigment granules
Pigment dispersing hormone (PDH)	Peptide[a]	Same	Chromatophores	Pigment granule dispersion and retinal light adaptation
Enkephalins	Peptide[a]	X-organ–sinus gland	Chromatophores	Concentrates red and black pigment granules
Metabolism				
Crustacean hyperglycemic hormone (CHH)	Peptide[a]	X-organ–sinus gland	Hepato-pancreas, abdominal muscles	Glycogenolysis and secretion
Myotropism				
Proctolin	Peptide[a]	Pericardial organ, neurons	Heart	Cardioexcitatory
Crustacean cardioactive peptide (CCAP)	Peptide[a]	Pericardial organ, abdominal ganglion	Heart, hindgut	Stimulatory
FLRFamide	Peptide[a]	Pericardial organ	Heart, muscle	Stimulatory
Orcokinin	Peptide[a]	Abdominal nerve cord	Hindgut	Stimulatory

[a] The exact structure is known.

B. Crustaceans and Molluscs

Many of the hormones in crustaceans are similar to those in insects (Table 3-5; 37,39–40). Those in mollusks appear to be quite different; it is not within the scope of this text to discuss many of them, although one is very interesting from an evolutionary point of view. *Insulin-like substance* is a molluscan peptide that is not only homologous to mammalian insulin but also has much the same function: it is made in the gut and associated structures and stimulates glycogen synthesis.

IV. Plant Hormones

A. Introduction

Although growth factors have often been relegated to the periphery of classical endocrinology, plant hormones have sometimes had a worse fate; some authorities even deny their existence. The controversy is both conceptual and technical. Conceptually, animals and plants are organized differently: animals are unitary creatures requiring a high degree of coordination to function. Coordination requires relatively central planning, the generation of precise instructions, a way to disseminate those instructions, and feedback. In animals, part of this coordination is provided by chemical signals, the hormones.

On the other hand, plants are modular organisms; for example, growth of various parts of the plant are determined as much by local environment as by any genetic plan. In addition to this apparent lack of central coordination, plant growth substances were thought to have very imprecise biological activities, were not thought to be transported, and were thought not to be subject to feedback regulation. Furthermore, hormone concentrations did not correlate with biological activity.

Some of these concerns are similar to those raised for vertebrate growth factors and can be dismissed if one takes a broader view of endocrinology as regulation at a local as well as an organismal level. Other concerns arise from technical problems involved in plant research; for example, plant hormones can now be measured accurately, revealing several systems in which hormone concentrations do correlate with biological activities. These techniques have also shown that many plant hormones are transported to other plant structures (Fig. 3-11). Therefore, the use of the term plant hormone is justified (41,42).

B. Growth Hormones

Auxins and *cytokinins* are major growth promoters and morphogens (Table 3-6, Fig. 3-12). Auxin, or *indoleacetic acid*, is synthesized in young leaves and developing seeds from the amino acid tryptophan. In this portion of the plant, auxin is responsible for apical dominance and opening stomata, pores

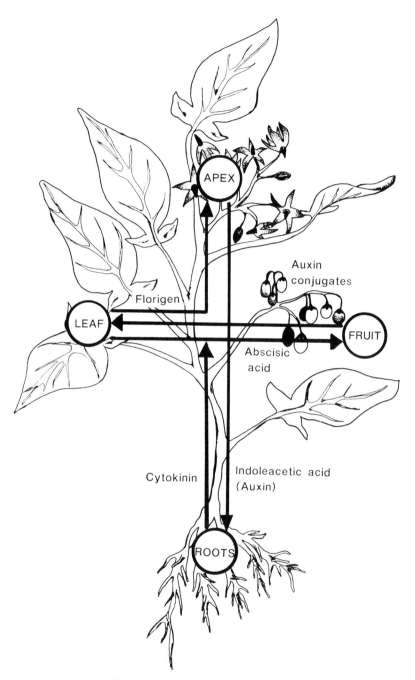

Fig. 3-11. Transport of plant hormones.

Table 3-6
The Major Plant Hormones

Hormones	Structure	Action
Auxin	Indoleacetic acid[a]	Stimulates shoot growth, root initiation, and xylem/phloem differentiation; responsible for apical dominance and photo- and gravitropism; opens stomata
Cytokinins	Substituted purines[a]	Cell division, bud induction, and leaf morphology; embryonic growth
Gibberellins	Diterpenes[a]	Germination, internodal elongation, and flowering
Abscisic acid	Terpenoid[a]	Dormancy; water conservation by stomatal closure; embryonic growth; accelerates senescence
Ethylene	Alkene[a]	Fruit ripening; abscission and dehiscence; wound responses; thigmotropism; induces macrocyst formation in certain fungi
Oligosaccharins	Oligosaccharides[a]	Elicits defense responses; morphogenesis, such as flower formation in tobacco (pectin)
Brassinosteroids	Sterol derivatives[a]	Elongation, curvature, and splitting of the internode, especially in seedlings
Traumatic acid	Dicarboxylic acid[a]	Abscission and adventitious bud formation, especially in response to wounding
Jasmonic acid	Cyclopentanone derivative[a]	Inhibits germination and promotes senescence, tuberization, and tendril coiling
Salicylic acid	2-Hydroxybenzoic acid[a]	Thermogenic in arum lilies; mediates pathogen resistance; induction of flowering

[a] The exact structure is known.

through which gaseous exchange takes place and water vapor is lost. Auxin also travels down the phloem to reach the roots. Growth is achieved by activating polysaccharide hydrolases that increase the extensibility of the cell wall, which allows for cell enlargement.

Cytokinins stimulate growth by inducing cell division. These adenine derivatives are synthesized in the root tips and travel up the xylem to the shoots. Cytokinin and auxin set up a gradient along the plant, and their ratios determine morphology (Fig. 3-13): a predominance of auxin favors root formation, whereas a high cytokinin-to-auxin ratio leads to shoot development (43). Low concentrations of both hormones will produce flowers.

Gibberellins stimulate another kind of growth: they promote internodal elongation and germination. These compounds are products of the isoprenoid or polyprenyl pathway, which also gives rise to steroids, retinoic acid, and juvenile hormone. They are synthesized in young shoots and developing seeds.

C. Stress Hormones

Abscisic acid is a derivative of carotene, another product of the isoprenoid pathway. It is synthesized in mature leaves in response to water stress; it

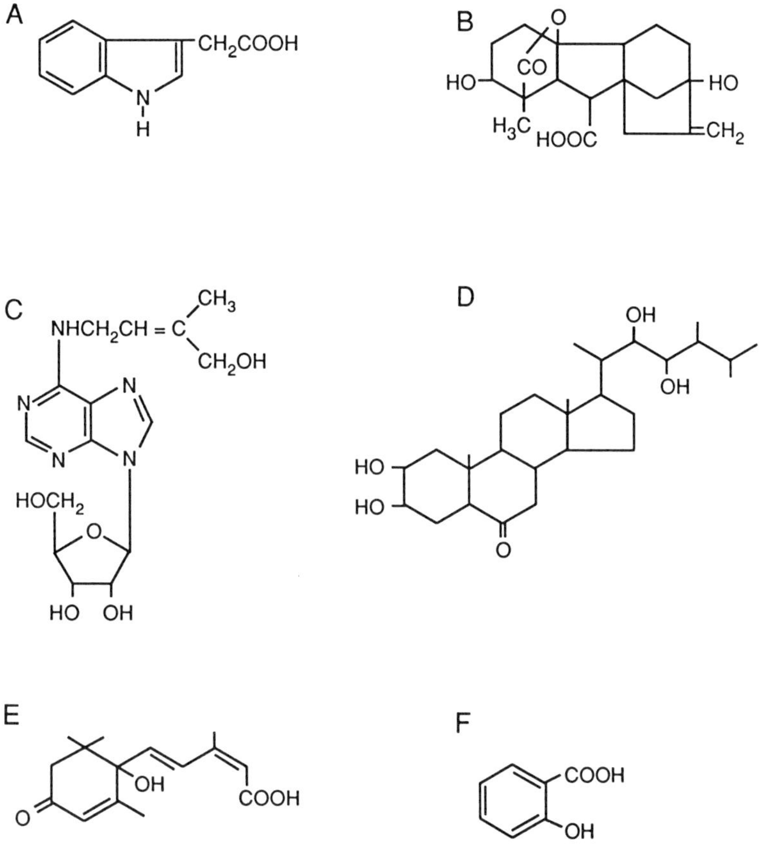

Fig. 3-12. Chemical structure of some plant hormones.

reduces water loss by closing the stomata. It also induces dormancy and accelerates senescence.

Ethylene is one of the few gaseous hormones in nature. It can be synthesized from the amino acid methionine by most tissues in response to stress (Fig. 3-14). The 1-aminocyclopropane-1-carboxylic acid synthase is the rate-limiting step and is highly regulated. Note that the pathway utilizes S-adenosylmethionine, an intermediate in polyamine metabolism. Since methionine is in limited supply in plants, the ethylene and polyamine pathways compete against one another for this compound; this parallels their antagonistic biological activities (see Chapter 15). Ethylene is responsible for the abscission and dehiscence of flowers, leaves, and fruit. It also induces fruit ripening and local wound responses.

Elicitor, or *oligosaccharins,* are oligosaccharides that are produced during infection or injury (44–45). They include β-glucan and chitin from fungal cell walls and pectin fragments from plant cell walls. The most active oligosaccharides have between 5- to 13-sugar monomers and are not transported

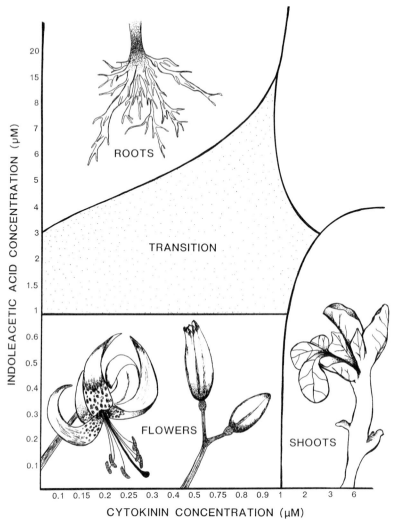

Fig. 3-13. Effect of indoleacetic acid–cytokinin ratios on plant explant morphology. Note that the scale is arbitrary. Adapted and reprinted by permission from Ref. 43. Copyright © 1989 the American Society of Plant Physiologists.

away from their site of production. Their effects include the induction of (i) β-glucanases and chitinases that degrade fungal cell walls, (ii) proteinase inhibitors to protect the plant, (iii) lignification (wood formation) to wall off the damage, (iv) ethylene, and (v) several isoprenoid pathway enzymes responsible for the synthesis of *phytoalexins*, compounds that are toxic to fungi and bacteria. Oligosaccharins may also affect normal growth and morphology.

Salicylic acid is probably best known as a thermogenic compound in

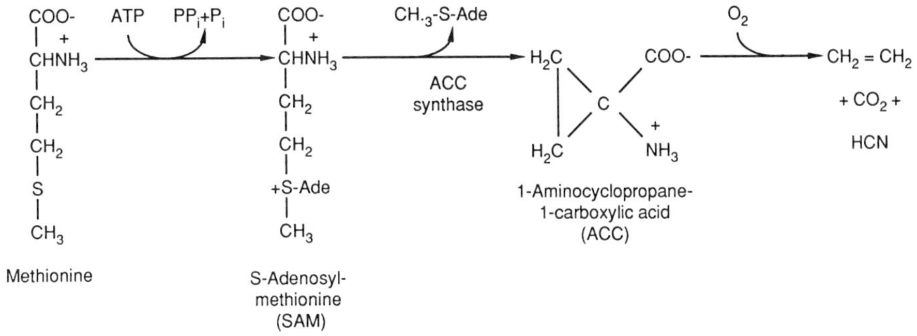

Fig. 3-14. Ethylene synthesis.

some species of *Arum* (46,47). These plants are pollinated by carrion-feeding insects that are attracted to the heat and pungent odor produced by these plants. Salicylic acid can also induce resistance to infections. For example, in the tobacco plant salicylic acid induces the hypersensitive response, in which cells adjacent to a viral infection die so that the infection is locally restricted. Salicylic acid is induced by infection and not just wounding.

Jasmonic acid, another gaseous hormone, inhibits germination, promotes senescence, and repartitions nitrogen in plant tissues, although some researchers have attributed its inhibitory effects to toxic doses (47–49). However, this molecule is far more interesting as a likely example of convergent chemical evolution (Fig. 3-15). Jasmonic acid is essentially a "prostaglandin" synthesized from linolenic acid; angiosperms do not have arachidonic acid, from which authentic prostaglandins are produced. Elicitors can elevate

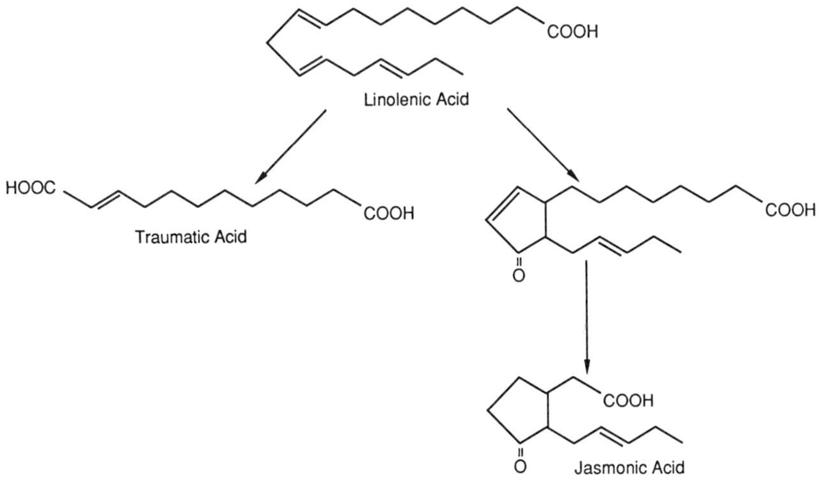

Fig. 3-15. Synthesis of traumatic and jasmonic acids.

jasmonic acid, which in turn can induce another stress hormone, *systemin* (47).

Systemin, an 18-amino-acid peptide, is the only known peptide hormone in plants. Despite its size, it has been shown to migrate throughout the plant where it induces protease inhibitors involved in defense mechanisms. Unlike salicylic acid, ethylene, jasmonic acid, and systemin are associated with both infection and wounding.

D. Miscellaneous Hormones

Brassinosteroids constitute a recent addition to the list of plant hormones and yet another product of the extremely versatile isoprenoid pathway (50). Their biological activity is very similar to that of the cytokinins: they stimulate the elongation, curvature, and splitting of the internodes. However, their greatest effect is in seedlings; indeed, although made in most tissues, the brassinosteroids are found in the highest concentrations in pollen and seeds.

Traumatic acid comes from the same pathway as jasmonic acid, but is not cyclized. As the name suggests, traumatic acid induces abscission and adventitious bud formation, especially in response to wounding.

V. Prospective

In the following parts of this text, the actions and relationships described in the first part are carried to the cellular and molecular levels. The topics are discussed in the same order that the biochemical information flows: the first thing that a hormone encounters during its interaction with a cell is its receptor (Part 2) and, if that receptor is membrane-bound, the information must be transferred to some other mediator, which can act directly on cellular processes (Part 3). These mediators, as well as the soluble receptors, can also act on the genome to induce transcription and affect other post-transcriptional processes (Part 4). Finally, several special topics are presented in Part 5.

References

General References

Gorbman, A., Dickhoff, W. W., Vigna, S. R., Clark, N. B., and Ralph, C. L. (1983). "Comparative Endocrinology." Wiley, New York.
Konopinska, D., Rosinski, G., and Sobótka, W. (1992). Insect peptide hormones, an overview of the present literature. *Int. J. Peptide Protein Res.* **39,** 1–11.
Meager, A. (1991). "Cytokines." Prentice Hall, Englewood Cliffs, New Jersey.
See also Refs. 6, 7, 10–12, 15, 17, 23, 24, 27, 35–41, and 46.

Cited References

1. Heldin, C. H., and Westermark, B. (1989). Growth factors as transforming proteins. *Eur. J. Biochem.* **184,** 487–496.
2. Nathan, C., and Sporn, M. (1991). Cytokines in context. *J. Cell Biol.* **113,** 981–986.
3. Derynck, R. (1988). Transforming growth factor-α. *Cell* **54,** 593–595.
4. Rizzino, A. (1988). Transforming growth factor-β: Multiple effects on cell differentiation and extracellular matrices. *Dev. Biol.* **130,** 411–422.
5. Miyazaki, K., and Horio, T. (1989). Growth inhibitors: Molecular diversity and roles in cell proliferation. *In Vitro Cell. Dev. Biol.* **25,** 866–872.
6. Barnard, J. A., Lyons, R. M., and Moses, H. L. (1990). The cell biology of transforming growth factor β. *Biochim. Biophys. Acta* **1032,** 79–87.
7. Fisher, D. A., and Lakshmanan, J. (1990). Metabolism and effects of epidermol growth factor and related growth factors in mammals. *Endocr. Rev.* **11,** 418–442.
8. Lyons, R. M., and Moses, H. L. (1990). Transforming growth factors and the regulation of cell proliferation. *Eur. J. Biochem.* **187,** 467–473.
9. Massagué, J. (1990). Transforming growth factor-α: A model for membrane-anchored growth factors. *J. Biol. Chem.* **265,** 21393–21396.
10. Centrella, M., Horowitz, M. C., Wozney, J. M., and McCarthy, T. L. (1994). Transforming growth factor-β gene family members and bone. *Endocr. Rev.* **15,** 27–39.
11. Kingsley, D. M. (1994). What do BMPs do in mammals? Clues from the mouse short-ear mutation. *Trends Genet.* **10,** 16–21.
12. Burgess, W. H., and Maciag, T. (1989). The heparin-binding (fibroblast) growth factor family of proteins. *Annu. Rev. Biochem.* **58,** 575–606.
13. Rifkin, D. B., and Moscatelli, D. (1989). Recent developments in the cell biology of basic fibroblast growth factor. *J. Cell Biol.* **109,** 1–6.
14. Holly, J. M. P., and Wass, J. A. H. (1989). Insulin-like growth factors; Autocrine, paracrine or endocrine? New perspectives of the somatomedin hypothesis in the light of recent developments. *J. Endocrinol.* **122,** 611–618.
15. Humbel, R. E. (1990). Insulin-like growth factors I and II. *Eur. J. Biochem.* **190,** 445–462.
16. Groopman, J. E., Molina, J. M., and Scadden, D. T. (1989). Hematopoietic growth factors: Biology and clinical applications. *N. Engl. J. Med.* **321,** 1449–1459.
17. Nicola, N. A. (1989). Hemopoietic cell growth factors and their receptors. *Annu. Rev. Biochem.* **58,** 45–77.
18. Pierce, J. H. (1989). Oncogenes, growth factors and hematopoietic cell transformation. *Biochim. Biophys. Acta* **989,** 179–208.
19. Whetton, A. D., and Dexter, T. M. (1989). Myeloid haemopoietic growth factors. *Biochim. Biophys. Acta* **989,** 111–132.
20. Harrison, L. C., and Campbell, I. L. (1988). Cytokines: An expanding network of immuno-inflammatory hormones. *Mol. Endocrinol.* **2,** 1151–1156.
21. Mizel, S. B. (1989). The interleukins. *FASEB J.* **3,** 2379–2388.
22. Paul, W. E. (1989). Pleiotrophy and redundancy: T cell-derived lymphokines in the immune response. *Cell* **57,** 521–524.
23. Arai, K., Lee, F., Miyajima, A., Miyatake, S., Arai, N., and Yokota, T. (1990). Cytokines: Coordinators of immune and inflammatory responses. *Annu. Rev. Biochem.* **59,** 783–836.

24. Fiers, W. (1991). Tumor necrosis factor: Characterization at the molecular, cellular and in vivo level. *FEBS Lett.* **285**, 199–212.
25. Vilcek, J., and Lee, T. H. (1991). Tumor necrosis factor: New insights into the molecular mechanisms of its multiple actions. *J. Biol. Chem.* **266**, 7313–7316.
26. Smith, W. L. (1989). The eicosanoids and their biochemical mechanisms of action. *Biochem. J.* **259**, 315–324.
27. Serhan, C. N. (1991). Lipoxins: Eicosanoids carrying intra- and intercellular messages. *J. Bioenerg. Biomembr.* **23**, 105–122.
28. Smith, G. D., and Griffin, J. F. (1978). Conformation of [Leu⁵]enkephalin from X-ray diffraction: Features important for recognition at opiate receptor. *Science* **199**, 1214–1216.
29. Dores, R. M., McDonald, L. K., Goldsmith, A., Deviche, P., and Rubin, D. A. (1993). The phylogeny of enkephalins: Speculations on the origins of opioid precursors. *Cell. Physiol. Biochem.* **3**, 231–244.
30. Gordon, L. J. (1986). Extracellular ATP: Effects, sources and fate. *Biochem. J.* **233**, 309–319.
31. Williams, M. (1987). Purine receptors in mammalian tissues: Pharmacology and functional significance. *Annu. Rev. Pharmacol. Toxicol.* **27**, 315–345.
32. Dubyak, G. R., and El-Moatassim, C. (1993). Signal transduction via P₂-purinergic receptors for extracellular ATP and other nucleotides. *Am. J. Physiol.* **265**, C577–C606.
33. Bendich, A., and Olson, J. A. (1989). Biological actions of cartenoids. *FASEB J.* **3**, 1927–1932.
34. Chao, W., and Olson, M. S. (1993). Platelet-activating factor: Receptors and signal transduction. *Biochem. J.* **292**, 617–629.
35. Venable, M. E., Zimmerman, G. A., McIntyre, T. M., and Prescott, S. M. (1993). Platelet-activating factor: A phospholipid autacoid with diverse actions. *J. Lipid Res.* **34**, 691–702.
36. Downer, R. G. H., and Laufer, H. (eds.) (1983). "Endocrinology of Insects." Liss, New York.
37. Epple, A., Scanes, C. G., and Stetson, M. H. (eds.) (1990). "Progress in Comparative Endocrinology." Wiley, New York.
38. Nagasawa, H. (1993). Recent advances in insect neuropeptides. *Comp. Biochem. Physiol.* **106C**, 295–300.
39. Laufer, H., and Downer, R. G. H. (eds.) (1988). "Endocrinology of Selected Invertebrate Types." Liss, New York.
40. Hasegawa, Y., Hirose, E., and Katakura, Y. (1993). Hormonal control of sexual differentiation and reproduction in crustacea. *Am. Zool.* **33**, 403–411.
41. Davies, P. J. (ed.) (1987). "Plant Hormones and Their Role in Plant Growth and Development." Martinus Nijhoff, Dordrecht, The Netherlands.
42. Palme, K., Hesse, T., Moore, I., Campos, N., Feldwisch, J., Garbers, C., Hesse, F., and Schell, J. (1991). Hormonal modulation of plant growth: The role of auxin perception. *Mech. Dev.* **33**, 97–106.
43. Eberhard, S., Doubrava, N., Marfà, V., Mohnen, D., Southwick, A., Darvill, A., and Albersheim, P. (1989). Pectic cell wall fragments regulate tobacco thin-cell-layer explant morphogenesis. *Plant Cell* **1**, 747–755.
44. Ryan, C. A. (1988). Oligosaccharides as recognition signals for the expression of defensive genes in plants. *Biochemistry* **27**, 8879–8883.
45. Fry, S. C., Aldington, S., Hetherington, P. R., and Aitken, J. (1993). Oligosaccharides as signals and substrates in the plant cell wall. *Plant Physiol.* **103**, 1–5.

46. Raskin, I. (1992). Salicylate, a new plant hormone. *Plant Physiol.* **99,** 799–803.
47. Enyedi, A. J., Yalpani, N., Silverman, P., and Raskin, I. (1992). Signal molecules in systemic plant resistance to pathogens and pests. *Cell* **70,** 879–886.
48. Staswick, P. E. (1992). Jasmonate, genes, and fragrant signals. *Plant Physiol.* **99,** 804–807.
49. Sembdner, G., and Parthier, B. (1993). The biochemistry and the physiological and molecular actions of jasmonates. *Annu. Rev. Plant Physiol. Plant Mol. Biol.* **44,** 569–589.
50. Mandava, N. B. (1988). Plant growth-promoting brassinosteroids. *Annu. Rev. Plant Physiol. Plant Mol. Biol.* **39,** 23–52.

PART 2

Receptors

CHAPTER **4**

Kinetics

CHAPTER OUTLINE

I. Introduction

The first step in the action of a hormone is its interaction with a specific binding protein in or on the target cell; such a protein is called a *receptor*. This chapter will describe the basic characteristics of these receptors and how to determine their number and affinity. The structure, function, and metabolism of the better-known receptors are discussed in the ensuing chapters: nuclear receptors are covered in Chapter 5 and membrane receptors in Chapter 6. Finally, mechanisms for the regulation of receptor activity are presented in Chapter 7.

What are some of the major characteristics of receptors? Because hormone concentrations are very low, the receptor should have a *high affinity*. A *high specificity* insures that closely related hormones will still preferentially bind to their own receptors and remain functionally distinct. Very closely related hormones may still cross-bind, but the affinity for the unintended ligand is usually low enough not to present any problems under physiological conditions. The receptor should be *saturable*, that is, there should be a finite number of them. This characteristic distinguishes receptor binding from nonspecific binding. The effects of hormones frequently decay rapidly following hormonal removal; this temporal pattern is a result of the *reversibility* of hormone–receptor binding. The receptor for a particular hormone should have a *tissue distribution* appropriate to the actions of that hormone; that is, it should be present in the target organs of that hormone and absent from the tissues unresponsive to the hormone. Finally, receptor binding should be correlated with some *biological effect*.

If a binding protein possesses these characteristics, it is probably a hormone receptor. However, there are always special circumstances that can make any individual case problematic. For example, the aldosterone receptor binds both aldosterone and cortisol with equal affinity, but the target cells for this mineralocorticoid only respond to aldosterone. Based on this loose binding specificity, one might assume that this protein was not the true aldosterone receptor. However, the specificity lies not with the receptor but with the metabolizing enzymes in the target cells. These tissues are rich in 11β-hydroxysteroid dehydrogenase, which inactivates cortisol; therefore, the nuclear receptor is normally never exposed to glucocorticoids and does not need to distinguish between them and mineralocorticoids (1,2). In another example, many target cells may not be responsive to hormones during some phase of their development, although they may still possess high-affinity specific receptors. In these cases, the receptors may be sequestered or uncoupled from transducers (see Chapter 7).

Historically, receptors were postulated by Langley as early as 1878 (3). In one experiment, he noted that curare could block the effects of nerve stimulation in muscle contraction but did not interfere with direct stimulation. He reasoned that curare could not be acting directly on the "chief substance" (that is, on those factors involved in contraction) but must act on something between the nerve stimulation and the chief substance; he called it the "receptive substance." He then universalized this mechanism for all hormones (4). In 1948, Ahlquist discovered that various adrenergic agonists exhibited two different orders of potency, depending on the tissue tested, and proposed the existence of two types of adrenergic receptors, α and β (5). However, the actual measurement of receptors did not come until 1962, when Jensen demonstrated intracellular receptors for estradiol (6). It was also in 1962 that Hunter and Greenwood developed an easy and reliable way of radioiodinating peptide hormones (7). Their intention was to use these hormones in radioimmunoassays, but in 1969 Lefkowitz used ^{125}I-labeled ACTH to demonstrate ACTH receptors in the adrenal gland (8). Since then, the literature has become sated with the measurement of receptors.

II. Receptor Assays

Receptors can be measured by three basic techniques: (i) nucleic acid hybridization, (ii) immunoassay, and (iii) kinetic analysis. Each assay has its advantages and disadvantages. The first two are easy and accurate; however, the hybridization assays actually determine receptor mRNA levels, which may not always correlate with the levels of receptor protein. The various immunoassays do measure receptor protein, but receptors can exist in inactive forms that cannot bind hormone (*cryptic* receptors), trigger a transduction system (*desensitized* receptors), or bind DNA (*untransformed* receptors) (see Chapters 5 and 6). Monoclonal antibodies may not be able to distinguish among these forms.

Kinetic analysis utilizes the binding of a radiolabeled ligand to detect the receptor. It has the advantage of not requiring that the receptor be purified or its gene cloned. It has the disadvantage of relying on several assumptions that some biological systems may not be able to satisfy (see Section III). The two most common types of kinetic measurement are (i) percentage of specific binding and (ii) receptor number and affinity. Percentage of specific binding is the easiest technique and merely consists of adding labeled hormone to a receptor sample and determining how much specifically binds. Unfortunately, molecules may nonspecifically adhere to almost anything, including other proteins and even the walls of the reaction vessel; total binding must be corrected for this phenomenon. Nonspecific binding can be determined in the presence of an excess of unlabeled hormone, because the latter will displace the labeled hormone from its receptors but not from nonspecific binding sites. Such a determination reveals that nonspecific binding is linear with respect to hormone concentration; it is also unsaturable (Fig. 4-1). Specific binding is then calculated by subtracting nonspecific binding from total binding; percentage of specific binding is the ratio of specific binding to total labeled hormone added.

The percentage of specific binding is a reflection of both receptor number and affinity. For example, assume that the percentage of total labeled hormone specifically bound to a tissue increases after some experimental treat-

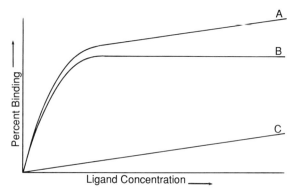

Fig. 4-1. Percentage of binding as a function of ligand concentration. Total binding (A) is a combination of both specific (B) and nonspecific (C) binding.

ment. The enhanced binding could be a result of (i) more receptors, (ii) a higher affinity of the same number of receptors, or (iii) an increase in both receptor number and affinity. Therefore, although the percentage of specific binding is easy to determine, the data are somewhat ambiguous.

III. Kinetics

A. Scatchard Analysis

The determination of receptor number and affinity involves analyses based on the laws of mass action; the hormone (H) and the receptor (R) bind in a reversible reaction:

$$H + R \rightleftharpoons HR$$

The rate of formation equals $k_f[H][R]$ and the rate of dissociation equals $k_r[HR]$. At equilibrium, the rate of formation equals the rate of dissociation:

$$k_f[H][R] = k_r[HR] \tag{1}$$

or

$$k_f/k_r = K_a = 1/K_d = [HR]/[H][R] \tag{2}$$

In equation (2), the two rate constants are combined into a single one, the association constant (K_a), or its reciprocal, the dissociation constant (K_d). The total number of receptors (n) is equal to the number of free receptors ([R]) plus the number bound to the hormone ([HR]). By solving for [R], one obtains the following relationship:

$$[R] = n - [HR] \tag{3}$$

This result is then substituted into equation (2):

$$K_a = [HR]/[H](n - [HR]) \tag{4}$$

This substitution is necessary because there is no way to measure free receptor. In contrast, the hormone can be radioactively labeled and free label represents free hormone (F = [H]), whereas bound label represents bound hormone (B = [HR]). For operational convenience, these new abbreviations will be used in equation (4) and both sides will be multiplied by $(n - B)$:

$$K_a = B/F(n - B) \tag{5}$$

or

$$K_a n - K_a B = B/F \tag{6}$$

This is the equation for a straight line where B/F is the ordinate and B is the abscissa (Fig. 4-2A). The x intercept (B/F = 0) is the total number of receptors (n), whereas the slope is the negative value of the association constant $(-K_a)$. This is the Scatchard plot. However, some authorities recommend rearranging equation (6) and performing a direct linear plot (Fig. 4-2B):

$$n/B - K_d/F = 1 \tag{7}$$

In this technique, B and F from each sample are plotted as separate points along the axes: B on the ordinate (0,B) and F on the abscissa $(-F,0)$. These two points are connected to give a straight line. There will be one such line for each sample and all these lines will intersect at a single point. The reflection of this intersecting point onto the ordinate (B) is the total number of receptors (n); the reflection onto the abscissa $(-F)$ is the dissociation constant (K_d). Table 4-1 contains actual data from the literature (10); these are the data plotted in Fig. 4-2B (10).

Others have advocated the Lineweaver–Burk plot [equation (8); Fig. 4-2C], the Hanes' plot [equation (9); Fig. 4-2D], or computer analysis of nontransformed nonlinear data:

$$1/B = K_d/nF + 1/n \tag{8}$$

$$F/B = K_d/n + F/n \tag{9}$$

As can be seen in Fig. 4-2, excellent data yield identical results by any method, but when data are less than perfect, some investigators claim that the Scatchard plot accentuates the error. In truth, no method is perfect. In a recent comparison of these methods (11), it was shown that the Lineweaver–Burk plot gave the best accuracy but the poorest reproducibility, whereas the Eadie–Hofstee plot, which is very similar to the Scatchard plot, gave the best reproducibility but the poorest accuracy.

B. Assumptions

Recently, the Scatchard analysis has come under some criticism, but most of this criticism is misplaced. The Scatchard plot is only the result of a mathematical derivation; the problem is that several assumptions must be made and most real systems do not satisfy all of them. Therefore, to appreciate the limitations of the Scatchard analysis, these assumptions and other cautions will be discussed in detail.

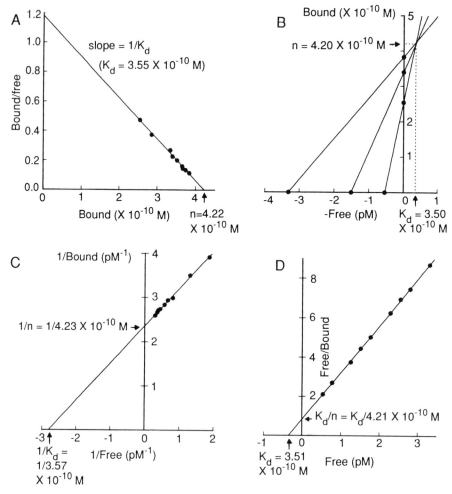

Fig. 4-2. Binding data for estradiol in rat uterine cytosol plotted by (A) the Scatchard, (B) the direct linear, (C) Lineweaver-Burk, or (D) the Hanes' method. The original data are given in Table 4-1; for clarity, only three data points are plotted in B: the first, the fourth, and the last. Plots A and B were adapted and reprinted by permission from Ref. 10. Copyright © 1976 Academic Press.

1. The labeled hormone is biologically identical to the native hormone. Most peptide hormones are iodinated with Na[^{125}I]; this rather large, electronegative atom can alter both the physical and the biological properties of the hormone. In addition, this isotope is a powerful gamma emitter that will progressively damage the hormone. Even tritiated hormones cannot be assumed to be indistinguishable from unmodified hormones; heavily tritiated steroids can have a significantly higher molecular weight than the endogenous hormone and the tritium could affect hydrogen bonding with the receptor. Further-

Table 4-1
Equilibrium Concentrations of Receptor-Bound and
Free 17β-Estradiol in Samples of Rat Uterine Cytosol

Bound (fM)	1/Bound (pM^{-1})	Free (fM)	1/Free (pM^{-1})	B/F	F/B
255	3.92	538	1.86	0.473	2.11
286	3.50	771	1.30	0.371	2.70
334	2.99	1252	0.80	0.267	3.75
340	2.94	1510	0.66	0.225	4.44
352	2.84	1763	0.57	0.199	5.03
365	2.74	2279	0.44	0.160	6.25
367	2.72	2541	0.39	0.144	6.94
374	2.67	2798	0.36	0.134	7.46
384	2.60	3312	0.30	0.115	8.70

more, tritiated compounds more than 2 months old have shown signs of degradation (12). Ideally, the labeled hormones should be tested in a sensitive biological assay to insure that the biological activity is preserved; then they should be periodically checked for damage and repurified as needed.

2. The labeled hormone is homogeneous. Although iodination conditions can be adjusted to give an "average" of one iodide atom per hormone molecule, the procedure actually generates a mixture of uniodinated, monoiodinated, and diiodinated species. Even monoiodinated hormones may have the iodide located on different tyrosines and each species may have different properties. For example, insulin has four tyrosines and iodination with chloramine T will yield a mixture of products, each with a different tyrosine labeled (13). As can be seen in Table 4-2 (13,14), these species have slightly different

Table 4-2
Kinetic and Biological Properties of Insulin Iodinated by Chloramine T[a]

Subunit and residue iodinated	Yield (%)	Receptor data		Biological activity[b]		Conclusion
		K_a (M)	n (nM)	Antilipolysis (%)	Glucose oxidation (%)	
A14	50	2.0×10^9	0.65	100	102	Same as native insulin
A19	30	1.2×10^9	0.43	75	—	Less active
B16	10	0.9×10^9	2.0	94	93	Slightly less active
B26	10	1.4×10^9	1.1	129	119	More active

[a] Data from Refs. 13 and 14.
[b] Versus unmodified insulin.

biological activities and each generates slightly different kinetic data. Similar results have also been shown for epidermal growth factor (EGF) (15), glucagon (16), and insulin-like growth factor I (17).

3. The receptor is homogeneous. Many receptors exist in multiple forms, such as the α- and β-adrenergic receptors (see Chapter 6). Fortunately, in most tissues one subtype predominates, but for new systems this possibility must always be eliminated. If both receptors are present in a sample and if their numbers and/or affinities are sufficiently different, the Scatchard analysis will yield a curvilinear plot (Fig. 4-3). Under these circumstances, statistical methods can dissect out each receptor component from the single concave curve.

4. The receptor acts independently. Many of the cytokines have receptors with multiple subunits; alone each subunit has a low to intermediate affinity, whereas only the intact complex has high affinity (see Chapter 6). In other cases, ligand binding will induce the receptor to form a homodimer that has a higher affinity than the monomer. In still other examples, receptors can exhibit negative cooperativity, which would result in a nonlinear Scatchard plot (see Chapter 7) similar to that produced by multiple receptor types (Fig. 4-3). Finally,

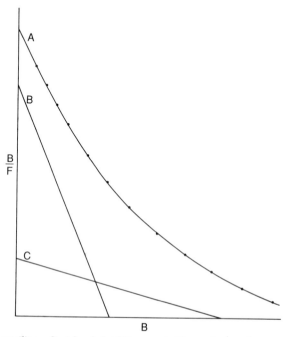

Fig. 4-3. A curvilinear Scatchard plot (A) generated by a mixture of receptors in the sample: (B) a high-affinity, low-capacity group and (C) a low-affinity, high-capacity group.

receptors can bind with accessory proteins that can then affect ligand affinity. For example, the β-adrenergic receptor interacts with a GTP-binding protein that can increase the affinity of that receptor for its ligand. Computer programs and mathematical models can be used to distinguish among these different types of aggregating systems (18).

5. The receptor is unoccupied. If some of the receptor is already occupied by endogenous hormone and if the affinity is sufficiently high to prevent dissociation during sample preparation, these occupied receptors will not be able to bind the labeled hormone. Such receptors are said to be "masked" and their existence results in an underestimation of n (19).

6. The reaction is at equilibrium. This assumption entails several other assumptions: (i) both the hormone and the receptor are stable; (ii) the reaction is reversible; and (iii) the equilibrium is not perturbed when F and B are separated. The destruction or loss of either the hormone or the receptor would decrease the concentration of the "reactants" and shift the equilibrium toward dissociation. Many peptide hormones, especially insulin and glucagon, are very susceptible to proteolysis and certain tissues, such as liver and fat, are very rich in such proteases. Therefore, protease inhibitors are frequently added to the assay tubes; the labeled hormone in the supernatant should always be checked for degradation. For steroids, a related problem exists: tissues that have estradiol receptors also have an enzyme that can convert estradiol into estrone. This conversion can be prevented by adding an excess of dihydrotestosterone, a competitive inhibitor. Steroid receptors are also very labile and must be stabilized by molybdenum salts or sulfhydryl-protecting reagents, depending on the system.

The measurement of membrane receptors in living cells is fraught with another problem: hormone binding to membrane receptors triggers the internalization and recycling of these receptors, and the hormone is destroyed (see Chapter 6). If the rate constants allow, incubations can be terminated before internalization begins. However, if equilibration requires a long time, the incubations can be performed at low temperatures, at which membrane recycling does not occur, or an antagonist can be used. However, although antagonists may not induce receptor internalization, their kinetic parameters may differ from those obtained with agonists. If membrane receptors are measured in broken cell preparations, another problem is encountered: the plasma membrane receptors will become contaminated with the intracellular receptors. In some systems, these latter receptors may represent 95% of the total receptors in the cell (20,21); they can be separated from the plasma membrane receptors by cell fractionation techniques.

Not even the assumption of reversibility is safe; about 5–10% of insulin becomes bound to its receptor by disulfide bonds (22).

Whether this event has any physiological importance or whether it is simply a result of random disulfide interchange is not known, but it obviously affects the equilibrium. EGF can also covalently bind to its receptor (23). In this case, the binding is an artifact of the chloramine T iodination. Chloramine T is a potent oxidizing agent (see subsequent discussion) that can activate several amino acids; this activation can then result in the formation of covalent bonds. In testicular membranes, the dissociation of labeled FSH is facilitated by inhibitors of transglutaminase, suggesting that some FSH molecules become cross-linked to the receptor by isopeptide bonds (24). Finally, this phenomenon has also been reported for steroids: 16α-hydroxyestrone, an estradiol metabolite, binds to a lysine in the estrogen receptor via a Schiff base with subsequent Heyns rearrangement (25).

Finally, to determine F and B they must be separated. For membrane receptors, the cells or membranes (B) can be centrifuged, leaving the free hormone (F) in the supernatant. For steroids, the receptors can be adsorbed onto one of several matrices. In either case, once the separation begins, a new equilibrium may become established; therefore, separations are usually performed rapidly and at reduced temperatures.

Binding studies can be performed by equilibrium dialysis, in which case separation is virtually instantaneous. This technique employs a cell with two chambers separated by a dialysis membrane whose pore size will allow the free passage of hormone but not of receptor. The receptor is placed in one chamber while the labeled hormone becomes freely distributed in both chambers. After equilibrium is reached, the solution in the receptor-free chamber is quickly evacuated and counted. The value of F is twice the measured counts (assuming the two chambers are of equal size) and that of B is the total number of counts added to the cell less the value of F. Unfortunately, this is an expensive technique when a large number of samples is being assayed. Furthermore, this method only works well when the receptor concentration is high relative to the ligand.

7. There is no specific nonreceptor binding. The classic way to determine specific binding is to incubate the receptor and labeled hormone with and without an excess of unlabeled hormone; specific binding is equated with receptor binding (see preceding discussion). Unfortunately, there are other nonreceptor proteins that can exhibit high affinity and specific binding for hormones. Degrading enzymes are examples: tissues containing receptors for catecholamines or acetylcholine are also rich in catechol-O-methyltransferase or acetylcholinesterase, respectively (26). Indeed, partly for this reason, the natural hormone cannot be used in binding studies [see assumption (6)]; instead, labeled agonists are employed. Although these substitutes are not degraded by these enzymes, they can still bind to them and do so with high affinity and specificity. Therefore, this enzyme binding

would show up experimentally as specific binding and complicate the interpretation of the results. Indeed, a putative auxin "receptor" isolated from henbane was recently shown to be glutathionine *S*-transferase, an enzyme that conjugates auxin (27). Other sources of specific nonreceptor binding are the serum binding globulins for steroids and thyroid hormones. When measuring these receptors in fresh tissue, care must be taken to remove as much blood as possible from the sample.

IV. Iodination

Several iodinated steroid and catecholamine derivatives are available commercially, but peptide hormones are still usually labeled by individual investigators. Only the most commonly used methods will be discussed. Central to most of these techniques is the oxidation of a radioisotope of iodide (I^-) to I^+, which then spontaneously incorporates into tyrosines (see Chapter 2). Three popular oxidizing agents are chloramine T, iodogen, and peroxide (Fig. 4-4).

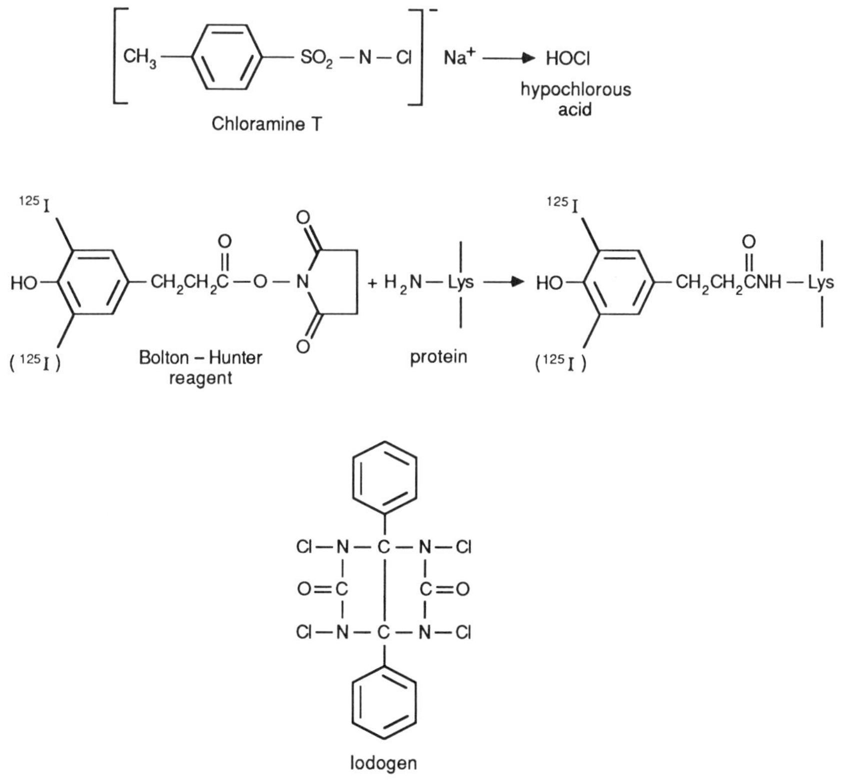

Fig. 4-4. Chemical structure of several iodinating reagents: Chloramine T, Bolton–Hunter reagent, and iodogen.

Chloramine T (*N*-monochloro-*p*-toluenesulfonamide) dissociates in water to form hypochlorous acid, the actual oxidizing agent; the reaction must be terminated by the addition of a reducing agent, sodium metabisulfite. This method is easy to perform but the strong oxidizing and reducing agents often damage proteins. Iodogen (1,3,4,6-tetrachloro-3*a*,6*a*-diphenylglycoluril) is very hydrophobic; it is usually dissolved in an organic solvent and coated onto the reaction vessel as the solvent evaporates. In essence, this is a solid-phase iodination, which can be terminated by simply decanting the supernatant. This method is reported to be less damaging to proteins. Finally, peroxide and lactoperoxidase can be used. This technique is also gentle because the enzyme allows the gradual use of the peroxide. In truth, hormones vary greatly in their susceptibility to damage by oxidation and the best method is usually determined by trial and error.

If a hormone is very sensitive to oxidation, so none of these techniques works, or if it lacks a tyrosine, or if the tyrosine is critically involved in receptor binding, an indirect iodination method is available. This technique uses a preiodinated compound that is basically a deaminated tyrosine whose carboxylic group is activated by succinylimide; this compound is the Bolton–Hunter reagent [*N*-succinylimidyl 3-(4-hydroxyphenyl)propionate], and is available in both the mono- and the diiodinated form (Fig. 4-4). This compound will react with any free amino group such as the amino terminus or the ε-amino group of lysine. The hormone is never exposed to an oxidizing agent; however, the reagent is relatively expensive.

V. Receptor Preparations

A. Membrane Receptors

Membrane receptors can be assayed from many different sources. Tissue fragments, freshly isolated cells, and established cell lines may all internalize the hormone–receptor complex [see assumption (6)]. Explants have the additional problems of having high nonspecific binding and of presenting the labeled hormone with a diffusion barrier. These problems can be circumvented by using freshly isolated cells, but these cells are obtained by treatment with collagenases contaminated with proteases. The latter enzymes have been shown to damage membrane receptors. Established cell lines lack all these problems, but data derived from them may not accurately reflect the situation in normal tissues.

These receptors can also be assayed in membrane fragments, but if there is a sizable intracellular pool of receptors, they will have to be removed by fractionation. The sensitivity of a cell is determined by its surface receptors, so the presence of contaminating, internally located receptors will give misleading results.

B. Steroid Receptors

Classically, steroid receptors were assayed in either the cytosol or the nucleus. Untransformed receptors resided in the cytoplasm; after steroid binding and activation, the hormone–receptor complex migrated to the nucleus. However, recent data suggest that most, if not all, steroid receptors are nuclear. In the absence of steroids, the receptors had a weak affinity for chromatin and homogenization leached them into the buffer-diluted cytosol. After steroid binding, the affinity increased and the complex remained in the nucleus even during homogenization; therefore, the hormone–receptor complex appeared to be translocated from the cytoplasm to the nucleus. This phenomenon is discussed further in Chapter 5.

VI. Summary

Receptors can be measured by several techniques; each has its advantages and disadvantages. Hybridization assays for receptor mRNA and immunoassays for the protein are easy and accurate but the former may not correlate with the actual number of receptors and the latter cannot give kinetic data and may not be able to distinguish among the different possible states that a receptor may occupy.

Receptors can also be determined by kinetics. Using the laws of mass action, one can derive equations that describe the interaction between a hormone and its receptor, from which one can calculate receptor number and affinity. However, there are several assumptions implicit in these derivations:

1. The labeled hormone is both homogeneous and biologically identical to the native hormone.

2. The receptor is homogeneous and acts independently.

3. The reaction is at equilibrium, that is, the hormone and receptor are stable, the reaction is reversible, and the equilibrium is not perturbed during the separation of F and B.

4. There is no specific nonreceptor binding.

The accuracy of the data derived from these equations is dependent on how well any given system satisfies these assumptions.

Membrane receptor determination in living cells may be complicated by receptor internalization, diffusion barriers, or receptor damage during the cell isolation procedure. Furthermore, receptor measurement in cell fragments is complicated by a heterogeneous membrane preparation, which should be fractionated before assay.

Iodination involves the oxidation of radioactive iodide and its incorporation into protein. The protein can be directly iodinated by chloramine T, iodogen, or peroxide and lactoperoxidase. The first is a harsher method than the other two. Proteins can also be indirectly iodinated by coupling them to a preiodinated species that reacts with amino groups; the Bolton–Hunter reagent is such a compound.

References

General References

Birnbaumer, L., and Swartz, T. (1984). Membrane receptors: Criteria and selected methods of study. *In* "Laboratory Methods Manual for Hormone Action and Molecular Endocrinology" (W. T. Schrader and B. W. O'Malley, eds.), 8th ed., pp. 3-1–3-33. Houston Biological Association, Houston.

Bylund, D. B., and Torws, M. L. (1993). Radioligand binding methods: Practical guide and tips. *Am. J. Physiol.* 265, L421–L429.

Kienhuis, C. B. M., Heuvel, J. J. T. M., Ross, H. A., Swinkels, L. M. J. W., Foekens, J. A., and Benraad, T. J. (1991). Six methods for direct radioiodination of mouse epidermal growth factor compared: Effect of nonequivalence in binding behavior between labeled and unlabeled ligand. *Clin. Chem.* 37, 1749–1755.

Laduron, P. M. (1984). Criteria for receptor sites in binding studies. *Biochem. Pharmacol.* 33, 833–839.

See also Refs. 11 and 17.

Cited References

1. Roy, A. K. (1992). Regulation of steroid hormone action in target cells by specific hormone-inactivating enzymes. *Proc. Soc. Exp. Biol. Med.* 199, 265–272.
2. Monder, C. (1991). Corticosteroids, receptors, and the organ-specific functions of 11β-hydroxysteroid dehydrogenase. *FASEB J.* 5, 3047–3054.
3. Langley, J. N. (1878). On the physiology of the salivary secretion. *J. Physiol. (London)* 1, 340–369.
4. Langley, J. N. (1905). On the reaction of cells and of nerve-endings to certain poisons, chiefly as regards the reaction of striated muscle to nicotine and curare. *J. Physiol. (London)* 33, 374–413.
5. Ahlquist, R. P. (1948). Study of adrenotropic receptors. *Am. J. Physiol.* 153, 586–600.
6. Jensen, E. V., and Jacobson, H. I. (1962). Basic guides to the mechanism of estrogen action. *Recent Prog. Horm. Res.* 18, 387–414.
7. Hunter, W. M., and Greenwood, F. C. (1962). Preparation of iodine-131 labelled human growth hormone of high specific activity. *Nature (London)* 194, 495–496.
8. Lefkowitz, R. J., Roth, J., Pricer, W., and Pastan, I. (1970). ACTH receptors in the adrenal. Specific binding of ACTH-^{125}I and its relations to adenyl cyclase. *Proc. Natl. Acad. Sci. U.S.A.* 65, 745–752.
9. Clark, J. H., Peck, E. J., and Markaverich, B. M. (1984). Steroid hormone receptors: Basic principles and measurement. *In* "Laboratory Methods Manual for Hormone Action and Molecular Endocrinology" (W. T. Schrader and B. W. O'Malley, eds.), 8th Ed., pp. 1-3–1-70. Houston Biological Association, Houston.
10. Woosley, J. T., and Muldoon, T. G. (1976). Use of the direct linear plot to estimate binding constants for protein-ligand interactions. *Biochem. Biophys. Res. Commun.* 71, 155–160.
11. Hall, H. (1992). Saturation analysis in receptor binding assays: An evaluation of six different calculation techniques. *Pharmacol. Toxicol.* 71, 45–51.
12. Le Goff, J. M., Berthois, Y., and Martin, P. M. (1988). Radioligand purification prior to routine receptor assays. *J. Steroid Biochem.* 31, 167–172.
13. Keefer, L. M., De Meyts, P., and Frank, B. H. (1982). Receptor binding properties

of the four isomers of ^{125}I-monoiodoinsulin. *Progr. Abstr. 64th Annu. Meet. Endocr. Soc.*, 333.

14. Peavy, D. E., Abram, J. D., Frank, B. H., and Duckworth, W. C. (1984). Receptor binding and biological activity of specifically labeled [^{125}I]- and [^{127}I]monoiodoinsulin isomers in isolated rat adipocytes. *Endocrinol. (Baltimore)* **114**, 1818–1824.
15. Matrisian, L. M., Planck, S. R., Finach, J. S., and Magun, B. E. (1985). Heterogeneity of ^{125}I-labeled epidermal growth factor. *Biochim. Biophys. Acta* **839**, 139–146.
16. Pingoud, V., and Thoule, H. (1987). Receptor binding of selectively labeled (Tyr-10) and (Tyr-13)-mono-^{125}I-glucagons and competition by homologous ^{127}I-labeled isomers. *Biochim. Biophys. Acta* **929**, 182–189.
17. Schäffer, L., Larsen, U. D., Linde, S., Hejnæs, K. R., and Skriver, L. (1993). Characterization of the three ^{125}I-iodination isomers of human insulin-like growth factor I (IGF1). *Biochim. Biophys. Acta* **1203**, 205–209.
18. Wofsy, C., and Goldstein, B. (1992). Interpretation of Scatchard plots for aggregating receptor systems. *Math. Biosci.* **112**, 115–154.
19. Kelly, P. A., Leblanc, G., and Djiane, J. (1979). Estimation of total prolactin-binding sites after *in vitro* desaturation. *Endocrinol. (Baltimore)* **104**, 1631–1638.
20. Posner, B. I., Josefsberg, Z., and Bergeron, J. J. M. (1979). Intracellular polypeptide hormone receptors: Characterization and induction of lactogen receptors in the Golgi apparatus of rat liver. *J. Biol. Chem.* **254**, 12494–12499.
21. Posner, B. I., Patel, B., Verma, A. K., and Bergeron, J. J. M. (1980). Uptake of insulin by plasmalemma and Golgi subcellular fractions of rat liver. *J. Biol. Chem.* **255**, 735–741.
22. Clark, S., and Harrison, L. C. (1982). Insulin binding leads to the formation of covalent (–S–S–) hormone receptor complexes. *J. Biol. Chem.* **257**, 12239–12244.
23. Linsley, P. S., Blifeld, C., Wrann, M., and Fox, C. F. (1979). Direct linkage of epidermal growth factor to its receptor. *Nature (London)* **278**, 745–748.
24. Grasso, P., and Reichert, L. E. (1992). Stabilization of follicle-stimulating hormone–receptor complexes may involve calcium-dependent transglutaminase activation. *Mol. Cell. Endocrinol.* **87**, 49–56.
25. Swaneck, G. E., and Fishman, J. (1991). Effects of estrogens on MCF-7 cells: Positive or negative regulation by the nature of the ligand–receptor complex. *Biochem. Biophys. Res. Commun.* **174**, 276–281.
26. Cuatrecasas, P. (1974). Membrane receptors. *Annu. Rev. Biochem.* **43**, 169–214.
27. Bilang, J., Macdonald, H., King, P. J., and Strum, A. (1993). A soluble auxin-binding protein from *Hyoscyamus muticus* is a glutathione S-transferase. *Plant Physiol.* **102**, 29–34.

CHAPTER **5**

Nuclear Receptors

CHAPTER OUTLINE

I. Introduction

As noted in Chapter 1, all hormones can be classified according to their water solubility. Hydrophobic hormones have direct access to the cellular interior, where they bind soluble proteins. These receptors are actually ligand-regulated transcription factors. As such, they will be covered in two chapters: in this chapter, their structure, classification, and metabolism will be examined; in Chapter 12, their transcriptional activity will be discussed. These proteins include the receptors for triiodothyronine, the retinoids, and the steroids and their derivatives.

II. Structure

The nuclear receptors are modular in construction, having four to five distinct domains: (i) an amino-terminal A/B region, (ii) a DNA-binding C region, (iii) a hinge D region, (iv) a ligand-binding E region, and occasionally (v) an F region extending beyond the E region (Fig. 5-1). This linear arrangement of functions is reflected in the structural organization: the receptor can be proteolytically cleaved into three pieces — the A/B, C, and E regions — suggesting separate structural domains. This hypothesis has been confirmed by electron microscopic studies showing that the glucocorticoid receptor is composed of two globular domains, presumably the A/B and E regions, separated by a tether, the C region (1). This structural independence is further reflected in the functional interaction between the domains: the various regions can be rearranged in recombinant molecules and the receptor will still retain its function (2,3).

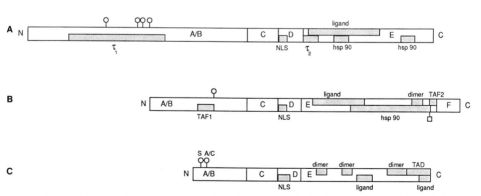

Fig. 5-1. Schematic representation of the (A) glucocorticoid, (B) estrogen, and (C) triiodo-thyronine receptors, showing the various functional domains. The receptors contain (A) 777, (B) 595, and (C) 456 amino acids. Circles represent serine or threonine phosphorylation sites (A, PKA; C, PKC; S, CKII); squares represent tyrosine phosphorylation sites. Hsp, Heat shock protein; NLS, nuclear localization signal; TAF and τ, transcription activation domains.

A. A/B Region

The amino terminus is the most variable part of the nuclear receptor; its major function is in transcription activation. In some receptors, the structural basis for this activity is known. For example, in the androgen receptor (AR), this function is localized in part to a stretch of glutamines that are known to activate transcription factors (see Chapter 12). A similar region is located in the rodent glucocorticoid receptor (GR) but not GRs of other species. The GR has another region that is very negatively charged; such acidic motifs are also known to activate transcription factors which has been demonstrated for the GR as well (4). However, the molecular basis for this activity in other receptors is still unknown.

In most nuclear receptors, there are actually two transcription activating domains: one in the A/B domain (τ_1 in GR or TAF1 in ER) and one in the E domain (τ_2 or TAF2). The two are quite different based on their dependence on cell type, promoter, hormone response element, receptor concentration, and hormones. For example, TAF1 from the estrogen receptor (ER) is active in yeast but not HeLa cells, whereas TAF2 works in HeLa cells but not yeast; both function in fibroblasts (4). Part of this difference may be related to the fact that TAF1 can act at simple promoters but TAF2 requires complex promoters (5). The number and type of DNA sequences that these receptors bind are also important; such sequences are generally called *hormone response elements* (HREs). Specific HREs are designated by replacing the H with the first letter of the particular hormone: for example, GRE is the glucocorticoid HRE and ERE is the estrogen HRE. TAF1 in ER requires multiple copies of the ERE for optimal activity (6); in addition, TAF1 is required for S2 gene transcription but not for vitellogenin gene activation (7). In another example, the A/B transcription activator in the retinoic acid receptor β (RARβ) is required for transcribing the cellular retinal binding protein II (CRBP II) gene but not the cellular retinoic acid binding protein II (CRABP II) gene (8). Finally, TAF1 of the ER is E_2 independent and requires high ER concentrations, whereas TAF2 is E_2 dependent and acts at lower ER levels (6).

Two other functions have frequently been attributed to the A/B domain, although both are strongly related to the transcriptional activity of this region: receptor synergism and gene selectivity. Receptor synergism refers to the phenomenon in which transcription activation by multiple HREs is greater than the sum of the effects of the individual HREs. In the GR, ER, and progesterone receptor (PgR), this synergism has been mapped to the τ_1/TAF1 region (9,10). The mechanism of transcription activation is thought to involve the binding of τ/TAF to transcription factors. This could easily explain the synergism: the more receptors bound near the gene, the more likely the necessary factors will be attracted and stably retained in the vicinity. Gene selectivity may reflect the fact that many induced genes have requirements for specific factors; therefore, the constellation of transcription factors bound by τ_1/TAF1 could activate a different set of genes than those bound by τ_2/TAF2.

B. C Region

The C region, or DNA-binding domain (DBD), consists of two zinc-binding sites (Fig. 5-2). Each zinc is coordinated by two pairs of cysteines located 10–15 amino acids apart. These structures were christened "zinc fingers" because it was thought that the peptide between the cysteine pairs would loop out like a finger and wrap around the DNA. The actual structure of the GR DBD has now been determined by X-ray crystallography (11), whereas that for the ER and RXR DBDs has been solved by nuclear magnetic resonance (NMR) (12,13); the results are in close agreement and differ considerably from the simple finger concept. As can be seen in Fig. 5-2, the structure is dominated by two α helices, one beginning in the carboxy-terminal knuckle of each finger and extending past the fingers. The amino-terminal helix lies in the major groove and makes sequence-specific contacts with the DNA bases, whereas the carboxy-terminal helix lies on top at right angles. As such, the structure resembles the helix–turn–helix transcription factors of prokaryotes. In the 9-*cis* retinoic acid receptor (RXR) there is an additional DNA-binding sequence, the A box, located 23–29 amino acids after the second finger. The A box binds the AT-rich region upstream from (5' to) the HRE (14). In the NMR structure, this A box forms an α helix whose amino terminus abuts the first helix and the zinc site. The basic residues in this helix

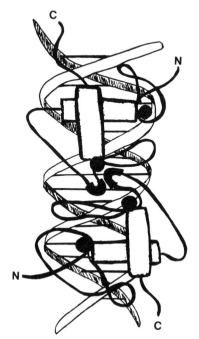

Fig. 5-2. Three-dimensional representation of the DNA-binding domains of two nuclear receptors. Part of the D box is thickened to highlight the dimerization interface.

make contact with the deoxyribose–phosphate backbone of the DNA and enhance DNA binding. The A box may also improve DNA binding by stabilizing the DBD, since some of its residues help form the hydrophobic core holding the first two helices together. Although this region is unstructured in GR and ER, functional studies indicate that an A box also exists in these steroid receptors (15,16). It is possible that elements outside the DBD are required to stabilize this structure in the GR and ER, or that it enhances DNA binding in an alternative manner. These nuclear receptors have DNA affinities in the range of $10^{-10} - 10^{-11}$ *M*.

The DBD also possesses a minor dimerization domain, the D box. This is located in the amino-terminal half of the second finger (thick line in Fig. 5-2). Each finger lines up in an antiparallel fashion to form hydrogen and ionic bonds (Fig. 5-3). This bonding is often too weak to stabilize the dimer in solution, but it may participate in cooperative binding on HREs. The members of the thyroid receptor (TR) family can bind direct repeats, suggesting that they dimerize head to tail. In this case, the D boxes would not juxtapose one another; rather, the D box of the RXR, which occupies the first repeat, interacts with the DR box, which is located within the first zinc finger of the dimerization partner of RXR (17,18). In addition, the DR box is responsible

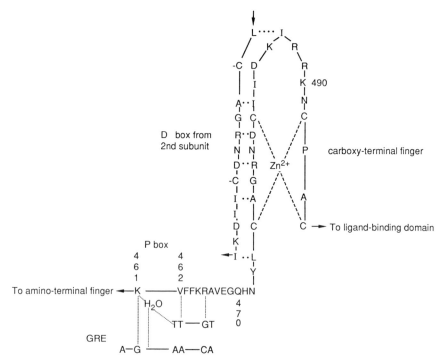

Fig. 5-3. Schematic representation of the P and D boxes in the DNA-binding domain of the glucocorticoid receptor. The dotted lines depict bonds either between the P box and the nucleotides of the GRE or between the two D boxes from separate GRs.

for spacing the dimers on direct repeats; another domain, the T box, which is located between the second zinc finger and the A box, is also involved in this function (19). In addition, the NMR structure of the RXR shows that the A box of the 3' RXR would abut the D box of the 5' RXR; functional studies demonstrate that the A box is necessary for cooperative DNA binding (13). Therefore, in these receptors, the A box would also represent a dimerization domain.

Several steroid receptors can repress the transcriptional activity of other factors (see Chapter 12 for details); this inhibition often requires the DBD but not DNA. In this case, it is thought that the zinc fingers are involved in binding directly to the other transcription factor, since similar metal-coordinated structures have been shown to be involved in protein–protein interactions (20). Finally, this region, in combination with the hinge region, is necessary for nuclear translocation in the PgR; however, this function is more closely associated with the D region (see subsequent discussion).

C. D Region

The D region is also known as the hinge because it is located between the DBD and the ligand-binding domain (LBD). Its major function is in nuclear localization. This task is accomplished by a specific sequence, the nuclear localization signal (NLS) $\{(+) - (+) - X_{10} - [(+)_{3-4}, X_{2-1}]\}$, which is recognized by an as yet uncharacterized nuclear transport system: [(+) represents a basic amino acid and X represents, any amino acid]. This sequence is often preceded by a casein kinase (CKII) site, whose phosphorylation accelerates nuclear translocation. There is still some controversy over whether the NLS is constitutively active or activated on ligand binding; this question is covered in Section IV.

Several other functions have also been associated with the hinge. Some ligand-binding determinants extend into the D region in the TR (21). This region is further involved in the heterodimerization of TR with the RAR or with the AP-1 transcription factor (see Chapter 12); homodimerization is localized to the E region. Some transcriptional stimulatory and inhibitory activities are found in the D region of TR as well (22). Finally, a synergistic function has been attributed to this region in the PgR.

D. E Region

Four major functions reside in the E region: (i) ligand binding, (ii) transcriptional activation, (iii) dimerization, and (iv) heat shock protein (hsp) binding. The ligand makes many contacts throughout the E region; however, naturally occurring mutants that disrupt ligand binding appear to cluster in two areas (23,24), suggesting that these domains contain major recognition sites (Fig. 5-4). The second transcriptional activation domain (TAD) is also located in the E region and was discussed earlier. The major dimerization site is found in the E region and is strong enough to stabilize receptor dimers in

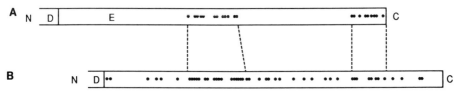

Fig. 5-4. Schematic representation of the ligand-binding domain of the (A) triiodothyronine and (B) androgen receptors. Each dot depicts a naturally occurring point mutation that disrupts ligand binding. The dashed lines demarcate the two regions in which these mutations are heavily clustered.

solution. Like the ligand-binding site, this domain is very diffuse; in fact, different regions of the LBD appear to mediate dimerization with different partners. Finally, various heat shock proteins have been associated with the unactivated nuclear receptor complex; their binding sites are also scattered throughout the E region.

In addition to these well-known functions, several other activities are thought to reside in this region including a second NLS in the GR, a site in GR that synergizes with a transcription factor, and transcription repressor activities located in the extreme ends of the TR E domain. Finally, it has been known for a long time that steroid receptors are very labile and can be stabilized by molybdate. It is now thought that this metal substitutes for a metal ion that normally binds to the E region.

III. Families

A. Glucocorticoid

The basic characteristics of the three major nuclear receptor families are given in Table 5-1. The most recently evolved and most closely related family is the glucocorticoid family, which includes the receptors for glucocorticoid, aldosterone, progesterone, and androgen. All four members have an identical P box; this is the sequence around the carboxy-terminal knuckle of the first finger and is responsible for recognizing the HRE (Fig. 5-3). Indeed, all four bind to the same HRE, which occurs as an inverted repeat or palindrome separated by 3 nucleotide base pairs (bps). Probably because of their recent evolutionary appearance, they have not yet diversified and only two isoreceptors are known. *Isoreceptors* are structurally and functionally distinct receptors for the same hormone; they may arise from separate genes or from the same gene via alternative processing. In chickens and humans, there are two progesterone receptors that are identical except that the short form (PgR A) lacks the amino-terminal 127–164 amino acids, depending on the species. It is still not clear whether PgR A is a result of the use of an alternative promoter for transcription (25) or the use of an alternative start site for translation (26). There is no difference between the two forms with respect to

Table 5-1
Characteristics of the Major Nuclear Receptor Families

Characteristic	Glucocorticoid	Estrogen	Thyroid
Members	GR II, MR (=GR I), PgR, AR	ER, ERRs, COUP/svp	TR, VDR, RAR, RXR, EcR, PPAR
Amino terminus	Long	Short–Medium	Short
Dimers	Homodimers[a]	Homodimers	Homo-/Heterodimers[b]
Isoreceptors	Rare[a]	No	Many
P-box sequence	CGSCKV	CEGCK(A/S)	CEGCKG
Hormone response element	Inverted repeat (TGTTCT) with 3-bp spacer	Inverted repeat (TGACCT) with 3-bp spacer	Solitary or repeat (inverted or direct) with variable spacer (TGACC, but variable)
Hsp 90	Yes	Yes[c]	No

[a] Heterodimerization between two PgRs with alternative transcription or translation start sites (PgR A and PgR B) is the only exception.
[b] Heterodimerization is not totally promiscuous, but all members of this family can at least dimerize with RXR.
[c] Not yet shown for COUP/svp.

ligand binding and tissue distribution; in fact, the two forms can heterodimerize. However, the long form, PgR B, is more active at a minimum promoter (27) and in the presence of multiple PREs (13).

The other isoreceptor is the mineralocorticoid receptor (MR), which binds cortisol as well as it does aldosterone. Since there is much more cortisol than aldosterone in the serum, the MR should be primarily regulated by cortisol. However, aldosterone target tissues contain an enzyme that degrades cortisol, preventing it from ever reaching the MR. In these tissues, the MR is truly an aldosterone receptor. In other tissues that possess an MR but lack this enzyme, the MR becomes a second GR. Furthermore, since the MR binds cortisol with an affinity 10 times that of the classical GR, the MR can function as a supersensitive GR; for this reason, the MR is sometimes referred to as GR I, whereas the classical GR becomes GR II. These two GRs allow the body to respond to cortisol over a 100-fold concentration range (28). These two isoreceptors act separately and do not heterodimerize.

There is a single AR for both testosterone and DHT, although its affinity for DHT is 10 times that for testosterone. As such, the AR is primarily a DHT receptor and functions as a testosterone receptor only in those tissues with high testosterone concentrations.

B. Thyroid

The members of the thyroid hormone receptor family are probably the oldest nuclear receptors, as reflected by their extreme heterogeneity. They are distinguished from the glucocorticoid family by having a short A/B region and a unique P box. They also have a high affinity for DNA and can often bind the HRE in the absence of a ligand. Finally, this group does not form stable complexes with the heat shock proteins, although some studies suggest that they may form a transient association during synthesis (29). Despite having the same P box, the HREs bound by this group are very diverse both in sequence and in arrangement; indeed, a single receptor may be capable of binding to several different HREs. Like all the other nuclear receptors, these receptors dimerize, but there must be considerable flexibility in this interaction since their HREs may occur as either direct or inverted repeats. Some receptors can even bind to a singlet or $\frac{1}{2}$HRE.

Most members of this family have multiple isoforms, usually as a result of separate genes or alternative splicing of mRNA. In some cases, these forms can have dramatically different tissue distributions, activities, or regulation. For example, TRα1 is primarily found in skeletal muscles and brown fat and is down-regulated by T_3. TRα2 is an alternatively spliced form of TRα1; TRα2 lacks part of the LBD region and cannot bind T_3. As a result, it cannot activate transcription and will actually repress gene induction by the intact form. It is found in the brain. TRβ1 is ubiquitous and its levels are generally unaffected by T_3. Finally, TRβ2 is predominantly found in the pituitary (30).

This group is also known for its promiscuous dimerization; not only can the isoreceptors heterodimerize, but totally different classes can interact. The RXR occupies a central position in this phenomenon, since it can dimerize with every other known member in this group. Some authorities think that RXR is an obligatory partner, that is, all active members in this family are heterodimers with RXR. However, it is not clear how absolute this requirement is. In most cases, the homodimer has a low activity that is significantly elevated if RXR is added to the reaction. Heretofore, this low activity had been attributed to endogenous RXR, but it can be reproduced in the yeast system in which there is no endogenous RXR (31). Furthermore, RXR dimers and non-RXR homodimers have different HRE preferences. For example, only vitamin D receptor (VDR) homodimers bind perfect repeats (32). These data suggest that RXRs are important modulators of receptor activity in this family but that they are not absolutely essential. When RXR is present, it usually binds to the first (5′) repeat; 9-cis retinoic acid is not required as a coagonist but its effect is often additive to that of the ligand for the other member of the receptor pair.

There are two other nuclear receptors whose family membership is unclear: the ecdysone receptor (EcR) in insects and the receptor for peroxisome proliferators (PPAR). Both have P boxes identical to that of the thyroid hormone receptors, but the EcR has a long A/B domain and prefers its HRE as an inverted repeat separated by a single bp (33). Despite this unique HRE, EcR must heterodimerize with RXR to induce transcription (34). The PPAR mediates the induction of cytochrome P450 IV and enzymes involved with the β-oxidation of long-chain fatty acids (35,36). Its ligand appears to include saturated and unsaturated fatty acids, especially arachidonic acid (37,38), which is a known hormone transducer (see Chapter 9). Therefore, PPAR may represent either an intracrine or a second messenger receptor. Its HRE is completely unrelated to those for the other members of this family, but it does require heterodimerization with the RXR for DNA binding (39).

C. Estrogen

The estrogen receptor appears to occupy a position intermediate between the glucocorticoid and thyroid hormone families. Although it has a unique P box, its sequence is closer to that for TR and it has the same HRE, except that the ERE is arranged as an inverted repeat with a 3-bp spacer. In fact, TR can bind to the ERE. However, like GR, it binds heat shock proteins, does not bind RXR, and its HRE is arranged similar to the GRE. This group also includes several estrogen receptor-related (ERR) sequences and the chicken ovalbumin upstream promoter (COUP) transcription factor. The latter is homologous to the seven-up (svp) transcription factor in *Drosophila*; for this reason, the factor is sometimes designated COUP/svp. The ligands for ERR and COUP are not known.

D. Orphans

Orphan receptors are proteins homologous to the nuclear receptors, but for whom no ligand has been identified. The ERRs and COUP are examples but their sequence is so close to that of the ER that it is possible to confidently place them in a particular family. However, most orphan receptors are too structurally diverse. In some cases, they may not even have a ligand; they may simply be transcription factors regulated developmentally or by post-translational modification rather than by ligand binding. Alternatively, they may be intracrine receptors whose ligands are cellular metabolites.

IV. Metabolism

A. Heat Shock Proteins

As the members of the GR and ER families are synthesized, they are incorporated into large complexes containing several heat shock proteins (hsps). Therefore, before discussing the activation and recycling of nuclear receptors, it would be worthwhile to examine these proteins. Heat shock proteins are so named because they are induced during heat shock or other stress. Since such conditions often denature proteins, it should not be surprising to discover that most of the heat shock proteins are involved in renaturing proteins: they may help refold them, rearrange their disulfide bonds, or disaggregate them (40–42). These proteins are simply designated by their molecular mass in kDa; the most important hsps for nuclear receptors are hsp 90, hsp 70, and hsp 56/59.

Hsp 90 is a homodimer whose subunits are each 90 kDa. It is a phosphoprotein that binds ATP and can autophosphorylate. However, the relevance of this phenomenon is uncertain since no other substrates are known and the level of this self-modification is only 1–2% (43,44). Although induced during stress, hsp 90 is quite abundant even under unstimulated conditions. It is found in both the cytoplasm and the nucleus, where it can associate with hsp 70 and hsp 56/59.

Several activities have been attributed to hsp 90. First, it is a protein chaperone that maintains proteins in a slightly unfolded state. Second, it binds microtubules. Third, it binds kinases; for example, it is a regulatory subunit for the eIF-2α kinase, which it activates when phosphorylated (45), and it activates CKII by preventing its aggregation. In contrast, it inhibits tyrosine kinases. Finally, it binds members of the GR and ER families: one hsp 90 dimer binds a single GR or PgR (46,47) but binds two ERs (48).

Several functions have been proposed for hsp 90 in these receptor complexes. First, it was thought that hsp 90 blocked the DBD in unactivated receptors; however, dissociation of hsp 90 alone is not sufficient to activate the receptor (49,50) and the MR can bind DNA with hsp 90 still attached (51). Second, it might be involved in the cytoplasmic retention of the unactivated GR by either blocking the NLS or tethering it to microtubules (52); but this mechanism would not apply to other nuclear receptors that are constitutively transported to the nucleus. Third, it may be concerned with receptor phosphorylation either directly or via another kinase that it may bind; however, its own kinase activity is very weak. Fourth, it might stabilize a partially unfolded GR or MR; this conformation is required for ligand binding (53,54), yet this unfolded state is not required for either the AR or the ER (55). Finally, it may be required for proper folding of nuclear receptors during translation (56). In the absence of hsp 90, GR aggregates during its synthesis; this tendency has been mapped to the LBD (57).

Some authorities have suggested that hsp 90 actually has no physiological function in these complexes and that its association with the GR and ER families is an artifact of the lability of these receptors: during processing, these receptors may attract hsp 90 because they begin to denature. Several pieces of evidence support this assumption: first, receptors and hsp 90 dissociate at 25°C; as a result, one would not expect this complex to form at the body temperature of mammals. Second, PgR and hsp 90 do not colocalize in the nucleus (58,59). Finally, hsp 90 binds other unrelated transcription factors such as AhR and MyoD1, suggesting a nonspecific interaction (60). Because hsp 90 does not associate with the thyroid hormone receptor family, complex formation, if real, appears to be a recent acquisition. It is possible that, because the GR family is the most highly evolved receptor group, it is also the most complex and now needs the help of protein chaperones. This hypothesis may explain why the best documented examples of physiological function are found in GR.

Hsp 70 is a 70-kDa ATPase that autophosphorylates during stress (61). Its major function is the assembly or dissociation of protein complexes (62–64). For example, it (i) facilitates ribosomal assembly, (ii) disrupts protein aggregation during heat shock, (iii) removes the clathrin coating from plasma membrane invaginations, (iv) facilitates the transport of proteins through endoplasmic reticular and mitochondrial membranes, probably by partially unfolding them, and (v) dissociates inhibitors from the DNA polymerase initiation complex so that DNA replication can occur.

Several functions have been proposed for hsp 70 in the GR family. First, it facilitates the transport of these receptors across the nuclear membrane. Second, it may enable hsp 90 to bind the complex during initial synthesis or recycling. Finally, it may be involved in the dissociation of hsp 90 after ligand binding.

Hsp 56/59 has also been found in complexes containing members of the GR and ER families; unlike the hsp 90 dimer, both hsp 56/59 and hsp 70 appear to be present as monomers (65). Hsp 56/59 is a peptidyl–prolyl isomerase that catalyzes the refolding of proteins (66); in addition, it is capable of binding and inhibiting the calcium-regulated phosphatase calcineurin (see Chapters 9 and 11). This heat shock protein is the target of several immunosuppressive drugs such as FK506; it is suspected that FK506 has a natural cellular counterpart that acts as a modulator of hsp 56/59 activity. Such a modulator might also affect steroid receptor complexes, but the data are conflicting. In one study, FK506 increased progesterone binding 2-fold and stimulated GR translocation to the nucleus (67,68), but another study could not find any effect of FK506 on glucocorticoid binding to GR, dissociation of the GR complex, nuclear transport of GR, or GR recycling (69). Hsp 56/59 alone is thought to facilitate the ligand-induced conformation change that appears to be responsible for receptor activation (see subsequent discussion).

Many other molecules have been found associated with steroid receptors. Chromatin acceptor proteins attract the receptors to DNA, an ether aminophosphoglyceride stabilizes the GR in an unactivated state (70,71), and an hsp 29 has been detected in the ER (72).

B. Activation and Recycling

During translation, nuclear receptors become associated with several heat shock proteins; as noted earlier, there is still controversy as to whether this interaction is stable or transient. Most authorities assume that the complex persists in members of the GR and ER families until activation; this discussion will assume so as well. This large complex was originally thought to remain in the cytoplasm until ligand binding and activation, when it was translocated to the nucleus. Later, immunofluorescent and nuclear extrusion studies indicated that these receptors were exclusively nuclear. The earlier studies were misleading because they always began with cell homogenization, and the unoccupied nuclear receptor has a very low affinity for chromatin; therefore, dilution by the homogenization buffer leached the receptor from the nucleus. After hormone binding and activation, the DNA affinity increased and the receptor remained on the chromatin so the complex appeared to be "translocated" from the cytoplasm to the nucleus. Now a more balanced view is emerging. The location of nuclear receptors reported by various laboratories is actually dependent on many factors: (i) the cell type under study (73), (ii) the techniques employed, particularly with respect to how much diffusion they allow, and (iii) receptor number. For example, in many transfection systems, the receptors are overexpressed; when there are large numbers of receptors, they inevitably make their way to the nucleus even in the absence of ligand (74). It appears that there is an equilibrium between cytoplasmic and nuclear receptors. This equilibrium is not identical for all receptors: the GR is almost exclusively located in the cytoplasm whereas many members of the thyroid hormone receptor family are predominantly nuclear.

The first step in activation is ligand binding, which has several effects. First, it triggers a change in conformation; the receptor becomes more compact and protease resistant (75,76). Second, it results in the dissociation of activation inhibitors, most notably hsp 90. However, other repressors may also exist; in transfected yeast cells, E_2 induces the release of an inhibitory protein, SSN6, from TAF1 (77). Third, it induces dimer formation. In the case of PgR, this is a direct result of the dissociation of hsp 90 (78), but in ERs E_2 plays a more direct role in promoting and stabilizing the dimer (79–80). Fourth, if the complex is predominantly cytoplasmic, the dimer is translocated into the nucleus. Finally, ligand binding results in receptor phosphorylation (see subsequent discussion). The temporal order of these effects is not known, nor have the cause-and-effect relationships been deciphered. A reasonable scenario might have the change in conformation cause hsp 90 to dissociate, exposing the NLS and dimerization domain. Phosphorylation in the exposed hinge would enhance the translocating ability of the NLS.

Once in the nucleus, the dimer would bind an HRE via its DBD and other transcription factors via TAD, leading to transcription activation. There is still controversy whether the ligand is directly involved in these later steps or whether the only function of the ligand is to remove inhibitors such as hsp 90. The fact that the isolated DBD is constitutively active would argue that the ligand is unnecessary (81–83). Unfortunately, these studies involve transfecting cells with the DBD fragment. As noted earlier, this process can result in very high receptor concentrations that have been shown to drive transcription when more physiological levels will not (84–86). In the presence of normal receptor levels, ligands can increase the specificity of DNA binding (87,88) and activate transcription (85,89).

When the ligand is withdrawn, the receptor complexes reappear faster than can be accounted for by de novo synthesis, demonstrating that the receptors must be recycled. This process is still an enigma, but growing evidence suggests that the receptor must be dephosphorylated. For example, if GR dephosphorylation is blocked, the GR will not recycle (90). Dephosphorylation may be required for exiting the nucleus and/or reassembly of the receptor complex.

Finally, there are several ways of activating nuclear receptors without ligand binding. The PgR can be translocated to the nucleus and activated by dopamine-induced phosphorylation (91). Although the kinase has not been identified, the site, located in the LBD, conforms to the calmodulin-dependent kinase II (see Chapter 9). Both the GR and the PgR can be activated by heat or chemical shock; the activation is not complete for the PgR, since progesterone is still required (92) but the GR is capable of stimulating transcription without cortisol (93,94). Also, the AR can be activated by cAMP-dependent protein kinase (PKA) in the absence of DHT (95). It is thought that nuclear receptors evolved from general transcription factors by the acquisition of an allosteric site for hydrophobic hormones. Prior to this step, these factors had to be regulated in some other way, for example, by phosphorylation or stress (see Chapter 12), and the just-mentioned effects may be vestiges of this regulation. On the other hand, this nonligand activation may still serve some physiological role. For example, the GR induces many genes related to the inflammatory response and its activation by stress may be an alternative means of triggering this response.

C. Phosphorylation

The literature on nuclear receptor phosphorylation is very confusing (96). Some of the problems are methodological, for example, many studies actually measure phosphate turnover rather than stoichiometry. Additional confusion arises from the fact that highly homologous receptors have totally different phosphorylation patterns and functions. The following is a brief summary of the present state of knowledge in this area (Table 5-2).

The heaviest phosphorylation in the GR is in τ_1 (97) at consensus sites for proline-directed protein kinases (see Chapter 11). Glucocorticoids increase phosphorylation 2 to 3-fold (98), whereas dephosphorylation occurs after nuclear binding, possibly associated with nuclear exiting (99–101). Phosphorylation of the GR does not affect DNA or ligand binding, and effects on transcription are minimal (102). It may affect binding to chromatin acceptor sites (96) and it appears to be involved in receptor recycling: if GR dephosphorylation is blocked, it cannot re-enter the nucleus (103).

Phosphorylation of the PgR has been reported in the A/B and D regions (104). Progesterone increases phosphorylation at both the A/B site (105,106) and the D site (107,108). The latter has been localized to serine 530 in the PgR B form (S-530B). Although the kinase has not been identified, phosphorylation at S-530B is preceded by phosphorylation at S-528B by PKA. The possible function of this phosphorylation on DNA binding and transcription is controversial. Progesterone-induced phosphorylation does not occur in the baculovirus expression system, but PgR binding to DNA is normal (109). Furthermore, the progesterone antagonist RU 486 stimulates phosphorylation but not transcription (106); however, it not not clear whether this phosphorylation occurs at the same sites modified by the agonist. Finally, the

Table 5-2

Phosphorylation of Nuclear Receptors

Receptor	Location	Regulation[a]	Possible function
FR	A/B (τ_1)	Cortisol; proline-directed kinase(s)	Recycling
PgR	A/B	Progesterone	
	D (S-530)	Progesterone; PKA (indirect)	DNA affinity, transcription, and/or dimer formation
	E (S-755)	Dopamine; calmodulin-dependent protein kinase II (?)	Nuclear translocation
	D/E	DNA-dependent protein kinase	DNA affinity or transcription
TRα1	A/B (S-12)	Casein kinase II	Unknown
	A/B (S-28 and S-29)	PKA and/or PKC	Required for full biological activity
VDR	C (S-51)	PKCβ	Decreases VDRE binding
	E (S-208)	1,25-DHCC; casein kinase II	Enhances transcription
	Unknown	PKA	Transcription
ER	A/B (TAF1)	Proline-directed protein kinase	DNA affinity; recycling; transcription
	E (Y-537)	Estradiol; calmodulin; tyrosine kinase	Hormone binding
	Unknown	PKA	Transcription without ligand
AR	A/B	Unknown	Unknown
	D	Dihydrotestosterone	High-affinity DNA binding
RARα	A/B	PKC	Inhibition of DNA binding
	Unknown	PKA	Transcription without ligand
RARβ	Unknown	RAR; tyrosine kinase	Unknown
RARγ	A/B and maybe D	PKA	Unknown

[a] PKA, Protein kinase A; PKC, protein kinase C; 1,25-DHCC, 1,25-dihydroxycholecalciferol; RAR, retinoic acid receptor.

isolated LBD can activate transcription although it is not phosphorylated (106), but the levels of the LBD in transfected cells may be unphysiologically high.

Other studies have found evidence favoring a physiological role for these modifications. For example, PgR phosphorylation is associated with hsp 90 dissociation and a 3-fold increase in DNA affinity (110); however, a cause-and-effect relationship was not proven. Second, stimulators of PKA, which indirectly triggers the phosphorylation of S-530B, mimic progesterone-induced transcription, whereas PKA inhibitors will block transcription (104,105). Finally, PgRs with S-530B mutations that prevent phosphorylation require four times the concentration of steroid for maximal transcription, which even then is reduced by 25–30% (111). No change in the affinity of PgR for DNA or ligand was noted. Mutations that introduce a negative charge at S-530B decrease the progesterone requirement for maximal effect by 90%. The difference between these studies and those cited earlier may reside in the experimental system; it has been shown that phosphorylation at different sites in the PgR can affect different promoters (112). Therefore, whether or not one sees an effect may depend on what promoter is being used. Also, there may be other sites and kinases more important in certain systems. For example, it has recently been shown that once the PgR has bound DNA it is subject to phosphorylation by a DNA-dependent kinase (113–115). The site for this modification is unknown but a consensus phosphorylation sequence for this kinase occurs in both the D (S-519B) and the E (S-692B) domains (116).

In addition to DNA binding and transcription, other functions have been attributed to the phosphorylation of the PgR. As noted earlier, dopamine can trigger the nuclear translocation of PgR by phosphorylating a site in the E domain (S-755B) (91) and hyperphosphorylated PgR cannot be down-regulated (106). Therefore, this modification appears to play a role in receptor processing. Finally, phosphorylation is associated with a stable dimer.

There are two phosphorylation sites on TRα1. The one at S-12 is a substrate of casein kinase II (CKII) and is not associated with any activity; it is not required for nuclear localization, DNA binding, or T$_3$ binding (117). The one at S-28/29 is a substrate for either PKA or a calcium-activated phospholipid-dependent protein kinase (PKC) and is required for full biological activity (118). TRβ1 is also phosphorylated, but the site and kinase are unknown. However, the modification enhances both transcription and DNA binding but, only in the presence of nuclear extracts (119). This result suggests that phosphorylation is facilitating the interaction between TR and other transcription factors.

The VDR is phosphorylated at three sites. Phosphorylation at the site in the E region of the molecule is induced by 1,25-DHCC and conforms to the consensus site for CKII (120,121); it enhances transcription, although it is not required for this process (122). PKCβ phosphorylation of S-51 in the DBD reduces the binding of VDR to its HRE, but mutation of this residue to alanine, which cannot be phosphorylated, is without effect (123). Therefore, PKC phosphorylation appears to repress VDR function. PKA can modify an unknown site that results in increased transcriptional activity, even in the absence of 1,25-DHCC; however, the presence of this ligand does result in further stimulation (124). In addition to phosphorylation, the VDR can undergo γ-carboxylation (125). This modification is more commonly associated with the calcium-dependent clotting factors and calcium-binding bone proteins, because the resulting γ-carboxyglutamic acid is an excellent calcium chelator. An inverse correlation between this modification and DNA binding has been noted, but a cause-and-effect relationship has not been proven.

The ER is one of the few nuclear receptors that is phosphorylated on tyrosines. This occurs in the E domain by a calcium–calmodulin-dependent tyrosine kinase (126). PKA can phosphorylate and activate ER even in the absence of a ligand; the site has not been identified (127). ER can also be phosphorylated in the A/B region by a proline-directed protein kinase (128). This latter modification appears to increase the affinity of the ER for the ERE

(129) and enhance transcription. As for the GR, dephosphorylation is required for recycling of the ER.

The nuclear, but not cytoplasmic, AR is also phosphorylated on tyrosines (130). In addition, two other sites, one in the A/B domain and one in the hinge, are phosphorylated by an unknown serine kinase in response to DHT (131,132). The latter is associated with high affinity DNA binding.

In summary, nuclear receptors are clearly phosphoproteins, but the enormous variation in location, timing, and kinases makes generalizations difficult. The most consistent finding is that the receptors must be dephosphorylated before they can be recycled, suggesting that this modification is important in receptor processing. Furthermore, there is considerable evidence that phosphorylation affects transcription, but the data are not conclusive. This problem is probably related to methodology. Other postulated effects, such as dimer stabilization, are still highly speculative.

V. Nongenomic Actions

A. Progesterone

There is now considerable evidence that in at least some tissues steroids may act more directly on cellular metabolism without the need for gene induction (133). One of the best documented examples is the action of progestins in gametes. The progesterone receptor in the *Xenopus* oocyte is a membrane protein rather than a soluble protein (134). The evidence is quite convincing: first, progesterone stimulates the oocyte to complete meiosis by raising intracellular calcium concentrations and by inhibiting the adenylate cyclase via a GTP-binding protein; both actions are classic functions for membrane receptors (Chapters 9 and 10). Second, no intracellular progesterone receptors can be detected. Third, progesterone bound to polymers that prevent the steroid from entering the cell still stimulates cell division, whereas the microinjected steroid is ineffective. Finally, photoaffinity labeling experiments demonstrate that progesterone binds to a membrane protein of 110 kDa. However, the affinity is quite low ($K_d = 10^{-6}M$) and the number of receptors on the oocyte is enormous (420×10^9); by comparison, there are only 10,000 insulin receptors on a fat cell. Part of the reason for the high number is the large size of the oocyte, which is 1.5 mm in diameter, whereas the adipocyte is only 70 μm. Nonetheless, after correction for this disparity in size, the difference is still impressive: 59,600 progesterone receptors/μm^2 of oocyte cell surface versus 0.65 insulin receptor/μm^2 of adipocyte cell surface. However, such numbers have been reported for other systems: there are 100,000 nicotinic ACh receptors/μm^2 on frog muscle. Furthermore, this low affinity correlates well with the high concentrations of progesterone required to elicit its biological activities.

Virtually the same data have been obtained for human sperm (135) and fish oocytes (136). In both cases, the only difference is that steroid specificity and affinity are much higher than in the *Xenopus* oocyte. In sperm, progesterone may be involved in the acrosome reaction.

Although the *Xenopus* progesterone receptor has not yet been sequenced, a putative membrane-bound estrogen receptor has (137): it is a tyrosine kinase that belongs to the EGF receptor family (see Chapter 6). The extracellular domain of this receptor has a sequence that is similar to the LBD of ER; as such, the receptor, called HER2, has a high affinity for estradiol and its kinase activity is stimulated by estradiol binding. The members of this family are similar to the *Xenopus* progesterone receptor in size, ability to affect cyclic nucleotide and calcium levels, and to stimulate mitogenesis; therefore, the *Xenopus* receptor may also belong to the EGF receptor family.

B. 1,25-Dihydroxycholecalciferol

Another well-known example is the effect of 1,25-dihydroxycholecalciferol (1,25-DHCC) on intracellular calcium levels (138–143): (i) the effect is very rapid, occurring within 5 seconds to 1 minute; (ii) it is associated with the elevation of several second messengers generated by membrane receptors; (iii) it can occur in isolated membranes; and (iv) the agonist–antagonist profile differs from that for the nuclear receptor. For example, $1\beta,25$-DHCC antagonizes the nongenomic, but not the genomic, effects of 1,25-DHCC (144). This extranuclear effect appears to be biologically relevant, since it occurs at concentrations of 1,25-DHCC as low as 10 pM. However, the mechanism does not seem to be the same in all tissues: in hepatocytes and chondrocytes, the elevation of intracellular calcium is mediated by activation of a phospholipase A_2 (see Chapter 9); in colon epithelium, osteoblasts, and parathyroid cells, it may be a result of phospholipase C stimulation; and in cardiac cells, cAMP elevation appears to trigger the phosphorylation and opening of a calcium channel. The nongenomic effects of 1,25-DHCC facilitate its transcriptional activity; for example, calcium elevation is required for the induction of osteocalcin by 1,25-DHCC (145)

C. Triiodothyronine

The nongenomic actions of T_3 are different because they involve a direct interaction between the hormone and enzymes. The first such enzyme was actually purified as a cytoplasmic T_3 receptor; only after sequence analysis was the "receptor" discovered to be protein disulfide isomerase (PDI) (146–149). This homodimer catalyzes disulfide bond formation during protein synthesis. However, PDI is very versatile: it also forms the β subunit of prolyl 4-hydroxylase, an enzyme that hydroxylates collagen, and is a subunit of the microsomal triacylglyceride transfer protein complex. In both enzyme complexes, it prevents the catalytic subunit from aggregating. It appears to be identical to recognin, which mediates adhesion and aggregation of retinal cells during embryogenesis. Finally, it is the glycosylation site binding protein in the complex that transfers N-linked sugars from dolichol phosphate to protein. In general, PDI appears to be acting either as a chaperone protein for post-translational modification or as a recognition subunit. Unfortunately, no one has been able to show that T_3 affects the activity of PDI, although T_3 does cause the protein to shift from the cytosol to actin; this migration is associated with a stimulation of actin polymerization (150). On the other hand, PDI is inhibited by estradiol in the nanomolar range (151), although E_2 binding has never been examined.

The other enzyme that T_3 binds is the M_2 isozyme of pyruvate kinase (152). The kinase monomer has only 5% of the activity of the tetramer; fructose 1,6-bisphosphate activates the enzyme by stabilizing the tetramer. In contrast, T_3 at nanomolar concentrations binds to and stabilizes the monomer.

D. Ion Channels

Finally, many ion channels have allosteric binding sites for steroids. The most thoroughly studied example is the effect of E_2 and progesterone on the $GABA_A$ receptor, a chloride channel (153). Both of these hormones will enhance the binding of γ-aminobutyric acid (GABA), which opens the channel. This effect can be demonstrated on isolated membranes and occurs at steroid concentrations in the nanomolar range. Progesterone can also bind and inhibit the neuronal nicotinic ACh receptor, a sodium channel (154).

VI. Summary

All known nuclear receptors consist of a single protein that is modular in construction. The amino terminus contains a transcriptional activation domain, the midsection binds DNA, and the hinge is responsible for nuclear localization. The carboxy terminus is the most complex: it contains the ligand-binding domain, the dimerization and heat shock protein-binding sites, and a second transcriptional activation motif.

The nuclear receptors are grouped into several families. The most recent to emerge is the glucocorticoid family, whose members are highly homologous, bind hsp 90, and recognize the same palindromic DNA sequence. In contrast, the thyroid family is probably the oldest because of the great diversity among its members. These receptors have many isoforms, exhibit promiscuous dimerization, do not bind hsp 90, and recognize a variety of DNA sequences, including direct repeats. The estradiol receptor seems to straddle these two families and too little is known about many orphan receptors to place them into a family.

The unoccupied receptor exists within a complex and cannot bind DNA. The composition may vary, but classically it contains a single receptor, an hsp 90 dimer, and one hsp 70 and/or hsp 56/59. After hormone binding, the components dissociate, the receptor dimerizes and undergoes phosphorylation, and then binds DNA, where it activates transcription. When the hormone is withdrawn, the receptor must be dephosphorylated before it can be recycled.

Steroids and related hormones may also have nongenomic actions mediated by hormone binding to membrane receptors, to enyzmes, or to allosteric sites on ion channels.

References

General References

Baniahmad, A., and Tsai, M. J. (1993). Mechanisms of transcriptional activation by steroid hormone receptors. *J. Cell. Biochem.* **51,** 151–156.

Freedman, L. P., and Luisi, B. F. (1993). On the mechanism of DNA binding by nuclear hormone receptors: A structural and functional perspective. *J. Cell. Biochem.* **51,** 140–150.

King, R. J. B. (1992). Effects of steroid hormones and related compounds on gene transcription. *Clin. Endocrinol.* **36,** 1–14.

Nemere, I., and Norman, A. W. (1991). Steroid hormone actions at the plasma membrane: Induced calcium uptake and exocytotic events. *Mol. Cell. Endocrinol.* **80,** C165–C169.

O'Malley, B. W., and Tsai, M. J. (1992). Molecular pathways of steroid receptor action. *Biol. Reprod.* **46,** 163–167.

Ortí, E., Bodwell, J. E., and Munck, A. (1992). Phosphorylation of steroid hormone receptors. *Endocr. Rev.* **13,** 105–128.

Parker, M. G. (ed.) (1991). "Nuclear Hormone Receptors: Molecular Mechanisms, Cellular Functions, Clinical Abnormalities." Academic Press, San Diego.

Pratt, W. B. (1993). The role of heat shock proteins in regulating the function, folding, and trafficking of the glucocorticoid receptor. *J. Biol. Chem.* **268,** 21455–21458.

Reichel, R. R., and Jacob, S. T. (1993). Control of gene expression by lipophilic hormones. *FASEB J.* **7,** 427–436.

Soboll, S. (1993). Thyroid hormone action on mitochondrial energy transfer. *Biochim. Biophys. Acta* **1144,** 1–16.

Smith, D. F., and Toft, D. O. (1993). Steroid receptors and their associated proteins. *Mol. Endocrinol.* **7,** 4–11.

Truss, M., and Beato, M. (1993). Steroid hormone receptors: Interaction with deoxyribonucleic acid and transcription factors. *Endocr. Rev.* **14,** 459–479.

Wehling, M., Eisen, C., and Christ, M. (1993). Aldosterone-specific membrane receptors and rapid non-genomic actions of mineralocorticoids. *Mol. Cell. Endocrinol.* **90,** C5–C9.

See also Refs. 4, 7, 28, 30, 40–42, 96, 104, and 149.

Cited References

1. Eriksson, P., Daneholt, B., and Wrange, Ö. (1991). The glucocorticoid receptor in homodimeric and monomeric form visualised by electron microscopy. *J. Struct. Biol.* **107,** 48–55.
2. Godowski, P. J., Picard, D., and Yamamoto, K. R. (1988). Signal transduction and transcriptional regulation by glucocorticoid receptor-LexA fusion proteins. *Science* **241,** 812–816.

3. Picard, D., Salser, S. J., and Yamamoto, K. R. (1988). A movable and regulable inactivation function within the steroid binding domain of the glucocorticoid receptor. *Cell* **54**, 1073–1080.
4. Gronemeyer, H. (1991). Transcription activation by estrogen and progesterone receptors. *Annu. Rev. Genet.* **25**, 89–123.
5. Metzger, D., Losson, R., Bornert, J. M., Lemoine, Y., and Chambon, P. (1992). Promoter specificity of the two transcriptional activation functions of the human oestrogen receptor in yeast. *Nucleic Acids Res.* **20**, 2813–2817.
6. Pierrat, B., Heery, D. M., Lemoine, Y., and Losson, R. (1992). Functional analysis of the human estrogen receptor using a phenotypic transactivation assay in yeast. *Gene* **119**, 237–245.
7. Godowski, P. J., and Picard, D. (1989). Steroid receptors: How to be both a receptor and a transcription factor. *Biochem. Pharmacol.* **38**, 3135–3143.
8. Nagpal, S., Saunders, M., Kastner, P., Durand, B., Nakshatri, H., and Chambon, P. (1992). Promoter context- and response element-dependent specificity of the transcriptional activation and modulating functions of retinoic acid receptors. *Cell* **70**, 1007–1019.
9. Wright, A. P. H., and Gustafsson, J.Å. (1991). Mechanism of synergistic transcriptional transctivation by the human glucocorticoid receptor. *Proc. Natl. Acad. Sci. U.S.A.* **88**, 8283–8287.
10. Leng, X., O'Malley, B. W., and Tsai, M. J. (1992). Regions required for cooperative binding of chicken progesterone receptor to multiple PREs. *FASEB J.* **6**, A70.
11. Luisi, B. F., Xu, W. X., Otwinowski, Z., Freedman, L. P., Yamamoto, K. R., and Sigler, P. B. (1991). Crystallographic analysis of the interaction of the glucocorticoid receptor with DNA. *Nature (London)* **352**, 497–505.
12. Schwabe, J. W. R., Neuhaus, D., and Rhodes, D. (1990). Solution structure of the DNA-binding domain of the oestrogen receptor. *Nature (London)* **348**, 458–461.
13. Lee, M. S., Kliewer, S. A., Provencal, J., Wright, P. E., and Evans, R. M. (1993). Structure of the retinoid X receptor α DNA binding domain: A helix required for homodimeric DNA binding. *Science* **260**, 1117–1121.
14. Wilson, T. E., Paulsen, R. E., Padgett, K. A., and Milbrandt, J. (1992). Participation of non-zinc finger residues in DNA binding by two nuclear orphan receptors. *Science* **256**, 107–110.
15. Mader, S., Chambon, P., and White, J. H. (1993). Defining a minimal estrogen receptor DNA binding domain. *Nucleic Acids Res.* **21**, 1125–1132.
16. El-Awady, M. K., Marschke, K. B., De Bellis, A., and Quigley, C. A. (1993). Natural and site-directed mutations in the zinc finger region of the human androgen receptor alter transcriptional activity. *Progr. Abstr. 75th Annu. Meet. Endocr. Soc.*, 203.
17. Perlmann, T., Rangarajan, P. N., Umesono, K., and Evans, R. M. (1993). Determinants for selective RAR and TR recognition of direct repeat HREs. *Genes Dev.* **7**, 1411–1422.
18. Kurokawa, R., Yu, V. C., Näär, A., Kyakumoto, S., Han, Z. H., Silverman, S., Rosenfeld, M. G., and Glass, C. K. (1993). Differential orientations of the DNA-binding domain and carboxy-terminal dimerization interface regulate binding site selection by nuclear receptor heterodimers. *Genes Dev.* **7**, 1423–1435.
19. Towers, T. L., Luisi, B. F., Asianov, A., and Freedman, L. P. (1993). DNA target

selectivity by the vitamin D_3 receptor: Mechanism of dimer binding to an asymmetric repeat element. *Proc. Natl. Acad. Sci. U. S. A.* **90,** 6310–6314.

20. Webster, L. C., and Ricciardi, R. P. (1991). *trans*-Dominant mutants of E1A provide genetic evidence that the zinc finger of the *trans*-activating domain binds a transcription factor. *Mol. Cell. Biol.* 11, 4287-4296.

21. Lin, K. H., Parkison, C., McPhie, P., and Cheng, S. (1991). An essential role of domain D in the hormone-binding activity of human $\beta 1$ thyroid hormone nuclear receptor. *Mol. Endocrinol.* **5,** 485–492.

22. Lee, Y., and Mahdavi, V. (1993). The D domain of the thyroid hormone receptor $\alpha 1$ specifies positive and negative transcriptional regulation functions. *J. Biol. Chem.* **268,** 2021–2028.

23. McPhaul, M. J., Marcelli, M., Zoppi, S., Wilson, C. M., Griffin, J. E., and Wilson, J. D. (1992). Mutations in the ligand-binding domain of the androgen receptor gene cluster in two regions of the gene. *J. Clin. Invest.* **90,** 2097–2101.

24. Mixson, A. J., Parrilla, R., Ransom, S. C., Wiggs, E. A., McClaskey, J. H., Hauser, P., and Weintraub, B. D. (1992). Correlations of language abnormalities with localization of mutations in the β-thyroid hormone receptor in 13 kindreds with generalized resistance to thyroid hormone: Identification of four new mutations. *J. Clin. Endocrinol. Metab.* **75,** 1039–1045.

25. Kastner, P., Krust, A., Turcotte, B., Stropp, U., Tora, L., Gronemeyer, H., and Chambon, P. (1990). Two distinct estrogen-regulated promoters generate transcripts encoding the two functionally different human progesterone receptor forms A and B. *EMBO J.* **9,** 1603–1614.

26. Conneely, O. M., Kettelberger, D. M., Tsai, M. J., Schrader, W. T., and O'Malley, B. W. (1989). The chicken progesterone receptor A and B isoforms are products of an alternate translation initiation event. *J. Biol. Chem.* **264,** 14062–14064.

27. Groyer-Picard, M. T., Vu-Hai, M. T., Jolivet, A., Milgrom, E., and Perrot-Applanat, M. (1990). Monoclonal antibodies for immunocytochemistry of progesterone receptors (PR) in various laboratory rodents, livestock, humans, and chickens: Identification of two epitopes conserved in PR of all these species. *Endocrinol. (Baltimore)* **126,** 1485–1491.

28. Evans, R. M. (1989). Molecular characterization of the glucocorticoid receptor. *Recent Prog. Horm. Res.* **45,** 1–22.

29. Privalsky, M. L. (1991). A subpopulation of the v-*erb* A oncogene protein, a derivative of a thyroid hormone receptor, associates with heat shock protein 90. *J. Biol. Chem.* **266,** 1456–1462.

30. Lazar, M. A. (1993). Thyroid hormone receptors: Multiple forms, multiple possibilities. *Endocr. Rev.* **14,** 184–193.

31. Heery, D. M., Zacharewski, T., Pierrat, B., Gronemeyer, H., Chambon, P., and Losson, R. (1993). Efficient transactivation by retinoic acid receptors in yeast requires retinoid X receptors. *Proc. Natl. Acad. Sci. U.S.A.* **90,** 4281–4285.

32. Nishikawa, J., Matsumoto, M., Sakoda, K., Kitaura, M., Imagawa, M., and Nishihara, T. (1993). Vitamin D receptor zinc finger region binds to a direct repeat as a dimer and discriminates the spacing number between each half-site. *J. Biol. Chem.* **268,** 19739–19743.

33. Koelle, M. R., Talbot, W. S., Segraves, W. A., Bender, M. T., Cherbas, P., and Hogness, D. S. (1991). The *Drosophila EcR* gene encodes an ecdysone receptor, a new member of the steroid receptor superfamily. *Cell* **67,** 59–77.

34. Thomas, H. E., Stunnenberg, H. G., and Stewart, A. F. (1993). Heterodimeriza-

tion of the *Drosophila* ecdysone receptor with retinoid X receptor and *ultraspiracle*. *Nature (London)* **362**, 471–475.

35. Issemann, I., and Green, S. (1990). Activation of a member of the steroid hormone superfamily by peroxisome proliferators. *Nature (London)* **347**, 645–650.

36. Keller, H., and Wahli, W. (1993). Peroxisome proliferator-activated receptors. *Trends Endocrinol. Metab.* **4**, 291–296.

37. Göttlicher, M., Widmark, E., Li, Q., and Gustafsson, J.Å. (1992). Fatty acids activate a chimera of the clofibric acid-activated receptor and the glucocorticoid receptor. *Proc. Natl. Acad. Sci. U.S.A.* **89**, 4653–4657.

38. Keller, H., Dreyer, C., Medin, J., Mahfoudi, A., Ozato, K., and Wahli, W. (1993). Fatty acids and retinoids control lipid metabolism through activation of peroxisome proliferator-activated receptor–retinoid X receptor heterodimers. *Proc. Natl. Acad. Sci. U.S.A.* **90**, 2160–2164.

39. Gearing, K. L., Göttlicher, M., Teboul, M., Widmark, E., and Gustafsson, J.Å. (1993). Interaction of the peroxisome-proliferator-activator receptor and retinoid X receptor. *Proc. Natl. Acad. Sci. U. S. A.* **90**, 1440–1444.

40. Pratt, W. B., Hutchison, K. A., and Scherrer, L. C. (1992). Steroid receptor folding by heat-shock proteins and composition of the receptor heterocomplex. *Trends Endocrinol. Metab.* **3**, 326–333.

41. Smith, D. F., and Toft, D. O. (1993). Steroid receptors and their associated proteins. *Mol. Endocrinol.* **7**, 4–11.

42. Becker, J., and Craig, E. A. (1994). Heat-shock proteins as molecular chaperones. *Eur. J. Biochem.* **219**, 11–23.

43. Csermely, P., and Kahn, C. R. (1991). The 90-kDa heat shock protein (hsp-90) possesses an ATP binding site and autophosphorylating activity. *J. Biol. Chem.* **266**, 4943–4950.

44. Nadeau, K., Das, A., and Walsh, C. T. (1993). Hsp90 chaperonins possess ATPase activity and bind heat shock transcription factors and peptidyl prolyl isomerases. *J. Biol. Chem.* **268**, 1479–1487.

45. Szyszka, R., Kramer, G., and Hardesty, B. (1989). The phosphorylation state of the reticulocyte 90-kDa heat shock protein affects its ability to increase phosphorylation of peptide initiation factor 2α subunit by the heme-sensitive kinase. *Biochemistry* **28**, 1435–1438.

46. Denis, M., Wikström, A. C., and Gustafsson, J.Å. (1988). Subunit composition of the molybdate-stabilized non-activated glucocorticoid receptor from rat liver. *J. Steroid Biochem.* **30**, 271–276.

47. Radanyi, C., Renoir, J. M., Sabbah, M., and Baulieu, E. E. (1989). Chick heat-shock protein of $M_r = 90,000$, free or released from progesterone receptor, is in a dimeric form. *J. Biol. Chem.* **264**, 2568–2573.

48. Giambiagi, N., and Pasqualini, J. R. (1990). Interaction of three monoclonal antibodies with the nonactivated and activated forms of the estrogen receptor. *Endocrinol. (Baltimore)* **126**, 1403–1409.

49. Bagchi, M. K., Tsai, S. Y., Tsai, M. J., and O'Malley, B. W. (1991). Progesterone enhances target gene transcription by receptor free of heat shock proteins hsp90, hsp56, and hsp70. *Mol. Cell. Biol.* **11**, 4998–5004.

50. Hutchison, K. A., Czar, M. J., and Pratt, W. B. (1992). Evidence that the hormone-binding domain of the mouse glucocorticoid receptor directly represses DNA binding activity in a major portion of receptors that are "misfolded" after removal of hsp90. *J. Biol. Chem.* **267**, 3190–3195.

51. Alnemri, E. S., Maksymowych, A. B., Robertson, N. M., and Litwack, G. (1991). Overexpression and characterization of the human mineralocorticoid receptor. *J. Biol. Chem.* **266**, 18072–18081.

52. Akner, G., Mossberg, K., Wikström, A. C., Sundqvist, K. G., and Gustafsson, J.Å. (1991). Evidence for colocalization of glucocorticoid receptor with cytoplasmic microtubules in human gingival fibroblasts, using two different monoclonal anti-GR antibodies, confocal laser scanning microscopy and image analysis. *J. Steroid Biochem. Mol. Biol.* **39**, 419–432.

53. Nemoto, T., Oharanemoto, Y., Sato, N., and Ota, M. (1993). Dual roles of 90-kDa heat shock protein in the function of the mineralocorticoid receptor. *J. Biochem. (Tokyo)* **113**, 769–775.

54. Bresnick, E. H., Dalman, F. C., Sanchez, E. R., and Pratt, W. B. (1989). Evidence that the 90-kDa heat shock protein is necessary for the steroid binding conformation of the L cell glucocorticoid receptor. *J. Biol. Chem.* **264**, 4992–4997.

55. Ohara-Nemoto, Y., Nemoto, T., and Ota, M. (1991). The M_r 90,000 heat shock protein-free androgen receptor has a high affinity for steroid, in contrast to the glucocorticoid receptor. *J. Biochem. (Tokyo)* **109**, 113–119.

56. Picard, D., Khursheed, B., Garabedian, M. J., Fortin, M. G., Lindquist, S., and Yamamoto, K. R. (1990). Reduced levels of hsp90 compromise steroid receptor action *in vivo*. *Nature (London)* **348**, 166–168.

57. Alnemri, E. S., and Litwack, G. (1993). The steroid binding domain influences intracellular solubility of the baculovirus overexpressed glucocorticoid and mineralocorticoid receptors. *Biochemistry* **32**, 5387–5393.

58. Pekki, A. K. (1991). Different immunoelectron microscopic locations of progesterone receptor and hsp90 in chick oviduct epithelial cells. *J. Histochem. Cytochem.* **39**, 1095–1101.

59. Tuohimaa, P., Pekki, A., Bläuer, M., Joensuu, T., Vilja, P., and Ylikomi, T. (1993). Nuclear progesterone receptor is mainly heat shock protein 90-free *in vivo*. *Proc. Natl. Acad. Sci. U. S. A.* **90**, 5848–5852.

60. Shaknovich, R., Shue, G., and Kohtz, D. S. (1992). Conformational activation of a basic helix–loop–helix protein (MyoD1) by the C-terminal region of murine HSP90 (HSP84). *Mol. Cell. Biol.* **12**, 5059–5068.

61. Leustek, T., Amirshapira, D., Toledo, H., Brot, N., and Weissbach, H. (1992). Autophosphorylation of 70 kDa heat shock proteins. *Cell. Mol. Biol.* **38**, 1–10.

62. Chiang, H. L., Terlecky, S. R., Plant, C. P., and Dice, J. F. (1989). A role for a 70-kilodalton heat shock protein in lysosomal degradation of intracellular proteins. *Science* **246**, 382–385.

63. Kost, S. L., Smith, D. F., Sullivan, W. P., Welch, W. J., and Toft, D. O. (1989). Binding of heat shock proteins to the avian progesterone receptor. *Mol. Cell. Biol.* **9**, 3829–3838.

64. Pelham, H. R. B. (1989). Heat shock and the sorting of luminal ER proteins. *EMBO J.* **8**, 3171–3176.

65. Tai, P. K. K., Albers, M. W., Chang, H., Faber, L. E., and Schreiber, S. L. (1992). Association of a 59-kilodalton immunophilin with the glucocorticoid receptor complex. *Science* **256**, 1315–1318.

66. Galat, A. (1993). Peptidylproline *cis-trans*-isomerases: Immunophilins. *Eur. J. Biochem.* **216**, 689–707.

67. Renoir, J. M., Radanyi, C., and Baulieu, E. E. (1992). Effect of the immunosuppressants FK506 and rapamycin on progesterone receptor function: The heat

shock protein-binding p59 immunophilin between immunological and hormonal activities. *C. R. Acad. Sci. Ser. III* **315**, 421–428.

68. Ning, Y. M., and Sánchez, E. R. (1993). Potentiation of glucocorticoid receptor-mediated gene expression by the immunophilin ligands FK506 and rapamycin. *J. Biol. Chem.* **268**, 6073–6076.

69. Hutchison, K. A., Scherrer, L. C., Czar, M. J., Ning, Y., Sanchez, E. R., Leach, K. L., Deibel, M. R., and Pratt, W. B. (1993). FK506 binding to the 56-kilodalton immunophilin (hsp56) in the glucocorticoid receptor heterocomplex has no effect on receptor folding or function. *Biochemistry* **32**, 3953–3957.

70. Hsu, T. C., Bodine, P. V., and Litwack, G. (1991). Endogenous modulators of glucocorticoid receptor function also regulate purified protein kinase C. *J. Biol. Chem.* **266**, 17573–17579.

71. Schulman, G., Bodine, P. V., and Litwack, G. (1992). Modulators of the glucocorticoid receptor also regulate mineralocorticoid receptor function. *Biochemistry* **31**, 1734–1741.

72. Mendelsohn, M. E., Zhu, Y., and O'Neill, S. (1991). The 29-kDa proteins phosphorylated in thrombin-activated human platelets are forms of the estrogen receptor-related 27-kDa heat shock protein. *Proc. Natl. Acad. Sci. U. S. A.* **88**, 11212-11216.

73. Jenster, G., Trapman, J., and Brinkmann, A. O. (1993). Nuclear import of the human androgen receptor. *Biochem. J.* **293**, 761–768.

74. Sanchez, E. R., Hirst, M., Scherrer, L. C., Tang, H. Y., Welsh, M. J., Harmon, J. M., Simons, S. S., Ringold, G. M., and Pratt, W. B. (1990). Hormone-free mouse glucocorticoid receptors overexpressed in chinese hamster ovary cells are localized to the nucleus and are associated with both hsp70 and hsp90. *J. Biol. Chem.* **265**, 20123–20130.

75. Allan, G. F., Leng, X., Tsai, S. Y., Weigel, N. L., Edwards, D. P., Tsai, M. J., and O'Malley, B. W. (1992). Hormone and antihormone induce distinct conformational changes which are central to steroid receptor activation. *J. Biol. Chem.* **267**, 19513–19520.

76. Andersson, M., Nordström, K., Demczuk, S., Harbers, M., and Vennström, B. (1992). Thyroid hormone alters the DNA binding properties of chicken thyroid hormone receptors α and β. *Nucleic Acids Res.* **20**, 4803–4810.

77. McDonnell, D. P., Vegeto, E., and O'Malley, B. W. (1992). Identification of a negative regulatory function for steroid receptors. *Proc. Natl. Acad. Sci. U. S. A.* **89**, 10563–10567.

78. DeMarzo, A. M., Beck, C. A., Oñate, S. A., and Edwards, D. P. (1991). Dimerization of mammalian progesterone receptors occurs in the absence of DNA and is related to the release of the 90-kDa heat shock protein. *Proc. Natl. Acad. Sci. U.S.A.* **88**, 72–76.

79. Sabbah, M., Redeuilh, G., and Baulieu, E. E. (1989). Subunit composition of the estrogen receptor: Involvement of the hormone-binding domain in the dimeric state. *J. Biol. Chem.* **264**, 2397–2400.

80. Medici, N., Nigro, V., Abbondanza, C., Moncharmont, B., Molinari, A. M., and Puca, G. A. (1991). *In vitro* binding of the purified hormone-binding subunit of the estrogen receptor to oligonucleotides containing natural or modified sequences of an estrogen-responsive element. *Mol. Endocrinol.* **5**, 555–563.

81. Ris-Stalpers, C., Kuiper, G. G. J. M., Faber, P. W., Schweikert, H. U., van Rooij, H. C. J., Zegers, N. D., Hodgins, M. B., Degenhart, H. J., Trapman, J., and Brinkmann, A. O. (1990). Aberrant splicing of androgen receptor mRNA results

in synthesis of a nonfunctional receptor protein in a patient with androgen insensitivity. *Proc. Natl. Acad. Sci. U. S. A.* **87,** 7866–7870.

82. Tzukerman, M., Zhang, X., Hermann, T., Wills, K. N., Graupner, G., and Pfahl, M. (1990). The human estrogen receptor has transcriptional activator and repressor functions in the absence of ligand. *New Biol.* **2,** 613–620.

83. Simental, J. A., Sar, M., Lane, M. V., French, F. S., and Wilson, E. M. (1991). Transcriptional activation and nuclear targeting signals of the human androgen receptor. *J. Biol. Chem.* **266,** 510–518.

84. McKenzie, E. A., Cridland, N. A., and Knowland, J. (1990). Activation of chromosomal vitellogenin genes in *Xenopus* oocytes by pure estrogen receptor and independent activation of albumin genes. *Mol. Cell. Biol.* **10,** 6674–6682.

85. McDonnell, D. P., Nawaz, Z., and O'Malley, B. W. (1991). *In situ* distinction between steroid receptor binding and transactivation at a target gene. *Mol. Cell. Biol.* **11,** 4350–4355.

86. Strait, K. A., Zou, L., and Oppenheimer, J. H. (1992). $\beta 1$ Isoform-specific regulation of a triiodothyronine-induced gene during cerebellar development. *Mol. Endocrinol.* **6,** 1874–1880.

87. Rodriguez, R., Carson, M. A., Weigel, N. L., O'Malley, B. W., and Schrader, W. T. (1989). Hormone-induced changes in the *in vitro* DNA-binding activity of the chicken progesterone receptor. *Mol. Endocrinol.* **3,** 356–362.

88. Brown, M., and Sharp, P. A. (1990). Human estrogen receptor forms multiple protein–DNA complexes. *J. Biol. Chem.* **265,** 11238–11243.

89. Kalff, M., Gross, B., and Beato, M. (1990). Progesterone receptor stimulates transcription of mouse mammary tumour virus in a cell-free system. *Nature (London)* **344,** 360–362.

90. Hsu, S., Qi, M., and DeFranco, D. B. (1992). Cell cycle regulation of glucocorticoid receptor function. *EMBO J.* **11,** 3457–3468.

91. Power, R. F., Mani, S. K., Codina, J., Conneely, O. M., and O'Malley, B. W. (1991). Dopaminergic and ligand-independent activation of steroid hormone receptors. *Science* **254,** 1636–1639.

92. Edwards, D. P., Estes, P. A., Fadok, V. A., Bona, B. J., Oñate, S., Nordeen, S. K., and Welch, W. J. (1992). Heat shock alters the composition of heteromeric steroid receptor complexes and enhances receptor activity in vivo. *Biochemistry* **31,** 2482–2491.

93. Sanchez, E. R. (1992). Heat shock induces translocation to the nucleus of the unliganded glucocorticoid receptor. *J. Biol. Chem.* **267,** 17–20.

94. Sánchez, E. R., and Zhong, S. (1992). Heat shock induction of glucocorticoid mediated transcription in mouse L929 cells stably expressing the pMAMneo-CAT reporter. *Progr. Abstr. 74th Annu. Meet. Endocr. Soc.,* 110.

95. McPhaul, M. J., and Deslypere, J. P. (1992). Ligand-dependent and independent activation of normal and mutant androgen receptors. *J. Cell. Biochem.* **16C** *[Suppl.],* 28.

96. Moudgil, V. K. (ed.) (1989). "Receptor Phosphorylation." CRC Press, Boca Raton, Florida.

97. Bodwell, J. E., Ortí, E., Coull, J. M., Pappin, D. J. C., Smith, L. I., and Swift, F. (1991). Identification of phosphorylated sites in the mouse glucocorticoid receptor. *J. Biol. Chem.* **266,** 7549–7555.

98. Hoeck, W., and Groner, B. (1990). Hormone-dependent phosphorylation of the glucocorticoid receptor occurs mainly in the amino-terminal transactivation domain. *J. Biol. Chem.* **265,** 5403–5408.

99. Hoeck, W., Rusconi, S., and Groner, B. (1989). Down-regulation and phosphorylation of glucocorticoid receptors in cultured cells: Investigations with a monospecific antiserum against a bacterially expressed receptor fragment. *J. Biol. Chem.* **264**, 14396–14402.

100. Ortí, E., Mendel, D. B., Smith, L. I., Bodwell, J. E., and Munck, A. (1989). A dynamic model of glucocorticoid receptor phosphorylation and cycling in intact cells. *J. Steroid Biochem.* **34**, 85–96.

101. Ortí, E., Mendel, D. B., Smith, L. I., and Munck, A. (1989). Agonist-dependent phosphorylation and nuclear dephosphorylation of glucocorticoid receptors in intact cells. *J. Biol. Chem.* **264**, 9728–9731.

102. Hoeck, W., Rusconi, S., and Groner, B. (1989). Down-regulation and phosphorylation of glucocorticoid receptors in cultured cells: Investigations with a monospecific antiserum against a bacterially expressed receptor fragment. *J. Biol. Chem.* **264**, 14396–14402.

103. DeFranco, D. B., Qi, M., Borror, K. C., Garabedian, M. J., and Brautigan, D. L. (1991). Protein phosphatase types 1 and/or 2A regulate nucleocytoplasmic shuttling of glucocorticoid receptors. *Mol. Endocrinol.* **5**, 1215–1228.

104. Takimoto, G. S., and Horwitz, K. B. (1993). Progesterone receptor phosphorylation: Complexities in defining a functional role. *Trends Endocrinol. Metab.* **4**, 1–7.

105. Sheridan, P. L., Evans, R. M., and Horwitz, K. B. (1989). Phosphotryptic peptide analysis of human progesterone receptors: New phosphorylated sites formed in nuclei after hormone treatment. *J. Biol. Chem.* **264**, 6520–6528.

106. Chauchereau, A., Loosfelt, H., and Milgrom, E. (1991). Phosphorylation of transfected wild type and mutated progesterone receptors. *J. Biol. Chem.* **266**, 18280–18286.

107. Denner, L. A., Schrader, W. T., O'Malley, B. W., and Weigel, N. L. (1990). Hormonal regulation and identification of chicken progesterone receptor phosphorylation sites. *J. Biol. Chem.* **265**, 16548–16555.

108. Denner, L. A., Weigel, N. L., Maxwell, B. L., Schrader, W. T., and O'Malley, B. W. (1990). Regulation of progesterone receptor-mediated transcription by phosphorylation. *Science* **250**, 1740–1743.

109. Christensen, K., Estes, P. A., Oñate, S. A., Beck, C. A., DeMarzo, A., Altmann, M., Lieberman, B. A., St. John, J., Nordeen, S. K., and Edwards, D. P. (1991). Characterization and functional properties of the A and B forms of human progesterone receptors synthesized in a baculovirus system. *Mol. Endocrinol.* **5**, 1755–1770.

110. Denner, L. A., Weigel, N. L., Schrader, W. T., and O'Malley, B. W. (1989). Hormone-dependent regulation of chicken progesterone receptor deoxyribonucleic acid binding and phosphorylation. *Endocrinol. (Baltimore)* **125**, 3051–3058.

111. Denner, L. A., Conneely, O. M., Schrader, W. T., and Weigel, N. L. (1991). Functional regulation of chicken progesterone receptor transcriptional activity by phosphorylation. *Progr. Abstr. 73rd Annu. Meet. Endocr. Soc.*, 32.

112. Takimoto, G. S., Tasset, D. M., Eppertt, A. C., and Horwitz, K. B. (1991). Transcription is regulated by phosphorylation of human progesterone receptors (hPR) following DNA binding. *Progr. Abstr. 73rd Annu. Meet. Endocr. Soc.*, 309.

113. Bagchi, M. K., Tsai, S. Y., Tsai, M. J., and O'Malley, B. W. (1992). Ligand and DNA-dependent phosphorylation of human progesterone receptor *in vitro*. *Proc. Natl. Acad. Sci. U. S. A.* **89**, 2664–2668.

114. Takimoto, G. S., Tasset, D. M., Eppert, A. C., and Horwitz, K. B. (1992).

Hormone-induced progesterone receptor phosphorylation consists of sequential DNA-independent and DNA-dependent stages: Analysis with zinc finger mutants and the progesterone antagonist ZK98299. *Proc. Natl. Acad. Sci. U. S. A.* **89,** 3050–3054.

115. Weigel, N. L., Carter, T. H., Schrader, W. T., and O'Malley, B. W. (1992). Chicken progesterone receptor is phosphorylated by a DNA-dependent protein kinase during *in vitro* transcription assays. *Mol. Endocrinol.* **6,** 8–14.

116. Carter, T. H., and Anderson, C. W. (1991). The DNA-activated protein kinase, DNA-PK. *Prog. Mol. Subcell. Biol.* **12,** 37–57.

117. Glineur, C., Bailly, M., and Ghysdael, J. (1989). The c-*erbA* α-encoded thyroid hormone receptor is phosphorylated in its amino terminal domain by casein kinase II. *Oncogene* **4,** 1247–1254.

118. Goldberg, Y., Glineur, C., Gesquière, J. C., Ricouart, A., Sap, J., Vennström, B., and Ghysdael, J. (1988). Activation of protein kinase C or cAMP-dependent protein kinase increases phosphorylation of the c-*erbA*-encoded thyroid hormone receptor and of the v-*erbA*-encoded protein. *EMBO J.* **7,** 2425–2433.

119. Lin, K., Ashizawa, K., and Cheng, S. (1992). Phosphorylation stimulates the transcriptional activity of the human β1 thyroid hormone nuclear receptor. *Proc. Natl. Acad. Sci. U. S. A.* **89,** 7737–7741.

120. Rochette-Egly, C., Gaub, M. P., Lutz, Y., Ali, S., Scheuer, I., and Chambon, P. (1992). Retinoic acid receptor-β: Immunodetection and phosphorylation on tyrosine residues. *Mol. Endocrinol.* **6,** 2197–2209.

121. Wiese, R. J., Uhland-Smith, A., Ross, T. K., Prahl, J. M., and DeLuca, H. F. (1992). Up-regulation of the vitamin D receptor in response to 1,25-dihydroxyvitamin D₃ results from ligand-induced stabilization. *J. Biol. Chem.* **267,** 20082–20086.

122. Jurutka, P. W., Hsieh, J. C., MacDonald, P. N., Terpening, C. M., Haussler, C. A., Haussler, M. R., and Whitfield, G. K. (1993). Phosphorylation of serine 208 in the human vitamin D receptor: The predominant amino acid phosphorylated by casein kinase II, *in vitro*, and identification as a significant phosphorylation site in intact cells. *J. Biol. Chem.* **268,** 6791–6799.

123. Hsieh, J. C., Jurutka, P. W., Nakajima, S., Galligan, M. A., Haussler, C. A., Shimizu, Y., Shimizu, N., Whitfield, G. K., and Haussler, M. R. (1993). Phosphorylation of the human vitamin D receptor by protein kinase C: Biochemical and functional evaluation of the serine 51 recognition site. *J. Biol. Chem.* **268,** 15118–15126.

124. Darwish, H. M., Burmester, J. K., Moss, V. E., and DeLuca, H. F. (1993). Phosphorylation is involved in transcriptional activation by the 1,25-dihydroxyvitamin D₃ receptor. *Biochim. Biophys. Acta* **1167,** 29–36.

125. Sergeev, I. N., and Norman, A. W. (1992). Vitamin K-dependent γ-carboxylation of the 1,25-dihydroxyvitamin D₃ receptor. *Biochem. Biophys. Res. Commun.* **189,** 1543–1547.

126. Castoria, G., Migliaccio, A., Green, S., Di Domenico, M., Chambon, P., and Auricchio, F. (1993). Properties of a purified estradiol-dependent calf uterus tyrosine kinase. *Biochemistry* **32,** 1740–1750.

127. Aronica, S. M., and Katzenellenbogen, B. S. (1993). Stimulation of estrogen receptor-mediated transcription and alteration in the phosphorylation state of the rat uterine estrogen receptor by estrogen, cyclic adenosine monophosphate, and insulin-like growth factor-I. *Mol. Endocrinol.* **7,** 743–752.

128. Le Goff, P., Montano, M. M., Schodin, D. J., and Katzenellenbogen, B. S. (1994).

Phosphorylation of the human estrogen receptor: Identification of hormone-regulated sites and examination of their influence on transcriptional activity. *J. Biol. Chem.* **269**, 4458–4466.

129. Denton, R. R., Koszewski, N. J., and Notides, A. C. (1992). Estrogen receptor phosphorylation: Hormonal dependence and consequence on specific DNA binding. *J. Biol. Chem.* **267**, 7263–7268.

130. Golsteyn, E. J., Goren, H. J., Lehoux, J. G., and Lefebvre, Y. A. (1990). Phosphorylation and nuclear processing of the androgen receptor. *Biochem. Biophys. Res. Commun.* **171**, 336–341.

131. van Laar, J. H., Berrevoets, C. A., Trapman, J., Zegers, N. D., and Brinkman, A. O. (1991). Hormone-dependent androgen receptor phosphorylation is accompanied by receptor transformation in human lymph node carcinoma of the prostate cells. *J. Biol. Chem.* **266**, 3734–3738.

132. Kuiper, G. G. J. M., de Ruiter, P. E., Trapman, J., Boersma, W. J. A., Grootegoed, J. A., and Brinkmann, A. O. (1993). Localization and hormonal stimulation of phosphorylation sites in the LNCaP-cell androgen receptor. *Biochem. J.* **291**, 95–101.

133. Griffing, G. T. (1993). Dinosaurs and steroids. *J. Clin. Endocrinol. Metab.* **77**, 1450–1451.

134. Maller, J. L., and Krebs, E. G. (1980). Regulation of oocyte maturation. *Curr. Top. Cell. Regul.* **16**, 271–311.

135. Blackmore, P. F. (1993). Rapid non-genomic actions of progesterone stimulate Ca^{2+} influx and the acrosome reaction in human sperm. *Cell. Signal.* **5**, 531–538.

136. Patiño, R., and Thomas, P. (1990). Characterization of membrane receptor activity for $17\alpha,20\beta,21$-trihydroxy-4-pregnen-3-one in ovaries of spotted seatrout (*Cynoscion nebulosus*). *Gen. Comp. Endocrinol.* **78**, 204–217.

137. Matsuda, S., Kadowaki, Y., Ichino, M., Akiyama, T., Toyoshima, K., and Yamamoto, T. (1993). 17β-Estradiol mimics ligand activity of the c-*erbB2* protooncogene product. *Proc. Natl. Acad. Sci. U.S.A.* **90**, 10803–10807.

138. Bourdeau, A., Atmani, F., Grosse, B., and Lieberherr, M. (1990). Rapid effects of 1,25-dihydroxyvitamin D_3 and extracellular Ca^{2+} on phospholipid metabolism in dispersed porcine parathyroid cells. *Endocrinol. (Baltimore)* **127**, 2738–2743.

139. Civitelli, R., Kim, Y. S., Gunsten, S. L., Fujimori, A., Huskey, M., Avioli, L. V., and Hruska, K. A. (1990). Nongenomic activation of the calcium message system by vitamin D metabolites in osteoblast-like cells. *Endocrinol. (Baltimore)* **127**, 2253–2262.

140. Wali, R. K., Baum, C. L., Sitrin, M. D., and Brasitus, T. A. (1990). 1,25$(OH)_2$ vitamin D_3 stimulates membrane phosphoinositide turnover, activates protein kinase C, and increases cytosolic calcium in rat colonic epithelium. *J. Clin. Invest.* **85**, 1296–1303.

141. Baran, D. T., Sorensen, A. M., Shalhoub, V., Owen, T., Oberdorf, A., Stein, G., and Lian, J. (1991). $1\alpha,25$-Dihydroxyvitamin-D_3 rapidly increases cytosolic calcium in clonal rat osteosarcoma cells lacking the vitamin-D receptor. *J. Bone Min. Res.* **6**, 1269–1275.

142. Selles, J., and Boland, R. (1991). Evidence on the participation of the 3′,5′-cyclic AMP pathway in the non-genomic action of 1,25-dihydroxy-vitamin D_3 in cardiac muscle. *Mol. Cell. Endocrinol.* **82**, 229–235.

143. Massheimer, V., and de Boland, A. R. (1992). Modulation of 1,25-dihydroxyvitamin D_3-dependent Ca^{2+} uptake in skeletal muscle by protein kinase C. *Biochem. J.* **281**, 349–352.

144. Norman, A. W., Bouillon, R., Farach-Carson, M. C., Bishop, J. E., Zhou, L. X., Nemere, I., Zhao, J., Muralidharan, K. R., and Okamura, W. H. (1993). Demonstration that $1\beta,25$-dihydroxyvitamin D_3 is an antagonist of the nongenomic but not genomic biological responses and biological profile of the three A-ring diasteromers of $1\alpha,25$-dihydroxyvitamin D_3. *J. Biol. Chem.* **268**, 20022–20030.

145. Baran, D. T., Sorensen, A. M., Shalhoub, V., Owen, T., Stein, G., and Lian, J. (1992). The rapid nongenomic actions of $1\alpha,25$-dihydroxyvitamin D_3 modulate the hormone-induced increments in osteocalcin gene transcription in osteoblast-like cells. *J. Cell. Biochem.* **50**, 124–129.

146. Freedman, R. B. (1989). Protein disulfide isomerase: Multiple roles in the modification of nascent secretory proteins. *Cell* **57**, 1069–1072.

147. Kivirikko, K. I., Myllylä, R., and Pihlajaniemi, T. (1989). Protein hydroxylation: Prolyl 4-hydroxylase, an enzyme with four cosubstrates and a multifunctional subunit. *FASEB J.* **3**, 1609–1617.

148. Rao, A. S. M. K., and Hausman, R. E. (1993). cDNA for R-cognin: Homology with a multifunctional protein. *Proc. Natl. Acad. Sci. U. S. A.* **90**, 2950–2954.

149. Noiva, R., and Lennarz, W. J. (1992). Protein disulfide isomerase: A multifunctional protein resident in the lumen of the endoplasmic reticulum. *J. Biol. Chem.* **267**, 3553–3556.

150. Safran, M., and Leonard, J. L. (1991). Characterization of a N-bromoacetyl-L-thyroxine affinity labeled 55-kilodalton protein as protein disulfide isomerase in cultured glial cells. *Endocrinol. (Baltimore)* **129**, 1876–1884.

151. Tsibris, J. C. M., Hunt, L. T., Ballejo, G., Barker, W. C., Toney, L. J., and Spellacy, W. N. (1989). Selective inhibition of protein disulfide isomerase by estrogens. *J. Biol. Chem.* **264**, 13967–13970.

152. Kato, H., Fukuda, T., Parkison, C., McPhie, P., and Cheng, S. Y. (1989). Cytosolic thyroid hormone-binding protein is a monomer of pyruvate kinase. *Proc. Natl. Acad. Sci. U. S. A.* **86**, 7861–7865.

153. Schumacher, M., and McEwen, B. S. (1989). Steroid and barbiturate modulation of the GABAa receptor: Possible mechanisms. *Mol. Neurobiol.* **3**, 275–304.

154. Valera, S., Ballivet, M., and Bertrand, D. (1992). Progesterone modulates a neuronal nicotinic acetylcholine receptor. *Proc. Natl. Acad. Sci. U. S. A.* **89**, 9949–9953.

CHAPTER **6**

Membrane Receptors

CHAPTER OUTLINE

I. Introduction

This chapter will describe the receptors for the hydrophilic hormones. Since these hormones cannot pass through the plasma membrane, their receptors are integral membrane proteins whose extracellular domains contain the hormone-binding activity. These receptors must also generate an output so the hormone signal can be transmitted into the interior of the cell. This chapter is concerned with the structure, synthesis, and metabolism of these receptors; several other related topics are also covered.

Because membranes are lipid bilayers, all membrane receptors must have one or more hydrophobic domains that can traverse the plasmalemma. These domains most commonly assume the form of an α helix, although β strands are thought to line the voltage-gated channels (see subsequent discussion). Note that the existence of transmembrane regions and other structural domains is often based solely on cDNA sequence analysis. Receptors are present in such low concentrations that the purification of enough protein for sequence and structural analysis is not feasible; rather, it is much easier to clone the cDNA for these receptors and infer structural and functional properties from these data. Unfortunately, not all the final characteristics of proteins can be determined from this approach: for example, one can only make intelligent guesses about where the signal sequence ends, where cleavage may take place, which asparagines (Asn, N) might be glycosylated, and which serines (Ser, S), threonines (Thr, T), and/or tyrosines (Tyr, Y) might be phosphorylated. Even the assignment of the transmembrane region can be difficult: four such domains were originally postulated for the nicotinic acetylcholine receptor (nAChR); later the sequence data were reinterpreted to show five transmembrane regions; then more complete data suggested that the original hypothesis of four helices was correct; now X-ray crystallographic data support the existence of both α-helical and β-strand transmembrane elements. In another example, the exact number of transmembrane helices for the ryanodine receptor family is still undetermined.

Receptors can be classified according to their output and structural relationships (Table 6-1): (i) those with inherent enzymatic activity, (ii) those that interact with G proteins, (iii) those that interact with soluble tyrosine kinases, (iv) those that form ion channels, and (v) those with an unknown output.

II. Enzyme-Linked Receptors

A. Tyrosine Kinase Receptors

All the enzyme-linked receptors have the same basic structural organization (Fig. 6-1): an extracellular amino terminus that binds the hormone, a single transmembrane domain, and an intracellular carboxy terminus that possesses the catalytic site. Cellular tyrosine kinases can be both membrane bound and soluble; the former are often referred to as receptor tyrosine kinases (RTKs).

Table 6-1

A Catalog of Membrane Receptors of Known Sequence[a]

Enzyme-linked receptors						Serpentine receptors				
EGF family	Insulin family	PDGF family	NGF family	Guanylate cyclases	Serine kinases	β-Type	M-Type	No homology		Neurokinin-type family
EGF	Insulin	PDGF	NGF	ANF	Activin	β_{1-3}	M_{1-5}	α mating factor	ACTH sub-family	Tachykinins
HER2	IGF-I	CSF-1	BDNF	NO	TGFβ	D_1 and D_5	α_2	a mating factor	ACTH	Neurokinin B (NK3)
HER3	HGF	FGF	NT-3	Guanylin	Anti-Müllerian hormone	H_2	D_{2-4}	Glutamate (metabotropic)	Cannabinoid (CB1 and CB2)	Neurokinin A (NK2)
HER4		KGF		Speract		α_1	A_{1-3}		MSH (MC1–MC3)	Substance P (NK1)
		SCF		Resact		5-HT$_2$ and 5-HT$_6$	H_1		IL-8 sub-family	Bombesin subfamily
		VEGF					Tyramine		AT_1–AT_3	Bombesin (GRP)
		Flt3					5-HT$_1$ and 5-HT$_5$		fMLP	ET$_A$, ET$_B$, ET$_C$
									GnRH	Neuromedin B
									IL-8 (α/A)	OT–VP subfamily
									MGSA (β/B)	Oxytocin
									MIP-1α	VP (V1a and V2)
									Neuropeptide Y (Y1)	CCK subfamily
									Opioid (δ, κ, μ)	CCK$_A$
									P_{2u} and P_{2Y}	CCK$_B$ – Gastrin
									PAF	Miscellaneous
									SRIF (ST_1–ST_4)	Bradykinin (B$_2$)
										C5a
										TRH

[a] See text or List of Abbreviations at the end of the book for definitions.

The latter have three regions that are found in many other proteins; because they were first discovered in the Src[1] tyrosine kinase, they are called Src homology (SH) domains (1). SH1 is the catalytic site that is shared by all these kinases; SH2 is a phosphotyrosine binding site and SH3 binds proline-rich sequences. The latter can affect localization by binding to various cytoskeletal elements (2). Both SH2 (3,4) and SH3 (5,6) domains are modular: they form compact "nodules" with their amino- and carboxy-terminal ends at one side so that they can be easily inserted into a protein without producing any major changes in the protein structure.

RTKs can autophosphorylate; these phosphotyrosines then become binding sites for proteins with SH2 domains. The binding is relatively specific between a particular phosphotyrosine and a given SH2 domain, because the amino acids surrounding the phosphotyrosine are also important for SH2

[1] By convention, the names of genes are designated by lower case letters, sometimes italicized, whereas the protein products of those genes are capitalized.

Nonneurokinin-type family	Fibronectin-like receptors			Ion channel receptors			Miscellaneous receptors
	Class I receptors		Class 2 receptors	Nicotinic family	Glutamate family	Ryanodine family	
	Simple	Complex					
Secretin subfamily	GHR	IL-6Rα	NGF (low	Nicotinic	AMPA (α	Ryanodine	Autocrine mobility fac-
Calcitonin	PRLR	NKSFRα	affinity)	Ach	subfamily)	IP$_a$	tor
CRF	IL-2Rβ	CNTFRα	TNFα and	GABA$_A$	Kainate (β/γ		IFNα-C3d-EBV
GHRH	IL-2Rγ	LIFRα	TNFβ	Glycine	subfamily)		IGF-II
GIP	IL-3Rα	G-CSFRβ	IFNα/β	Serotonin	NMDA (ε/ζ		IL-1
GLP-1		β$_c$	and	(5-	subfamily)		
Glucagon	IL-4Rα	IL-6β/	IFNγ	HT$_3$)			
PACAP		LIFRβ/	IL-10				
Parathormone	IL-5Rα	CNTFRβ					
Secretin							
VIP$_1$ and VIP$_2$	IL-7Rα						
Glycohormones							
FSH	IL-9Rα						
LH							
TSH	EPOR						
Eicosanoids							
PGE (EP$_1$–EP$_3$)							
PGF$_{2\alpha}$							
TXA$_2$							
Miscellaneous							
cAMP							
Thrombin							

recognition (Table 6-2) (7–9). Essentially, the substrate has a binding site for the enzyme and not vice versa. Several commonly recognized protein groups interact with the RTKs through SH2 domains (9). Many of these proteins will be covered in greater detail under transduction (Part 3), but a brief description is provided here.

Phospholipase Cγ hydrolyzes polyphosphatidylinositol into two second messengers that are involved in calcium signaling. Its binding to phosphotyrosine allows the RTK to phosphorylate it and stimulate its phospholipase activity. On the other hand, GAP is inhibited by phosphorylation; GAP is a component of the small GTP-binding protein signaling pathway. Small GTP-binding proteins act like molecular switches that are "on" when GTP is bound and "off" when GDP is bound. GAP is a GTPase-activating protein that turns the switch off by assisting in the hydrolysis of GTP to GDP. In addition, both Raf kinase and phosphatidylinositol 3-kinase (PI3K) bind RTKs but are not phosphorylated, suggesting that activation is allosteric or

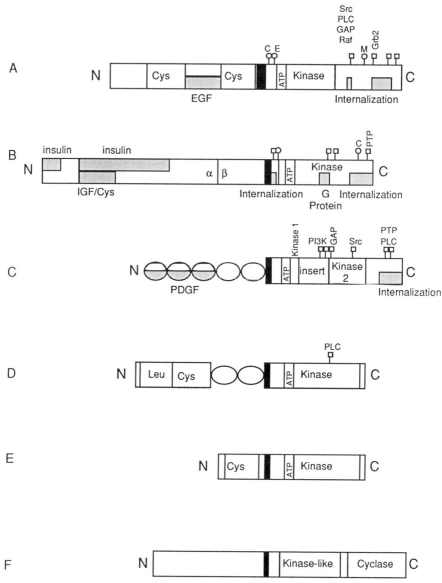

Fig. 6-1. Enzyme-linked receptors (A) EGF receptor, (B) insulin/IGF-I receptor, (C) PDGF receptor, (D) NGF receptor, (E) TGFβ receptor, and (F) ANF receptor. These receptors have a single transmembrane region (black), with the amino terminus (N) extracellular and the carboxy terminus (C) cytoplasmic. Immunoglobulin-like loops are represented by ovals, functional domains are shaded and labeled, and phosphorylation sites are depicted as either circles (serine or threonine) or squares (tyrosine). The responsible kinases are: A, PKA; C, PKC; E, MAPK; G, PKG; M, CaMKII; P, GSK-3; S, CKII. The receptors contain (A) 1186, (B) 1343, (C) 1067, (D) 790, (E) 542, and (F) 1029 amino acids. GAP, GTPase activating protein; PI3K, phosphatidylinositol 3-kinase; PLC, phospholipase C.

Table 6-2
Sequence Specificity for SH2 Domains from Various Proteins[a]

Sequence	Binding proteins
Y–E–E–I	Src, Lck, Fyn, Fgr[b]
Y–(-)–π–P	Crk,[c] Nck,[c] Abl[b]
Y–φ–X–M	Regulatory subunit of PI3K
Y–φ–X–φ	PLCγ, PTP
Y–X–X–L	Lck, ZAP–70[b]
P–X–Y–(V/I)–N–(V/I)	Grb2[c]

[a] φ, Hydrophobic amino acids; π, hydrophilic amino acids; PTP, protein tyrosine phosphatase; X, any amino acid.
[b] Soluble tyrosine kinase.
[c] Adaptor.

that the binding merely serves to bring the kinases together with their substrates. PI3K can also bind the SH3 motif in several soluble tyrosine kinases (11). Raf kinase is a protein serine kinase and PI3K phosphorylates a phospholipid; both are associated with mitogenesis. The SH2-containing protein tyrosine phosphatases (PTPs) are other proteins that can bind phosphorylated tyrosines. Finally, RTKs bind small peptides that are composed solely of SH2 and SH3 domains; these peptides are thought to act like bridges between RTKs and their substrates. They are called adaptors and include Crk, Nck, Grb2 (*growth factor receptor-bound protein 2*), and Shc (*SH2-containing protein*).

Because they are intrinsic components of the membrane receptor, RTKs are most directly associated with hormone action. However, soluble tyrosine kinases can also function in transduction and can associate with both RTKs and cytokine receptors (Table 6-3) (12). These kinases, such as Src and Fyn, are stimulated when the inhibitory carboxy termini are phosphorylated or when the kinases bind SH2 groups that displace the carboxy termini from the catalytic sites (13).

The biological activity of any given RTK will depend on what substrates it attracts and activates. Table 6-4 shows the different constellations of second messengers that each RTK can bind.

1. EGF Receptor Family

The EGF receptor family is characterized by two clusters of cysteines in the extracellular domain, an uncleaved protein, and an intact kinase domain (Fig. 6-1) (14). The major members of this family include EGFR, which binds EGF, and several human EGF-like receptors (HERs). The ligand for HER2 (also called Neu) is controversial. Initially, heregulin (also called Neu differentiation factor) was identified as the ligand for HER2 (15–16); EGF and heregulin are homologous. However, other researchers claim that heregulin actually binds HER4, while estradiol binds HER2 (17). A third receptor, HER3, has also been cloned but its ligand is still unknown. The ligand-bind-

Table 6-3
Structural and Functional Characteristics of Soluble Tyrosine Kinases

Family	Members	Size (kDa)	Structure[a] Kinase	SH2	SH3	Possible function
Src	Blk, Fgr, Fyn, Hck, Lyn, Src, Yes, Yrk	53–64	1	1	1	Transduction by antigens, RTKs, and cytokine receptors
Jak	Jak1, Jak2	130	2	0	0	Cytokine receptor transduction
Syk	Syk, Zap	70–72	1	2	0	Antigen transduction
Fak	Fak	125	1	0	0	Integrin transduction
Abl	Abl, Arg	150	1	1	1	Cytoskeletal–nuclear transduction
Itk	Bpk, Itk, Tec	62–77	1	1	1	Lymphocyte differentiation
Csk	Csk	50	1	1	1	Phosphorylation and inhibition of Src and Lck
Fes	Fer, Fes	92–98	1	1	0	Unknown

[a] Number of kinase, SH2, and SH3 domains in each family.

ing domain of the EGFR has been localized between the two cysteine-rich domains; in fact, this isolated peptide can bind EGF by itself (18). The EGFR dimerizes on ligand binding but the extracellular region responsible for this event has not been determined yet.

The transmembrane domain appears to serve only as a membrane anchor, since it can tolerate considerable mutations without affecting the function of the receptor (19). However, a natural point mutation in this region in HER2 favors dimerization and results in the constitutive activation of the kinase. Since dimerization is associated with EGFR activation (see subsequent discussion), the native transmembrane domain may not favor oligomerization in the absence of ligand to maintain a low basal activity.

Table 6-4
SH2-Containing Proteins Bound by Various RTKs

Hormone receptor[a]	Phospholipase Cγ	PI-3 kinase	Raf kinase	GAP
EGF	Very weak	Weak	+	+
HER2 (Neu)	+	+	0	+
Insulin	0	Weak	Weak	Weak
IGF I	?	Weak	?	?
PDGF	+	+	+	+
CSF-1 (M-CSF)	0	+	+	+
SCF (Kit)	Weak	+	Weak	Weak
FGF	+	?	?	0
HGF	+	+	?	+
NGF (Trk)	+	+	+	+

[a] Spectrum of activity may vary depending upon the particular isoreceptor.

The intracellular region adjacent to the membrane, the juxtamembrane domain, has several critical phosphorylation sites. Phosphorylation by PKC inhibits the kinase activity (20,21), whereas the MAP kinase sites are required for receptor internalization (22,23). This region is also involved in mitogenesis (24), perhaps by affecting substrate specificity (25). Finally, both the phosphatidylinositol and the phosphatidylinositol 4-phosphate kinases, as well as calmodulin, bind in this domain; calmodulin inhibits tyrosine kinase activity (26), but the binding of the kinases does not affect either their own activity or that of the EGFR (27).

The ATP-binding and kinase domains follow. In the remaining carboxy terminus are several very important phosphorylation sites. S-1046 and S-1047 are phosphorylated by calmodulin-dependent kinase II (CaMKII); this modification reduces the tyrosine kinase activity by half and is, in part, responsible for agonist-induced desensitization (28). Y-992 is the binding site for PLCγ (29,30) and probably GAP and Raf (31–33); Y-1068 binds an adaptor, known as Grb2 (34). A cluster of tyrosines around 1100 is associated with internalization. The role of tyrosine phosphorylation in the biological activity of all RTKs is often confused by conflicting reports that mutation of a given tyrosine to phenylalanine does or does not impair such activity. Researchers now know that RTKs have latent phosphorylation sites that can become modified if the primary site is mutated. Since these new sites can often partially replace the original ones, the investigator may erroneously conclude that the original site is unimportant. Therefore, tyrosine phosphorylation is critical to most of the biological activities of RTKs. For example, in the EGFR, autophosphorylation is required for the phosphorylation of PLCγ and the stimulation of PI3K but not for mitogenesis (35).

Ligand binding triggers receptor dimerization, which is associated with both high affinity and kinase activity. Homodimers of either EGFR or HER2 can only bind their respective ligands, but heterodimers can bind and be activated by either ligand (36,37). As noted earlier, the primary output for this family is tyrosine phosphorylation, but this is not the only output. Some EGFR binding proteins, like PI3K and Raf, are not phosphorylated and may be activated allosterically or by translocation to the membrane, where their substrates are found. Finally, the EGFRs exert some activities through GTP-binding proteins, known more simply as G proteins. Researchers have long known that in some systems EGF can potentiate cAMP accumulation, a major output of G protein activation (38), but whether or not this was a direct effect was not clear. However, G proteins can be coprecipitated with EGFR antibodies (39) and EGF can activate G protein in isolated membranes (40), suggesting that the effect may be direct.

2. Insulin Receptor Family

Like the EGFR, members of the insulin receptor family have clustered cysteines in the ligand-binding region and an intact kinase domain; however, these receptors are cleaved in the extracellular domain to give rise to a membrane-bound subunit (β) attached by disulfide bonds to an exclusively extracellular subunit (α) (41). The members of this family include the receptors for insulin, IGF-I, and hepatocyte growth factor (HGF; also called scatter factor).

Electron microscopy shows that the extracellular domain forms two long arms (42), each of which binds one insulin (43). The actual binding region is centered around the single cysteine cluster (44–46) that appears to recognize a common core structure in both insulin and IGF-I. The IGF-I receptor (IGF-IR) has additional determinants in this region to specify IGF-I; as such, the cysteine cluster is sufficient for specifically recognizing IGF-I. However, the insulin receptor requires additional sequences outside this region to recognize and exclusively bind insulin (Fig. 6-1).

As in the EGFR, the transmembrane region of the insulin receptor only acts as a membrane anchor (47). The juxtamembrane domain is required for internalization, glycogen synthase activation, MAP kinase stimulation, and mitogenesis (48–50). In addition, several phosphorylation sites are important for the stimulation of PI3K (51,52) and the binding of IRS-1, an adaptor for the insulin receptor (53). The ATP-kinase domain that follows also contains several important phosphorylation sites. Y-1162 and Y-1163 are required for immediate internalization, insulin-stimulated kinase activity, glucose transport, and diacylglycerol production (54,55), whereas Y-1146 participates in internalization and growth, but not in metabolic activity (56). Again, the reader is warned that most of these data come from mutation studies; as noted earlier, the substitution of a particular tyrosine may activate latent phosphorylation sites. In addition, cell lines, transfection techniques, level of mutant receptors, and other methodological variation can contribute to conflicting results (57).

The carboxy terminus may affect substrate specificity. Deletion of the last 43 amino acids eliminates metabolic activity and the activation of protein phosphatase 1 (58) but markedly enhances MAP kinase activation (59) and mitogenesis (60). This region may form part of the substrate-binding pocket that selects metabolic messengers over mitogenic ones; its deletion would allow mitogenic substrates access to the catalytic site. The carboxy terminus is also important in internalization. The extreme carboxy terminus (residues 978–1300) is required for microaggregation on the plasma membrane, whereas the adjacent region (residues 944–965) is involved in the migration to coated pits and internalization (61).

The major output of the insulin receptor is tyrosine phosphorylation; its major substrate is an 180- to 185-kDa protein (pp180 or IRS-1, insulin receptor substrate 1). This protein is an adaptor for PI3K and Grb2. The insulin receptor phosphorylates itself in response to ligand binding; IRS-1, which has SH2 groups, is attracted to the receptor and is phosphorylated by it. The modified IRS-1 then binds to the regulatory subunit of PI3K and allosterically activates the enzyme (62–64); interaction with Grb2 eventually leads to the activation of Ras (see Chapter 8). Other potential outputs are the G proteins: the insulin receptor can bind G proteins and stimulate GTP binding (65,66). Finally, insulin action has been associated with the liberation of oligosaccharide second messengers (67; see also Chapter 10). Either of these alternative pathways may explain the ability of kinase-inactivated insulin receptors to stimulate pyruvate dehydrogenase. This activity resides in the carboxy-terminal 112 amino acids (68,69), which may represent the binding site for a G protein or an oligosaccharide-releasing enzyme.

Although the EGFR forms dimers only on ligand binding, the insulin and IGF-I receptors form a stable "dimer" between two $\alpha\beta$ pairs; this tetramer is linked by disulfide bonds. Whether the HGF receptor also forms covalently linked tetramers is not known. In addition to "homodimers," an insulin receptor $\alpha\beta$ pair can form a "heterodimer" with an IGF-IR $\alpha\beta$ (70,71); this hybrid binds and is activated by both ligands, although IGF-I is more potent (72).

3. PDGF Receptor Family

Several characteristics set the PDGF receptor family apart from the other RTKs (Fig. 6-1,73,74): (i) the cysteines in the amino terminus are scattered rather than clustered, (ii) the protein is uncleaved, (iii) the kinase domain is split, and (iv) the extracellular domain consists of a series of immunoglobulin-like loops. The known members include receptors for PDGF, FGF, CSF-1 (also called macrophage colony stimulating factor, M-CSF), stem cell factor (SCF, whose receptor is called Kit), keratinocyte growth factor (KGF), and vascular endothelial growth factor (VEGF; also called vascular permeability factor, VPF). Many of these receptors have multiple forms. The PDGF receptor (PDGFR) has two major isoforms, the A and B receptors, that are products of distinct genes. The FGF isoreceptors (FGFRs) are the result of both variable mRNA splicing and separate genes.

The extracellular region consists entirely of immunoglobulin-like domains: the number varies from two in some FGFR variants to seven in the VEGF receptor. The PDGFR has five such domains, but only the first three are required for ligand binding; both Kit and CSF-1R also require the first three loops for binding (75–76). The complete FGFR has three such domains, but many mRNA splicing variants lack the first loop without losing any binding activity. Although the other two loops are necessary for maximum affinity, specificity of binding resides primarily in the carboxy half of the third loop and in an acidic domain between the first two loops (77). The FGF2R has two separate exons encoding this part of the third loop: one exon produces a receptor that binds only FGF whereas the other one generates a receptor that binds KGF (78–80). The function of the remaining loops is unclear; the fourth loop in Kit may participate in dimerization (75), whereas the fourth and fifth loops in CSF-1R may be inhibitory to maintain the receptor in a low basal state (76). FGF and VEGF binding to their respective receptors requires heparin as a cofactor (81,82). Heparin binds both FGF and its receptor; the binding site in the latter has been mapped to an acidic domain between the first two loops and extends into the amino terminus of the second loop (83). However, it is not clear whether heparin only facilitates FGF binding or also actually participates in transduction. In addition, a third binding protein for FGF has recently been isolated (84); its extracellular region consists of 16 repeating cysteine-rich domains whereas its intracellular region is only 13 amino acids long. Such a receptor is unlikely to transduce a signal and, like heparin, may serve to concentrate FGF. These accessory receptors are not uncommon; as will be seen later, many other hormones also use proteoglycans (TGFβ) or cysteine-rich proteins (NGF) in their transduction complex.

Unlike the members of the EGF and insulin RTKs, mutations in the transmembrane region of PDGFR render the receptor inactive, suggesting that this domain may participate in dimer formation. The ATP-kinase domain that follows is split by intervening sequences of unknown function. These sequences frequently contain phosphorylated tyrosines that bind to substrates containing SH2 motifs, but there is no obvious reason why these amino acids could not have been located elsewhere. The SH2 binding sites in PDGFR have been thoroughly mapped and the phosphotyrosines bound by PI3K, GAP (85–87), PLCγ (32,88,89), and Src (88) have been determined (Fig. 6-1). Similar mapping has been done for the CSF-1R (90) and the FGFR (32). Surprisingly, the sites for any given SH2 protein do not always occur in the same region of these different RTKs. Furthermore, note that most of these proteins contain two SH2 domains and their binding sites can be mapped to two closely spaced phosphotyrosines, suggesting that both SH2 sites are active in binding to the RTK. As in all the other RTKs, the carboxy terminus and a juxtamembrane phosphotyrosine are involved in internalization (91).

As for the EGFR family, activation occurs when the ligand binds its RTK and induces dimerization (92–96); heterodimerization can occur within a given family. For example, their are two isoforms of PDGF, A and B, that can form three possible hormones: AA, AB, and BB. There are also two isoreceptors, A and B, that can form three possible receptors: AA, AB, and BB. PDGF-AA will only induce PDGFR-AA formation; PDGF-AB will trigger the dimerization of both PDGFR-AA and -BB; PDGF-BB can bind to all three receptor types (97,98).

4. NGF Receptor Family

The NGF receptor family is difficult to classify: the kinase domain is most closely related to that of the insulin receptor family (99–101) and it appears to activate PI3K indirectly via an adaptor, as the insulin receptor does (102), but the kinase domain is split by a short insert and the extracellular region is composed, in part, of immunoglobulin-like loops, like the PDGFR family. It has been proposed that these RTKs are actually chimeras between an insulin receptor-like ancestor and an immunoglobulin-like molecule. Another characteristic of this family is a very short carboxy-terminal tail following the kinase domain. All the members of this family are involved in growth and differentiation of the nervous system and include the receptors for NGF, brain-derived neurotrophic factor (BDNF), and several neurotropins (NTs). The receptors for these hormones are designated Trk, TrkB, and TrkC, respectively.

The amino-terminal half of the extracellular domain consists of a leucine-rich region flanked by cysteine clusters; however, these cysteine clusters are not as large or as dense as in the insulin receptor. The carboxy-terminal half contains two immunoglobulin-like loops. As noted earlier, the kinase domain has an insert of only 14–15 amino acids (not shown in Fig. 6-1 because of its very short length). In some isoforms, this insert is variable and determines, in part, the substrate specificity; for example, Trk isoreceptors with longer inserts will not phosphorylate PLCγ (103). As do the other RTKs, the NGF receptor dimerizes (104).

In addition to the RTKs, all these neurotropic hormones bind a common low-affinity NGF receptor, LNGFR. This molecule will be covered in greater detail under the class 2 fibronectin-like receptor family (see subsequent discussion), but its relationship to the Trk family will be discussed here. Basically, there are two perspectives: some individuals say LNGFR forms an integral and essential part of the NGF receptor complex and others deny any critical role for LNGFR. Those supporting a role for LNGFR present the following evidence: first, cells transfected with only Trk do not have high-affinity receptors (105). Second, NGF lacking the first 9 amino acids has a 300-fold reduced affinity for Trk but only a 5- to 10-fold reduced affinity for LNGFR, yet the biological activity is lowered merely 50-fold, less than one might expect if only the Trk were transducing a signal (106). Finally, a targeted mutation of LNGFR produces a sensory deficit in animals (107), indicating a critical role for this receptor in sensory neuron development. The opponents of this view also have evidence: first, other NGF mutants will not bind LNGFR but do bind Trk normally and have full biological activity (108–109). Second, these investigators claim that cells transfected with only Trk do have high-affinity receptors (110). Third, Trk and LNGFR cannot be co-immunoprecipitated, suggesting that there is no tight association between the two molecules (100). Fourth, the same targeted mutation in LNGFR noted earlier has no effect at all on sympathetic neurons (107). Finally, chimeric receptors with the extracellular domain of the tumor necrosis factor receptor (TNFR) and the transmembrane and cytoplasmic region of Trk are fully activated by TNF in target cells (111). TNF would not stimulate LNGFR, thereby eliminating it from the transduction pathway.

Several roles have been postulated for this low-affinity receptor: (i) it may combine with Trk to form a high affinity state; (ii) it may mediate some of the biological activities of these neurotropic hormones, especially in a tissue-specific manner; (iii) it may concentrate the ligand for Trk, like heparin does for the FGFR; and (iv) it may be a clearance receptor responsible for internalization of the receptor complex. The lack of co-immunoprecipitation and the relatively slow rate of LNGFR internalization (112) would argue against the last possibility. On the other hand, the close association between LNGFR and a serine–threonine kinase suggests that LNGFR may have a transduction function (113); for example, LNGFR is responsible for mediating the effects of NGF on programmed cell death, or apoptosis, in neurons (114).

B. Serine Kinase Receptors

The serine kinase receptors are very similar to the RTKs: they have an extracellular amino terminus, a single transmembrane helix, and a carboxy-terminal kinase domain. However, in these receptors, the kinase phosphorylates serines and threonines rather than tyrosines. The TGFβ (115,116), the activin (117), and the anti-Müllerian hormone (118) receptors belong to this family. The amino terminus binds the hormone and is cysteine-rich but does not resemble either the EGFR or immunoglobulins.

The kinase domain has two short inserts of unknown function. Its major output is serine phosphorylation, although the only characterized substrate is itself. The TGFβ receptor can also activate small and trimeric G proteins (119,120; see also Chapter 8). The TGFβ receptor is actually a complex of three different binding components: the type I and II receptors are both homologous serine kinases (121). Some type I receptors are shared among several members of this family (122–124). This is possible because the type I receptor does not bind hormones by itself but does increase the affinity of the individual type II receptors for their particular ligands (125). In addition, each subunit appears to couple to separate tranducers: the type I receptor mediates growth inhibition and induces the hypophosphorylation of Rb, an anti-oncogene (see Chapter 16); the type II receptor stimulates the synthesis of the extracellular matrix and Jun, a transcription factor (126). Despite this bifurcation, these receptors are not independent; both are required for biological activity (127). The type III receptor is a proteoglycan called betaglycan; it increases the affinity and broadens the binding specificity of the type II receptor (125). Betaglycan does not generate a transduction signal.

C. Guanylate Cyclases

Like all the enzyme-linked receptors, the membrane-bound guanylate cyclases traverse the membrane once: the amino termini are extracellular and the cyclase domains are intracellular (128,129). In addition, there is a homologous soluble guanylate cyclase that acts as a cytoplasmic receptor for nitric oxide (NO) and carbon monoxide (CO).

1. Membrane-Bound

Guanylate cyclases A and B (GC-A and GC-B) are very closely related and bind different forms of the atrial natriuretic factor: GC-A binds ANF from the heart and GC-B binds CNF from the brain. The intracellular domain actually consists of two regions homologous to the catalytic site in kinases; the carboxy-terminal one is the guanylate cyclase but no enzymatic activity has been associated with the amino-terminal one. However, deletion of this region increases cyclase activity, suggesting that it represents a regulatory domain that represses cyclase activity. The cyclase activity also has an absolute requirement for ATP (130), whose binding site has been localized to this pseudokinase site (131). Therefore, it appears that the ligand induces ATP to bind to this site and relieve the inhibition of the cyclase. The ATP also reduces the affinity of the receptor for hormone (132).

Ligand binding activates the cyclase and induces oligomerization (133), reported as either dimers or tetramers (134). The receptor can also be regulated by serine kinases. GC is a substrate for PKA, PKG, and PKC; phosphorylation by the latter inhibits cyclase activity (135). Ligand binding also results in GC dephosphorylation, which reduces GC activity by 80%; this dephosphorylation represents a major part of agonist-induced desensitization (136). Finally, cyclase activity can be stimulated by calcium and calmodulin (137), although high calcium is inhibitory. The latter effect is probably mediated by PKC which is activated, in part, by calcium.

GC-C is similar in structural organization to GC-A and GC-B except for a 60- to 65-amino-acid carboxy-terminal extension; however, its amino acid sequence is considerably more divergent (138,139). The ATP-binding site is not perfectly conserved and the cyclase activity is not absolutely dependent on ATP, although this nucleotide will still enhance cyclase activity (129,140). GC-C was initially identified as the receptor for a bacterial endotoxin that triggers fluid secretion via chloride channels. Recently, an endogenous peptide, *guanylin*, was isolated based on its ability to bind and activate the GC-C (141).

ANF-R2 is homologous to GC-A and GC-B in the extracellular region, but its cytoplasmic region is extremely short and lacks a cyclase domain. It binds another isoform of ANF called BNF. Because this receptor does not appear to have an intracellular region long enough to transduce a signal, it has been postulated that ANF-R2 is a clearance receptor, that is, it merely internalizes hormone for degradation. However, it may be coupled to cAMP inhibition in platelets (142), and has been associated with smooth muscle proliferation, although it does not affect cyclic nucleotide levels in this tissue (143).

2. Soluble

The soluble guanylate cyclase has no membrane-spanning region; it consists of a carboxy-terminal cyclase domain and an amino-terminal heme-binding domain (144). Cyclase activity requires a dimer between two homologous but nonidentical subunits (145–147). The enzyme is activated when either NO or CO binds to the heme moiety and displaces it from the enzyme; as such, regulation of this enzyme can be best understood by examining the regulation of the generation of these two ligands. NO is produced from arginine by NO synthase, an NADPH-dependent monoxygenase. NO synthase is totally dependent on calcium and calmodulin (148), so any hormone activating this pathway will stimulate NO production (Fig. 6-2). The synthase is also phosphorylated by PKA, PKC, and CaMKII; the only general agreement is that PKC inhibits synthase activity (148). CaMKII has been reported to inhibit, and PKA to activate, NO synthase but these results are controversial (149,150). One possible explanation for these disparate results is that phosphorylation has functions other than altering enzymatic

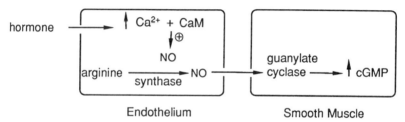

Fig. 6-2. Nitric oxide pathway. Hormones elevate cytosolic calcium levels in the endothelial cell. The calcium activates calmodulin (CaM), which in turn stimulates nitric oxide (NO) synthase.

activity; for example, phosphorylation has been reported to shift the location of NO synthase from the membrane to the cytosol (151). In addition to acute regulation, the type II isozyme of NO synthase can be induced; types I and III are constitutively synthesized. CO is produced from the degradation of heme by heme oxygenase in the liver (type 1 isozyme) or brain (type 2); the former enzyme is responsible for the bulk degradation of heme whereas the latter generates CO for GC activation. The regulation of heme oxygenase 2 has not yet been fully studied. A final aspect of regulation is the extreme lability of NO itself, although some authorities suggest that its half-life may be prolonged by reversibly S-nitrosylating proteins (152).

III. Serpentine Receptors

A. General Characteristics

The next family of receptors is one of the oldest and probably one of the largest groups. Several names have been given to this group: since one of their distinguishing characteristics is that they pass through the membrane seven times (Fig. 6-3), they have been labeled the *seven-transmembrane-segment* (7-TMS) receptors. Because they assume a snake-like appearance as they weave through the membrane, they are also known as the *serpentine* receptors. Finally, they have no intrinsic enzymatic activity; instead they bind to and activate G proteins. Therefore, they have been referred to as the *G protein-coupled* receptors. Because serpentine is the least cumbersome term, it will be used in this text.

The first member of this family to be studied in detail was rhodopsin, the light-sensitive protein in the retina. Indeed, this family is as important in sensory preception as in hormone recognition, since it is involved in the detection of odor and taste as well as light. In rhodopsin, many of the transmembrane helices are kinked because of the presence of proline residues; this creates a basket, in which resides the light-absorbing pigment retinal. In the hormone receptors, this basket becomes the ligand-binding site. The critical residues in this binding pocket have been determined for the

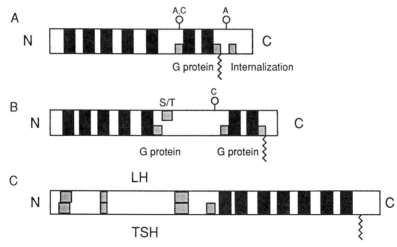

Fig. 6-3. Serpentine receptors: (A) β-type receptor, (B) muscarinic-type receptor, and (C) glycohormone receptor. These receptors have seven transmembrane helices (black) and are often palmitoylated (the zig-zag line). Other markings are defined in the legend to Fig. 6-1. S/T, A serine–threonine-rich region.

most common of the ligands, small amines with attached aromatic rings (153,154). The amino group is neutralized by an aspartate in helix 3; this ion pair is stabilized by a surrounding cluster of aromatic rings (Fig. 6-4). Additional aromatic residues in helices 5 and 6 interact with the aromatic ring of the ligand, which usually contains hydroxyl groups. These latter groups form hydrogen bonds with serines in helix 5. Obviously, these relationships will be modified to fit the particular structure of the ligand; Fig. 6-4 schematically depicts some of these adaptations. The most dramatic modifications are seen with the large peptide or protein ligands (see subsequent discussion).

As noted earlier, these receptors are coupled to G proteins; the G proteins, in turn, bind to and modulate several critical enzymes in second messenger pathways. G_s stimulates adenylate cyclase to generate cAMP, whereas G_i inhibits this cyclase; G_q activates a phospholipase C that triggers a cascade that eventually elevates cellular calcium and activates certain protein kinases (see Chapters 8 and 9). Different sites on the serpentine receptors interact with different G proteins; most of these sites occur in the third intracellular loop between helices 5 and 6 and in the juxtamembrane segment of the carboxy terminus. Coupling to G_s and G_i requires the carboxy-terminal 10–20 amino acids of the third loop as well as the juxtamembrane segment of the carboxy terminus (155–157); the interaction with G_q also requires the amino-terminal 10–20 amino acids of the third loop (159–160). In general, the segments in the third loop are believed to couple with the G protein, whereas the carboxy terminus activates it (161). The amazing fact is that these critical regions show very little, if any, homology among the different serpentine receptors; apparently the overall three-dimensional structure is more important than a particular amino acid sequence. Indeed, all

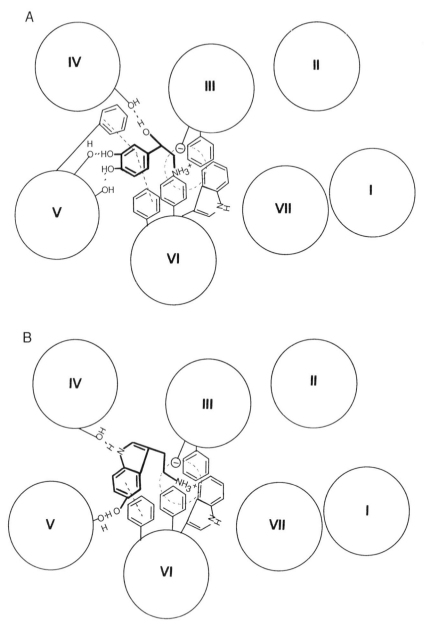

Fig. 6-4. The ligand-binding site in serpentine receptors. (A) β-adrenergic receptor, (B) 5-hydroxytryptamine (serotonin) receptor; (C) histamine receptor; (D) muscarinic acetylcholine receptor. The large circles containing Roman numerals are transmembrane helices; the dashed circle represents the hydrophobic box that encloses the ammonium ion; straight dashed lines depict van der Waals interactions.

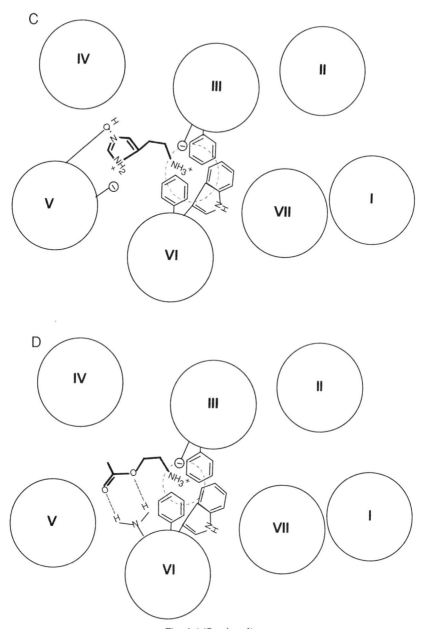

Fig. 6-4 *(Continued)*.

these segments can form amphipathic helices; these isolated helices can, at very high concentrations, activate G proteins.

Another output for the serpentine receptors is tyrosine phosphorylation. These receptors have no kinase domain and no known G protein can directly activate a tyrosine kinase. Because tyrosine phosphorylation occurs within 5 seconds and often does not require calcium or many of the serine kinases normally activated by G proteins (162–164), a direct interaction between these receptors and soluble tyrosine kinases has been postulated, but no such physical link has yet been demonstrated. Alternatively, tyrosine kinases could be indirectly activated via a cascade that begins with a serine–threonine kinase or as a result of changes in cell shape: a cytoskeleton-associated tyrosine kinase, Fak, is frequently activated by many of the hormones that bind these receptors (165,166); this stimulation may be a result of the associated alterations in cell morphology. Identified tyrosine-phosphorylated substrates include MAP kinase (167) and PLCγ (168,169).

The two other notable characteristics of serpentine receptors are serine–threonine-rich regions and palmitoylation. The serine–threonine-rich domain is located in the carboxy terminus of the β-adrenergic receptors and in the third loop of the muscarinic receptors. These amino acids, when phosphorylated, are responsible for uncoupling the receptor from G proteins; this dissociation is part of the process of desensitization (170,171). Those receptors lacking such regions undergo desensitization very slowly (172). Also related to this phenomenon is a highly conserved cysteine in the juxtamembrane region of the carboxy terminus. This residue is covalently attached to palmitic acid, which is presumably buried in the membrane. This creates an additional cytoplasmic loop that interferes with the phosphorylation of the adjacent serine–threonine-rich domain in β-adrenergic receptors (173). Agonist binding increases the turnover of this modification and allows phosphorylation and desensitization to occur (174). However, in muscarinic and α_2 receptors, the serine–threonine-rich region is located in the third loop; in this receptor class, palmitoylation is not required for biological activity (175,176).

B. Classification

1. β-Type Receptors

The β-type receptors are named after the prototypical receptor in this group: the β-adrenergic receptor (βAR). This class also includes certain isoforms of the α-adrenergic, histamine (H), dopamine (D), and serotonin or 5-hydroxytryptamine (5-HT) receptors[2] (Table 6-1). All these receptors elevate either cAMP or calcium. They have a very short amino terminus with two highly conserved N-glycosylation sites. The third loop is modest in length and the serine–threonine-rich region is located in the long carboxy terminus.

---

[2] This text uses the 5-HT nomenclature proposed by Humphrey *et al.* (177).

2. Muscarinic-Type Receptors

This family is named after its model receptor: the muscarinic acetylcholine receptor. This groups includes the muscarinic (M), adenosine (A), and tyramine receptors, as well as certain isoforms of the α-adrenergic, histamine, dopamine, and 5-HT receptors. All these receptors either lower cAMP or elevate calcium. The serine–threonine-rich region is shifted from the carboxy terminus to the third cytoplasmic loop; this results in a large third loop and a small carboxy terminus.

3. Neurokinin-Type Receptors

Most of the other receptors are extremely heterogeneous. There is no consensus classification scheme for these receptors; the one used in this text is based on amino acid sequence analyses in selected regions of these proteins (178). The ligands for these receptors are usually peptides and proteins that could not possibly fit into the transmembrane binding pocket. In general, other parts of these receptors are also involved in ligand binding. For example, the tachykinins are a family of hormones with a common carboxy terminus; this region is believed to bind to the transmembrane helices and activate the receptor. The amino terminus and first extracellular loop also appear to be involved in recognizing a common motif of the tachykinins, whereas the second and third extracellular loops bind hormone-specific regions that distinguish among the different tachykinins (179–182). The general division of labor appears to hold for many of these receptors: common structural motifs bind the transmembrane helices and activate the receptors, whereas extracellular segments provide specificity. Many of these receptors affect the same second messenger pathways as the β-type and M-type receptors but their coupling must be somewhat different. For example, the gonadotropin-releasing hormone (GnRH) receptor has no carboxy terminus (183,184); neither does an alternatively spliced form of the metabotropic glutamate receptor (185,186). However, the prostaglandin E receptor does use its carboxy terminus to activate G_i (187). The third intracellular loop is another major site for transduction, but this region in the neurokinin-like receptors is very short. In the formyl peptide (fMLP) receptor it is only 15 amino acids long and does not play a major role in elevating calcium levels (188).

4. Nonneurokinin-Type Receptors

These receptors appear to be structurally organized like the neurokinin-like receptors. For example, the glycoprotein hormone receptors have exceedingly long amino termini that are sufficient by themselves to bind ligands with high affinity and specificity (189–191). However, high concentrations of LH can activate an LH receptor (LHR) lacking almost all of the amino terminus; transduction must be occurring through the transmembrane helices (192,193). However, FSH can elevate cAMP using a chimeric LHR receptor having the amino terminus of the FSHR (194). Therefore, the helices lack specificity. Researchers think that the amino terminus and several extracellular loops bind the glycoprotein hormones with high affinity and specificity, whereas the helices bind some common motif with low affinity. The affinity is not a problem, since the amino terminus concentrates the hormone for presentation to the helices.

The structural requirements for transduction have not been as well studied as in the β- and M-type receptors. However, desensitization and internalization appear to be mediated by the carboxy terminus (195,196).

Two unusual members of this family deserve special comment, the first of which is the thrombin receptor (197). Thrombin is a serine protease in the blood coagulation pathway, but it is also capable of interacting with a membrane receptor (see Chapter 3). It turns out that the actual ligand for the thrombin receptor is located in the middle of the amino terminus of the receptor. Thrombin removes the amino-terminal 16–17 amino acids and exposes the peptide agonist that then binds to the receptor. The binding specificity for thrombin resides exclusively in the cleavage site; once cleavage has occurred, thrombin is no longer needed. This is beautifully illustrated by changing the sequence at this site to one recognized by enterokinase; this mutated receptor is now activated by enterokinase instead of thrombin (198). This system has several unique features: first, the agonist is tethered to its receptor to provide continuous activation after cleavage; second, receptor activation is irreversible. The system can be turned off by either metabolizing or inactivating the receptor (199).

A second unusual member of this group, the calcitonin receptor, belongs to the secretin subfamily. Calcitonin is secreted when calcium levels are elevated, and interaction with its receptor triggers a series of events that will eventually lower the concentration of this cation (see Chapter 1). However, calcium itself can also directly stimulate the calcitonin receptor; therefore, this membrane protein acts as a dual receptor, binding to either calcitonin or calcium (200).

5. Miscellaneous Receptors

Finally, several hormone receptors have seven transmembrane helices but have no sequence homology at all to the serpentine receptors. They include the yeast mating factor receptors, the metabotropic glutamate receptor (mGluR), and another calcium sensor used by the parathyroid gland (201). Yeast cells of opposite mating type each produce a short peptide hormone that prepares the other cell for sexual reproduction. Although their receptors have unique sequences, their topology, linkage to G proteins, and regulation by serine–threonine-rich regions in their carboxy termini strongly suggest that they are members of the serpentine group (202,203). A similar situation exists with the glutamate receptor. Glutamate is a major excitatory neurotransmitter in the brain, where it binds to ion channels (see subsequent discussion). However, it can also have metabolic effects that are mediated by a seven-transmembrane-helical protein, the mGluR. This receptor has a very long amino terminus, whose coding region is separated from that for the transmembrane helices by an intron; furthermore, part of this amino terminus is homologous to the amino terminus of the ion channel receptor (204,205). As such, the mGluR may have arisen by exon shuffling in which the exons encoding the amino terminus of the ion channel became associated with exons for the body of a serpentine receptor (see Chapter 15).

IV. Fibronectin-Like Receptors

Fibronectin is an extracellular matrix protein that is important in cell adhesion and migration. Structurally it is composed of three repeating modules, each of which has specific binding properties. The type III repeat consists of seven β strands organized into a sandwich; this forms a binding surface for cells or heparin. This type III domain is also found in the most recently characterized group of receptors. These receptors have almost no sequence homology at all, but they do cross the membrane once, have type III repeats in the extracellular domain, and have a similar genomic organization. Finally, alternative processing is frequent; the most common variations are receptors lacking large portions of their intracellular, and sometimes transmembrane, regions. The latter results in the production of soluble receptors, which may have important regulatory functions (206; see also Chapter 7).

A. Cytokine (Class 1) Family

1. General Characteristics

The cytokine, or class 1, family has two type III repeats modified in a highly characteristic way (207). First, two small disulfide loops are inserted into the amino terminus of the first repeat; second, a WS box appears near the membrane at the carboxy terminus of the second motif. The WS box is a sequence of $W-S-X-W-S$, where X represents any amino acid. In contrast to the general lack of overall sequence homology, the WS box is highly conserved; the only known exceptions are sequences of $L-S-X-W-S$ in the IL-3Rα and $Y-G-X-F-S$ in the GHR.

The three-dimensional structure of the extracellular domain of the GHR has been determined (208,209): the two type III repeats are oriented at right angles with their ends forming half of a binding pocket (Fig. 6-5). Like all cytokine receptors, the GHR is a dimer and both receptors participate in creating the ligand-binding site. GH, which consists of four α helices in a bundle, sits in the notch between these dimers and forms contacts with residues along the sides of its helices. The major point of interaction is with the sides of this pocket (210), although this may vary depending on the particular hormone–receptor complex. For example, IL-3 and IL-6 bind primarily to the floor of the pocket (211,212). Note that all the cytokines whose three-dimensional structures are known are α-helical bundles; the type III repeats may be ideally suited to binding this kind of protein motif.

The function of the WS box is unknown and the reported data are conflicting. For example, mutations in this motif disrupt ligand binding in the

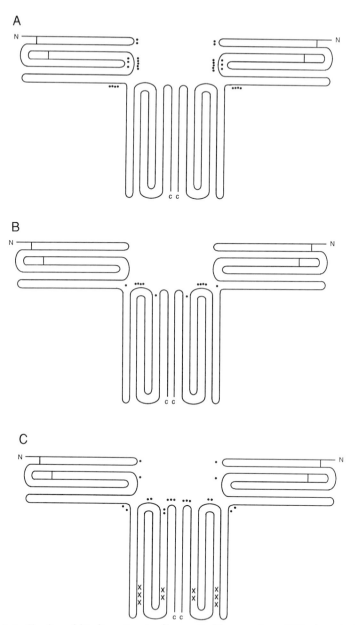

Fig. 6-5. The ligand-binding sites in fibronectin-like receptors. Critical contact points between the class 1 receptors and their ligands are depicted by dots for the (A) GH, (B) IL-3, and (C) IL-6 receptors. In addition, the residues involved in signal transmission in the latter are marked with Xs. (D) Two of the three finger-like extracellular domains of the TNFR (a class 2 receptor) are depicted with asterisks to denote contact points with the centrally enclosed TNF molecule.

D

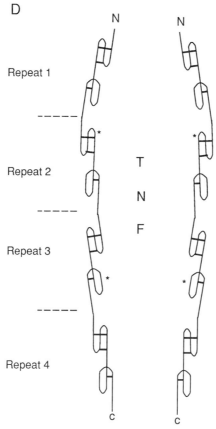

Repeat 1

Repeat 2

Repeat 3

Repeat 4

Fig. 6-5 (Continued).

IL-2βR but not the G-CSFR. It is difficult to visualize how the box could directly affect ligand binding, since it is not in the pocket. It may affect it indirectly through dimerization; all these receptors must form homo- or heterodimers for high-affinity binding and transduction. However, in the GHR dimer, the WS boxes do not appear to interact with each other. However, the serines are involved in intrastrand hydrogen bonds that may be critical for maintaining the receptor in a conformation required for ligand binding or dimerization (213). Finally, the WS box may be required for receptor processing; when the WS box in the erythropoietin (EPO) receptor is mutated, the EPOR is retained in the endoplasmic reticulum and never terminally glycosylated (214).

These receptors function as oligomers (215). Transduction is accomplished by a full-length receptor which must dimerize to be active. Classically, this is called the β subunit, although the nomenclature of these receptors has not been standardized. Sometimes, this β dimer is adequate for hormone binding, but more often an additional homologous subunit is required for high-affinity binding. This component is usually called the α subunit; because it usually does not function in signaling, the cytoplasmic domain is short. In the extreme situation, the α subunit may even be soluble. Several hormones may share a β dimer and use unique α subunits to provide binding specificity.

2. Simple Cytokine Subfamily

There is little homology in the cytoplasmic domains of these receptors, but several common motifs are recognized by their amino acid composition rather than sequence. The function of these regions has been most thoroughly studied in the IL-2R. Therefore, this receptor will be discussed in detail as a prototype for the cytokine receptors.

Like most cytokines, IL-2 has four α helices arranged in a bundle (216) but it binds a heterotetramer ($\alpha\beta_2\gamma$) rather than a homodimer; the β and γ subunits are homologous and belong to the cytokine receptor family (217). Because the latter subunit is common to several other receptor complexes, it is also known as γ_c. In addition, a nonhomologous α dimer forms part of this complex. With only 10 amino acids in the intracellular region, the α subunits are not likely to have transducing functions but they do affect ligand binding. Basically, the β subunit is more important for binding whereas the γ subunit functions in transduction; for example, the γ subunit contains an SH2 domain that is involved in the activation of soluble tyrosine kinases (218). The α subunit boosts the ligand binding of the $\beta\gamma$ complex from intermediate (4.6 nM) to high (0.08 nM) affinity.

Intracellularly, several short serine–threonine-proline-rich regions are common to many of these receptors (Fig. 6-6); they are essential for triggering mitogenesis, although the mechanism is not clear (219). This region is followed by an acidic domain that binds Lck, a soluble tyrosine kinase (220). This association appears to mediate many of the biological activities of IL-2 and other cytokines (221–222). For example, IL-2 binding stimulates Lck activity 5- to 6-fold, resulting in the phoshorylation of IL-2R. The phosphorylated IL-2Rβ then binds Raf which is, in turn, phosphorylated and activated by Lck (223). The phosphorylated IL-2R can also associate with and activate PI3K (224). Many of the cytokine receptors stimulate soluble tyrosine kinases: the IL-3R activates Lyn and Jak, but not Lck, Hck, Fyn, or Yes (225–227); the GM-CSFR activates Lyn, Yes, and Jak (227,228); IFN receptor activates Tyk2 (229); and the EPOR and GHR activate Jak (213). However, there is considerable overlap among these pathways and the basis for biological specificity is unclear. Each of these soluble tyrosine kinases has a different spectrum of substrate specificity (230): for example, Blk and Lyn bind MAP kinase 10 times better than Fyn does, whereas Fyn and Lyn bind PI3K but Blk does not. These kinases are constitutively bound to the cytokine receptors and are activated by receptor oligomerization (231–232).

IL-2Rβ and IL-2Rγ represent the simplest cytokine receptor structures: a

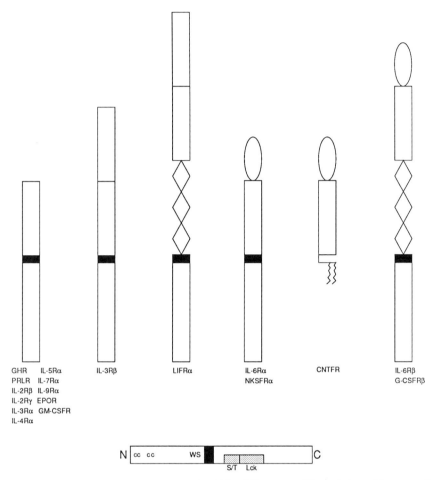

Fig. 6-6. Cytokine (class 1) receptors. *(Top)* The different possible variations. The rectangle above the black transmembrane helix represents the cytokine domain; diamonds represent fibronectin type III regions; ovals represent immunoglobulin-like loops. CNTFR is anchored in the membrane by the covalent attachment to a phospholipid. *(Bottom)* The IL-2R shown in more detail. The conserved cysteines (small Cs), WSXWS sequence (WS), serine–threonine–rich region (S/T), and Lck-binding site are depicted.

single cytokine motif at the amino terminus. The IL-4Rα and the IL-7Rα are other simple cytokine receptors that also share γ$_c$ (233–235). The GHR and the EPOR belong to this class and appear to homodimerize. The IL-3Rα and the GM-CSFRα are additional members but they heterodimerize to a subunit with a duplicated cytokine motif, the IL-3Rβ/IL-5Rβ/GM-CSFRβ subunit, called β$_c$ (Fig. 6-6). IL-5R, like IL-2R, is a trimer; an IL-5Rα homodimer associates with the common β$_c$ subunit (236). How the prolactin receptor oligomerizes is not known.

3. Complex Cytokine Subfamily

Other cytokine receptors are structurally more complex. As noted earlier, the cytokine motif can be duplicated. Alternatively, it may be combined with an immunoglobulin-like loop and/or extra fibronectin type III domains (Fig. 6-6). The function of these extra pieces is not clear. The G-CSFRβ has both an immunoglobulin loop and three type III domains, and neither is required for ligand binding or transduction (237). The IL-6Rα, the natural killer cell stimulatory factor receptor α (NKSFRα), the ciliary neurotropic factor receptor α (CNTFRα), and the leukemia inhibitory factor receptor α (LIFRα) share the same β subunits — the IL-6Rβ dimer — and the G-CSFRβ forms a homodimer. In those receptors in which it has been examined, oligomerization is required for high affinity and biological activity; this aggregation is induced by ligand binding for the GHR (238), IL-6R (239), and CNTFR (240).

The most interesting of these variations is the CNTFR. First, CNTFR is an oligomer composed of the CNTFRα, LIFRα, and the IL-6Rβ subunits (200). Second, CNTFRα has no transmembrane or cytoplasmic domain; instead, it is held to the membrane via a covalently attached phospholipid (241) called phosphatidylinositol-glycan (PI-glycan) (see Chapter 10). However, not even this anchor is necessary, since soluble CNTFRα is still active (242). Signal transduction is mediated by the other two subunits and CNTFRα merely associates with the extracellular domains of LIFRα and IL-6Rβ to alter their ligand specificity. As noted earlier, the function of the α subunits is often restricted to their extracellular domains, even if a cytoplasmic tail is present; for example, the IL-6Rα, stripped of its transmembrane and cytosolic regions, is still sufficient for activity when it is recombined with IL-6Rβ (243).

B. TNF/IFN (Class 2) Family

In class 2 receptors, the FNIII unit appears to have undergone some degeneracy, since only five of the original seven strands are discernible. This domain was then duplicated twice to give four homologous regions. These domains are arranged differently than those in the class 1 receptors: in the latter, the β structures abut each other at right angles to form a niche for hormone binding (Fig. 6-5). In class 2 receptors, the domains line up end-to-end to form long fingers that wrap around the hormone (244). Interestingly, the major contact points remain at the terminal loops, especially those in the second and third domains; however, all four cysteine-rich regions are required for ligand binding (245). This structure is found in the TNFR, the IFNγ-R, the IL-1OR, and the LNGFR. The receptors for IFNα and IFNβ underwent a further duplication of the extracellular domain.

The LNGFR has a low affinity for all the neurotropic hormones; its relevance was discussed earlier (Section II,A,4). The receptor has four cysteine-rich domains followed by a serine–threonine-rich domain in the extracellular region. Only the cysteine-rich domains, especially the third and fourth, are involved in NGF binding (246,247). The intracellular region has no distinguishing characteristics.

Two TNFRs have been cloned that are simply known by their molecular weights; p70 and p55. Recent data suggest that p70 does not transduce a signal; rather, it may only increase the local concentration of TNF for p55 (248). Like the LNGFR, each has four cysteine-rich regions but in p70 the first domain appears to be of critical importance (249). The intracellular region is rich in serines and threonines, like the class 1 receptors. Several characteristics of these receptors are interesting. First, TNFs are trimers that bind to three p70 or p55 receptors (250). Second, like the GHR, these receptors are ubiquitinated (251). *Ubiquitin* is a peptide that is attached via an isopeptide bond to other proteins destined for destruction (see Chapter 13). Its presence suggests that these receptors have a high turnover rate. Finally, its output appears to involve the activation of several lipases, such as sphingomyelinase and phospholipase A_2 (252,253), that have only recently been associated with signal transduction (see Chapter 9). Coupling may be achieved by a G protein (254).

The IFN subfamily consists of two receptors, one for IFNα and β and another for IFNγ. Although IFNα and β are homologous, IFNγ has a unique sequence; nonetheless, the three-dimensional structures of the hormones are very similar (255). In addition, their receptors share sequence homology, at least in the extracellular domain. The cysteines in this region are arranged in a motif that occurs once in the IFNγR but is duplicated in the IFNα/β receptor (256,257). There is no similarity in their intracellular domains. The IFNα/β receptor has a serine–threonine-rich domain and acts, in part, through soluble tyrosine kinases that are members of the Jak family (229). IFNγR also has a serine–threonine-rich region that can be phosphorylated in response to IFNγ; this phosphorylation is correlated with biological activity (258). Unlike TNF, both IFNγ and its receptor are dimers (259).

V. Miscellaneous Membrane Receptors

There are four other receptors that do not fit into any of the already-mentioned groups; all have a single transmembrane helix. Two homologous receptors for IL-1 have been cloned; they have three immunoglobulin-like loops in the extracellular domain. Like the TNFR, they activate sphingomyelinase (260), probably via a G protein (261). Another miscellaneous receptor is an IFNα receptor unrelated to the class 2 fibronectin-like receptor just described. This receptor has a high affinity for IFNα, but also binds the complement component C3d (262,263). It mediates the effects of C3d, but its role in transducing IFNα activity is not clear. The extracellular region consists of 16 repeating units, whereas its intracellular domain binds casein kinase II (264) and a tumor-inhibiting protein or anti-oncogene called p53 (265; see also Chapter 16). The autocrine motility factor (AMF) enhances the motility of the cell that produces it and may be involved in tumor metastasis. The structure of its receptor is unremarkable except for a purported similarity to the anti-oncogene, p53 (266).

The last miscellaneous receptor is the IGF-II receptor (IGF-IIR). The extracellular domain consists of 15 repeating units containing 8 cysteines each and binds IGF II, mannose 6-phosphate, and any protein containing this sugar. Indeed, this protein was first characterized as a cation-independent mannose 6-phosphate receptor responsible for transporting mannose 6-phosphate-containing proteins to the lysosome. IGF-II and the sugar bind to different sites; the latter interacts at two separate regions comprising repeats 1–3 and 7–10 (267). Although these two ligands bind separately, mannose 6-phosphate does synergize with IGF-II in generating second messengers (268). The extreme carboxy terminus binds to an inhibitory G protein (269) adjacent to a region phosphorylated by casein kinase II (270); this phosphorylation is required for the receptor to be transported to the prelysosome. The intracellular domain is also palmitoylated (271).

Because IGF-II can act through the IGF-IR and because the IGF-IIR serves other functions, the relevance of the IGF-IIR for mediating the biological activities of IGF-II has been questioned. First, the IGF-IIR constitutively recycles, suggesting a housekeeping rather than a signaling function (272). Second, the IGF-II/mannose 6-phosphate receptor from chicken and *Xenopus* does not bind IGF-II, although IGF-II is biologically active in these species (273–275). Third, during rat embryogenesis IGF-II is abundant, but only the IGF-IR is present; therefore, IGF-II must act through the IGF-IR (276). Fourth, mutant IGF-IIs that prefer either the IGF-IR or IGF-IIR have been constructed, and biological activity always correlates with IGF-IR binding (277). Finally, overexpression of IGF-IR enhances IGF-II activity, whereas mutated IGF-IRs that are dominant inhibitors block IGF-II effects (278). In contrast, overexpression of IGF-IIR actually inhibits the response to IGF-II, suggesting that the IGF-IIR acts like a sink to trap IGF-II (279).

There are also arguments in support of a role for the IGF-IIR in IGF-II action. First, stimulating antibodies specific for the IGF-IIR induce thymidine uptake and calcium fluxes (280). Second, the IGF-IIR appears to bind an inhibitory G protein; such coupling is normally associated with signal transduction (281,282). Finally, an agonist specific the IGF-IIR mimics the effect of IGF-II on cell motility; this effect is not blocked by antibodies against the IGF-IR (283). Based on the data from other vertebrates (273–275), the cation-independent mannose 6-phosphate receptor recently acquired the ability to bind IGF-II. It is quite possible that this protein in now in a state of functional flux as it begins to assume new roles. This may explain why in some systems it appears to mediate some of the actions of IGF-II, whereas in other systems it is dispensable. Alternatively, the IGF-IIR may either concentrate IGF-II for the IGF-IR or sequester this hormone, thereby indirectly affecting its biological activity.

VI. Ion Channel Receptors

The last group of receptors to be considered in this chapter is composed of the ion channels. The first two families are ligand-gated channels, that is,

they are ion pores that are regulated in response to hormones or neurotransmitters. The last two families are regulated by second messengers. However,
because the basic principles are the same, they will all be discussed together.

A. Nicotinic Acetylcholine Receptor Family

The ligand-gated channels have four transmembrane helices and both termini are extracellular (Figs. 6-7 and 6-8). The second helix (M2) from each of
five separate subunits forms the channel wall. Each second helix is believed
to be flanked by the first and third helices; however, the X-ray crystallographic structure has not been solved to a resolution sufficient to follow the
peptide backbone. As such, these transmembrane regions have been identified from hydropathy plots of the amino acid sequence. The four-helix model
is the generally accepted model, although other models have also been
proposed (284).

Acetylcholine has two types of receptors: (i) the muscarinic acetylcholine
receptor is a serpentine receptor, and was discussed already, and (ii) the
nicotinic acetylcholine receptor (nAChR) is a ligand-gated sodium channel.
Like acetylcholine, serotonin (5-hydroxytryptamine) has receptors in both of
the structural groups; the 5-HT$_3$ receptor is a divalent cation channel. Other
members of this family include the receptors for inhibitory neurotransmitters, γ-aminobutyric acid (GABA$_A$), and glycine; both form chloride channels
(285,286). The GABA$_B$ receptor is thought to be a serpentine receptor but it
has not yet been cloned.

In these receptors, the five subunits are homologous but not identical: in
the muscle nAchR, the subunit structure is $\alpha_2\beta\gamma\delta$. However, this can vary
depending on the particular isoreceptor or the developmental stage of the
organism. For example, the neuronal nAChR has a simpler composition,
$\alpha_2\beta_3$; in the adult, the γ subunit of the muscle nAChR is replaced by the ϵ
subunit. Some functional specialization has occurred among these subunits:
the γ/ϵ subunit stabilizes the closed state, thereby desensitizing the nAChR
(287); the δ subunit is involved in channel closing and voltage gating
(288,289). Both α subunits in the nAChR represent the major acetylcholine
binding sites, but the γ/ϵ and δ subunits also contribute (290). The binding
site may straddle subunits: the α subunits provide hydrophobic pockets,
whereas the γ/ϵ and δ subunits provide counterions in the form of negatively
charged amino acids (291). Finally, a 43-kDa peripheral protein appears to
overlie pairs of receptors at the β subunit and is involved in receptor clustering, as occurs at synapses (292).

Structural and functional analyses have identified several rings within
the ion channel (Fig. 6-8) (293). Beginning on the extracellular side, there is
an outer anion ring in the nAChR. This ring provides a hydrophilic environment for ions and may begin the process of selectivity, since this ring is basic
or neutral in the chloride channels. This is followed by two hydrophobic
rings: first a ring of valine and then one of leucine. Because hydrophobic
amino acids would impede the movement of ions, these rings may block ion
flow in the closed state, that is, they may represent the gating mechanism. If

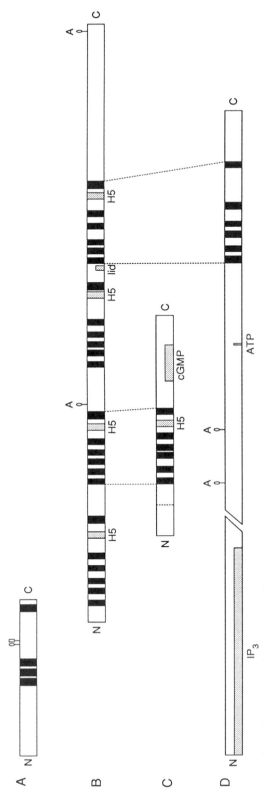

Fig. 6-7. Ion channels: (A) the nACh receptor, (B) the voltage-gated calcium channel, (C) the cGMP-gated channel, and (D) the IP₃ receptor. The (B) L-type voltage-gated channel (C) cGMP-gated channel, and the (D) IP₃ receptor are aligned to show their presumed relatedness. H5 denotes the β-loop that lines the channel; other markings are defined in the legend to Fig. 6-1.

178

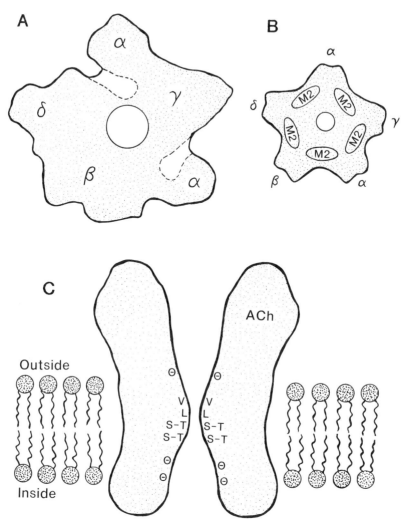

Fig. 6-8. The nicotinic acetylcholine receptor. (A) A transverse cross section through the nAChR above the plasma membrane as viewed from overhead. The low density areas in the α subunits (dashed lines) are thought to represent ligand-binding pockets. (B) A transverse cross section at the level of the plasmalemma showing the second transmembrane helix (M2) that lines the channel. (C) A longitudinal section showing the rings forming the ion channel.

these amino acids are replaced by hydrophilic ones, the channel becomes leaky, suggesting that these rings do indeed act as gates (294). This region is followed by two serine–threonine rings, although only one of these rings is conserved in the chloride channels. They may act as ion binding and transport sites and may participate in ion selectivity by size, since this region and the leucine ring above it represent the narrowest part of the pore. This constriction appears to be a result of an M2 kink that points toward the center of the pore (295). The intermediate anion ring is located below the serine–threonine rings and may represent the major mechanism for ion selectivity. Not only is it narrow but it is negatively charged in the nAchR and positively charged in the chloride channels. The inner anion ring is on the cytoplasmic side of the channel and appears merely to provide a hydrophilic environment at the pore opening.

The mechanism of ligand-induced gating is not clear. The acetylcholine binding site is located in the amino terminus around the vicinal cysteines; in three dimensions, this site is 20–30 Å above the surface of the membrane and 50 Å from the narrowest part of the channel. The ligand may transmit a signal between these sites but the distance is substantial. The facts that all known ligand-gated receptors bind two ligands and that these sites appear to straddle subunits in the nAchR suggest that ligand binding may alter the orientation between the subunits. For example, ligand binding may cause the subunits to spread apart or to twist and widen the pore.

The nAChR is regulated not just by ligand binding but also by phosphorylation. Both PKA and PKC can phosphorylate the large intracellular loops in the γ and δ subunits; this is associated with desensitization and the prevention of subunit assembly (296). In the latter case, dephosphorylation must take place before the receptor can be assembled after synthesis. Tyrosine phosphorylation of this same loop in the β, γ, and δ subunits is associated with synapse formation (297). Phosphorylation by PKA and PKC also occurs in the other members of this family, but the effects are controversial (298–300).

B. Glutamate Receptor Family

The glutamate receptor (GluR) family has the same topology as the nAChR family; but because there is no sequence homology, it is placed into its own family (301). In addition to the four transmembrane helices, the GluRs have much longer amino and carboxy termini; for example, the amino terminus is 450–500 amino acids long compared with the aproximately 200 residues in the nAChR family. This extension may accommodate other binding sites; for example, some of these receptors have coagonists or bind allosteric modulators. The second helix still forms the channel wall, but some of the rings are slightly modified; for example, leucine is replaced by phenylalanine in the hydrophobic ring and there is an extra asparagine–glutamine ring between the outer anion ring and the hydrophobic ring. This amide ring is critical for the calcium selectivity of these channels.

Three families were initially identified by agonist binding but are now classified structurally. The α subfamily specifically binds α-amino-3-hydroxy-5-methyl-4-isoxazole propionic acid (AMPA). It can be phosphorylated at two site by PKA; this modification potentiates the agonist-induced calcium fluxes (302). The β/γ subfamily specifically binds kainate and can also be phosphorylated; PKA and CaMKII increase calcium fluxes and PKC induces long-term potentiation (303–305). In addition to directly affecting ion fluxes, the kainate receptor appear to interact with a G protein (306), although the physiological results of this coupling are unknown. The ϵ/ζ subfamily specifically binds N-methyl-D-aspartate (NMDA) and has several unique properties: (i) it requires glycine as a coagonist, (ii) it is activated by polyamines, which enhance glycine binding (307); (iii) it is potentiated by arachidonic acid, which binds in the amino terminus (308), and (iv) it has a slower response time than the first two GluRs. As noted earlier, both the mGluR and the GluRs have homologous amino termini (205); in the NMDA receptor, this region is duplicated and may be responsible for binding each of the coagonists, glutamate and glycine.

The nature and function of the phosphorylation of the NMDA receptor is controversial: modification by either PKC or CaMKII increases calcium fluxes (309); but the PKC site is in the carboxy terminus, which it is presumed to be extracellular (310). Furthermore, other groups claim that PKC acts indirectly (311).

C. Voltage-Gated Family

The voltage-gated ion channels consist of four domains (312–314). Each domain contains six transmembrane helices and a β loop (H5) between helices 5 and 6 (Fig. 6-7). The β loops from each of the four domains create an 8-stranded β barrel that forms the wall of the channel. The fourth helix is positively charged and acts as the voltage sensor; the intracellular loop between the fourth and fifth helices blocks the channel. On depolarization, the positively charged fourth helix is attracted to the negatively charged outer surface. The amino acid side-chain interactions prevent a straightforward outward movement; instead, the helix rotates 60° as it elevates 5 Å. This movement disrupts the adjacent intracellular loop and the channel becomes unblocked.

The four domains described already may exist on either separate proteins or a single, large one. The former condition is believed to be the ancestral prototype and persists today in the potassium channel. In time, gene duplication with fusion occurred to produce the voltage-gated sodium and calcium channels. This structural difference affects the mechanism of fast inactivation. The channel can be closed by simply reversing the movement of the fourth helix, but this is relatively slow. In the potassium channel, the extreme amino terminus is rich in basic and hydrophobic amino acids. When the channel opens, negative charges are exposed and attract the amino terminus; the hydrophobic residues then plug the pore. However, the sodium channel only has a single amino terminus because the four domains are fused. In this channel, a cluster of hydrophobic amino acids between the third and fourth domains flips shut over intracellular opening (315). Finally, as channels became regulated by factors other than voltage, the fourth voltage-sensitive helix and other nonessential helices were eliminated. The inward rectifying potassium channel is an example of this modification; essentially, it is a miniature potassium channel that only possesses the last two helices and the intervening β loop (316). Some of these channels are regulated by G proteins (317).

In photoreceptors, darkness generates an electrical current whereas light turns the current off. Light accomplishes this by activating a cGMP phosphodiesterase that lowers cGMP levels; cGMP is necessary to keep open a cation channel that carries this dark current. Therefore, cGMP hydrolysis inactivates the channel and terminates the dark current. The channel diverged early from the potassium channel branch; as such, it consists of four separate subunits, each with six transmembrane helices and an H5 region (Fig. 6-7; 318,319). In addition, a cGMP-binding domain is located in the carboxy terminus. Other cyclic nucleotide-gated channels have also been discovered and those in olfactory and aortic epithelia are homologous to the one in the photoreceptors (320).

D. Ryanodine Receptor Family

The ion channels discussed so far are located on the plasma membrane; the members of the ryanodine receptor family are located on calcium-containing intracellular organelles such as the sarcoplasmic reticulum of muscle. They are difficult to classify because they share no homology with any of the other channels; even the number of their transmembrane segments is uncertain. Some characteristics, such as the spacing of the helices, resemble the voltage-gated channels; for this reason, this text depicts them as having six transmembrane helices (Fig. 6-7).

In muscle, the action potential at the plasma membrane and T-tubules results in the release of calcium from the sarcoplasmic reticulum; this calcium, in turn, triggers contraction. The ryanodine receptor couples these two membranes. The hydrophobic helices are embedded in the sarcoplasmic reticulum, where they form a calcium channel; the extremely long amino terminus acts as a physical bridge to the plasma membrane, where it contacts a typical voltage-gated calcium channel. Apparently, the depolarization brought about by the action potential activates the voltage-gated calcium channel, which then opens the ryanodine receptor, presumably by transmitting a signal through the amino terminus of this receptor. Recently, this receptor has been found in nonmuscle tissue. Furthermore, the ability of cyclic ADP–ribose, an NAD^+ metabolite, to open these channels has suggested that they may be regulated by second messengers (321).

Another member of this family the inositol 1,4,5-trisphosphate (IP_3) receptor (322,323), is clearly activated by a second messenger. IP_3 is one of several mediators generated by the hydrolytic activity of phospholipase C (see Chapter 9). It diffuses from the plasma membrane, where it is liberated, to the endoplasmic reticulum, where it activates its receptor, a calcium channel. The IP_3 receptor is a noncovalently linked tetramer that forms a 25-nm square (324,325). Each subunit binds one IP_3 at the extreme amino terminus and binding is cooperative. If the IP_3 receptor is like the ryanodine receptor, the channel is straight as it traverses the membrane, but then splits into four channels that bend 90° and exit the amino-terminal domain laterally (326). As such, it resembles a rotating sprinkler head, where the water comes up the stem and then is ejected laterally through the spinning arms. This analogy applies only to the three-dimensional structure; there is no evidence that the IP$_3$ receptor rotates. This lateral dispersion may facilitate the rapid diffusion of the calcium ions into the cytoplasm. In addition to ligand gating, the IP$_3$ receptor is allosterically regulated by ATP and calcium; it is also phosphorylated by several kinases. These controls are discussed in Chapter 9.

VII. Receptor Metabolism

A. Synthesis

Membrane receptors are proteins and are synthesized in the same manner as all other proteins. However, some variations can have a major impact on the ultimate function of the receptor. Protein synthesis actually begins with transcription of the gene followed by processing of the resulting mRNA. Exon 11 in the insulin receptor mRNA encodes 12 amino acids located near the carboxy terminus of the α subunit. In some molecules, this exon is spliced out, resulting in a shorter receptor with a higher affinity for insulin and a more rapid rate of internalization (327–329). This may be physiologically important; the longer less-sensitive form occurs in the liver, which receives blood directly from the pancreas via the hepatic portal system and is exposed to high concentrations of insulin. The lower affinity receptor may protect the liver from overstimulation. In the FGF2R, there are two alternative exons that encode the carboxy half of the third immunoglobulin-like loop (78–80): one exon produces a receptor that binds only FGF, whereas the other generates a receptor that binds KGF.

Translation occurs on membrane-bound ribosomes: membrane insertion is initiated by the signal sequence and is stopped by a pair of basic residues at the end of the hydrophobic helix. As for all membrane proteins, the extracellular domain is glycosylated. The function of this carbohydrate has been investigated by several techniques: (i) stripping the mature protein of sugars by glycosidases, (ii) blocking the addition of carbohydrate by either a specific inhibitor such as tunicamycin, or (iii) blocking glycosylation by mutation of the asparagine acceptor site. In general, stripping the mature receptor has no effect on ligand binding or signal transduction; however, preventing the addition of sugars during translation does impair both functions. In the latter case, the receptors appear to be misfolded and are retained in the endoplasmic reticulum. Therefore, glycosylation seems to be necessary for protein processing, such as folding and membrane targeting, but not for ligand binding or signal transduction (330–334). Many receptors also undergo another post-translational modification: palmitoylation. Palmitic acid is added in the Golgi; however, its high turnover rate suggests that mechanisms to remove and reattach this fatty acid also exist in the cytosol. Its role in the desensitization of serpentine receptors was discussed earlier.

Finally, multisubunit receptors must be assembled. The insulin receptor represents the simplest case, since the α and β subunits are part of a single polyprotein. Therefore, the subunits are necessarily synthesized stoichiometrically and are physically attached until cleavage. Pulse–chase experiments show that this cleavage does not take place until the receptor is at least core glycosylated (Fig. 6-9; 335). The nAChR represents a more complex example; the assembly of subunits is initially prevented by phosphorylation (296). After dephosphorylation, $\alpha\gamma$ (or $\alpha\epsilon$) and $\alpha\delta$ dimers form first (336,337); this interaction is mediated by the amino termini (338). Then each dimer binds a β subunit to create the final pentamer. Alternative pathways have also been postulated based on different methodologies. In one, an $\alpha\beta\gamma$ trimer forms first; the δ and ϵ subunits are then inserted sequentially (339). Finally, several of the subunits are tyrosine phosphorylated; this appears to attract the 43-kDa peripheral protein that is responsible for aggregating the receptors at synapses (297).

B. Clustering

After hormone binding, the hormone–receptor complex is processed; this helps terminate the signal and may also be involved in the mechanism of action of the hormone. Cells actually contain two functionally distinct classes of receptors: one for hormones and one for nutrients. Examples of the nutrient class include the low-density lipoproteins, which carry triglycerides and cholesterol; intrinsic factor, which carries vitamin B_{12}; and transferrin, which carries iron. Like the peptide hormones, these nutrient carriers are too large to pass through the plasma membrane; therefore, they too must be internalized by endocytosis. Although there is some overlap in the way each group is processed, there are some general differences that can distinguish the two (Table 6-5).

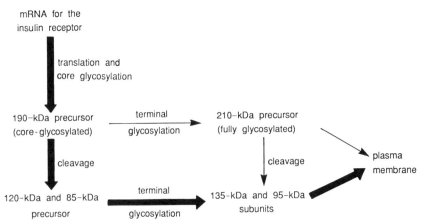

Fig. 6-9. Synthetic pathway for the insulin receptor. The major pathway is shown with bold arrows.

Table 6-5

Comparison of the Nutrient and Hormone Processing Pathways

Characteristic	Nutrient pathway	Hormone pathway
Examples	Low-density lipoprotein; intrinsic factor; transferrin	Hormones
Clustering	Usually preclustered	Usually diffuse
Possible mechanism	Transglutaminases	Noncovalent
Internalization	Continuous	Discontinuous
Recycling	Short loop	Long loop

Immediately after hormone binding, the hormone–receptor complexes begin to aggregate into coated pits. These pits are plasma membrane invaginations 50–150 nm in diameter and surrounded by a basket or cage of polygonal units. The basic unit of this cage is a triskelion (Fig. 6-10; 340) containing three 180-kDa clathrin molecules and three 33- to 36-kDa light chains, or clathrin-associated proteins; the former form the legs whereas the latter act as glue. The legs are 445 Å long with a bend 190 Å from the vertex; the legs align with each other to form hexagons and pentagons (Fig. 6-10). The tips of the legs turn in to form struts that bind adaptors in the plasma membrane. These adaptors recognize a tyrosine in the carboxy terminus; the tyrosine is located on a loop and is surrounded by basic residues (341,342).

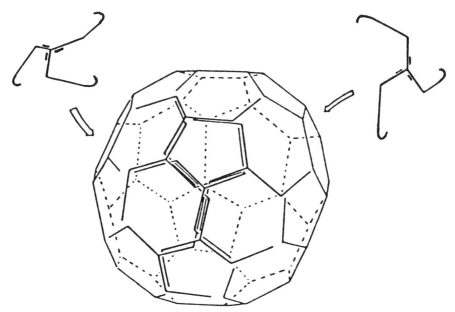

Fig. 6-10. Clathrin trimers (triskelions) and their packing organization. Reprinted by permission from Ref. 340. Copyright © 1983 Cell Press.

After aggregation, the pits bud off and quickly lose their clathrin coat. The role of this coat is unknown; however, the injection of anti-clathrin antibodies into cells inhibits endocytosis (343). Note that the presence and nature of clustering is highly variable: (i) preaggregation of receptors inside or outside coated pits, (ii) aggregation outside coated pits, and (iii) no aggregation at all have been reported for various hormones and tissues.

Why do the receptors cluster? The mechanism has still not been determined, but the following facts are known:

1. Clustering does not require energy.

2. Clustering is not affected by drugs that disrupt the cytoskeleton.

3. There may or may not be segregation of ligands. For example, insulin and EGF receptors will aggregate within the same pit (344), but the β_2R and α_2R are sequestered into different vesicles (345).

Therefore, clustering appears to be the result of simple diffusion associated with a change in receptor conformation that favors mutual binding. This binding may be covalent and involve isopeptide bonds or disulfide linkages. Transglutaminases will form a peptide (amide) bond between the lysine of one peptide and the glutamine of another:

$$R(CH_2)_4NH_2 + H_2NCO(CH_2)_2R' \longrightarrow R(CH_2)_4NHCO(CH_2)_2R' + NH_3$$

In the nutrient pathways, dansylcadaverine and bacitracin can inhibit both the enzyme and clustering, suggesting a cause-and-effect relationship; however, in the hormone systems, this correlation is generally poor (346,347). Because of the high content of cysteines in the receptors with tyrosine kinase activity, disulfide bonds were considered a more likely possibility in the hormone pathway. However, covalent linkages have rarely been documented and the aggregation of hormone receptors is believed to be due to noncovalent interactions.

What is the function of clustering? In several systems, aggregation appears to be essential for the biological activity of the hormone. For example, certain antibodies against the insulin receptor can mimic the action of insulin only if the antibodies remain intact; their bivalent nature induces clustering (348). If they are cleaved in half so they are monovalent, both clustering and biological activity are lost. If the cleaved halves are reunited by a second antibody directed against the first, both clustering and biological activity are restored. The EGFR can be induced to cluster by a variety of agents utilizing several different mechanisms; in this case, activity is always associated with oligomerization, independent of the methodology (349). Therefore in these systems, clustering, even in the absence of the hormone, is sufficient for biological activity.

What is the molecular basis for this clustering-induced biological activity? The answer may reside in the structure of the RTKs: they have only a single transmembrane helix connecting the hormone-binding site and the tyrosine kinase domain. It is difficult to imagine how any type of conformational change could be transmitted through an α helix, particularly one embedded within a membrane. This problem could be overcome by lateral transduction instead of transmembrane transduction: hormone binding induces a conformational change in the cysteine-rich extracellular region, which aggregates. The cytoplasmic domains are passively carried along, but when they meet, an allosteric stimulation of the tyrosine kinase occurs.

C. Internalization and Processing

In the nutrient pathway, the receptors are being continuously internalized and recycled, even when unoccupied. Apparently, nutrients are present in the internal environment in high enough concentrations to make such a system worthwhile. However, in the hormone pathway, internalization is ligand-induced; for example, EGF increases internalization 10-fold over baseline rates without EGF.

The two pathways also differ in their processing of the internalized ligand–receptor complex. In the nutrient pathway, the endocytotic vesicle, called an *endosome* or *receptosome*, becomes acidified via an ATP-dependent mechanism. At about the same time, slender tubules begin to emerge from the surface of the vesicle; this entire complex has been called CURL (compartment for *u*ncoupling *r*eceptors and *l*igands). This acidification disrupts ligand–receptor binding and the unoccupied receptors migrate into the tubules while the free ligand remains in the vesicle (Fig. 6-11). Actually, the entire process of segregation may be passive; the geometry of these structures is such that 90% of the surface area is in the tubules, although 90% of the volume is in the vesicle. Since receptors are membrane bound and ligands are soluble, their distribution could be entirely explained by simple diffusion. However, some evidence suggests that this separation also involves more active processes (350). The tubules then detach and return to the plasma membrane, where the receptors are recycled. Finally, the vesicle fuses with lysosomes and the ligand is degraded. This pathway is known as the short loop (351).

Hormone–receptor complexes are treated in a similar manner except that the liberated receptors first go to the Golgi apparatus before returning to the plasma membrane; this is called the long loop (352). The reason for this detour is not known; temporary storage, repair, and/or purification from other membrane components have all been postulated. In another less common variation, some hormone receptors are not recycled at all: for example, the EGF receptor is totally degraded in many tissues. This destruction may be related to the tyrosine kinase activity of the receptor: mutant receptors without such activity are internalized normally but are recycled instead of degraded (353,354). In addition, this phenomenon shows tissue specificity: insulin receptors in the liver are recycled, but those in adipocytes are not. The purpose of this variation is to induce a refractory period in the target tissue after hormone stimulation; the occupied receptors are destroyed and the

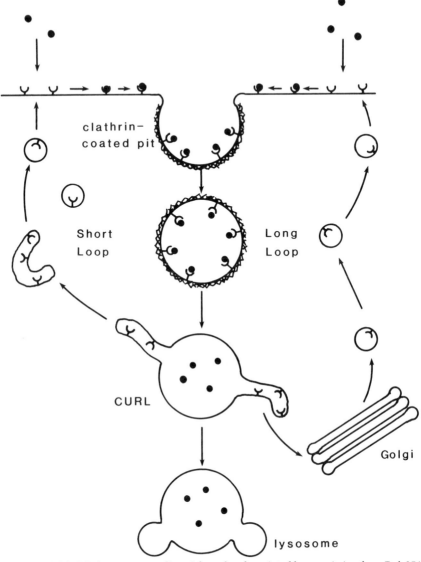

Fig. 6-11. Model of receptor recycling. Adapted and reprinted by permission from Ref. 351. Copyright © 1983 Cell Press.

tissue becomes less sensitive to additional hormone until new receptors can be synthesized (see Chapter 7).

D. Relevance

One of the most controversial issues to arise over receptor metabolism is its relevance to the biological activity of hormones (Table 6-6). One school holds

Table 6-6
Summary of the Arguments for and against the Importance of Internalization in Hormone Action

Yes	Counterargument	No	Counterargument
Intracellular receptors exist	Those in the endoplasmic reticulum and Golgi apparatus are probably precursors	Hormones linked to Sepharose are fully active	Hormones may be leaking from the matrix
Direct actions: hormone stimulation of nucleoside triphosphatase, phosphoprotein phosphatase, RNA polymerase I, PKC, and DNase	Possible contaminating plasmalemma may be generating second messengers	Some receptor antibodies can mimic the hormones	This statement assumes that the hormone is the effector instead of the receptor, as well as that the binding and effector sites of the hormone differ; neither assumption may be true
Lysosomatropic alkylamines inhibit EGFR processing and EGF-induced DNA synthesis	These same compounds are ineffective in other systems, for example, insulin-induced amino acid transport	Internal hormones are ineffective: microinjection, fusion, or deletion of signal sequence	The hormones are on the wrong side of the membrane
FGF lacks a signal sequence and accumulates in the nucleus	Activity of FGF can be greatly increased by adding a signal sequence	Mutant receptors unable to internalize have normal activity Temporally, second messengers are generated before receptor aggregation and internalization	Not all the biological activities of the hormones have been measured May not be sufficient for long-term responses such as mitogenesis

that the second messenger is generated at the time of hormone binding or receptor clustering and that all events thereafter are only involved in hormone degradation and receptor recycling. The other school believes that internalization is a means for delivering the hormone and/or receptor to the cell interior, where it directly exerts some of its biological activity (355).

The latter group notes that both hormones and their receptors do exist intracellularly (356). However, since these receptors appear to be identical to those in the plasma membrane (357), they may only represent newly synthesized, stored, or recycling receptors. This group also claims that hormones and/or receptors can have direct actions on enzymes (358–361) or on DNA (362). These reports are often countered by the suggestion that these preparations are not pure: contaminating plasma membranes may generate a second messenger in the presence of the hormone, whereas contaminating enzymes may give rise to spurious activities. Another argument supporting a functional role for processing comes from experiments using lysosomatrophic alkylamines, which are alkaline compounds taken up by lysosomes (363). These agents block the acidification of the endosome and prevent processing of the hormone–receptor complex. If the biological signal were generated at the cell surface, the inhibition of processing should have no effect on hormone action. On the contrary, these agents do inhibit the activity of some hormones such as EGF. Unfortunately, these same compounds are ineffective or only partially effective in other systems. The most interesting example of the latter group is angiotensin II, whose acute release of a second messenger is unaffected by these agents; however, the sustained accumulation of the same mediator is blocked (364). Therefore, in some systems, internalization may help prolong the effects of a hormone. Finally, it is noted that FGF lacks a signal sequence (365) and accumulates in the nucleus (366). Opponents suggest that FGF lacks a signal sequence, not because it is active internally but because it is a wound hormone that may be released only during cell injury. In support of this counterargument, they point to the fact that FGF is much more active when it has been genetically engineered to have a signal sequence (367).

The opposing group also has its arguments. For example, some hormones covalently bound to Sepharose are fully active. Sepharose is a large cross-linked polysaccharide that cannot enter the cell; therefore, the coupled hormone must be acting at the cell surface. However, it is now known that these bonds are very labile and that sufficient hormone can leak off the matrix to account for the observed biological activity (368). Other evidence against a functional role for processing includes the phenomenon of stimulating antibodies. As noted earlier, certain receptor antibodies can bind the receptor and mimic hormone action. Obviously, the hormone does not have to be internalized to act, since there is no hormone present at all. However, this conclusion is based on tenuous assumptions. First, it assumes that the hormone itself is the biologically active agent. Perhaps the only role for the hormone is to trigger the internalization of the receptor, which then executes the appropriate functions; this mechanism would be analogous to that previously proposed for steroid receptors. Second, it assumes that the hormone has one site for receptor binding and membrane transduction and another site for internal biological activity; since the antibody only has the binding site, there can be no internal activity. However, if the internal site of action has the same structural constraints as the receptor, an antibody should have no problems interacting with either. An elegant series of experiments provides additional ammunition for the opponents: hormones introduced into the cytoplasm of the cell have no activity. This can be accomplished by microinjection (369), by cell fusion with hormone-laden erythrocyte ghosts (370), or by deletion of the signal sequence (371). However, the binding site of receptors is oriented toward the extracellular environment or toward the interior of endosomes; none face the cytoplasm. Therefore, the hormone has been introduced into the cell on the wrong side of the membrane and cannot bind to its receptor. This experiment might eliminate the possibility that free hormone is directly affecting cellular processes, but it does not address the role of an internalized hormone–receptor complex in hormone action.

In yet another argument, it is noted that mutant insulin and EGF receptors that are incapable of internalization are biologically active (372,373). However, not all the biological activities were measured. For example, at 4°C the GM-CSFR does not internalize, yet soluble tyrosine kinases are still activated, although Raf is not (374). Therefore, internalization may be required for some but not all biological activities. Finally, the EGFR can stimulate phospholipid breakdown and calcium fluxes before aggregation occurs (375), but again there may be other second messengers that are not generated until after internalization.

In addition to mediating some biological activities, internalization may have another function. The PDGFR has been shown to remain active for up to 10 minutes after internalization (376) and to be co-internalized with PI3K, one of its effectors (377). Therefore, even if internalization is not required for a particular activity, it may be important in prolonging the effect.

VIII. Miscellaneous Topics

A. Spare Receptors

Very early in the study of membrane receptors, an apparent discrepancy between hormone activity and receptor binding was noted: maximal activity occurred when only a small fraction of the receptors was occupied. For example, hCG maximally stimulated testosterone synthesis in Leydig cells when only 0.3% of the receptors were bound; insulin maximally stimulated glucose oxidation in adipocytes with a receptor occupancy level of 2%; similar results have been reported for glucagon and the catecholamines. The reverse phenomenon has also been observed: 80% of the insulin receptors on mammary tumor cells can be destroyed by trypsin while insulin-induced glucose transport decreases by only 13%. Initially, two hypotheses were formulated to explain this discrepancy. One postulated that specific hormone binding was composed of two fractions: a small pool of true receptors coupled to a transduction system and a large pool of receptors with no known function. The ANF clearance receptor might represent an example of the latter. The other, more popular hypothesis claimed that most receptors were simply spare receptors.

Further work has suggested two more hypotheses that seem more logical. According to the first, spare receptors are an artifact produced when only one biological activity is monitored, that is, different responses may require different degrees of receptor occupancy (348). As noted earlier, many actions of insulin occur when receptor binding is low: these include glucose transport and oxidation, inhibition of lipolysis, and alterations in protein phosphorylation. However, the stimulation of amino acid transport and RNA synthesis requires nearly maximal binding, and other activities occur at intermediate occupancy levels; these latter effects include the stimulation of glycogen synthase, acetyl coenzyme A carboxylase, pyruvate dehydrogenase, tyrosine aminotransferase, and protein synthesis. In general, activities requiring protein synthesis need higher levels of receptor occupancy.

The other hypothesis claims that these spare receptors modulate the hormone sensitivity of the cell (378). The kinetics of hormone–receptor binding follow the laws of mass action (see Chapter 4):

$$H + R \rightleftharpoons HR \longrightarrow \text{biological response}$$

The critical concentration is that for HR which, in turn, is determined by the concentrations of both the hormone and the receptor. By increasing the concentration of R, the reaction can be driven to the right or, to put it another way, the higher R is, the less H is required to reach the same concentration of HR. The cell is therefore more sensitive to H. One could also increase hormone sensitivity by increasing the affinity, but there are two drawbacks to this option (379). First, increasing the affinity would decrease hormone–receptor dissociation, resulting in a slower response time. Second, a higher affinity would saturate the receptor at lower hormone concentrations and the system would no longer be responsive to these high ligand levels. As such, "spare receptors" are an elegant way to increase hormone sensitivity while preserving a fast response time and sensitivity to a wide range of hormone concentrations.

B. Isoreceptors

Isoreceptors are structurally and functionally distinct receptors for the same hormone; such receptors frequently have different tissue distributions, second messengers, and functions (Table 6-7). Since all the receptors in a single class recognize the same natural hormone, other ligands must be used to distinguish among them. In this respect, pharmacologists have been very helpful; they have provided researchers with numerous agonists, some of which may be highly specific for one particular isoreceptor. For example, nicotine preferentially binds to the acetylcholine receptor on skeletal muscle, whereas muscarine is more specific for those receptors in the parasympathetic nervous system; these isoreceptors are now named for their respective agonists. Although isoreceptors are very common, some hormones such as insulin and EGF, have only one receptor except for possible slight variations in glycosylation.

Why would one hormone have multiple receptors? Isoreceptors allow a hormone to have widely diverse, even opposite, effects in different tissues. The adrenergic receptors provide an excellent example (Table 6-7). Catecholamines, like many hormones, have numerous actions that are related to a single overall function, in this case the "flight-or-fight" response (see Chapter 2). Smooth muscle *contracts* in the bladder sphincter to prevent voiding

Table 6-7

Examples of Isoreceptors for Selected Hormones

Hormone	Isoreceptor	Mediator	Location	Function
Acetylcholine	Nicotinic (muscle)	Sodium	Skeletal muscle	Contraction
	Nicotinic (neural)	Sodium	Nervous system	Neurotransmission
	Muscarinic (M1)	Calcium	Parasympathetic nervous system	Neurotransmission
	Muscarinic (M2)	Decreased cAMP	Parasympathetic nervous system	Neurotransmission
Vasopressin	V1	Calcium	Liver; arterioles	Glycogenolysis; contraction
	V2	cAMP	Kidney	Water resorption
Histamine	H1	Calcium	Bronchioles; arterioles; gut	Contraction
	H2	cAMP	Stomach	Acid secretion
	H3	Lower calcium	Brain; arterioles; bronchioles	Presynaptic inhibition; relaxation
Epinephrine and norepinephrine	α_1	Calcium	Liver; smooth muscle of blood vessels, gut, and urinary system	Glycogenolysis; contraction
	α_2	Decreased cAMP	Fat; platelets; smooth muscle of gut	Lipolysis; platelet aggregation; relaxation
	β_1	cAMP	Fat; heart; smooth muscle of gut	Lipolysis; tachycardia; relaxation
	β_2	cAMP	Skeletal muscle; smooth muscle of blood vessels, bronchioles, and urinary system	Glycogenolysis; relaxation
Dopamine	D1	cAMP	Central nervous system; retina; parathyroid gland; vascular smooth muscle	PTH secretion; relaxation
	D2	Decreased cAMP	Sympathetic and central nervous system; pituitary gland	Inhibition of PRL and MSH secretion
Opiate peptides	μ	Potassium, calcium, cAMP	Hypothalamus	Euphoria; decrease gut motility
	δ	Potassium, calcium, cAMP	Limbic system; basal ganglia	Analgesia; hyperthermia
	κ	Potassium, calcium, cAMP	Substantia nigra; neurohypophysis	Sedation; dysphoria; anorexia

and in the mesenteric arterioles to shift blood to the skeletal muscles; how-ever, smooth muscle must *relax* in the airways to increase oxygenation and in the intestines, since digestion is being deferred. Furthermore, catecholamines affect not only smooth muscle, but also metabolism and cardiovascular activity. These diverse actions would be difficult to elicit using a single receptor and second messenger.

Isoreceptors could also extend the dose response of a system; for exam-ple, fat cells contain β_1, β_2, and β_3 receptors, all of which mediate lipolysis (380). However, their hormone responsiveness differs: the β_1AR is most sensitive, whereas the β_3AR is least sensitive. These isoreceptors allow the fat cell to respond to a wide range of catecholamine concentrations.

C. Cryptic Receptors

The concept of cryptic receptors is derived from numerous observations in which the number of receptors suddenly increases without an obvious ex-planation. Presumably, these receptors already existed in some latent form incapable of hormone binding, that is, they were *cryptic receptors*. The in-ducing factor is envisioned as merely stimulating the conversion of a latent to an overt receptor. There are several possible mechanisms. First, the receptor could undergo a change in conformation: phosphorylation and cleavage are obvious examples. GnRH receptor can be unmasked by the former (381) and cleavage of the insulin receptor may be an example of the latter. However, peptide cleavage is not the only possibility; both gonadotropin receptors can be exposed by partial deglycosylation (382,383). Perturbations of the envi-ronment of receptors can also increase the total number of binding sites in the absence of protein synthesis: detergents, phospholipases (384), and phospholipid methylation (385) have all been reported to induce this phe-nomenon. The ionic environment is equally important; basic compounds can expose EGFRs (386). Finally, energy depletion is another circumstance that can lead to the appearance of additional receptors (387). The mechanism for the latter effect is unknown. These membrane proteins may represent a ready reservoir of receptors for rapid cellular responses.

IX. Summary

Membrane receptors are of four types: (i) enzyme-linked, (ii) serpentine, (iii) fibronectin-like, and (iv) ion channels. All the RTKs cross the plasmalemma once and have their amino terminus extracellularly, where the hormone binds. The carboxy terminus is intracellular, and contains the tyrosine kinase domain and critical tyrosine phosphorylation sites that are responsible for substrate binding. The extreme carboxy terminus is required for receptor internalization. The EGFR subfamily has two cysteine clusters in the amino terminus and an intact kinase domain, and is uncleaved. The insulin receptor subfamily has a single cysteine cluster and an intact kinase domain, and is cleaved into α and β subunits. The PDGFR subfamily has immunoglobulin loops in the amino terminus and a split kinase domain, and is uncleaved. Finally, the NGFR subfamily also has immunoglobulin-like loops in the amino terminus, but the kinase domain is most like that of the insulin receptor. Other enzyme-linked receptors are the serine kinases and the guanylate cyclases. The former are identical in structural organization to the RTKs; they only differ in substrate specificity. However, the cyclases do have one major difference: they have two catalytic sites intracellularly. The carboxy-terminal one is the cyclase, whereas the amino-terminal one has evolved into a regulatory domain. A soluble form of the cyclase is activated by NO and CO via a heme-containing amino terminus.

The serpentine receptors are smaller, cross the plasma membrane seven times, and interact with GTP-binding proteins. The M-type receptors have a longer cytoplasmic loop between helices 5 and 6 and a shorter carboxy terminus than the peptide or the β-type receptors. The ligands primarily bind to the transmembrane helices, although the amino terminus and extracellular loops can also bind when the ligand is large. Transduction occurs through the juxtamembrane portion of the carboxy terminus and the cytoplasmic loop between helices 5 and 6.

The fibronectin-like receptors have modified fibronectin type III repeats and an intracellular domain that lacks sequence homology but is rich in serines, threonines, prolines, and acidic residues. Their biological effects are probably mediated through the activation of soluble tyrosine kinases.

The ion channel receptors are of two types. The nAChR and glutamate receptor families consist of five homologous subunits containing four transmembrane helices each. The second helix of each subunit forms the channel wall. The voltage-gated channels have four subunits, or one protein with four fused domains; each subunit or domain contains six transmembrane helices. The channel wall is formed from a β loop between helices 5 and 6. Several members of this family are regulated by second messengers: the cyclic nucleotide-gated ion channels and the IP_3 receptor.

After hormone binding, the receptors cluster into coated pits and are internalized. Acidification of these vesicles disrupts hormone–receptor binding; the hormone remains within the central cavity while the receptors migrate into tubules that bud off the vesicle. The tubules break off, are routed through the Golgi apparatus, and then are recycled to the plasma membrane. The vesicles containing the hormone fuse with lysosomes and the ligand is degraded. Clustering may allow allosteric interaction among receptors, whereas internalization and processing help terminate the hormone signal while conserving receptors.

Although only a small number of receptors is occupied, even during maximal stimulation, the spare receptors are still important in determining the hormonal sensitivity of a cell. Furthermore, not all receptors for a given hormone are identical; many can be divided into several subgroups. These isoreceptors permit a hormone to have different actions in different tissues. Finally, some receptors are incapable of binding their ligands until some additional event takes place; these cryptic receptors may represent a silent reservoir of binding proteins.

References

General References

Bolen, J. B. (1993). Nonreceptor tyrosine protein kinases. *Oncogene* **8**, 2025–2031.

Brown, B. L., and Dobson, P. R. M. (eds.) (1993). "Cell Signalling: Biology and Medicine of Signal Transduction." Raven Press, New York.

Collins, S. (1993). Recent perspectives on the molecular structure and regulation of the β_2-adrenoceptor. *Life Sci.* **52**, 2083–2091.

Hadcock, J. R., and Malbon, C. C. (1993). Agonist regulation of gene expression of adrenergic receptors and G proteins. *J. Neurochem.* **60**, 1–9.

Ormandy, C. J., and Sutherland, R. L. (1993). Mechanisms of prolactin receptor regulation in mammary gland. *Mol. Cell. Endocrinol.* **91**, C1–C6.

Schmidt, H. H. H. W., Lohmann, S. M., and Walter, U. (1993). The nitric oxide and cGMP signal transduction system: Regulation and mechanism of action. *Biochim. Biophys. Acta* **1178**, 153–175.

Sorkin, A., and Waters, C. M. (1993). Endocytosis of growth factor receptors. *Bioessays* **15**, 375–382.

Tian, W. N., and Deth, R. C. (1993). Precoupling of G_i/G_o-linked receptors and its allosteric regulation by monovalent cations. *Life Sci.* **52**, 1899–1907.

See also Refs. 1, 3, 10, 12–14, 34, 41, 53, 57, 65, 67, 93, 99, 100, 121, 128, 129, 141, 144, 148, 166, 178, 207, 215, 217, 221, 222, 228, 256, 264, 284, 286, 287, 293, 300, 301, 307, 312–314, 322, 323, 340, 355, 365, 378 and 379.

Cited References

1. Pawson, T., and Schlessinger, J. (1993). SH2 and SH3 domains. *Curr. Biol.* **3**, 434–442.
2. Bar-Sagi, D., Rotin, D., Batzer, A., Mandiyan, V., and Schlessinger, J. (1993). SH3 domains direct cellular localization of signaling molecules. *Cell* **74**, 83–91.
3. Margolis, B. (1992). Proteins with SH2 domains: Transducers in the tyrosine kinase signaling pathway. *Cell Growth Diff.* **3**, 73–80.
4. Overduin, M., Rios, C. B., Mayer, B. J., Baltimore, D., and Cowburn, D. (1992). Three-dimensional solution structure of the *src* homology 2 domain of c-abl. *Cell* **70**, 697–704.
5. Musacchio, A., Noble, M., Pauptit, R., Wierenga, R., and Saraste, M. (1992). Crystal structure of a Src-homology 3 (SH3) domain. *Nature (London)* **359**, 851–855.
6. Yu, H., Rosen, M. K., Shin, T. B., Seidel-Dugan, C., Brugge, J. S., and Schreiber, S. L. (1992). Solution structure of the SH3 domain of src and identification of its ligand-binding site. *Science* **258**, 1665–1668.
7. Songyang, Z., Shoelson, S. E., Chaudhuri, M., Gish, G., Pawson, T., Haser, W. G., King, F., Roberts, T., Ratnofsky, S., Lechleider, R. J., Neel, B. G., Birge, R. B., Fajardo, J. E., Chou, M. M., Hanafusa, H., Schaffhausen, B., and Cantley, L. C. (1993). SH2 domains recognize specific phosphopeptide sequences. *Cell* **72**, 767–778.

8. Piccione, E., Case, R. D., Domchek, S. M., Hu, P., Chaudhuri, M., Backer, J. M., Schlessinger, J., and Shoelson, S. E. (1993). Phosphatidylinositol 3-kinase p85 SH2 domain specificity defined by direct phosphopeptide/SH2 domain binding. *Biochemistry* **32**, 3197–3202.

9. Weiss, A. (1993). T cell antigen receptor signal transduction: A tale of tails and cytoplasmic protein-tyrosine kinases. *Cell* **73**, 209–212.

10. Mayer, B. J., and Baltimore, D. (1993). Signalling through SH2 and SH3 domains. *Trends Cell Biol.* **3**, 8–13.

11. Prasad, K. V. S., Janssen, O., Kapeller, R., Raab, M., Cantley, L. C., and Rudd, C. E. (1993). Src-homology 3 domain of protein kinase p59^{fyn} mediates binding to phosphatidylinositol 3-kinase in T cells. *Proc. Natl. Acad. Sci. U.S.A.* **90**, 7366–7370.

12. Bolen, J. B. (1993). Nonreceptor tyrosine protein kinases. *Oncogene* **8**, 2025–2031.

13. Cooper, J. A., and Howell, B. (1993). The when and how of Src regulation. *Cell* **73**, 1051–1054.

14. Hernández-Sotomayor, S. M. T., and Carpenter, G. (1992). Epidermal growth factor receptor: Elements of intracellular communication. *J. Membr. Biol.* **128**, 81–89.

15. Holmes, W. E., Sliwkowski, M. X., Akita, R. W., Henzel, W. J., Lee, J., Park, J. W., Yansura, D., Abadi, N., Raab, H., Lewis, G. D., Shepard, H. M., Kuang, W. J., Wood, W. I., Goeddel, D. V., and Vandlen, R. L. (1992). Identification of heregulin, a specific activator of p185^{erbB}. *Science* **256**, 1205–1210.

16. Wen, D., Peles, E., Cupples, R., Suggs, S. V., Bacus, S. S., Luo, Y., Trail, G., Hu, S., Silbiger, S. M., Levy, R. B., Koski, R. A., Lu, H. S., and Yarden, Y. (1992). Neu differentiation factor: A transmembrane glycoprotein containing an EGF domain and an immunoglobulin homology unit. *Cell* **69**, 559–572.

17. Matsuda, S., Kadowaki, Y., Ichino, M., Akiyama, T., Toyoshima, K., and Yamamoto, T. (1993). 17β-Estradiol mimics ligand activity of the c-*erbB*2 protooncogene product. *Proc. Natl. Acad. Sci. U.S.A.* **90**, 10803–10807.

18. Kohda, D., Odaka, M., Lax, I., Kawasaki, H., Suzuki, K., Ullrich, A., Schlessinger, J., and Inagaki, F. (1993). A 40-kDa epidermal growth factor/transforming growth factor α-binding domain produced by limited proteolysis of the extracellular domain of the epidermal growth factor receptor. *J. Biol. Chem.* **268**, 1976–1981.

19. Carpenter, C. D., Ingraham, H. A., Cochet, C., Walton, G. M., Lazar, C. S., Sowadski, J. M., Rosenfeld, M. G., and Gill, G. N. (1991). Structural analysis of the transmembrane domain of the epidermal growth factor receptor. *J. Biol. Chem.* **266**, 5750–5755.

20. Countaway, J. L., McQuilkin, P., Girons, N., and Davis, R. J. (1990). Multisite phosphorylation of the epidermal growth factor receptor: Use of site-directed mutagenesis to examine the role of serine/threonine phosphorylation. *J. Biol. Chem.* **265**, 3407–3416.

21. Decker, S. J., Ellis, C., Pawson, T., and Velu, T. (1990). Effects of substitution of threonine 654 of the epidermal growth factor receptor on epidermal growth factor-mediated activation of phospholipase C. *J. Biol. Chem.* **265**, 7009–7015.

22. Heisermann, G. J., Wiley, H. S., Walsh, B. J., Ingraham, H. A., Fiol, C. J., and Gill, G. N. (1990). Mutational removal of the Thr^{669} and Ser^{671} phosphorylation sites alters substrate specificity and ligand-induced internalization of the epidermal growth factor receptor. *J. Biol. Chem.* **265**, 12820–12827.

23. Northwood, I. C., Gonzalez, F. A., Wartmann, M., Raden, D. L., and Davis, R. J. (1991). Isolation and characterization of two growth factor-stimulated protein kinases that phosphorylate the epidermal growth factor receptor at threonine 669. *J. Biol. Chem.* **266,** 15226–15276.

24. Segatto, O., Lonardo, F., Wexler, D., Fazioli, F., Pierce, J. H., Bottaro, D. P., White, M. F., and Di Fiore, P. P. (1991). The juxtamembrane regions of the epidermal growth factor receptor and gp185^{erbB-2} determine the specificity of signal transduction. *Mol. Cell. Biol.* **11,** 3191–3202.

25. Di Fiore, P. P., Helin, K., Kraus, M. H., Pierce, J. H., Artrip, J., Segatto, O., and Bottaro, D. P. (1992). A single amino acid substitution is sufficient to modify the mitogenic properties of the epidermal growth factor receptor to resemble that of gp185^{erbB}. *EMBO J.* **11,** 3927–3933.

26. José, E. S., Benguría, A., Geller, P., and Villalobo, A. (1992). Calmodulin inhibits the epidermal growth factor receptor tyrosine kinase. *J. Biol. Chem.* **267,** 15237–15245.

27. Cochet, C., Filhol, O., Payrastre, B., Hunter, T., and Gill, G. N. (1991). Interaction between the epidermal growth factor receptor and phosphoinositide kinases. *J. Biol. Chem.* **266,** 637–644.

28. Countaway, J. L., Nairn, A. C., and Davis, R. J. (1992). Mechanism of desensitization of the epidermal growth factor receptor protein–tyrosine kinase. *J. Biol. Chem.* **267,** 1129–1140.

29. Rotin, D., Margolis, B., Mohammadi, M., Daly, R. J., Daum, G., Li, N., Fischer, E. H., Burgess, W. H., Ullrich, A., and Schlessinger, J. (1992). SH2 domains prevent tyrosine dephosphorylation of the EGF receptor: Identification of Tyr992 as the high-affinity binding site for SH2 domains of phospholipase Cγ. *EMBO J.* **11,** 559–567.

30. Vega, Q. C., Cochet, C., Filhol, O., Chang, C. P., Rhee, S. G., and Gill, G. N. (1992). A site of tyrosine phosphorylation in the C-terminus of the epidermal growth factor receptor is required to activate phospholipase C. *Mol. Cell. Biol.* **12,** 128–135.

31. Margolis, B., Li, N., Koch, A., Mohammadi, M., Hurwitz, D. R., Zilberstein, A., Ullrich, A., Pawson, T., and Schlessinger, J. (1990). The tyrosine phosphorylated carboxyterminus of the EGF receptor is a binding site for GAP and PLC-γ. *EMBO J.* **9,** 4375–4380.

32. App, H., Hazan, R., Zilberstein, A., Ullrich, A., Schlessinger, J., and Rapp, U. (1991). Epidermal growth factor (EGF) stimulates association and kinase activity of Raf-1 with the EGF receptor. *Mol. Cell. Biol.* **11,** 913–919.

33. Hsu, C. Y. J., Hurwitz, D. R., Mervic, M., and Zilberstein, A. (1991). Autophosphorylation of the intracellular domain of the epidermal growth factor receptor results in different effects on its tyrosine kinase activity with various peptide substrates: Phosphorylation of peptides representing Tyr(P) sites of phospholipase C-γ. *J. Biol. Chem.* **266,** 603–608.

34. Schlessinger, J., and Ullrich, A. (1992). Growth factor signaling by receptor tyrosine kinases. *Neuron* **9,** 383–391.

35. Decker, S. J. (1993). Transmembrane signaling by epidermal growth factor receptors lacking autophosphorylation sites. *J. Biol. Chem.* **268,** 9176–9179.

36. Wada, T., Qian, X., and Greene, M. I. (1990). Intermolecular association of the p185^{neu} protein and EGF receptor modulates EGF receptor function. *Cell* **61,** 1339–1347.

37. Qian, X., Decker, S. J., and Greene, M. I. (1992). p185^{c-neu} and epidermal growth

factor receptor associate into a structure composed of activated kinases. *Proc. Natl. Acad. Sci. U.S.A.* **89,** 1330–1334.

38. Ball, R. L., Tanner, K. D., and Carpenter, G. (1990). Epidermal growth factor potentiates cyclic AMP accumulation in A-431 cells. *J. Biol. Chem.* **265,** 12836–12845.
39. Yang, L., Baffy, G., Rhee, S. G., Manning, D., Hansen, C. A., and Williamson, J. R. (1991). Pertussis toxin-sensitive G_i protein involvement in epidermal growth factor-induced activation of phospholipase C-q in rat hepatocytes. *J. Biol. Chem.* **266,** 22451–22458.
40. Budnik, L. T., and Mukhopadhyay, A. K. (1991). Epidermal growth factor, a modulator of luteal adenylate cyclase: Characterization of epidermal growth factor receptors and its interaction with adenylate cyclase system in bovine luteal cell membrane. *J. Biol. Chem.* **266,** 13908–13913.
41. Ellis, L., Tavaré, J. M., and Levine, B. A. (1991). Insulin receptor tyrosine kinase structure and function. *Biochem. Soc. Trans.* **19,** 426–432.
42. Schaefer, E. M., Erickson, H. P., Federwisch, M., Wollmer, A., and Ellis, L. (1992). Structural organization of the human insulin receptor ectodomain. *J. Biol. Chem.* **267,** 23393–23402.
43. Yip, C. C., and Jack, E. (1992). Insulin receptors are bivalent as demonstrated by photoaffinity labeling. *J. Biol. Chem.* **267,** 13131–13134.
44. Schumacher, R., Mosthaf, L., Schlessinger, J., Brandenburg, D., and Ullrich, A. (1991). Insulin and insulin-like growth factor-1 binding specificity is determined by distinct regions of their cognate receptors. *J. Biol. Chem.* **266,** 19288–19295.
45. Zhang, B., and Roth, R. A. (1991). Binding properties of chimeric insulin receptors containing the cysteine-rich domain of either the insulin-like growth factor I receptor or the insulin receptor related receptor. *Biochemistry* **30,** 5113–5117.
46. Schumacher, R., Soos, M. A., Schlessinger, J., Brandenburg, D., Siddle, K., and Ullrich, A. (1993). Signaling-competent receptor chimeras allow mapping of major insulin binding domain determinants. *J. Biol. Chem.* **268,** 1087–1094.
47. Frattali, A. L., Treadway, J. L., and Pessin, J. E. (1991). Evidence supporting a passive role for the insulin receptor transmembrane domain in insulin-dependent signal transduction. *J. Biol. Chem.* **266,** 9829–9834.
48. McClain, D. A. (1990). Endocytosis of insulin receptors is not required for activation or deactivation of the hormone response. *J. Biol. Chem.* **265,** 21363–21367.
49. Myers, M. G., Backer, J. M., Siddle, K., and White, M. F. (1991). The insulin receptor functions normally in chinese hamster ovary cells after truncation of the C terminus. *J. Biol. Chem.* **266,** 10616–10623.
50. Kaburagi, Y., Momomura, K., Yamamoto-Honda, R., Tobe, K., Tamori, Y., Sakura, H., Akanuma, Y., Yazaki, Y., and Kadowaki, T. (1993). Site-directed mutagenesis of the juxtamembrane domain of the human insulin receptor. *J. Biol. Chem.* **268,** 16610–16622.
51. Kapeller, R., Chen, K. S., Yoakim, M., Schaffhausen, B. S., Backer, J., White, M. F., Cantley, L. C., and Ruderman, N. B. (1991). Mutations in the juxtamembrane region of the insulin receptor impair activation of phosphatidylinositol 3-kinase by insulin. *Mol. Endocrinol.* **5,** 769–777.
52. Backer, J. M., Schroeder, G. G., Kahn, C. R., Myers, M. G., Wilden, P. A., Cahill, D. A., and White, M. F. (1992). Insulin stimulation of phosphatidylinositol 3-kinase activity maps to insulin receptor regions required for endogenous substrate phosphorylation. *J. Biol. Chem.* **267,** 1367–1374.

53. Myers, M. G., and White, M. F. (1993). The new elements of insulin signaling: Insulin receptor substrate-1 and proteins with SH2 domains. *Diabetes* **42,** 643–650.

54. Cherqui, G., Reynet, C., Caron, M., Melin, B., Wicek, D., Clauser, E., Capeau, J., and Picard, J. (1990). Insulin receptor tyrosine residues 1162 and 1163 control insulin stimulation of myristoyl-diacylglycerol generation and subsequent activation of glucose transport. *J. Biol. Chem.* **265,** 21254–21261.

55. Zhang, B., Tavaré, J. M., Ellis, L., and Roth, R. A. (1991). The regulatory role of known tyrosine autophosphorylation sites of the insulin receptor kinase domain: An assessment by replacement with neutral and negatively charged amino acids. *J. Biol. Chem.* **266,** 990–996.

56. Wilden, P. A., Backer, J. M., Kahn, C. R., Cahill, D. A., Schroeder, G. J., and White, M. F. (1990). The insulin receptor with phenylalanine replacing tyrosine-1146 provides evidence for separate signals regulating cellular metabolism and growth. *Proc. Natl. Acad. Sci. U.S.A.* **87,** 3358–3362.

57. Tavaré, J. M., and Siddle, K. (1993). Mutational analysis of insulin receptor function: Consensus and controversy. *Biochim. Biophys. Acta* **1178,** 21–29.

58. Begum, N., Olefsky, J. M., and Draznin, B. (1993). Mechanism of impaired metabolic signaling by a truncated human insulin receptor: Decreased activation of protein phosphatase 1 by insulin. *J. Biol. Chem.* **268,** 7917–7922.

59. Ando, A., Momomura, K., Tobe, K., Yamamoto-Honda, R., Sakura, H., Tamori, Y., Kaburagi, Y., Koshio, O., Akanuma, Y., Yazaki, Y., Kasuga, M., and Kadowaki, T. (1992). Enhanced insulin-induced mitogenesis and mitogen-activated protein kinase activities in mutant insulin receptors with substitution of two COOH-terminal tyrosine autophosphorylation sites by phenylalanine. *J. Biol. Chem.* **267,** 12788–12796.

60. Thies, R. S., Ullrich, A., and McClain, D. A. (1989). Augmented mitogenesis and impaired metabolic signaling mediated by a truncated insulin receptor. *J. Biol. Chem.* **264,** 12820–12825.

61. Smith, R. M., Sasaoka, T., Shah, N., Takata, Y., Kusari, J., Olefsky, J. M., and Jarett, L. (1993). A truncated human insulin receptor missing the COOH-terminal 365 amino acid residues does not undergo insulin mediated receptor migration or aggregation. *Endocrinol. (Baltimore)* **132,** 1453–1462.

62. Backer, J. M., Myers, M. G., Shoelson, S. E., Chin, D. J., Sun, X. J., Miralpeix, M., Hu, P., Margolis, B., Skolnik, E. Y., Schlessinger, J., and White, M. F. (1992). Phosphatidylinositol 3'-kinase is activated by association with IRS-1 during insulin stimulation. *EMBO J.* **11,** 3469–3479.

63. Folli, F., Saad, M. J. A., Backer, J. M., and Kahn, C. R. (1992). Insulin stimulation of phosphatidylinositol 3-kinase activity and association with insulin receptor substrate 1 in liver and muscle of the intact rat. *J. Biol. Chem.* **267,** 22171–22177.

64. Myers, M. G., Backer, J. M., Sun, X. J., Shoelson, S., Hu, P., Schlessinger, J., Yoakim, M., Schaffhausen, B., and White, M. F. (1992). IRS-1 activates phsophatidylinositol 3'-kinase by associating with *src* homology 2 domains of p85. *Proc. Natl. Acad. Sci. U.S.A.* **89,** 10350–10354.

65. Ives, H. E. (1991). GTP binding proteins and growth factor signal transduction. *Cell. Signal.* **3,** 491–499.

66. Kellerer, M., Obermaier-Kusser, B., Pröfrock, A., Schleicher, E., Seffer, E., Mushack, J., Ermel, B., and Häring, H. U. (1991). Insulin activates GTP binding to a 40 kDa protein in fat cells. *Biochem. J.* **276,** 103–108.

67. Saltiel, A. R. (1991). The role of glycosyl-phosphoinositides in hormone action. *J. Bioenerg. Biomembr.* **23**, 29–41.

68. Gottschalk, W. K. (1991). The pathway mediating insulin's effects on pyruvate dehydrogenase bypasses the insulin receptor tyrosine kinase. *J. Biol. Chem.* **266**, 8814–8819.

69. Gottshalk, W. K., Lammers, R., and Ullrich, A. (1992). The carboxy terminal 110 amino acid portion of the insulin receptor is important for insulin signalling to pyruvate dehydrogenase. *Biochem. Biophys. Res. Commun.* **189**, 906–911.

70. Moxham, C. P., Duronio, V., and Jacobs, S. (1989). Insulin-like growth factor I receptor β-subunit heterogeneity: Evidence for hybrid tetramers composed of insulin-like growth factor I and insulin receptor heterodimers. *J. Biol. Chem.* **264**, 13238–13244.

71. Treadway, J. L., Morrison, B. D., Goldfine, I. D., and Pessin, J. E. (1989). Assembly of insulin/insulin-like growth factor-1 hybrid receptors *in vitro*. *J. Biol. Chem.* **264**, 21450–21453.

72. Frattali, A. L., and Pessin, J. E. (1993). Relationship between α subunit ligand occupancy and β subunit autophosphorylation in insulin/insulin-like growth factor-1 hybrid receptors. *J. Biol. Chem.* **268**, 7393–7400.

73. Heldin, C. H., and Westermark, B. (1990). Signal transduction by the receptors for platelet-derived growth factor. *J. Cell Sci.* **96**, 193–196.

74. Givol, D., and Yayon, A. (1992). Complexity of FGF receptors: Genetic basis for structural diversity and functional specificity. *FASEB J.* **6**, 3362–3369.

75. Blechman, J. M., Lev, S., Givol, D., and Yarden, Y. (1993). Structure–function analyses of the Kit receptor for the Steel factor. *Stem Cells* **11** *(Suppl 2)*, 12–21.

76. Wang, Z., Myles, G. M., Brandt, C. S., Lioubin, M. N., and Rohrschneider, L. (1993). Identification of the ligand-binding regions in the macrophage colony-stimulating factor receptor extracellular domain. *Mol. Cell. Biol.* **13**, 5348–5359.

77. Chaudhuri, M. M., Moscatelli, D., and Basilico, C. (1993). Involvement of the conserved acidic amino acid domain of FGF receptor 1 in ligand-receptor interaction. *J. Cell. Physiol.* **157**, 209–216.

78. Werner, S., Duan, D. S. R., de Vries, C., Peters, K. G., Johnson, D. E., and Williams, L. T. (1992). Differential splicing in the extracellular region of fibroblast growth factor receptor 1 generates receptor variants with different ligand-binding specificities. *Mol. Cell. Biol.* **12**, 82–88.

79. Miki, T., Bottaro, D. P., Fleming, T. P., Smith, C. L., Burgess, W. H., Chan, A. M. L., and Aaronson, S. A. (1992). Determination of ligand-binding specificity by alternative splicing: Two distinct growth factor receptors encoded by a single gene. *Proc. Natl. Acad. Sci. U.S.A.* **89**, 246–250.

80. Yayon, A., Zimmer, Y., Guo-Hong, S., Avivi, A., Yarden, Y., and Givol, D. (1992). A confined variable region confers ligand specificity on fibroblast growth factor receptors: Implications for the origin of the immunoglobulin fold. *EMBO J.* **11**, 1885–1890.

81. Klagsbrun, M., and Baird, A. (1991). A dual receptor system is required for basic fibroblast growth factor activity. *Cell* **67**, 229–231.

82. Gitay-Goren, H., Soker, S., Vlodavsky, I., and Neufeld, G. (1992). The binding of vascular endothelial growth factor to its receptors is dependent on cell surface-associated heparin-like molecules. *J. Biol. Chem.* **267**, 6093–6098.

83. Kan, M., Wang, F., Xu, J., Crabb, J. W., Hou, J., and McKeehan, W. L. (1993). An essential heparin-binding domain in the fibroblast growth factor receptor kinase. *Science* **259**, 1918–1921.

84. Burrus, L. W., Zuber, M. E., Lueddecke, B. A., and Olwin, B. B. (1992). Identification of a cysteine-rich receptor for fibroblast growth factors. *Mol. Cell. Biol.* **12**, 5600–5609.

85. Fantl, W. J., Escobedo, J. A., Martin, G. A., Turck, C. W., del Rosario, M., McCormick, F., and Williams, L. T. (1992). Distinct phosphotyrosines on a growth factor receptor bind to specific molecules that mediate different signaling pathways. *Cell* **267**, 413–423.

86. Kashishian, A., Kazlauskas, A., and Cooper, J. A. (1992). Phosphorylation sites in the PDGF receptor with different specificities for binding GAP and PI3 kinase *in vivo*. *EMBO J.* **11**, 1373–1382.

87. Kazlauskas, A., Kashishian, A., Cooper, J. A., and Valius, M. (1992). GTPase-activating protein and phosphatidylinositol 3-kinase bind to distinct regions of the platelet-derived growth factor receptor β subunit. *Mol. Cell. Biol.* **12**, 2534–2544.

88. Rönnstrand, L., Mori, S., Arridsson, A. K., Eriksson, A., Wernstedt, C., Hellman, U., Claesson-Welsh, L., and Heldin, C. H. (1992). Identification of two C-terminal autophosphorylation sites in the PDGF β-receptor: Involvement in the interaction with phospholipase C-γ. *EMBO J.* **11**, 3911–3919.

89. Valius, M., Bazenet, C., and Kazlauskas, A. (1993). Tyrosines 1021 and 1009 are phosphorylation sites in the carboxy terminus of the platelet-derived growth factor receptor β subunit and are required for binding of phospholipase Cγ and a 64-kilodalton protein, respectively. *Mol. Cell. Biol.* **13**, 133–143.

90. Reedijk, M., Liu, X., van der Geer, P., Letwin, K., Waterfield, M. D., Hunter, T., and Pawson, T. (1992). Tyr721 requlates specific binding of the CSF-1 receptor kinase insert to PI 3'-kinase SH2 domains: A model for SH2-mediated receptor-target interactions. *EMBO J.* **11**, 1365–1372.

91. Mori, S., Claesson-Welsh, L., and Heldin, C. H. (1991). Identification of a hydrophobic region in the carboxyl terminus of the platelet-derived growth factor β-receptor which is important for ligand-mediated endocytosis. *J. Biol. Chem.* **266**, 21158–21164.

92. Claesson-Welsh, L., Eriksson, A., Westermark, B., and Heldin, C. H. (1989). cDNA cloning and expression of the human A-type platelet-derived growth factor (PDGF) receptor establishes structural similarity to the B-type PDGF receptor. *Proc. Natl. Acad. Sci. U.S.A.* **86**, 4917–4921.

93. Heldin, C. H., and Westermark, B. (1989). Platelet-derived growth factor: Three isoforms and two receptor types. *Trends Genet.* **5**, 108–111.

94. Seifert, R. A., Hart, C. E., Phillips, P. E., Forstrom, J. W., Ross, R., Murray, M. J., and Bowen-Pope, D. F. (1989). Two different subunits associate to create isoform-specific platelet-derived growth factor receptors. *J. Biol. Chem.* **264**, 8771–8778.

95. Blume-Jensen, P., Claesson-Welsh, L., Siegbahn, A., Zsebo, K. M., Westermark, B., and Heldin, C. H. (1991). Activation of the human c-*kit* product by ligand-induced dimerization mediates circular actin reorganization and chemotaxis. *EMBO J.* **10**, 4121–4128.

96. de Vries, C., Escobedo, J. A., Ueno, H., Houck, K., Ferrara, N., and Williams, L. T. (1992). The *fms*-like tyrosine kinase, a receptor for vascular endothelial growth factor. *Science* **255**, 989–991.

97. Bishayee, S., Majumdar, S., Khire, J., and Das, M. (1989). Ligand-induced dimerization of the platelet-derived growth factor receptor: Monomer–dimer interconversion occurs independent of receptor phosphorylation. *J. Biol. Chem.* **264**, 11699–11705.

98. Kanakaraj, P., Raj, S., Khan, S. A., and Bishayee, S. (1991). Ligand-induced interaction between α- and β-type platelet-derived growth factor (PDGF) receptors: Role of receptor heterodimers in kinase activations. *Biochemistry* **30**, 1761–1767.
99. Barker, P. A., and Murphy, R. A. (1992). The nerve growth factor receptor: A multicomponent system that mediates the actions of the neurotrophin family of proteins. *Mol. Cell. Biochem.* **110**, 1–15.
100. Meakin, S. O., and Shooter, E. M. (1992). The nerve growth factor family of receptors. *Trends Neurosci.* **15**, 323–331.
101. Glass, D. J., and Yancopoulos, G. D. (1993). The neurotrophins and their receptors. *Trends Cell Biol.* **3**, 262–268.
102. Ohmichi, M., Decker, S. J., and Saltiel, A. R. (1992). Activation of phosphatidy-linositol-3 kinase by nerve growth factor involves indirect coupling of the *trk* proto-oncogene with src homology 2 domains. *Neuron* **9**, 769–777.
103. Lamballe, F., Tapley, P., and Barbacid, M. (1993). *trk*C encodes multiple neurotrophin-3 receptors with distinct biological properties and substrate specificities. *EMBO J.* **12**, 3083–3094.
104. Hartman, D. S., McCormack, M., Schubenel, R., and Hertel, C. (1992). Multiple trkA proteins in PC12 cells bind NGF with a slow association rate. *J. Biol. Chem.* **267**, 24516–24522.
105. Soppet, D., Escandon, E., Maragos, J., Middlemas, D. S., Reid, S. W., Blair, J., Burton, L. E., Stanton, B. R., Kaplan, D. R., Hunter, T., Nikolics, K., and Parada, L. F. (1991). The neutrophic factors brain-derived neurotrophic factor and neurotrophin-3 are ligands for the *trk*B tyrosine kinase receptor. *Cell* **65**, 895–903.
106. Kahle, P., Burton, L. E., Schmelzer, C. H., and Hertel, C. (1992). The amino terminus of nerve growth factor is involved in the interaction with the receptor tyrosine kinase p140^{trkA}. *J. Biol. Chem.* **267**, 22707–22710.
107. Lee, K. F., Li, E., Huber, L. J., Landis, S. C., Sharpe, A. H., Chao, M. V., and Jaenisch, R. (1992). Targeted mutation of the gene encoding the low affinity NGF receptor p75 leads to deficits in the peripheral sensory nervous system. *Cell* **69**, 737–749.
108. Drinkwater, C. C., Suter, U., Angst, C., and Shooter, E. M. (1991). Mutation of tryptophan-21 in mouse nerve growth factor (NGF) affects binding to the fast NGF receptor but not induction of neurites on PC12 cells. *Proc. R. Soc. London B* **246**, 307–313.
109. Ibáñez, C. F., Ebendal, T., Barbany, G., Murray-Rust, J., Blundell, T. L., and Persson, H. (1992). Disruption of the low affinity receptor-binding site in NGF allows neuronal survival and differentiation by binding to the *trk* gene product. *Cell* **69**, 329–341.
110. Squinto, S. P., Stitt, T. N., Aldrich, T. H., Davis, S., Bianco, S. M., Radziejewski, C., Glass, D. J., Masiakowski, P., Furth, M. E., Valenzuela, D. M., DiStefano, P. S., and Yancopoulos, G. D. (1991). *trk*B encodes a functional receptor for brain-derived neurotrophic factor and neurotrophin-3 but not nerve growth factor. *Cell* **65**, 885–893.
111. Rovelli, G., Heller, R. A., Canossa, M., and Shooter, E. M. (1993). Chimeric tumor necrosis factor-TrkA receptors reveal that ligand-dependent activation of the TrkA tyrosine kinase is sufficient for differentiation and survival of PC12 cells. *Proc. Natl. Acad. Sci. U.S.A.* **90**, 8717–8721.
112. Jing, S., Tapley, P., and Barbacid, M. (1992). Nerve growth factor mediates signal transduction through trk homodimer receptors. *Neuron* **9**, 1067–1079.
113. Volonte, C., Ross, A. H., and Greene, L. A. (1993). Association of a purine-ana-

logue-sensitive protein kinase activity with p75 nerve growth factor receptors. *Mol. Biol. Cell* **4**, 71–78.

114. Rabizadeh, S., Oh, J., Zhong, L., Yang, J., Bitler, C. M., Butcher, L. L., and Bredesen, D. E. (1993). Induction of apoptosis by the low-affinity NGF receptor. *Science* **261**, 345–348.

115. Lin, H. Y., Wang, X. F., Ng-Eaton, E., Weinberg, R. A., and Lodish, H. F. (1992). Expression cloning of the TGF-β type II receptor, a functional transmembrane serine/threonine kinase. *Cell* **68**, 775–785.

116. Ebner, R., Chen, R. H., Shum, L., Lawler, S., Zioncheck, T. F., Lee, A., Lopez, A. R., and Derynck, R. (1993). Cloning of a type I TGF-β receptor and its effect on TGF-β binding to the type II receptor. *Science* **260**, 1344–1348.

117. Mathews, L. S., and Vale, W. W. (1991). Expression cloning of an activin receptor, a predicted transmembrane serine kinase. *Cell* **65**, 973–982.

118. Baarends, W. M., van Helmond, M. J. L., van der Schoot, P. J. C. M., Hooger-brugge, J. W., de Winter, J. P., Wilming, L. G., Meijers, J. H. C., Themmen, A. P. N., and Grootegoed, J. A. (1993). A novel member of the activin and TGF-β type II receptor gene family encodes the putative anti-müllerian hormone receptor. *Progr. Abstr. 75th Annu. Meet. Endocr. Soc.*, 299.

119. Mulder, K. M., and Morris, S. L. (1992). Activation of p21^{ras} by transforming growth factor β in epithelial cells. *J. Biol. Chem.* **267**, 5029–5031.

120. Pellegrini, S., and Schindler, C. (1993). Early events in signalling by interferons. *Trends Biochem. Sci.* **18**, 338–342.

121. Segarini, P. R. (1993). TGF-β receptors: A complicated system of multiple binding proteins. *Biochim. Biophys. Acta* **1155**, 269–275.

122. Attisano, L., Cárcamo, J., Ventura, F., Weis, F. M. B., Massagué, J., and Wrana, J. L. (1993). Identification of human activin and TGFβ type I receptors that form heterodimeric kinase complexes with type II receptors. *Cell* **75**, 671–680.

123. Ebner, R., Chen, R. H., Lawler, S., Zioncheck, T., and Derynck, R. (1993). Determination of type I receptor specificity by the type II receptors fro TGF-β or activin. *Science* **262**, 900–902.

124. Franzén, P., ten Dijke, P., Ichijo, H., Yamashita, H., Schulz, P., Heldin, C. H., and Miyazono, K. (1993). Cloning of a TGFβ type I receptor that forms a heteromeric complex with the TGFβ type II receptor. *Cell* **75**, 681–692.

125. López-Casillas, F., Wrana, J. L., and Massagué, J. (1993). Betaglycan presents ligand to the TGFβ signaling receptor. *Cell* **73**, 1435–1444.

126. Chen, R. H., Ebner, R., and Derynck, R. (1993). Inactivation of the type II receptor reveals two receptor pathways for the diverse TGF-β activities. *Science* **260**, 1335–1338.

127. Wrana, J. L., Attisano, L., Cárcamo, J., Zentella, A., Doody, J., Liaho, M., Wang, X. F., and Massagué, J. (1992). TGFβ signals through a heteromeric protein kinase receptor complex. *Cell* **71**, 1003–1014.

128. Koesling, D., Böhme, E., and Schultz, G. (1991). Guanylyl cyclases, a growing family of signal-transducing enzymes. *FASEB J.* **5**, 2785–2791.

129. Wong, S. K. F., and Garbers, D. L. (1992). Receptor guanylyl cyclases. *J. Clin. Invest.* **90**, 299–305.

130. Chinkers, M., Singh, S., and Garbers, D. L. (1991). Adenine nucleotides are required for activation of rat atrial natriuretic peptide receptor/guanylyl cyclase expressed in a baculovirus system. *J. Biol. Chem.* **266**, 4088–4093.

131. Goraczniak, R. M., Duda, T., and Sharma, R. K. (1992). A structural motif that

defines the ATP-regulatory module of guanylate cyclase in atrial natriuretic factor signalling. *Biochem. J.* **282**, 533–537.

132. Jewett, J. R. S., Koller, K. J., Goeddel, D. V., and Lowe, D. G. (1993). Hormonal induction of low affinity receptor guanylyl cyclase. *EMBO J.* **12**, 769–777.

133. Lowe, D. G. (1992). Human natriuretic peptide receptor-A guanylyl cyclase is self-associated prior to hormone binding. *Biochemistry* **31**, 10421–10425.

134. Iwata, T., Uchida-Mizuno, K., Katafuchi, T., Ito, T., Hagiwara, H., and Hirose, S. (1991). Bifunctional atrial natriuretic peptide receptor (type A) exists as a disulfide-linked tetramer in plasma membranes of bovine adrenal cortex. *J. Biochem. (Tokyo)* **110**, 35–39.

135. Larose, L., Rondeau, J. J., Ong, H., and De Léan, A. (1992). Phosphorylation of atrial natriuretic factor R_1 receptor by serine/threonine protein kinases: Evidences for receptor regulation. *Mol. Cell. Biochem.* **115**, 203–211.

136. Potter, L. R., and Garbers, D. L. (1992). Dephosphorylation of the guanylyl cyclase-A receptor causes desensitization. *J. Biol. Chem.* **267**, 14531–14534.

137. Sekiya, M., Vaugh, J., Shigematsu, Y., Frohlich, E. D., and Cole, F. E. (1991). Calcium and calmodulin regulate atrial natriuretic factor stimulation of cGMP in a human renal cell line. *Peptides* **12**, 1127–1133.

138. Schulz, S., Green, C. K., Yuen, P. S. T., and Garbers, D. L. (1990). Guanylyl cyclase is a heat-stable entertoxin receptor. *Cell* **63**, 941–948.

139. de Sauvage, F. J., Camerato, T. R., and Goeddel, D. V. (1991). Primary structure and functional expression of the human receptor for *Escherichia coli* heat-stable enterotoxin. *J. Biol. Chem.* **266**, 17912–17918.

140. Vaandrager, A. B., Schulz, S., De Jonge, H. R., and Garbers, D. L. (1993). Guanylyl cyclase C is an *N*-linked glycoprotein receptor that accounts for multiple heat-stable enterotoxin-binding proteins in the intestine. *J. Biol. Chem.* **268**, 2174–2179.

141. Schulz, S., Yuen, P. S. T., and Garbers, D. L. (1991). The expanding family of guanylyl cyclases. *Trends Pharmacol. Sci.* **12**, 116–120.

142. Anand-Srivastava, M. B., Sairam, M. R., and Cantin, M. (1990). Ring-deleted analogs of atrial natriuretic factor inhibit adenylate cyclase/cAMP system: Possible coupling of clearance atrial natriuretic factors receptors to adenylate cyclase/cAMP signal transduction system. *J. Biol. Chem.* **265**, 8566–8572.

143. Cahill, P. A., and Hassid, A. (1991). Clearance receptor-binding atrial natriuretic peptides inhibit mitogenesis and proliferation of rat aortic smooth muscle cells. *Biochem. Biophys. Res. Commun.* **179**, 1606–1613.

144. Schmidt, H. H. H. W., Lohmann, S. M., and Walter, U. (1993). The nitric oxide and cGMP signal transduction system: Regulation and mechanism of action. *Biochim. Biophys. Acta* **1178**, 153–175.

145. Harteneck, C., Koesling, D., Söling, A., Schultz, G., and Böhme, E. (1990). Expression of soluble guanylyl cyclase: Catalytic activity requires two enzyme subunits. *FEBS Lett.* **272**, 221–223.

146. Nakane, M., Arai, K., Saheki, S., Kuno, T., Buechler, W., and Murad, F. (1990). Molecular cloning and expression of cDNAs coding for soluble guanylate cyclase from rat lung. *J. Biol. Chem.* **265**, 16841–16845.

147. Buechler, W. A., Nakane, M., and Murad, F. (1991). Expression of soluble guanylate cyclase activity requires both enzyme subunits. *Biochem. Biophys. Res. Commun.* **174**, 351–357.

148. Knowles, R. G., and Moncada, S. (1992). Nitric oxide as a signal in blood vessels. *Trends Biochem. Sci.* **17**, 399–402.

149. Nakane, M., Mitchell, J., Förstermann, U., and Murad, F. (1991). Phosphorylation by calcium calmodulin-dependent protein kinase II and protein kinase C modulates the activity of nitric oxide synthase. *Biochem. Biophys. Res. Commun.* **180**, 1396–1402.

150. Bredt, D. S., Ferris, C. D., and Snyder, S. H. (1992). Nitric oxide synthase regulatory sites: Phosphorylation by cyclic AMP-dependent protein kinase, protein kinase C, and calcium/calmodulin protein kinase; identification of flavin and calmodulin binding sites. *J. Biol. Chem.* **267**, 10976–10981.

151. Michel, T., Li, G. K., and Busconi, L. (1993). Phosphorylation and subcellular translocation of endothelial nitric oxide synthase. *Proc. Natl. Acad. Sci. U.S.A.* **90**, 6252–6256.

152. Stamler, J. S., Jaraki, O., Osborne, J., Simon, D. I., Keaney, J., Vita, J., Singel, D., Valeri, C. R., and Loscalzo, J. (1992). Nitric oxide circulates in mammalian plasma primarily as an *S*-nitroso adduct of serum albumin. *Proc. Natl. Acad. Sci. U.S.A.* **89**, 7674–7677.

153. Hibert, M. F., Trumpp-Kallmeyer, S., Bruinvels, A., and Hoflack, J. (1991). Three-dimensional models of neurotransmitter G-binding protein-coupled receptors. *Mol. Pharmacol.* **40**, 8–15.

154. Oprian, D. D. (1992). The ligand-binding domain of rhodopsin and other G protein-linked receptors. *J. Bioenerg. Biomembr.* **24**, 211–217.

155. Kobilka, B. K., Kobilka, T. S., Daniel, K., Regan, J. W., Caron, M. G., and Lefkowitz, R. J. (1988). Chimeric α_2-, β_2-adrenergic receptors: Delineation of domains involved in effector coupling and ligand binding specificity. *Science* **240**, 1310–1316.

156. O'Dowd, B. F., Hnatowich, M., Regan, J. W., Leader, W. M., Caron, M. G., and Lefkowitz, R. J. (1988). Site-directed mutagenesis of the cytoplasmic domains of the human β_2-adrenergic receptor: Localization of regions involved in G protein–receptor coupling. *J. Biol. Chem.* **263**, 15985–15992.

157. Liggett, S. B., Caron, M. G., Lefkowitz, R. J., and Hnatowich, M. (1991). Coupling of a mutated form of the human β_2-adrenergic receptor to G_i and G_s: Requirement for multiple cytoplasmic domains in the coupling process. *J. Biol. Chem.* **266**, 4816–4821.

158. Shapiro, R. A., and Nathanson, N. M. (1989). Deletion analysis of the mouse m1 muscarinic acetylcholine receptor: Effects on phosphoinositide metabolism and down-regulation. *Biochemistry* **28**, 8946–8950.

159. Kubo, T., Bujo, H., Akiba, I., Nakai, J., Mishina, M., and Numa, S. (1988). Location of a region of the muscarinic acetylcholine receptor involved in selective effector coupling. *FEBS Lett.* **241**, 119–125.

160. Cotecchia, S., Exum, S., Caron, M. G., and Lefkowitz, R. J. (1990). Regions of the α_1-adrenergic receptor involved in coupling to phosphatidylinositol hydrolysis and enhanced sensitivity of biological function. *Proc. Natl. Acad. Sci. U.S.A.* **87**, 2896–2900.

161. Münch, G., Dees, C., Hekman, M., and Palm, D. (1991). Multisite contacts involved in coupling of the β-adrenergic receptor with the stimulatory guanine-nucleotide-binding regulatory protein: Structural and functional studies by β-receptor-site-specific synthetic peptides. *Eur. J. Biochem.* **198**, 357–364.

162. Zachary, I., Gil, J., Lehmann, W., Sinnett-Smith, J., and Rozengurt, E. (1991). Bombesin, vasopressin, and endothelin rapidly stimulate tyrosine phosphorylation in intact Swiss 3T3 cells. *Proc. Natl. Acad. Sci. U.S.A.* **88**, 4577–4581.

163. Zachary, I., Sinnett-Smith, J., and Rozengurt, E. (1991). Stimulation of tyrosine

kinase activity in anti-phosphotyrosine immune complexes of Swiss 3T3 cell lysates occurs rapidly after addition of bombesin, vasopressin, and endothelin to intact cells. *J. Biol. Chem.* **266**, 24126–24133.

164. Taniguchi, T., Kitagawa, H., Yasue, S., Yanagi, S., Sakai, K., Asahi, M., Ohta, S., Takeuchi, F., Nakamura, S., and Yamamura, H. (1993). Protein-tyrosine kinase p72^{syk} is activated by thrombin and is negatively regulated through Ca^{2+} mobilization in platelets. *J. Biol. Chem.* **268**, 2277–2279.

165. Gutkind, J. S., and Robbins, K. C. (1992). Activation of transforming G protein-coupled receptors induces rapid tyrosine phosphorylation of cellular proteins, including p125^{FAK} and the p130 v-*src* substrate. *Biochem. Biophys. Res. Commun.* **188**, 155–161.

166. Zachary, I., and Rozengurt, E. (1992). Focal adhesion kinase (p125^{FAK}): A point of convergence in the action of neuropeptides, integrins, and oncogenes. *Cell* **71**, 891–894.

167. Molly, C. J., Taylor, D. S., and Weber, H. (1993). Angiotensin II stimulation of rapid protein tyrosine phosphorylation and protein kinase activation in rat aortic smooth muscle cells. *J. Biol. Chem.* **268**, 7338–7345.

168. Kosugi, S., Okajima, F., Ban, T., Hidaka, A., Shenker, A., and Kohn, L. D. (1992). Mutation of alanine 623 in the third cytoplasmic loop of the rat thyrotropin (TSH) receptor results in a loss in the phosphoinositide but not cAMP signal induced by TSH and receptor autoantibodies. *J. Biol. Chem.* **267**, 24153–24156.

169. Guinebault, C., Payrastre, B., Sultan, C., Mauco, G., Breton, M., Levy-Toledano, S., Plantavid, M., and Chap, H. (1993). Tyrosine kinases and phosphoinositide metabolism in thrombin-stimulated human platelets. *Biochem. J.* **292**, 851–856.

170. Bouvier, M., Hausdorff, W. P., De Blasi, A., O'Dowd, B. F., Kobilka, B. K., Caron, M. G., and Lefkowitz, R. J. (1988). Removal of phosphorylation sites from the β_2-adrenergic receptor delays onset of agonist-promoted desensitization. *Nature (London)* **333**, 370–373.

171. Lameh, J., Philip, M., Sharma, Y. K., Moro, O., Ramachandran, J., and Sadée, W. (1992). Hm1 muscarinic cholinergic receptor internalization requires a domain in the third cytoplasmic loop. *J. Biol. Chem.* **267**, 13406–13412.

172. Nantel, F., Bonin, H., Emorine, L. J., Zilberfarb, V., Strosberg, A. D., Bouvier, M., and Marullo, S. (1993). The human β_3-adrenergic receptor is resistant to short term agonist-promoted desensitization. *Mol. Pharmacol.* **43**, 548–555.

173. Moffett, S., Mouillac, B., Bonin, H., and Bouvier, M. (1993). Altered phosphorylation and desensitization patterns of a human β_2-adrenergic receptor lacking the palmitoylated Cys341. *EMBO J.* **12**, 349–356.

174. Mouillac, B., Caron, M., Bonin, H., Dennis, M., and Bouvier, M. (1992). Agonist-modulated palmitoylation of β_2-adrenergic receptor in Sf9 cells. *J. Biol. Chem.* **267**, 21733–21737.

175. Vankoppen, C. J., and Nathanson, N. M. (1991). The cysteine residue in the carboxyl-terminal domain of the M2 muscarinic acetylcholine receptor is not required for receptor-mediated inhibition of adenylate cyclase. *J. Neurochem.* **57**, 1873–1877.

176. Kennedy, M. E., and Limbird, L. E. (1993). Mutations of the α_{2A}-adrenergic receptor that eliminate detectable palmitoylation do not perturb receptor-G-protein coupling. *J. Biol. Chem.* **268**, 8003–8011.

177. Humphrey, P. P. A., Hartig, P., and Hoyer, D. (1993). A proposed new nomenclature for 5-HT receptors. *Trends Pharmacol. Sci.* **14**, 233–236.

178. Burbach, J. P. H., and Meijer, O. C. (1992). The structure of neuropeptide receptors. *Eur. J. Pharmacol. Mol. Pharmacol.* **227,** 1–18.
179. Fong, T. M., Huang, R. R. C., and Strader, C. D. (1992). Localization of agonist and antagonist binding domains of the human neurokinin-1 receptor. *J. Biol. Chem.* **267,** 25664–25667.
180. Fong, T. M., Yu, H., Huang, R. R. C., and Strader, C. D. (1992). The extracellular domain of the neurokinin-1 receptor is required for high-affinity binding of peptides. *Biochemistry* **31,** 11806–11811.
181. Yokota, Y., Akazawa, C., Ohkubo, H., and Nakanishi, S. (1992). Delineation of structural domains involved in the subtype specificity of tachykinin receptors through chimeric formation of substance P/substance K receptors. *EMBO J.* **11,** 3585–3591.
182. Fong, T. M., Yu, H., and Strader, C. D. (1992). Molecular basis for the species selectivity of the neurokinin-1 receptor antagonists CP-96,345 and RP67580. *J. Biol. Chem.* **267,** 25668–25671.
183. Reinhart, J., Mertz, L. M., and Catt, K. J. (1992). Molecular cloning and expression of cDNA encoding the murine gonadotropin-releasing hormone receptor. *J. Biol. Chem.* **267,** 21281–21284.
184. Tsutsumi, M., Zhou, W., Millar, R. P., Mellon, P. L., Roberts, J. L., Flanagan, C. A., Dong, K., Gillo, B., and Sealfon, S. C. (1992). Cloning and function expression of a mouse gonadotropin-releasing hormone receptor. *Mol. Endocrinol.* **6,** 1163–1169.
185. Houamed, K. M., Kuijper, J. L., Gilbert, T. L., Haldeman, B. A., O'Hara, P. J., Mulvihill, E. R., Almers, W., and Hagen, F. S. (1991). Cloning, expression, and gene structure of a G protein-coupled glutamate receptor from rat brain. *Science* **252,** 1318–1321.
186. Masu, M., Tanabe, Y., Tsuchida, K., Shigemoto, R., and Nakanishi, S. (1991). Sequence and expression of a metabotropic glutamate receptor. *Nature (London)* **349,** 760–765.
187. Sugimoto, Y., Negishi, M., Hayashi, Y., Namba, T., Honda, A., Watabe, A., Hirata, M., Narumiya, S., and Ichikawa, A. (1993). Two isoforms of the EP_3 receptor with different carboxyl-terminal domains: Identical ligand binding properties and different coupling properties with G_i proteins. *J. Biol. Chem.* **268,** 2712–2718.
188. Prossnitz, E. R., Quehenberger, O., Cochrane, C. G., and Ye, R. D. (1993). The role of the third intracellular loop of the neutrophil N-formyl peptide receptor in G protein coupling. *Biochem. J.* **294,** 581–587.
189. Sprengel, R., Braun, T., Nikolics, K., Segaloff, D. L., and Seeburg, P. H. (1990). The testicular receptor for follicle stimulating hormone: Structure and functional expression of cloned cDNA. *Mol. Endocrinol.* **4,** 525–530.
190. Tsai-Morris, C. H., Buczko, E., Wang, W., and Dufau, M. L. (1990). Intronic nature of the rat luteinizing hormone receptor gene defines a soluble receptor subspecies with hormone binding activity. *J. Biol. Chem.* **265,** 19385–19388.
191. Xie, Y. B., Wang, H., and Segaloff, D. L. (1990). Extracellular domain of lutropin/choriogonadotropin receptor expressed in transfected cells binds choriogonadotropin with high affinity. *J. Biol. Chem.* **165,** 21411–21414.
192. Ji, I., and Ji, T. H. (1991). Exons 1-10 of the rat LH receptor encode a high affinity hormone binding site and exon 11 encodes G-protein modulation and a potential second hormone binding site. *Endocrinol. (Baltimore)* **128,** 2648–2650.
193. Ji, I., and Ji, T. H. (1991). Human choriogonadotropin binds to a lutropin

receptor with essentially no N-terminal extension and stimulates cAMP synthesis. *J. Biol. Chem.* **266**, 13076–13079.

194. Sprengel, R., and Seeburg, P. H. (1991). Engineering gonadotropin receptors with altered hormone specificity. *Progr. Abstr. 73rd Annu. Meet. Endocr. Soc.*, 159.

195. Sánchez-Yagüe, J., Rodríguez, M. C., Segaloff, D. L., and Ascoli, M. (1992). Truncation of the cytoplasmic tail of the lutropin/choriogonadotropin receptor prevents agonist-induced uncoupling. *J. Biol. Chem.* **267**, 7217–7220.

196. Nussenzveig, D. R., Heinflink, M., and Gershengorn, M. C. (1993). Agonist-stimulated internalization of the thyrotropin-releasing hormone receptor is dependent on two domains in the receptor carboxyl terminus. *J. Biol. Chem.* **268**, 2389–2392.

197. Vu, T. K. H., Hung, D. T., Wheaton, V. I., and Coughlin, S. R. (1991). Molecular cloning of a functional thrombin receptor reveals a novel proteolytic mechanism of receptor activation. *Cell* **64**, 1057–1068.

198. Vu, T. K. H., Wheaton, V. I., Hung, D. T., Charo, I., and Coughlin, S. R. (1991). Domains specifying thrombin-receptor interaction. *Nature (London)* **353**, 674–677.

199. Hoxie, J. A., Ahuja, M., Belmonte, E., Pizarro, S., Parton, R., and Brass, L. F. (1993). Internalization and recycling of activated thrombin receptors. *J. Biol. Chem.* **268**, 13756–13763.

200. Stroop, S. D., Thompson, D. L., Kuestner, R. E., and Moore, E. E. (1993). A recombinant human calcitonin receptor functions as an extracellular calcium sensor. *J. Biol. Chem.* **268**, 19927–19930.

201. Brown, E. M., Gamba, G., Riccardi, D., Lombardi, M., Butters, R., Kifor, O., Sun, A., Hediger, M. A., Lytton, J., and Hebert, S. C. (1993). Cloning and characterization of an extracellular Ca^{2+}-sensing receptor from bovine parathyroid. *Nature (London)* **366**, 575–580.

202. Konopka, J. B., Jenness, D. D., and Hartwell, L. H. (1988). The C-terminus of the *S. cerevisiae* α-pheromone receptor mediates an adaptive response to pheromone. *Cell* **54**, 609–620.

203. Reneke, J. E., Blumer, K. J., Courchesne, W. E., and Thorner, J. (1988). The carboxy-terminal segment of the yeast α-factor receptor is a regulatory domain. *Cell* **55**, 221–234.

204. Houamed, K. M., Kuijper, J. L., Gilbert, T. L., Haldeman, B. A., O'Hara, P. J., Mulvihill, E. R., Almers, W., and Hagen, F. S. (1991). Cloning, expression, and gene structure of a G protein-coupled glutamate receptor from rat brain. *Science* **252**, 1318–1321.

205. O'Hara, P. J., Sheppard, P. O., Thøersen, H., Venezia, D., Haldeman, B. A., McGrane, V., Houamed, K. M., Thomsen, C., Gilbert, T. L., and Mulvihill, E. R. (1993). The ligand-binding domain in metabotropic glutamate receptors is related to bacterial periplasmic binding proteins. *Neuron* **11**, 41–52.

206. Heaney, M. L., and Golde, D. W. (1993). Soluble hormone receptors. *Blood* **82**, 1945–1948.

207. Taga, T., and Kishimoto, T. (1992). Cytokine receptors and signal transduction. *FASEB J.* **6**, 3387–3396.

208. de Vos, A. M., Ultsch, M., and Kossiakoff, A. A. (1992). Human growth hormone and extracellular domain of its receptor: Crystal structure of the complex. *Science* **255**, 306–312.

209. Beattie, J. (1993). Structural and functional aspects of the interaction between growth hormone and its receptor. *Biochim. Biophys. Acta* **1203**, 1–10.

210. Bass, S. H., Mulkerrin, M. G., and Wells, J. A. (1991). A systematic mutational analysis of hormone-binding determinants in the human growth hormone receptor. *Proc. Natl. Acad. Sci. U.S.A.* **88,** 4498–4502.
211. Wang, H. M., Ogorochi, T., Arai, K., and Miyajima, A. (1992). Structure of mouse interleukin 3 (IL-3) binding protein (AIC2A): Amino acid residues critical for IL-3 binding. *J. Biol. Chem.* **267,** 979–983.
212. Yawata, H., Yasukawa, K., Natsuka, S., Murakami, M., Yamasaki, K., Hibi, M., Taga, T., and Kishimoto, T. (1993). Structure-function analysis of human IL-6 receptor: Dissociation of amino acid residues required for IL-6-binding and for IL-6 signal transduction through gp130. *EMBO J.* **12,** 1705–1712.
213. Duriez, B., Sobrier, M. L., Duquesnoy, P., Tixier-Boichard, M., Decuypere, E., Coquerelle, G., Zeman, M., Goossens, M., and Amselem, S. (1993). A naturally occurring growth hormone receptor mutation: *In vivo* and *in vitro* evidence for the functional importance of the WS motif common to all members of the cytokine receptor superfamily. *Mol. Endocrinol.* **7,** 806–814.
214. Yoshimura, A., Zimmers, T., Neumann, D., Longmore, G., Yoshimura, Y., and Lodish, H. F. (1992). Mutations in the Trp-Ser-X-Trp-Ser motif of the erythropoietin receptor abolish processing, ligand binding, and activation of the receptor. *J. Biol. Chem.* **267,** 11619–11625.
215. Stahl, N., and Yancopoulos, G. D. (1993). The alphas, betas, and kinases of cytokine receptor complexes. *Cell* **74,** 587–590.
216. Milburn, M. V., Hassell, A. M., Lambert, M. H., Jordan, S. R., Proudfoot, A. E. I., Graber, P., and Wells, T. N. C. (1993). A novel dimer configuration revealed by the crystal structure at 2.4 Å resolution of human interleukin-5. *Nature (London)* **363,** 172–176.
217. Minami, Y., Kono, T., Yamada, K., and Taniguchi, T. (1992). The interleukin-2 receptors: Insights into a complex signalling mechanism. *Biochim. Biophys. Acta* **1114,** 163–177.
218. Asao, H., Takeshita, T., Ishii, N., Kumaki, S., Nakamura, M., and Sugamura, K. (1993). Reconstitution of functional interleukin 2 receptor complexes on fibroblastoid cells: Involvement of the cytoplasmic domain of the q chain in two distinct signaling pathways. *Proc. Natl. Acad. Sci. U.S.A.* **90,** 4127–4131.
219. Hatakeyama, M., Mori, H., Doi, T., and Taniguchi, T. (1989). A restricted cytoplasmic region of IL-2 receptor β chain is essential for growth signal transduction but not for ligand binding and internalization. *Cell* **59,** 837–845.
220. Hatakeyama, M., Kono, T., Kobayashi, N., Kawahara, A., Levin, S. D., Perlmutter, R. M., and Taniguchi, T. (1991). Interaction of the IL-2 receptor with the src-family kinase p56^{lck}: Identification of novel intermolecular association. *Science* **252,** 1523–1528.
221. Tsygankov, A., and Bolen, J. (1993). The Src family of tyrosine protein kinases in hemopoietic signal transduction. *Stem Cells* **11,** 371–380.
222. Kishimoto, T., Taga, T., and Akira, S. (1994). Cytokine signal transduction. *Cell* **76,** 253–262.
223. Maslinski, W., Remillard, B., Hadro, E., and Strom, T. B. (1991). Interleukin-2 induces translocation of active serine/threonine kinase Raf-1 from IL-2 receptor beta chain to cytosol. *J. Cell Biol.* **115,** 273a.
224. Remillard, B., Petrillo, R., Maslinski, W., Tsudo, M., Strom, T. B., Cantley, L., and Varticovski, L. (1991). Interleukin-2 receptor regulates activation of phosphatidylinositol 3-kinase. *J. Biol. Chem.* **266,** 14167–14170.
225. Otani, H., Siegel, J. P., Erdos, M., Gnarra, J. R., Toledano, M. B., Sharon, M.,

Mostowski, H., Feinberg, M. B., Pierce, J. H., and Leonard, W. J. (1992). Interleukin (IL)-2 and IL-3 induce distinct but overlapping responses in murine IL-3-dependent 32D cells transduced with human IL-2 receptor β chain: Involvement of tyrosine kinase(s) other than p56^{lck}. *Proc. Natl. Acad. Sci. U.S.A.* **89,** 2789–2793.

226. Torigoe, T., O'Connor, R., Fagard, R., Fischer, S., Santoli, D., and Reed, J. C. (1992). Regulation of SRC-family protein tyrosine kinases by interleukins, IL-2, and IL-3. *Leukemia* **6,** S94–S97.

227. Witthuhn, B. A., Quelle, F. W., Silvennoinen, O., Yi, T., Tang, B., Miura, O., and Ihle, J. N. (1993). JAK2 associates with the erythropoietin receptor and is tyrosine phosphorylated and activated following stimulation with erythropoietin. *Cell* **74,** 227–236.

228. Bolen, J. B., Rowley, R. B., Spana, C., and Tsygankov, A. Y. (1992). The Src family of tyrosine protein kinases in hemopoietic signal transduction. *FASEB J.* **6,** 3403–3409.

229. Velazquez, L., Fellous, M., Stark, G. R., and Pellegrini, S. (1992). A protein tyrosine kinase in the interferon α/β signaling pathway. *Cell* **70,** 313–322.

230. Pleiman, C. M., Clark, M. R., Gauen, L. K. T., Winitz, S., Coggeshall, K. M., Johnson, G. L., Shaw, A. S., and Cambier, J. C. (1993). Mapping of sites on the Src family protein tyrosine kinases p55^{blk}, p59^{fyn}, and p56^{lyn} which interact with the effector molecules phospholipase C-γ2, microtubule-associated protein kinase, GTPase-activating protein, and phosphatidylinositol 3-kinase. *Mol. Cell. Biol.* **13,** 5877-5887.

231. Lütticken, C., Wegenka, U. M., Yuan, J., Buschmann, J., Schindler, C., Ziemiecki, A., Harpur, A. G., Wilks, A. F., Yasukawa, K., Taga, T., Kishimoto, T., Barbieri, G., Pellegrini, S., Sendtner, M., Heinrich, P. C., and Horn, F. (1994). Association of transcription factor APRF and protein kinase Jak1 with the interleukin-6 signal transducer gp130. *Science* **263,** 89–92.

232. Stahl, N., Boulton, T. G., Farruggella, T., Ip, N. Y., Davis, S., Witthuhn, B. A., Quelle, F. W., Silvennoinen, O., Barbieri, G., Pellegrini, S., Ihle, J. N., and Yancopoulos, G. D. (1994). Association and activation of Jak-Tyk kinases by CNTF-LIF-OSM-IL-6 β receptor components. *Science* **263,** 92–95.

233. Kondo, M., Takeshita, T., Ishii, N., Nakamura, M., Watanabe, S., Arai, K., and Sugamura, K. (1993). Sharing of the interleukin-2 (IL-2) receptor γ chain between receptors for IL-2 and IL-4. *Science* **262,** 1874–1877.

234. Noguchi, M., Nakamura, Y., Russell, S. M., Ziegler, S. F., Tsang, M., Cao, X., and Leonard, W. J. (1993). Interleukin-2 receptor γ chain: A functional component of the interleukin-7 receptor. *Science* **262,** 1877–1880.

235. Russell, S. M., Keegan, A. D., Harada, N., Nakamura, Y., Noguchi, M., Leland, P., Friedmann, M. C., Miyajima, A., Puri, R. K., Paul, W. E., and Leonard, W. J. (1993). Interleukin-2 receptor γ chain: A functional component of the interleukin-4 receptor. *Science* **262,** 1880–1883.

236. Devos, R., Guisez, Y., Cornelis, S., Verhee, A., Van der Heyden, J., Manneberg, M., Lahm, H. W., Fiers, W., Tavernier, J., and Plaetinck, G. (1993). Recombinant soluble human interleukin-5 (hIL-5) receptor molecules: Cross-linking and stoichiometry of binding to IL-5. *J. Biol. Chem.* **268,** 6581–6587.

237. Fukunaga, R., Ishizaka-Ikeda, E., Pan, C. X., Seto, Y., and Nagata, S. (1991). Functional domains of the granulocyte colony-stimulating factor receptor. *EMBO J.* **10,** 2855–2865.

238. Cunningham, B. C., Ultsch, M., de Vos, A. M., Mulkerrin, M. G., Clauser, K. R.,

and Wells, J. A. (1991). Dimerization of the extracellular domain of the human growth hormone receptor by a single hormone molecule. *Science* **254**, 821–825.

239. Murakami, M., Hibi, M., Nakagawa, N., Nakagawa, T., Yasukawa, K., Yamanishi, K., Taga, T., and Kishimoto, T. (1993). IL-6-induced homodimerization of gp130 and associated activation of a tyrosine kinase. *Science* **260**, 1808–1810.

240. Davis, S., Aldrich, T. H., Stahl, N., Pan, L., Taga, T., Kishimoto, T., Ip, N. Y., and Yancopoulos, G. D. (1993). LIFRβ and gp130 as heterodimerizing signal transducers of the tripartite CNTF receptor. *Science* **260**, 1805–1808.

241. Davis, S., Aldrich, T. H., Valenzuela, D. M., Wong, V., Furth, M. E., Squinto, S. P., and Yancopoulos, G. D. (1991). The receptor for ciliary neurotrophic factor. *Science* **253**, 59–63.

242. Davis, S., Aldrich, T. H., Ip, N. Y., Stahl, N., Scherer, S., Farruggella, T., DiStefano, P. S., Curtis, R., Panayotatos, N., Gascan, H., Chevalier, S., and Yancopoulos, G. D. (1993). Released form of CNTF receptor α component as a soluble mediator of CNTF responses. *Science* **259**, 1736–1739.

243. Suzuki, H., Yasukawa, K., Saito, T., Narazaki, M., Hasegawa, A., Taga, T., and Kishimoto, T. (1993). Serum soluble interleukin-6 receptor in MRL/lpr mice is elevated with age and mediates the interleukin-6 signal. *Eur. J. Immunol.* **23**, 1078–1082.

244. Banner, D. W., D'Arcy, A., Janes, W., Gentz, R., Schoenfeld, H. J., Broger, C., Loetscher, H., and Lesslauer, W. (1993). Crystal structure of the soluble human 55 kd TNF receptor-human TNFβ complex: Implications for TNF receptor activation. *Cell* **73**, 431–445.

245. Hsu, K. C., and Chao, M. V. (1993). Differential expression and ligand binding properties of tumor necrosis factor receptor chimeric mutants. *J. Biol. Chem.* **268**, 16430–16436.

246. Welcher, A. A., Bitler, C. M., Radeke, M. J., and Shooter, E. M. (1991). Nerve growth factor binding domain of the nerve growth factor receptor. *Proc. Natl. Acad. Sci. U.S.A.* **88**, 159–163.

247. Baldwin, A. N., Bitler, C. M., Welcher, A. A., and Shooter, E. M. (1992). Studies on the structure and binding properties of the cysteine-rich domain of rat low affinity nerve growth factor receptor (p75^{NGFR}). *J. Biol. Chem.* **267**, 8352–8359.

248. Tartaglia, L. A., Pennica, D., and Goeddel, D. V. (1993). Ligand passing: The 75-kDa tumor necrosis factor (TNF) receptor recruits TNF for signaling by the 55-kDa TNF receptor. *J. Biol. Chem.* **268**, 18542–18548.

249. Marsters, S. A., Frutkin, A. D., Simpson, N. J., Fendly, B. M., and Ashkenazi, A. (1992). Identification of cysteine-rich domains of the type 1 tumor necrosis factor receptor involved in ligand binding. *J. Biol. Chem.* **267**, 5747-5750.

250. Zhang, X. M., Weber, I., and Chen, M. J. (1992). Site-directed mutational analysis of human tumor necrosis factor-α receptor binding site and structure–functional relationship. *J. Biol. Chem.* **267**, 24069–24075.

251. Loetscher, H., Schlaeger, E. J., Lahm, H. W., Pan, Y. C., Lesslauer, W., and Brockhaus, M. (1990). Purification and partial amino acid sequence analysis of two distinct tumor necrosis factor receptors from HL60 cells. *J. Biol. Chem.* **265**, 20131–20138.

252. Wiegmann, K., Schütze, S., Kampen, E., Himmler, A., Machleidt, T., and Krönke, M. (1992). Human 55-kDa receptor for tumor necrosis factor coupled to signal transduction cascades. *J. Biol. Chem.* **267**, 17997–18001.

253. Yanaga, F., and Watson, S. P. (1992). Tumor necrosis factor α stimulates sphingomyelinase through the 55 kDa receptor in HL-60 cells. *FEBS Lett.* **314**, 297–300.

254. Hayakawa, M., Hori, T., Shibamoto, S., Tsujimoto, M., Oku, N., and Ito, F. (1991). Solubilization of human placental tumor necrosis factor receptors as a complex with a guanine nucleotide-binding protein. *Arch. Biochem. Biophys.* **286,** 323–329.

255. Ealick, S. E., Cook, W. J., Vijay-Kumar, S., Carson, M., Nagabhushan, T. L., Trotta, P. P., and Bugg, C. E. (1991). Three-dimensional structure of recombinant human interferon-γ. *Science* **252,** 698–702.

256. Bazan, J. F. (1990). Shared architecture of hormone binding domains in type I and II interferon receptors. *Cell* **61,** 753–754.

257. Gaboriaud, C., Uzé, G., Lutfalla, G., and Mogensen, K. (1990). Hydrophobic cluster analysis reveals duplication in the external structure of human α-interferon receptor and homology with γ-interferon receptor external domain. *FEBS Lett.* **269,** 1–3.

258. Hershey, G. K. K., McCourt, D. W., and Schreiber, R. D. (1990). Ligand-induced phosphorylation of the human interferon-q receptor: Dependence on the presence of a functionally active receptor. *J. Biol. Chem.* **265,** 17868–17875.

259. Fountoulakis, M., Zulauf, M., Lustig, A., and Garotta, G. (1992). Stoichiometry of interaction between interferon γ and its receptor. *Eur. J. Biochem.* **208,** 781–787.

260. Mathias, S., Younes, A., Kan, C. C., Orlow, I., Joseph, C., and Kolesnick, R. N. (1993). Activation of the sphingomyelin signaling pathway in intact EL4 cells and in a cell-free system by IL-1β. *Science* **259,** 519–522.

261. O'Neill, L. A. J., Bird, T. A., Gearing, A. J. H., and Saklatvala, J. (1990). Interleukin-1 signal transduction: Increased GTP binding and hydrolysis in membranes of a murine thymoma line (EL4). *J. Biol. Chem.* **265,** 3146–3152.

262. Moore, M. D., Cooper, N. R., Tack, B. F., and Nemerow, G. R. (1987). Molecular cloning of the cDNA encoding the Epstein–Barr virus/C3d receptor (complement receptor type 2) of human B lymphocytes. *Proc. Natl. Acad. Sci. U.S.A.* **84,** 9194–9198.

263. Delcayre, A. X., Salas, F., Mathur, S., Kovats, K., Lotz, M., and Lernhardt, W. (1991). Epstein–Barr virus/complement C3d receptor is an interferon α receptor. *EMBO J.* **10,** 919–926.

264. Williams, B. R. G. (1991). Transcriptional regulation of interferon-stimulated genes. *Eur. J. Biochem.* **200,** 1–11.

265. Frade, R., Gauffre, A., Hermann, J., and Barel, M. (1992). EBV/C3d receptor (CR2) interacts by its intracytoplasmic carboxy-terminal domain and two distinct binding sites with the p53 anti-oncoprotein and the p68 calcium-binding protein. *J. Immunol.* **149,** 3232–3238.

266. Watanabe, H., Carmi, P., Hogan, V., Raz, T., Silletti, S., Nabi, I. R., and Raz, A. (1991). Purification of human tumor cell autocrine motility factor and molecular cloning of its receptor. *J. Biol. Chem.* **266,** 13442–13448.

267. Westlund, B., Dahms, N. M., and Kornfeld, S. (1991). The bovine mannose 6-phosphate/insulin-like growth factor II receptor: Localization of mannose 6-phosphate binding sites to domains 1-3 and 7-11 of the extracytoplasmic region. *J. Biol. Chem.* **266,** 23233–23239.

268. Rogers, S. A., and Hammerman, M. R. (1989). Mannose 6-phosphate potentiates insulin-like growth factor II-stimulated inositol trisphosphate production in proximal tubular basolateral membranes. *J. Biol. Chem.* **264,** 4273–4276.

269. Okamoto, T., Katada, T., Murayama, Y., Ui, M., Ogata, E., and Nishimoto, I. (1990). A simple structure encodes G protein-activating function of the IGF-II/mannose 6-phosphate receptor. *Cell* **62,** 709–717.

270. Méresse, S., Ludwig, T., Frank, R., and Hoflack, B. (1990). Phosphorylation of the cytoplasmic domain of the bovine cation-independent mannose 6-phosphate receptor: Serines 2421 and 2492 are the targets of a casein kinase II associated to the Golgi-derived HAI adaptor complex. *J. Biol. Chem.* **265,** 18833–18842.

271. Westcott, K. R., and Rome, L. H. (1988). Cation-independent mannose 6-phosphate receptor contains covalently bound fatty acid. *J. Cell. Biochem.* **38,** 23–33.

272. Dahms, N. M., Lobel, P., and Kornfeld, S. (1989). Mannose 6-phosphate receptors and lysosomal enzyme targeting. *J. Biol. Chem.* **264,** 12115–12118.

273. Canfield, W. M., and Kornfield, S. (1989). The chicken liver cation-independent mannose 6-phosphate receptor lacks the high affinity binding site for insulin-like growth factor II. *J. Biol. Chem.* **264,** 7100–7103.

274. Clairmont, K. B., and Czech, M. P. (1989). Chicken and *Xenopus* mannose 6-phosphate receptors fail to bind insulin-like growth factor II. *J. Biol. Chem.* **264,** 16390–16392.

275. Yang, Y. W. H., Robbins, A. R., Nissley, S. P., and Rechler, M. M. (1991). The chick embryo fibroblast cation-independent mannose 6-phosphate receptor is functional and immunologically related to the mammalian insulin-like growth factor-II (IGF-II)/Man 6-P receptor but does not bind IGF-II. *Endocrinol. (Baltimore)* **128,** 1177–1189.

276. Bondy, C. A., Werner, H., Roberts, C. T., and LeRoith, D. (1990). Cellular pattern of insulin-like growth factor-I (IGF-I) and type I IGF receptor gene expression in early organogenesis: Comparison with IGF-II gene expression. *Mol. Endocrinol.* **4,** 1386–1398.

277. Sakano, K., Enjoh, T., Numata, F., Fujiwara, H., Marumoto, Y., Higashihashi, N., Sato, Y., Perdue, J. F., and Fujita-Yamaguchi, Y. (1991). The design, expression, and characterization of human insulin-like growth factor II (IGF-II) mutants specific for either the IGF-II/cation-independent mannose 6-phosphate receptor or IGF-I receptor. *J. Biol. Chem.* **266,** 20626–20635.

278. Weber, M. M., Melmed, S., Rosenbloom, J., Yamasaki, H., and Prager, D. (1992). Rat somatotroph insulin-like growth factor-II (IGF-II) signaling: Role of the IGF-I receptor. *Endocrinol. (Baltimore)* **131,** 2147–2153.

279. Francis, G. L., Aplin, S. E., Milner, S. J., McNeil, K. A., Wallace, J. C., and Ballard, F. J. (1993). Why is IGF-II generally less potent than IGF-I? *Progr. Abstr. 75th Annu. Meet. Endocr. Soc.*, 173.

280. Kojima, I., Nishimoto, I., Iiri, T., Ogata, E., and Rosenfeld, R. (1988). Evidence that type II insulin-like growth factor receptor is coupled to calcium gating system. *Biochem. Biophys. Res. Commun.* **154,** 9–19.

281. Nishimoto, I., Murayama, Y., Katada, T., Ui, M., and Ogata, E. (1989). Possible direct linkage of insulin-like growth factor-II receptor with guanine nucleotide-binding proteins. *J. Biol. Chem.* **264,** 14029–14038.

282. Okamoto, T., Nishimoto, I., Murayama, Y., Ohkuni, Y., and Ogata, E. (1990). Insulin-like growth factor-II/mannose 6-phosphate receptor is incapable of activating GTP-binding proteins in response to mannose 6-phosphate, but capable in response to insulin-like growth factor-II. *Biochem. Biophys. Res. Commun.* **168,** 1201–1210.

283. Minniti, C. P., Kohn, E. C., Grubb, J. H., Sly, W. S., Oh, W., Müller, H. L., Rosenfeld, R. G., and Helman, L. J. (1992). The insulin-like growth factor II (IGF-II)/mannose 6-phosphate receptor mediates IGF-II-induced motility in human rhabdomyosarcoma cells. *J. Biol. Chem.* **267,** 9000–9004.

284. Unwin, N. (1993). Neurotransmitter action: Opening of ligand-gated ion channels. *Cell* **72** *(Suppl.)*, 31–41.
285. Langosch, D., Becker, C. M., and Betz, H. (1990). The inhibitory glycine receptor: A ligand-gated chloride channel of the central nervous system. *Eur. J. Biochem.* **194**, 1–8.
286. DeLorey, T. M., and Olsen, R. W. (1992). γ-Aminobutyric acid$_A$ receptor structure and function. *J. Biol. Chem.* **267**, 16747–16750.
287. Galzi, J. L., Revah, F., Bessis, A., and Changeux, J. P. (1991). Functional architecture of the nicotinic acetylcholine receptor: From electric organ to brain. *Annu. Rev. Pharmacol.* **31**, 37–72.
288. Imoto, K., Konno, T., Nakai, J., Wang, F., Mishina, M., and Numa, S. (1991). A ring of uncharged polar amino acids as a component of channel constriction in the nicotinic acetylcholine receptor. *FEBS Lett.* **289**, 193–200.
289. Golino, M. D., and Hamill, O. P. (1992). Subunit requirements for *Torpedo* AChR channel expression: A specific role for the δ-subunit in voltage-dependent gating. *J. Membr. Biol.* **129**, 297–309.
290. Sine, S. M., and Claudio, T. (1991). γ- and δ-subunits regulate the affinity and the cooperativity of ligand binding to the acetylcholine receptor. *J. Biol. Chem.* **266**, 19369–19377.
291. Czajkowski, C., Kaufmann, C., and Karlin, A. (1993). Negatively charged amino acid residues in the nicotinic receptor δ subunit that contribute to the binding of acetylcholine. *Proc. Natl. Acad. Sci. U.S.A.* **90**, 6285–6289.
292. Froehner, S. C. (1991). The submembrane machinery for nicotinic acetylcholine receptor clustering. *J. Cell Biol.* **114**, 1–7.
293. Devillers-Thiery, A., Galzi, J. L., Eiselé, J. L., Bertrand, S., Bertrand, D., and Changeux, J. P. (1993). Functional architecture of the nicotinic acetylcholine receptor: A prototype of ligand-gated ion channels. *J. Membr. Biol.* **136**, 97–112.
294. Revah, F., Bertrand, D., Galzi, J. L., Devillers-Thiéry, A., Mulle, C., Hussy, N., Bertrand, S., Ballivet, M., and Changeux, J. P. (1991). Mutations in the channel domain alter desensitization of a neuronal nicotinic receptor. *Nature (London)* **353**, 846–849.
295. Unwin, N. (1993). Nicotinic acetylcholine receptor at 9 Å resolution. *J. Mol. Biol.* **229**, 1101–1124.
296. Green, W. N., Ross, A. F., and Claudio, T. (1991). Acetylcholine receptor assembly is stimulated by phosphorylation of its γ subunit. *Neuron* **7**, 659–666.
297. Mei, L., and Huganir, R. L. (1991). Purification and characterization of a protein tyrosine phosphatase which dephosphorylates the nicotinic acetylcholine receptor. *J. Biol. Chem.* **266**, 16063–16072.
298. Kellenberger, S., Malherbe, P., and Sigel, E. (1992). Function of the $\alpha1\beta2\gamma2S$ γ-aminobutyric acid type A receptor is modulated by protein kinase C via multiple phosphorylation sites. *J. Biol. Chem.* **267**, 25660–25663.
299. Moss, S. J., Smart, T. G., Blackstone, C. D., and Huganir, R. L. (1992). Functional modulation of GABA$_A$ receptors by cAMP-dependent protein phosphorylation. *Science* **257**, 661–665.
300. Swope, S. L., Moss, S. J., Blackstone, C. D., and Huganir, R. L. (1992). Phosphorylation of ligand-gated ion channels: A possible mode of synaptic plasticity. *FASEB J.* **6**, 2514–2523.
301. Nakanishi, S. (1992). Molecular diversity of glutamate receptors and implications for brain function. *Science* **258**, 597–603.
302. Keller, B. U., Hollmann, M., Heinemann, S., and Konnerth, A. (1992). Calcium

influx through subunits GluR1/GluR3 of kainate/AMPA receptor channels is regulated by cAMP dependent protein kinase. *EMBO J.* **11**, 891–896.

303. Egebjerg, J., Bettler, B., Hermans-Borgmeyer, I., and Heinemann, S. (1991). Cloning of a cDNA for a glutamate receptor subunit activated by kainate but not AMPA. *Nature (London)* **351**, 745–748.
304. Werner, P., Voigt, M., Keinänen, K., Wisden, W., and Seeburg, P. H. (1991). Cloning of a putative high-affinity kainate receptor expressed predominantly in hippocampal CA3 cells. *Nature (London)* **351**, 742–744.
305. McGlade-McCulloh, E., Yamamoto, H., Tan, S. E., Brickey, D. A., and Soderling, T. R. (1993). Phosphorylation and regulation of glutamate receptors by calcium/calmodulin-dependent protein kinase II. *Nature (London)* **362**, 640–642.
306. Willard, J. M., and Oswald, R. E. (1992). Interaction of the frog brain kainate receptor expressed in Chinese hamster ovary cells with a GTP-binding protein. *J. Biol. Chem.* **267**, 19112–19116.
307. Scott, R. H., Sutton, K. G., and Dolphin, A. C. (1993). Interactions of polyamines with neuronal ion channels. *Trends Neurosci.* **16**, 153–160.
308. Petrou, S., Ordway, R. W., Singer, J. J., and Walsh, J. V. (1993). A putative fatty acid-binding domain of the NMDA receptor. *Trends Biochem. Sci.* **18**, 41–42.
309. Kitamura, Y., Miyazaki, A., Yamanaka, Y., and Nomura, Y. (1993). Stimulatory effects of protein kinase C and calmodulin kinase II on N-methyl-D-aspartate receptor/channels in the postsynaptic density of rat brain. *J. Neurochem.* **61**, 100–109.
310. Tingley, W. G., Roche, K. W., Thompson, A. K., and Huganir, R. L. (1993). Regulation of NMDA receptor phosphorylation by alternative splicing of the C-terminal domain. *Nature (London)* **364**, 70–73.
311. Durand, G. M., Bennett, M. V. L., and Zukin, R. S. (1993). Splice variants of the N-methyl-D-aspartate receptor NR1 identify domains involved in regulation by polyamines and protein kinase C. *Proc. Natl. Acad. Sci. U.S.A.* **90**, 6731–6735.
312. Armstrong, C. M. (1992). Voltage-dependent ion channels and their gating. *Physiol. Rev.* **72** *(Suppl. 4)*, S5–S13.
313. Catterall, W. A. (1992). Cellular and molecular biology of voltage-gated sodium channels. *Physiol. Rev.*. **72** *(Suppl. 4)*, S15–S48.
314. Pongs, O. (1992). Molecular biology of voltage-dependent potassium channels. *Physiol. Rev.* **72** *(Suppl. 4)*, S69–S88.
315. West, J. W., Patton, D. E., Scheuer, T., Wang, Y., Goldin, A. L., and Catterall, W. A. (1992). A cluster of hydrophobic amino acid residues required for fast Na^+-channel inactivation. *Proc. Natl. Acad. Sci. U.S.A.* **89**, 10910–10914.
316. Kubo, Y., Baldwin, T. J., Jan, Y. N., and Jan, L. Y. (1993). Primary structure and functional expression of a mouse inward rectifier potassium channel. *Nature (London)* **362**, 127–133.
317. Kubo, Y., Reuveny, E., Slesinger, P. A., Jan, Y. N., and Jan, L. Y. (1993). Primary structure and functional expression of a rat G-protein-coupled muscarinic potassium channel. *Nature (London)* **364**, 802–806.
318. Goulding, E. H., Ngai, J., Kramer, R. H., Colicos, S., Axel, R., Siegelbaum, S. A., and Chess, A. (1992). Molecular cloning and single-channel properties of the cyclic nucleotide-gated channel from catfish olfactory neurons. *Neuron* **8**, 45–58.
319. Goulding, E. H., Tibbs, G. R., Liu, D., and Siegelbaum, S. A. (1993). Role of H5 domain in determining pore diameter and ion permeation through cyclic nucleotide-gated channels. *Nature (London)* **364**, 61–64.

320. Biel, M., Altenhofen, W., Hullin, R., Ludwig, J., Freichel, M., Flockerzi, V., Dascal, N., Kaupp, U. B., and Hofmann, F. (1993). Primary structure and functional expression of a cyclic nucleotide-gated channel from rabbit aorta. *FEBS Lett.* **329,** 134–138.
321. Takasawa, S., Nata, K., Yonekura, H., and Okamoto, H. (1993). Cyclic ADP-ribose in insulin secretion from pancreatic β cells. *Science* **259,** 370–373.
322. Taylor, C. W., and Richardson, A. (1991). Structure and function of inositol trisphosphate receptors. *Pharmacol. Ther.* **51,** 97–137.
323. Berridge, M. J. (1993). Inositol trisphosphate and calcium signalling. *Nature (London)* **361,** 315–325.
324. Chadwick, C. C., Saito, A., and Fleischer, S. (1990). Isolation and characterization of the inositol trisphosphate receptor from smooth muscle. *Proc. Natl. Acad. Sci. U.S.A.* **87,** 2132–2136.
325. Maeda, N., Niinobe, M., and Mikoshiba, K. (1990). A cerebellar Purkinje cell marker P_{400} protein is an inositol 1,4,5-trisphosphate ($InsP_3$) receptor protein. Purification and characterization of $InsP_3$ receptor complex. *EMBO J.* **9,** 61–67.
326. Wagenknecht, T., Grassucci, R., Frank, J., Saito, A., Inui, M., and Fleischer, S. (1989). Three-dimensional architecture of the calcium channel/foot structure of sarcoplasmic reticulum. *Nature (London)* **338,** 167–170.
327. Mosthaf, L., Grako, K., Dull, T. J., Coussens, L., Ullrich, A., and McClain, D. A. (1990). Functionally distinct insulin receptors generated by tissue-specific alternative splicing. *EMBO J.* **9,** 2409–2413.
328. Vogt, B., Carrascosa, J. M., Ermel, B., Ullrich, A., and Häring, H. U. (1991). The two isotypes of the human insulin receptor (HIR-A and HIR-B) follow different internalization kinetics. *Biochem. Biophys. Res. Commun.* **177,** 1013–1018.
329. Yamaguchi, Y., Flier, J. S., Yokota, A., Benecke, H., Backer, J. M., and Moller, D. E. (1991). Functional properties of two naturally occurring isoforms of the human insulin receptor in Chinese hamster ovary cells. *Endocrinol. (Baltimore)* **129,** 2058–2066.
330. Rands, E., Candelore, M. R., Cheung, A. H., Hill, W. S., Strader, C. D., and Dixon, R. A. F. (1990). Mutational analysis of β-adrenergic receptor glycosylation. *J. Biol. Chem.* **265,** 10759–10764.
331. Strader, C. D., Sigal, I. S., and Dixon, A. F. (1990). Mapping the functional domains of the β-adrenergic receptor. *Am. J. Resp. Cell Mol. Biol.* **1,** 81–86.
332. Bottaro, D. P., Rubin, J. S., Faletto, D. L., Chan, A. M. L., Kmiecik, T. E., Vande Woude, G. F., and Aaronson, S. A. (1991). Identification of the hepatocyte growth factor receptor as the c-*met* proto-oncogene product. *Science* **251,** 802–804.
333. Delorme, E., Lorenzini, T., Giffin, J., Martin, F., Jacobsen, F., Boone, T., and Elliott, S. (1992). Role of glycosylation on the secretion and biological activity of erythropoietin. *Biochemistry* **31,** 9871–9876.
334. Bastian, W., Zhu, J., Way, B., Lockwood, D., and Livingston, J. (1993). Glycosylation of Asn^{397} or Asn^{418} is required for normal insulin receptor biosynthesis and processing. *Diabetes* **42,** 966–974.
335. Hedo, J. A., and Simpson, I. A. (1985). Biosynthesis of the insulin receptor in rat adipose cells: Intracellular processing of the M_r-190,000 pro-receptor. *Biochem. J.* **232,** 71–78.
336. Gu, Y., Forsayeth, J. R., Verrall, S., Yu, X. M., and Hall, Z. W. (1991). Assembly of the mammalian muscle acetylcholine receptor in transfected 307 cells. *J. Cell Biol.* **114,** 799–807.

337. Yu, X. M., and Hall, Z. W. (1991). Extracellular domains mediating ϵ subunit interactions of muscle acetylcholine receptor. *Nature (London)* **352**, 64–67.
338. Verrall, S., and Hall, Z. W. (1991). The N-terminal domains of acetylcholine receptor subunits contain the recognition signal for heterodimer formation. *J. Cell Biol.* **115**, 323a.
339. Green, W. N., and Claudio, T. (1993). Acetylcholine receptor assembly: Subunit folding and oligomerization occur sequentially. *Cell* **74**, 57–69.
340. Harrison, S. C., and Kirchhausen, T. (1983). Clathrin, cages, and coated vesicles. *Cell* **33**, 650–652.
341. Ktistakis, N. T., Thomas, D., and Roth, M. G. (1990). Characteristics of the tyrosine recognition signal for internalization of transmembrane surface glycoproteins. *J. Cell Biol.* **111**, 1393–1407.
342. Canfield, W. M., Johnson, K. F., Ye, R. D., Gregory, W., and Kornfeld, S. (1991). Localization of the signal for rapid internalization of the bovine cation-independent mannose 6-phosphate/insulin-like growth factor-II receptor to amino acids 24-29 of the cytoplasmic tail. *J. Biol. Chem.* **266**, 5682–5688.
343. Doxsey, S. J., Brodsky, F. M., Blank, G. S., and Helenius, A. (1987). Inhibition of endocytosis by anti-clathrin antibodies. *Cell* **50**, 453–463.
344. Maxfield, F. R., Schlessinger, J., Shechter, Y., Pastan, I., and Willingham, M. C. (1978). Collection of insulin, EGF and α_2-macroglobulin in the same patches on the surface of cultured fibroblasts and common internalization. *Cell* **14**, 805–810.
345. von Zastrow, M., Link, R., Daunt, D., Barsh, G., and Kobilka, B. (1993). Subtype-specific differences in the intracellular sorting of G protein-coupling receptors. *J. Biol. Chem.* **268**, 763–766.
346. Chuang, D. M. (1984). β-Adrenergic receptor internalization and processing: Role of transglutaminase and lysosomes. *Mol. Cell. Biochem.* **58**, 79–89.
347. Davies, P. J. A., and Murtaugh, M. P. (1984). Transglutaminase and receptor-mediated endocytosis in macrophages and cultured fibroblasts. *Mol. Cell. Biochem.* **58**, 69–77.
348. Kahn, C. R., Baird, K. L., Flier, J. S., Grunfeld, C., Harmon, J. T., Harrison, L. C., Karlsson, F. A., Kasuga, M., King, G. L., Lang, U. C., Polskalny, M., and van Obberghen, E. (1981). Insulin receptors, receptor antibodies, and the mechanism of insulin action. *Recent Prog. Horm. Res.* **37**, 477–533.
349. Mohammadi, M., Honegger, A., Sorokin, A., Ullrich, A., Schlessinger, J., and Hurwitz, D. R. (1993). Aggregation-induced activation of the epidermal growth factor protein tyrosine kinase. *Biochemistry* **32**, 8742–8748.
350. Geuze, H. J., Slot, J. W., and Schwartz, A. L. (1987). Membranes of sorting organelles display lateral heterogeneity in receptor distribution. *J. Cell. Biol.* **104**, 1715–1723.
351. Geuze, H. J., Slot, J. W., Strous, J. A. M., Lodish, H. F., and Schwartz, A. L. (1983). Intracellular site of asialoglycoprotein receptor-ligand uncoupling: Double-label immunoelectron microscopy during receptor-mediated endocytosis. *Cell* **32**, 277–287.
352. Brown, M. S., Anderson, R. G. W., and Goldstein, J. L. (1983). Recycling receptors: The round-trip itinerary of migrant membrane proteins. *Cell* **32**, 663–667.
353. Honegger, A. M., Dull, T. J., Felder, S., Van Obberghen, E., Bellot, F., Szapary, D., Schmidt, A., Ullrich, A., and Schlessinger, J. (1987). Point mutation at the

ATP binding site of EGF receptor abolishes protein-tyrosine kinase activity and alters cellular routing. *Cell* **51**, 199–209.

354. Sorkin, A., Kornilova, E., Teslenko, L., Sorokin, A., and Nikolsky, N. (1989). Recycling of epidermal growth factor–receptor complexes in A431 cells. *Biochim. Biophys. Acta* **1011**, 88–96.

355. Burwen, S. J., and Jones, A. L. (1987). The association of polypeptide hormones and growth factors with the nuclei of target cells. *Trends Biochem. Sci.* **12**, 159–162.

356. Goldfine, I. D. (1981). Interaction of insulin, polypeptide hormones, and growth factors with intracellular membranes. *Biochim. Biophys. Acta* **650**, 53–67.

357. Wong, K. Y., Hawley, D., Vigneri, R., and Goldfine, I. R. (1988). Comparison of solubilized and purified plasma membrane and nuclear insulin receptors. *Biochemistry* **27**, 375–379.

358. Purrello, F., Vigneri, R., Clawson, G. A., and Goldfine, I. D. (1982). Insulin stimulation of nucleoside triphosphatase activity in isolated nuclear envelopes. *Science* **216**, 1005–1007.

359. Reyl, F. J., and Lewin, M. J. M. (1982). Intracellular receptor for somatostatin in gastric mucosal cells: Decomposition and reconstitution of somatostatin-stimulated phosphoprotein phosphatases. *Proc. Natl. Acad. Sci. U.S.A.* **79**, 978–982.

360. Buckley, A. R., Crowe, P. D., and Russell, D. H. (1988). Rapid activation of protein kinase C in isolated rat liver nuclei by prolactin, a known hepatic mitogen. *Proc. Natl. Acad. Sci. U.S.A.* **85**, 8649–8653.

361. Nakanishi, Y., Kihara, K., Mizuno, K., Masamune, Y., Yoshitake, Y., and Nishikawa, K. (1992). Direct effect of basic fibroblast growth factor on gene transcription in a cell-free system. *Proc. Natl. Acad. Sci. U.S.A.* **89**, 5216–5220.

362. Rakowicz-Szulczynska, E. M., Rodeck, U., Herlyn, M., and Koprowski, H. (1986). Chromatin binding of epidermal growth factor, nerve growth factor, and platelet-derived growth factor in cells bearing the appropriate surface receptors. *Proc. Natl. Acad. Sci. U.S.A.* **83**, 3728–3732.

363. King, A. C., and Cuatrecasas, P. (1982). Exposure of cells to an acidic environment reverses the inhibition by methylamine of the mitogenic response to epidermal growth factor. *Biochem. Biophys. Res. Commun.* **106**, 479–485.

364. Griendling, K. K., Delafontaine, P., Rittenhouse, S. E., Gimbrone, M. A., and Alexander, R. W. (1987). Correlation of receptor sequestration with sustained diacylglycerol accumulation in angiotensin II-stimulated cultured vascular smooth muscle cells. *J. Biol. Chem.* **262**, 14555–14562.

365. Burgess, W. H., and Maciag, T. (1989). The heparin-binding (fibroblast) growth factor family of proteins. *Annu. Rev. Biochem.* **58**, 575–606.

366. Bouche, G., Gas, N., Prats, H., Baldin, V., Tauber, J. P., Teissié, J., and Amalric, F. (1987). Basic fibroblast growth factor enters the nucleolus and stimulates the transcription of ribosomal genes in ABAE cells undergoing $G_0 \rightarrow G_1$ transition. *Proc. Natl. Acad. Sci. U.S A.* **84**, 6770–6774.

367. Heldin, C. H., and Westermark, B. (1989). Growth factors as transforming proteins. *Eur. J. Biochem.* **184**, 487–496.

368. Davidson, M. B., Van Herle, A. J., and Gerschenson, L. E. (1973). Insulin and Sepharose insulin effects on tyrosine transaminase levels in cultured rat liver cells. *Endocrinol. (Baltimore)* **92**, 1442–1446.

369. Philpott, H. G., and Petersen, O. H. (1979). Extracellular but not intracellular

application of peptide hormones activates pancreatic acinar cells. *Nature (London)* **281**, 684–686.

370. Heumann, R., Schwab, M., and Thoenen, H. (1981). A second messenger required for nerve growth factor biological activity? *Nature (London)* **292**, 838–840.

371. Davis, J. A., and Linzer, D. I. H. (1988). Autocrine stimulation of Nb2 cell proliferation by secreted, but not intracellular, prolactin. *Mol. Endocrinol.* **2**, 740–746.

372. Wells, A., Welsh, J. B., Lazar, C. S., Wiley, H. S., Gill, G. N., and Rosenfeld, M. G. (1990). Ligand-induced transformation by a noninternalizing epidermal growth factor receptor. *Science* **247**, 962–964.

373. Yamasaki, H., Prager, D., and Melmed, S. (1993). Structure-function of the human insulin-like growth factor-I receptor: A discordance of somatotroph internalization and signaling. *Mol. Endocrinol.* **7**, 681–685.

374. Okuda, K., Druker, B., Kanakura, Y., Koenigsmann, M., and Griffin, J. D. (1991). Internalization of the granulocyte-macrophage colony-stimulating factor receptor is not required for induction of protein tyrosine phosphorylation in human myeloid cells. *Blood* **78**, 1928–1935.

375. Carraway, K. L., and Cerione, R. A. (1991). Comparison of epidermal growth factor (EGF) receptor-receptor interactions in intact A431 cells and isolated plasma membranes: Large scale receptor micro-aggregation is not detected during EGF-stimulated early events. *J. Biol. Chem.* **266**, 8899–8906.

376. Sorkin, A., Eriksson, A., Heldin, C. H., Westermark, B., and Claesson-Welsh, L. (1993). Pool of ligand-bound platelet-derived growth factor β-receptors remain activated and tyrosine phosphorylated after internalization. *J. Cell. Physiol.* **156**, 373–382.

377. Kapeller, R., Chakrabarti, R., Cantley, L., Fay, F., and Corvera, S. (1993). Internalization of activated platelet-derived growth factor receptor–phosphatidylinositol-3' kinase complexes: Potential interactions with the microtubule cytoskeleton. *Mol. Cell. Biol.* **13**, 6052–6063.

378. Kahn, C. R., Smith, R. J., and Chin, W. W. (1992). Mechanism of action of hormones that act at the cell surface. *In* "Textbook of Endocrinology" (J. D. Wilson and D. W. Foster, eds.), 8th Ed., pp. 91-134. Saunders, Philadelphia.

379. Taylor, C. W. (1990). The role of G proteins in transmembrane signalling. *Biochem J* **272**, 1–13.

380. Galitzky, J., Reverte, M., Portillo, M., Carpéné, C., Lafontan, M., and Berlan, M. (1993). Coexistence of β_1-, β_2-, and β_3-adrenoceptors in dog fat cells and their differential activation by catecholamines. *Am. J. Physiol.* **264**, E403–E412.

381. Leblanc, P., L'Héritier, A., and Kordon, C. (1992). A Ca^{2+} calmodulin dependent kinase rather than protein kinase C is involved in up-regulation of the LHRH receptor. *Biochem. Biophys. Res. Commun.* **183**, 666–671.

382. Nishimori, K., Yamoto, M., and Nakano, R. (1989). *In vitro* membrane desialylation in porcine granulosa cells unmasks functional receptors for follicle-stimulating hormone. *Endocrinol. (Baltimore)* **124**, 2659–2665.

383. VuHai-LuuThi, M. T., Misrahi, M., Houllier, A., Jolivet, A., and Milgrom, E. (1992). Variant forms of the pig lutropin/choriogonadotropin receptor. *Biochemistry* **31**, 8377–8383.

384. Cuatrecasas, P. (1971). Unmasking of insulin receptors in fat cell membranes: Perturbation of membrane lipids. *J. Biol. Chem.* **246**, 6532–6542.

385. Bhattacharya, A., and Vonderhaar, B. K. (1979). Phospholipid methylation

stimulates lactogenic binding in mouse mammary gland membranes. *Proc. Natl. Acad. Sci. U.S.A.* **76,** 4489–4492.

386. Lokeshwar, V. B., Huang, S. S., and Huang, J. S. (1989). Protamine enhances epidermal growth factor (EGF)-stimulated mitogenesis by increasing cell surface EGF receptor number: Implications for existence of cryptic EGF receptors. *J. Biol. Chem.* **264,** 19318–19326.

387. Costlow, M. E., and Hample, A. (1982). Prolactin receptors in cultured rat mammary tumor cells. *J. Biol. Chem.* **257,** 6971–6977.

CHAPTER 7

Receptor Regulation

I. Introduction

Because hormone–receptor binding obeys the laws of mass action, the number of receptors determines, in part, the sensitivity of the cell to the hormone (see Chapter 6, Section VIII,A). However, sensitivity can also be influenced by other receptor characteristics, such as receptor affinity or location. These potential molecular mechanisms are discussed here using specific examples of both homologous and heterologous regulation. *Homologous regulation* is the control of a receptor by its own ligand; conversely, *heterologous regulation* is the control of a receptor by a hormone that does not bind to that receptor.

II. Receptor Number

A. Synthesis and Stability

The concentration of any molecule will be a result of the balance between synthesis and degradation; synthesis, in turn, is a product of both transcription and translation. This chapter will not be concerned with the mechanisms of synthesis, except to warn the reader that increased receptor mRNA is not necessarily reflected in the amount of translated receptor.

   The insulin receptor has been one of the most thoroughly studied systems, and several investigators have reported on the mechanisms involved in the regulation of this receptor by glucocorticoids. This is an example of heterologous control. In most of these experiments, cells are exposed to amino acids containing heavy isotopes (^2H, ^{13}C, and ^{15}N). These heavy amino acids will be incorporated only into the newly synthesized receptors, which can then be separated from the pre-existing receptors by density gradient centrifugation. This procedure allows one to determine both the synthetic rate and the turnover rate of insulin receptors. In hepatocytes, dexamethasone, a synthetic glucocorticoid, increases the insulin receptor number 5-fold (Table 7-1; 1). This effect is due exclusively to an increase in the rate of synthesis, which is also elevated 5-fold, whereas the half-life is unchanged.

   In adipocytes, the mechanism is different. The stimulatory effect of dexamethasone is a result of increasing the receptor half-life instead of its synthesis (2). The reciprocal effect is observed with insulin, which lowers it own receptor abundance by shortening its receptor half-life. Neither the affinity of the receptor nor its cellular distribution is altered during the experiment. Tissue-specific differences are quite common and should always be considered when reading the literature. In fact, not only can mechanisms be different, but a hormone may have opposite effects in different tissues. For example, estradiol elevates the PgR in the stroma and muscularis of the uterus and oviduct, whereas it inhibits it in the epithelium (3). In another example, GH can lower its own receptor in adipocytes while increasing it in muscle (4).

   The same kind of regulation is seen for steroid receptors. Estradiol stim-

Table 7-1
Regulation of Receptor Synthesis and Stability

Receptor	Tissue	Hormone treatment	Receptor number (%)	Half-life (hr)	Synthetic rate (%)
Insulin	Hepatocytes	Control	100	9.0	100
		Dexamethasone[a]	517	9.4	474
	Adipocytes	Control	100	10.2	100
		Dexamethasone[a]	213	18.2	115
		Insulin	43	4.2	110
Progesterone	Breast cancer	Control	100	21	100
	cells	Estradiol	1000	21	700[b]
		R5020[c]	15	6	<10
Glucocorticoid	Pituitary	Control	100	22.5	100
	cells	Triamcinolone[a]	51	10.2	100
1,25-DHCC[d]	Fibroblasts	Control	100	4	100[b]
	and intes-	1,25-DHCC	300	8	100[b]
	tinal cells				

[a] Synthetic glucocorticoid.
[b] mRNA synthesis.
[c] Synthetic progestin.
[d] 1,25-Dihydroxycholecalciferol.

ulates the PgR in breast cancer cells 10-fold by elevating receptor synthesis (5). This system also illustrates the fact that there does not have to be a single mechanism: R5020, a progesterone agonist, decreases the PgR by both inhibiting synthesis and shortening the receptor half-life (6). Homologous regulation of the GR and VDR are examples of steroid receptor regulation exclusively through receptor stability. Triamcinolone, another synthetic glucocorticoid, halves GR number in a pituitary cell line by reducing the half-life (7) whereas 1,25-DHCC triples its own receptor in fibroblasts and intestinal cells by prolonging the half-life (8).

These examples were chosen deliberately because of their straight-forward data: either only one mechanism is utilized or, if both receptor synthesis and stability are affected, the two mechanisms reinforce one another. It is possible to have both mechanisms activated but in opposite directions: EGF increases its own receptor mRNA 5-fold but also increases EGFR degradation (9–11). The net effect is determined by the balance between these two processes. Initially, degradation predominates as the EGFR is down-regulated; then synthesis becomes preeminent as the receptors are replenished. The βARs show a different time course: β-agonists initially stimulate βAR levels as a result of increased transcription, but continuous receptor activation leads to down-regulation by decreasing the βAR mRNA half-life from 12 to 5 hours (12–13).

Mechanisms for affecting gene expression and mRNA stability will be discussed in Chapters 12 and 14. Protein half-life is often regulated by proteolytic mechanisms; one such pathway is ubiquitination. As discussed in Chapter 6, ubiquitin is a peptide that is covalently coupled to proteins destined for degradation. Ubiquitination of the GH, TNF, SCF, and PDGF receptors has been detected (14–17); this modification of the SCF and PDGF receptors is induced by ligand binding and is associated with down-regulation. LH binding to its receptor activates a different pathway, one involving an ectoprotease that cleaves the extracellular domain near the membrane (18). Heterologous regulation has also been reported: PKC can stimulate the release of the Kit LBD (19) and glucocorticoids lower serum levels of the soluble IL-2R (20), although the precise effects of the steroids may be influenced by the duration of the treatment and the physiological state of the animal.

B. Activation

Receptors are normally activated by the binding of their ligands. However, as mentioned in Chapter 6, some receptors may be nonfunctional; these are the cryptic receptors. The recruitment of these receptors into the responsive pool is another mechanism by which the number of *functional* receptors can be increased. This mechanism can be very rapid, since protein synthesis is not required.

Another way of increasing the number of functioning receptors without ligand binding is by heterologous activation. RTKs are activated by autophosphorylation; however, some RTKs can phosphorylate and activate closely related, but unoccupied, RTKs. For example, the insulin receptor can phosphorylate and activate empty IGF-IRs (21). Receptor aggregation per se also favors allosteric kinase activation and autophosphorylation. This is more clearly observed with polyvalent antibodies (Chapter 6) or polycations (22). Whether there is any physiological correlate of this phenomenon is not known.

Steroid receptors can also undergo heterologous activation. The PgR can be phosphorylated and activated by dopamine stimulation (23). The GnRH is another activator of the PgR; although this stimulation is cAMP-dependent, no actual phosphorylation of the PgR has been demonstrated yet (24).

C. Compartmentalization

Finally, receptors may be physically present and functional, but not accessible to their ligands. Because the ligands for membrane receptors are hydrophilic, they cannot traverse the plasmalemma; therefore, receptors located on internal membrane structures cannot bind their ligands. Translocation of the receptors from these structures to the plasma membrane would be another way of increasing the number of receptors.

The IGF-IIR undergoes translocation to the plasmalemma in response to insulin, EGF, IGF-I, or IGF-II (25,26). This mechanism can increase the number of IGF-IIRs at the cell surface by 50–100% within 10–15 minutes. This shift can be blocked by β-agonists, whose effects are largely mediated by a cAMP-dependent protein kinase (PKA). This antagonism suggests that phosphorylation may determine receptor location in the IGF-IIR system. Another possible mechanism for translocation involves carbohydrate residues, which are known to be important in intracellular targeting of proteins. The LHR precursor is heavily glycosylated and located within the cell (27). Although reduction in the carbohydrate content of the LHR precedes its appearance at the plasmalemma, no causal relationship has been proven. However, such a relatioship is suggested by the fact that a homologous receptor, the FSHR, can be unmasked by desialylation (28).

If moving receptors to the cell surface increases the sensitivity of the cell to hormones, then moving the receptors back inside should render the cells less responsive. Indeed, this mechanism was thought to play an important role in the desensitization of cells to β-agonists: after binding β-agonists, the βAR internalizes in a process called sequestration. This shift is associated with the loss of cell responsiveness. However, the association appears to be fortuitous: first, careful temporal studies have shown that desensitization precedes internalization (29). Second, mutant βARs incapable of internalization can still be desensitized (30). Therefore, sequestration merely appears to be a means for dephosphorylating the βAR during recycling, rather than a mechanism for reducing the hormonal responsiveness of a cell. However, internalization may still be an important mechanism for regulating the sensitivity of the cell to hormones whose receptors do not recycle, including the EGF and PAF receptors (31).

III. Receptor Affinity and Specificity

The other major receptor characteristic that determines the responsiveness of a cell to hormones is affinity. Many of the factors that affect receptor affinity also affect its ligand specificity; therefore, both topics will be addressed in this section.

A. Covalent Modification

Phosphorylation is a major means of regulating the substrate affinity of enzymes, so it should not be surprising that it also affects receptor affinity. EGF- or PDGF-induced tyrosine phosphorylation of the EGFR reduces its affinity for EGF (32), whereas a similar modification of the GnRH receptor by the EGFR enhances receptor affinity (33).

B. Allosterism

Another mechanism for altering receptor affinity is allosterism; this can occur via either small regulatory molecules or subunit oligomerization. An example of the former is the guanylate cyclase receptor for ANF; the association of ANF with its receptor leads to the binding of ATP to the membrane proximal kinase-like domain. The ATP binding is necessary for cyclase activity and is also responsible for inducing a low-affinity state of the receptor (34).

Oligomerization can either be homogeneous or heterogeneous. For example, EGFR dimerization represents homogeneous aggregation and results in a higher affinity for EGF than in the EGFR monomer (35,36). Homogeneous oligomerization may also decrease the receptor affinity in a process called *negative cooperativity*. It was originally thought that the insulin receptor exhibited this phenomenon because insulin binding data generate a curvilinear Scatchard plot (see Chapter 4). Such a plot could represent multiple isoreceptors with different affinities or negative cooperativity; since only one insulin receptor gene had been found, negative cooperativity appeared to be the best interpretation. This conclusion was further supported by dissociation experiments (37): the dissociation of labeled insulin from its receptor was faster in the presence of excess unlabeled hormone than in its absence. The excess of unlabeled hormone kept the receptor occupancy at a high level, thereby maintaining a low affinity and promoting rapid dissociation. In the absence of this excess hormone, the receptor affinity would increase as insulin dissociated and receptor occupancy fell; this higher affinity would retard further dissociation.

However, this concept has been vigorously challenged and is still controversial. For example, the dissociation experiment may be explained by the *mobile receptor* hypothesis (38). This idea has been developed mathematically, but only a conceptual presentation will be given here. The hypothesis claims that a hormone may bind to either its receptor alone or to the receptor–effector complex; furthermore, the affinity of the latter for the hormone is greater. In fact, this has been shown for several of the serpentine receptors, which can be precoupled to G proteins. Hormone dissociation, therefore, would be slower from the receptor–effector complex than from the receptor alone. If an excess of unlabeled hormone were present, it would bind to the free receptors and, because of its abundance, would outcompete the labeled hormone–receptor complex for effector binding. Without an attached effector, the labeled hormone would now dissociate more rapidly. Again, this is exactly what is observed for the βAR, despite the fact that this receptor yields a linear Scatchard plot, indicating no allosterism. The curvilinear plot for insulin may be a result of hormone degradation, which gives rise to fragments with a spectrum of receptor affinities. This event occurs in the liver. When the data are corrected for this degradation, the Scatchard plot becomes linear.

Oligomerization can also be heterogeneous. Most cytokine receptors consist of at least two nonidentical, although homologous, subunits (Chapter 6); either subunit can only bind its ligand with low to intermediate affinity, whereas both components bind hormone with high affinity. Receptor affinity may also be affected by interacting with a nonbinding subunit; as noted earlier, many serpentine receptors are precoupled to G proteins and this association increases the affinity of the attached receptor for its ligand (39). Finally, different receptors can associate and generate new binding specificities. The EGFR and HER2 can heterodimerize to produce a hybrid receptor with very high affinity for EGF, although the HER2 dimer itself will not bind EGF (40). Similarly, an insulin/IGF-I receptor hybrid has binding properties distinct from those of either component (41).

C. Alternative Splicing

Alternative splicing of the receptor mRNA is another way of affecting receptor affinity and specificity. Exon 11 of the insulin receptor encodes for 12 amino acids in the extracellular domain close to the membrane (42). The intact receptor has half the insulin affinity of the one lacking these amino acids. This variation may have physiological significance, since the long form is found in liver, which is exposed to high concentrations of insulin secreted from the pancreas. The lower affinity may protect the liver from overstimulation. The FGFR2 can also undergo alternative splicing involving the carboxy half of the third immunoglobulin loop: FGFR2 binds only FGF, whereas the variant binds both FGF and KGF (43–45).

IV. Endogenous Antagonists

A. Ligand Antagonists

Given a fixed receptor number, affinity, and location, receptor function can be influenced by the presence of hormone antagonists. One normally thinks of antagonists as synthetic compounds originating from pharmacology laboratories, but many organisms produce their own hormone antagonists to further regulate receptor activity. For example, an IL-1 antagonist is homologous to IL-1α and IL-1β and binds to, but does not activate, their receptor (46). The IL-1 antagonist arises from a unique gene, but antagonists can also be generated by alternative splicing from the same gene as the agonist. For example, an alternatively spliced HGF is truncated in the second kringle domain; sufficient structure is preserved to allow it to bind to the HGFR, but it cannot activate the receptor (47).

B. Receptor Antagonists

Receptor antagonists are of two kinds: (i) soluble receptors and (ii) membrane-bound receptors. All known receptor antagonists are modifications of normal receptors. The soluble receptors represent the extracellular domains of membrane-bound receptors; they are usually generated by alternative splicing, although some may be released by proteolysis. These proteins dampen hormone effects, presumably by sequestering the hormone and preventing it from reaching the intact receptor (48). Other receptors may be truncated beyond the membrane domain or may lack critical autophosphorylation sites as a result of alternative splicing (49); such proteins are still membrane bound and can dimerize but have no transducing activity. Since the biological activity of RTKs and cytokine receptors is dependent on the dimerization of functional proteins, a heterodimer containing an intact and a truncated receptor is inactive. Essentially, the truncated receptor binds an intact receptor and removes it from the pool of potentially active receptors. Truncated receptors have been reported for IL-4 (50), HGF (51), prolactin (52), PDGF (53), GH (54), VEGF (55), and FGF (56); but inhibitory effects have only been demonstrated for the latter four. Not all soluble receptors are inhibitory: soluble IL-6Rα is active in combination with IL-6Rβ.

V. Transduction Uncoupling

Receptors without any intrinsic activity must couple to a transducer; these include the serpentine receptors that activate G proteins and the cytokine receptors that activate soluble tyrosine kinases. The former have been studied more intensively and will be the major subject matter for this section. The serpentine receptor can be uncoupled by changes in either the receptor or the G protein; the former will be discussed here whereas the latter will be discussed in Chapter 8.

A. Receptor Phosphorylation

The major mechanism for rapid reversible uncoupling is phosphorylation. Homologous uncoupling of the βAR can be mediated by two different kinases depending on the concentration of the agonist. In the presence of low agonist concentrations, G protein activation leads to the elevation of cAMP and the stimulation of PKA. PKA will then phosphorylate the βAR in the carboxy half of the third cytoplasmic loop and in the juxtamembrane portion of the carboxy terminus (57). Any hormone elevating cAMP can stimulate the phosphorylation of any other receptor similarly coupled to G$_s$, even if the hormones for those other receptors are not present; this is known as *class sensitization*. However, phosphorylation is more rapid when the βAR is occupied. The PKA effect is slow, requiring about 3.5 minutes, and does not lead to receptor internalization (58).

High agonist concentrations activate a second kinase, the *β-adrenergic receptor kinase* (βARK) (59). This kinase exhibits some substrate specificity; it will phosphorylate the β_2AR, α_2AR, M$_2$R, and the substance P receptor, but not the β_1AR or the α_1AR. Its target is the serine–threonine-rich region in the carboxy terminus of the β_2AR and the third cytoplasmic loop of the α_2AR (60). The phosphorylation per se does not uncouple the β_2AR from G$_s$; rather, the modified site binds another molecule, *β-arrestin*, which is the actual uncoupler (61). This phosphorylation occurs rapidly, requiring less than 15 seconds, and leads to receptor internalization. As noted earlier, sequestration

is not part of the desensitization process but is necessary for dephosphorylation and recycling.

The α_1AR uses a different transduction system that elevates calcium and
phospholipid metabolites (see Chapter 9); one of its major outputs is yet
another kinase, protein kinase C (PKC). As one might expect, PKC can
phosphorylate the α_1AR and uncouple it from its transducer (62). As is true
for the β_2AR, this modification proceeds twice as rapidly in the presence of
agonist as in its absence (63). Heterologous regulation by bradykinin, which
uses the same transducer, has the same effect; this would be another example
of class desensitization. However, bradykinin does not induce internalization
because the α_1AR is not occupied. The α_1AR is internalized when it is
stimulated by its own agonist, norepinephrine.

Desensitization can also cross classes; for example, PKC increases 5-fold
the concentration of β-agonist necessary to activate adenylate cyclase. However, the phosphorylation state of the β_2AR is unchanged (64). In this case,
PKC appears to act at the G protein or adenylate cyclase (65). Conversely,
PKA phosphorylates a site in the third cytoplasmic loop of the M_1R, leading
to its desensitization (66). Finally, insulin can induce the tyrosine phosphorylation of the β_2AR and reduce coupling efficiency by 50% (67). Since direct
stimulation of the transducers was normal, it was assumed that the receptor
modification was the cause for the uncoupling.

The actual mechanism of coupling is unknown, but it appears to be a
functional, rather than a physical, uncoupling. For example, the desensitized
muscarinic acetylcholine receptor is internalized with its G protein (68).
Furthermore, the affinity of the uncoupled muscarinic receptor is still increased in the presence of its G protein (69), indicating that the two can
physically interact.

B. Other Mechanisms

Another mechanism that can affect coupling to transducers is alternative
splicing; this mechanism is slower and would have more long-term effects
than phosphorylation. There are two dopamine 2 receptors: the $D_{2A}R$ has 29
more amino acids in the third intracellular loop than the $D_{2B}R$ (70). Both
isoreceptors elevate calcium but the $D_{2B}R$ inhibits cAMP levels twice as
effectively as the $D_{2A}R$. In other words, the additional amino acids appear to
interfere with the coupling of the D_2R to G_i.

In a second example, alternative splicing of the PGE receptor, EP3, gives
rise to a protein with four different carboxy termini influence G protein
coupling (71). Isoform A activates G_i or G_o; isoforms B stimulates G_s; isoform
C activates G_s but inhibits G_o; and isoform D stimulates G_i, G_s, and G_q. The
PACAP receptor is also subject to alternative splicing; in this case, the
varying sequences occur in the third cytoplasmic loop and influence G
protein activation (72).

Receptor–effector coupling can also affect and be affected by the lipid
composition of the membrane. β-Adrenergic agonists increase the phospha-

tidylcholine content of membranes, thereby increasing their fluidity (73). This, in turn, is thought to facilitate the coupling of the receptor to G_s (see Chapter 9). This hypothesis is further supported by studies in which the fluidity of the membrane was experimentally altered: lipids that increase fluidity enhance β-agonist-induced adenylate cyclase activity, whereas lipids that decrease fluidity have the opposite effect (74,75). In addition to coupling with transducers, membrane lipids can also affect receptor oligomerization; for example, gangliosides impair PDGF dimer formation (76). Finally, cholesterol and negatively charged phospholipids enhance ion-gating in the nAChR; the mechanism for this effect is unknown (77).

VI. Developmental Regulation

Many cellular processes are so complex that several hormones are involved, in which case the regulation of their receptors is frequently coordinated. The mammary gland is an excellent example (78). In the nonpregnant mouse, the mammary epithelium is poorly developed; although the ducts extend throughout the fat pad, they are widely spaced and there are no alveoli. During pregnancy, the epithelium rapidly proliferates under the influence of estrogens and progesterone; EGF may play an ancillary role. After parturition, growth ceases and lactation begins; in the mouse, milk production requires insulin, cortisol, and PRL. Growth and differentiation are generally mutually exclusive events; for example, progesterone and EGF stimulate epithelial proliferation but inhibit milk protein synthesis. Figure 7-1 schematically shows the tissue concentration of these receptors in the mammary gland during pregnancy and lactation; all the data are from studies of mice except those for the PRL receptor, which are from rat studies (79–84). Data for other hormone receptors in the mammary gland are less complete but follow the same general pattern; for example, both the GHR (85) and the IGF-IR (86) are elevated during pregnancy and decrease with lactation. It is clear that the concentrations of receptors for the growth promoters are high during pregnancy but fall near parturition. The levels of receptors for the differentiative hormones, however, do not rise until late pregnancy and are maximal during lactation.

Furthermore, these hormones influence each other's receptors in a way that generally reinforces the developmental pattern (Table 7-2; 87). Insulin, cortisol, and PRL are required for the normal maintenance of each other's receptors and may even elevate their levels. The effects of estrogen and progesterone are more complex. Progesterone may stimulate or inhibit both the PRL and insulin receptors, depending on the system; estradiol stimulates the release of PRL, which can then elevate its own receptor. It is quite possible that these sex steroids act as triggers that lead to the eventual rise in the level of receptors for the lactational hormones.

Many of the mechanisms discussed here can also be used for the developmental regulation of receptors. First, because developmental changes take

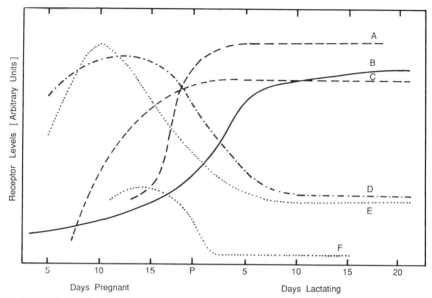

Fig. 7-1. Developmental regulation of the mammary gland receptors for (A) cortisol, (B) PRL, (C) insulin, (D) estrogen, (E) EGF, and (F) progesterone. All data are from studies of mice except those for PRL receptors, which are from studies of rats.

a relatively long time to occur, gene induction is often fast enough to produce the necessary modulations in receptor levels. Alternative splicing is another mechanism: although a truncated LHR mRNA is transcribed in the immature rat ovary, it cannot be translated (88). The intact mRNA is not synthesized and translated until 7 days postpartum. Finally, compartmentalization has also been documented in a developmental system. The EPOR is present in many myeloid precursors but these cells are unresponsive to EPO, because

Table 7-2

Hormonal Regulation of Hormone Receptors

Receptor	Hormone							
	Insulin	Cortisol	PRL	E_2	Progesterone	Testoterone	GH	T_3
PRL	+	+	+	+	±	−	+	+
Cortisol		+	+					
Insulin			+		±			
E_2			+	+		−		
Progesterone			0	+	−			

a Data are combined from studies of rat and/or mouse mammary gland and/or liver and include both *in vivo* and *in vitro* studies.

b Symbols: (+), the indicated hormone either stimulates or is required for the maintenance of a given receptor; (−), the receptor levels are decreased; (0), the receptor levels are not affected; no entry, no information is available.

the EPORs are intracellular. These receptors migrate to the plasma membrane in the precursors destined to enter the erythrocyte lineage (89).

VII. Summary

The types of receptor regulation discussed in this chapter are summarized in Table 7-3. Actual receptor number can be changed by altering either synthesis or degradation, whereas the number of functional receptors can be changed by activation or migration between cellular compartments. Receptor affinity can be changed acutely by phosphorylation or allosterism; a slower but longer effect can be achieved by changing the structure of the receptor, for example, by alternative splicing. One could also view endogenous antagonist as a means of altering receptor affinity, since their presence increases the concentration of hormone required for a given response. A ligand antagonists can either be a pure antagonist transcribed from a unique gene or an alternatively spliced agonist that can still bind the receptor but cannot activate it. Receptor antagonists are either soluble receptors that sequester the hormone or kinase-defective molecules that bind with intact receptors to produce a nonfunctional dimer. Finally, the receptor may be uncoupled from its transducer. In the serpentine receptors, this desensitization is accomplished by receptor phosphorylation.

Table 7-3
General Mechanisms for Hormone Receptor Regulation[a]

Mechanism	Example
Change number	
Synthesis	Insulin receptor induction by glucocorticoids in hepatocytes
Stability	Insulin receptor induction by glucocorticoids in adipocytes
Activation	IGF-IR phosphorylation by the insulin receptor
Compartmentalization	Shift of IGF-IIR to plasmalemma by insulin
Change affinity	
Phosphorylation	EGFR autophosphorylation
Allosterism	Guanylate cyclase by ATP; EGFR dimerization
Alternate splicing	Insulin receptor ± exon 11
Antagonists	
Ligand	IL-1 antagonist; HGF alternative splicing
Receptor	Soluble TNFR; membrane-bound, truncated PDGFR
Alter coupling with transducer:	
Phosphorylation	β_2AR phosphorylation by PKA or βARK
Alternative splicing	Alternative carboxy termini of EP3
Membrane properties	Lipid composition and the βAR

[a] See text or List of Abbreviations at the end of the book for definitions.

References

General References

Collins, S. (1993). Recent perspectives on the molecular structure and regulation of the β_2-adrenoceptor. *Life Sci.* **52**, 2083–2091.

Hadcock, J. R., and Malbon, C. C. (1993). Agonist regulation of gene expression of adrenergic receptors and G proteins. *J. Neurochem.* **60**, 1–9.

Lohse, M. J. (1993). Molecular mechanisms of membrane receptor desensitization. *Biochim. Biophys. Acta* **1179**, 171–188.

Ormandy, C. J., and Sutherland, R. L. (1993). Mechanisms of prolactin receptor regulation in mammary gland. *Mol. Cell. Endocrinol.* **91**, C1–C6.

Tian, W. N., and Deth, R. C. (1993). Precoupling of G_i/G_o-linked receptors and its allosteric regulation by monovalent cations. *Life Sci.* **52**, 1899–1907.

See also Refs. 24, 31, 39, 59, 73, 75, 78, and 87.

Cited References

1. Salhanick, A. L., Krupp, M. N., and Amatruda, J. M. (1983). Dexamethasone stimulates insulin receptor synthesis in cultured rat hepatocytes. *J. Biol. Chem.* **258**, 14130–14135.

2. Knutson, V. P., Ronnett, G. V., and Lane, M. D. (1982). Control of insulin receptor level in 3T3 cells: Effect of insulin-induced down-regulation and dexamethasone-induced up-regulation on rate of receptor inactivation. *Proc. Natl. Acad. Sci. U.S.A.* **79**, 2822–2826.

3. Hyde, B. A., Blaustein, J. D., and Black, D. L. (1989). Differential regulation of progestin receptor immunoreactivity in the rabbit oviduct. *Endocrinol. (Baltimore)* **125**, 1479–1483.

4. Frick, G. P., Leonard, J. L., and Goodman, H. M. (1990). Effect of hypophysectomy on growth hormone receptor gene expression in rat tissues. *Endocrinol. (Baltimore)* **126**, 3076–3082.

5. Nardulli, A. M., Greene, G. L., O'Malley, B. W., and Katzenellenbogen, B. S. (1988). Regulation of progesterone receptor messenger ribonucleic acid and protein levels in MCF-7 cells by estradiol: Analysis of estrogen's effect on progesterone receptor synthesis and degradation. *Endocrinol. (Baltimore)* **122**, 935–944.

6. Nardulli, A. M., and Katzenellenbogen, B. S. (1988). Progesterone receptor regulation in T47D human breast cancer cells: Analysis by density labeling of progesterone receptor synthesis and degradation and their modulation by progesterone. *Endocrinol. (Baltimore)* **122**, 1532–1540.

7. McIntyre, W. R., and Samuels, H. H. (1983). Triamcinolone acetonide regulates glucocorticoid receptor levels by decreasing the half-life of the activated nuclear receptor form. *Progr. Abstr. 65th Annu. Meet. Endocr. Soc.*, 228.

8. Wiese, R. J., Uhland-Smith, A., Ross, T. K., Prahl, J. M., and DeLuca, H. F. (1992). Up-regulation of the vitamin D receptor in response to 1,25-dihydroxyvitamin D_3 results from ligand-induced stabilization. *J. Biol. Chem.* **267**, 20082–20086.

9. Clark, A. J. L., Ishii, S., Richert, N., Merling, G. T., and Pastan, I. (1985). Epidermal growth factor regulates the expression of its own receptor. *Proc. Natl. Acad. Sci. U.S.A.* **82**, 8374–8378.

10. Earp, H. S., Austin, K. S., Blaisdell, J., Rubin, R. A., Nelson, K. G., Lee, L. W., and

Grisham, J. W. (1986). Epidermal growth factor (EGF) stimulates EGF receptor synthesis. *J. Biol. Chem.* **261**, 4777–4780.

11. Bjorge, J. D., and Kudlow, J. E. (1987). Epidermal growth factor receptor synthesis is stimulated by phorbol ester and epidermal growth factor. *J. Biol. Chem.* **262**, 6615–6622.

12. Collins, S., Bouvier, M., Bolanowski, M. A., Caron, M. G., and Lefkowitz, R. J. (1989). cAMP stimulates transcription of the β_2-adrenergic receptor gene in response to short-term agonist exposure. *Proc. Natl. Acad. Sci. U.S.A.* **86**, 4853–4857.

13. Hadcock, J. R., Wang, H., and Malbon, C. C. (1989). Agonist-induced destabilization of β-adrenergic receptor mRNA: Attenuation of glucocorticoid-induced up-regulation of β-adrenergic receptors. *J. Biol. Chem.* **264**, 19928–19933.

14. Leung, D. W., Spencer, S. A., Cachianes, G., Hammonds, R. G., Collins, C., Henzel, W. J., Barnard, R., Waters, M. J., and Wood, W. I. (1987). Growth hormone receptor and serum binding protein: Purification, cloning and expression. *Nature (London)* **330**, 537–543.

15. Loetscher, H., Schlaeger, E. J., Lahm, H. W., Pan, Y. C., Lesslauer, W., and Brockhaus, M. (1990). Purification and partial amino acid sequence analysis of two distinct tumor necrosis factor receptors from HL60 cells. *J. Biol. Chem.* **265**, 20131–20138.

16. Mori, S., Heldin, C. H., and Claesson-Welsh, L. (1993). Ligand-induced ubiquitination of the platelet-derived growth factor β-receptor play a negative role in its mitogenic signaling. *J. Biol. Chem.* **268**, 577–583.

17. Miyazama, K., Toyama, K., Gotoh, A., Hendrie, P. C., Mantel, C., and Broxmeyer, H. E. (1994). Ligand-dependent polyubiquitination of c-*kit* gene product: A possible mechanism of receptor down modulation in M07e cells. *Blood* **83**, 137–145.

18. West, A. P., and Cooke, B. A. (1991). Regulation of the truncation of luteinizing hormone receptors at the plasma membrane is different in rat and mouse Leydig cells. *Endocrinol. (Baltimore)* **128**, 363–370.

19. Yee, N. S., Langen, H., and Besmer, P. (1993). Mechanism of kit ligand, phorbol ester, and calcium-induced down-regulation of c-*kit* receptors in mast cells. *J. Biol. Chem.* **268**, 14189–14201.

20. Sauer, J., Rupprecht, M., Arzt, E., Stalla, G. K., and Rupprecht, R. (1993). Glucocorticoids modulate soluble interleukin-2 receptor levels in vivo depending on the state of immune activation and the duration of glucocorticoid exposure. *Immunopharmacology* **25**, 269–276.

21. Tartare, S., Ballotti, R., and Van Obberghen, E. (1991). Interaction between heterologous receptor tyrosine kinases: Hormone-stimulated insulin receptors activate unoccupied IGF-I receptors. *FEBS Lett.* **295**, 219–222.

22. Xu, Q. Y., Li, S. L., LeBon, T. R., and Fujita-Yamaguchi, Y. (1991). Aggregation of IGF-I receptors or insulin receptors and activation of their kinase activity are simultaneously caused by the presence of polycations or K-*ras* basic peptides. *Biochemistry* **30**, 11811–11819.

23. Power, R. F., Mani, S. K., Codina, J., Conneely, O. M., and O'Malley, B. W. (1991). Dopaminergic and ligand-independent activation of steroid hormone receptors. *Science* **254**, 1636–1639.

24. Turgeon, J. L., and Waring, D. W. (1992). Functional cross-talk between receptors for peptide and steroid hormones. *Trends Endocrinol. Metab.* **3**, 360–365.

25. Lönnroth, P., Appell, K. C., Wesslau, C., Cushman, S. W., Simpson, I. A., and

Smith, U. (1988). Insulin-induced subcellular redistribution of insulin-like growth factor II receptors in the rat adipose cell: Counterregulatory effects of isoproterenol, adenosine, and cAMP analogues. *J. Biol. Chem.* **263**, 15386–15391.

26. Braulke, T., Tippmer, S., Neher, E., and von Figura, K. (1989). Regulation of the mannose 6-phosphate/IGF II receptor expression at the cell surface by mannose 6-phosphate, insulin like growth factors and epidermal growth factor. *EMBO J.* **8**, 681–686.

27. VuHai-LuuThi, M. T., Misrahi, M., Houllier, A., Jolivet, A., and Milgrom, E. (1992). Variant forms of the pig lutropin/choriogonadotropin receptor. *Biochemistry* **31**, 8377–8383.

28. Nishimori, K., Yamoto, M., and Nakano, R. (1989). *In vitro* membrane desialylation in porcine granulosa cells unmasks functional receptors for follicle-stimulating hormone. *Endocrinol. (Baltimore)* **124**, 2659–2665.

29. Yu, S. S., Lefkowitz, R. J., and Hausdorff, W. P. (1993). β-Adrenergic receptor sequestration: A potential mechanism of receptor resensitization. *J. Biol. Chem.* **268**, 337–341.

30. Hausdorff, W. P., Campbell, P. T., Ostrowski, J., Yu, S. S., Caron, M. G., and Lefkowitz, R. J. (1991). A small region of the β-adrenergic receptor is selectively involved in its rapid regulation. *Proc. Natl. Acad. Sci. U.S.A.* **88**, 2979–2983.

31. Chao, W., and Olson, M. S. (1993). Platelet-activating factor: receptors and signal transduction. *Biochem. J.* **292**, 617–629.

32. Walker, F., and Burgess, A. W. (1991). Reconstitution of the high affinity epidermal growth factor receptor on cell-free membranes after transmodulation by platelet-derived growth factor. *J. Biol. Chem.* **266**, 2746–2752.

33. Liebow, C., Lee, M. T., Kamer, A. R., and Schally, A. V. (1991). Regulation of luteinizing hormone-releasing hormone receptor binding by heterologous and autologous receptor-stimulated tyrosine phosphorylation. *Proc. Natl. Acad. Sci. U.S.A.* **88**, 2244–2248.

34. Jewett, J. R. S., Koller, K. J., Goeddel, D. V., and Lowe, D. G. (1993). Hormonal induction of low affinity receptor guanylyl cyclase. *EMBO J.* **12**, 769–777.

35. Defize, L. H. K., Boonstra, J., Meisenhelder, J., Kruijer, W., Tertoolen, L. G. J., Tilly, B. C., Hunter, T., van Bergen en Hegegouwen, P. M. P., Moolenaar, W. H., and de Laat, S. W. (1989). Signal transduction by epidermal growth factor occurs through the subclass of high affinity receptors. *J. Cell Biol.* **109**, 2495–2507.

36. Canals, F. (1992). Signal transmission by epidermal growth factor receptor: Coincidence of activation and dimerization. *Biochemistry* **31**, 4495–4501.

37. De Meyts, P., Roth, J., Neville, D. M., Gavin, J. R., and Lesniak, M. A. (1973). Insulin interaction with its receptors: Experimental evidence for negative cooperativity. *Biochem. Biophys. Res. Commun.* **55**, 154–161.

38. Jacobs, S., and Cuatrecases, P. (1976). The mobile receptor hypothesis and "cooperativity" of hormone binding: Application to insulin. *Biochim. Biophys. Acta* **433**, 482–495.

39. Levitzki, A. (1986). β-Adrenergic receptors and their mode of coupling to adenylate cyclase. *Physiol. Rev.* **66**, 819–854.

40. Qian, X., Decker, S. J., and Greene, M. I. (1992). p185$^{c\text{-}neu}$ and epidermal growth factor receptor associate into a structure composed of activated kinases. *Proc. Natl. Acad. Sci. U.S.A.* **89**, 1330–1334.

41. Treadway, J. L., Morrison, B. D., Goldfine, I. D., and Pessin, J. E. (1989). Assembly of insulin/insulin-like growth factor-1 hybrid receptors *in vitro*. *J. Biol. Chem.* **264**, 21450–21453.

42. Mosthaf, L., Grako, K., Dull, T. J., Coussens, L., Ullrich, A., and McClain, D. A. (1990). Functionally distinct insulin receptors generated by tissue-specific alternative splicing. *EMBO J.* **9**, 2409–2413.
43. Miki, T., Bottaro, D. P., Fleming, T. P., Smith, C. L., Burgess, W. H., Chan, A. M. L., and Aaronson, S. A. (1992). Determination of ligand-binding specificity by alternative splicing: Two distinct growth factor receptors encoded by a single gene. *Proc. Natl. Acad. Sci. U.S.A.* **89**, 246–250.
44. Werner, S., Duan, D. S. R., de Vries, C., Peters, K. G., Johnson, D. E., and Williams, L. T. (1992). Differential splicing in the extracellular region of fibroblast growth factor receptor 1 generates receptor variants with different ligand-binding specificities. *Mol. Cell. Biol.* **12**, 82–88.
45. Yayon, A., Zimmer, Y., Guo-Hong, S., Avivi, A., Yarden, Y., and Givol, D. (1992). A confined variable region confers ligand specificity on fibroblast growth factor receptors: Implications for the origin of the immunoglobulin fold. *EMBO J.* **11**, 1885–1890.
46. Eisenberg, S. P., Brewer, M. T., Verderber, E., Heimdal, P., Brandhuber, B. J., and Thompson, R. C. (1991). Interleukin 1 receptor antagonist is a member of the interleukin 1 gene family: Evolution of a cytokine control mechanism. *Proc. Natl. Acad. Sci. U.S.A.* **88**, 5232–5236.
47. Chan, A. M. L., Rubin, J. S., Bottaro, D. P., Hirschfield, D. W., Chedid, M., and Aaronson, S. A. (1991). Identification of a competitive HGF antagonist encoded by an alternative transcript. *Science* **254**, 1382–1385.
48. Smith, C. A., Davis, T., Wignall, J. M., Din, W. S., Farrah, T., Upton, C., McFadden, G., and Goodwin, R. G. (1991). T2 open reading frame from the Shope Fibroma Virus encodes a soluble form of the TNF receptor. *Biochem. Biophys. Res. Commun.* **176**, 335–342.
49. Shi, E., Kan, M., Xu, J., Wang, F., Hou, J., and McKeehan, W. L. (1993). Control of fibroblast growth factor receptor kinase signal transduction by heterodimerization of combinatorial splice variants. *Mol. Cell. Biol.* **13**, 3907–3918.
50. Mosley, B., Beckman, M. P., March, C. J., Idzerda, R. L., Gimpel, S. D., VandenBos, T., Friend, D., Alpert, A., Anderson, D., Jackson, J., Wignall, J. M., Smith, C., Gallis, B., Sims, J. E., Urdal, D., Widmer, M. B., Cosman, D., and Park, L. S. (1989). The murine interleukin-4 receptor: Molecular cloning and characterization of secreted and membrane bound forms. *Cell* **59**, 335–348.
51. Prat, M., Crepaldi, T., Gandino, L., Giordano, S., Longati, P., and Comoglio, P. (1991). C-Terminal truncated forms of Met, the hepatocyte growth factor receptor. *Mol. Cell. Biol.* **11**, 5954–5962.
52. Lesueur, L., Edery, M., Ali, S., Paly, J., Kelly, P. A., and Djiane, J. (1991). Comparison of long and short forms of the prolactin receptor on prolactin-induced milk protein gene transcription. *Proc. Natl. Acad. Sci. U.S.A.* **88**, 824–828.
53. Ueno, H., Colbert, H., Escobedo, J. A., and Williams, L. T. (1991). Inhibition of PDGF β receptor signal transduction by coexpression of a truncated receptor. *Science* **252**, 844–848.
54. Hansen, B. S., Hjorth, S., Welinder, B. S., Skriver, L., and De Meyts, P. (1993). The growth hormone (GH)-binding protein cloned from human IM-9 lymphocytes modulates the down-regulaton of GH receptors by 22- and 20-kilodalton human GH in IM-9 lymphocytes and the biological effects of the hormone in Nb_2 lymphoma cells. *Endocrinol. (Baltimore)* **133**, 2809–2817.
55. Kendall, R. L., and Thomas, K. A. (1993). Inhibition of vascular endothelial cell

growth factor activity by an endogenously encoded soluble receptor. *Proc. Natl. Acad. Sci. U.S.A.* **90,** 10705–10709.

56. Ueno, H., Gunn, M., Dell, K., Tseng, A., and Williams, L. (1992). A truncated form of fibroblast growth factor receptor 1 inhibits signal transduction by multiple types of fibroblast growth factor receptor. *J. Biol. Chem.* **267,** 1470–1476.

57. Hausdorff, W. P., Bouvier, M., O'Dowd, B. F., Irons, G. P., Caron, M. G., and Lefkowitz, R. J. (1989). Phosphorylation sites on two domains of the β_2-adrenergic receptor are involved in distinct pathways of receptor desensitization. *J. Biol. Chem.* **264,** 12657–12665.

58. Roth, N. S., Campbell, P. T., Caron, M. G., Lefkowitz, R. J., and Lohse, M. J. (1991). Comparative rates of desensitization of β-adrenergic receptors by the β-adrenergic receptor kinase and the cyclic AMP-dependent protein kinase. *Proc. Natl. Acad. Sci. U.S.A.* **88,** 6201–6204.

59. Inglese, J., Freedman, N. J., Koch, W. J., and Lefkowitz, R. J. (1993). Structure and mechanism of the G protein-coupled receptor kinases. *J. Biol. Chem.* **268,** 23735–23738.

60. Liggett, S. B., Ostrowski, J., Chestnut, L. C., Kurose, H., Raymond, J. R., Caron, M. G., and Lefkowitz, R. J. (1992). Sites in the third intracellular loop of the α_{2A}-adrenergic receptor confer short term agonist-promoted desensitization: Evidence for a receptor kinase-mediated mechanism. *J. Biol. Chem.* **267,** 4740–4746.

61. Lohse, M. J., Benovic, J. L., Codina, J., Caron, M. G., and Lefkowitz, R. J. (1990). β-Arrestin: A protein that regulates β-adrenergic receptor function. *Science* **248,** 1547–1550.

62. Leeb-Lundberg, L. M. F., Cotecchia, S., Deblasi, A., Caron, M. G., and Lefkowitz, R. J. (1987). Regulation of adrenergic receptor function by phosphorylation: I. Agonist-promoted desensitization and phosphorylation of α_1-adrenergic receptors coupled to inositol phospholipid metabolism in DDT1 MF-2 smooth muscle cells. *J. Biol. Chem.* **262,** 3098–3105.

63. Bouvier, M., Leeb-Lundberg, L. M. F., Benovic, J. L., Caron, M. G., and Lefkowitz, R. J. (1987). Regulation of adrenergic receptor function by phosphorylation: II. Effects of agonist occupancy on phosphorylation of α_1- and β_2-adrenergic receptors by protein kinase C and the cyclic AMP-dependent protein kinase. *J. Biol. Chem.* **262,** 3106–3113.

64. Johnson, J. A., Clark, R. B., Friedman, J., Dixon, R. A. F., and Strader, C. D. (1990). Identification of a specific domain in the β-adrenergic receptor required for phorbol ester-induced inhibition of catecholamine-stimulated adenylyl cyclase. *Mol. Pharmacol.* **38,** 289–293.

65. Bouvier, M., Guilbault, N., and Bonin, H. (1991). Phorbol-ester-induced phosphorylation of the β_2-adrenergic receptor decreases its coupling to G_s. *FEBS Lett.* **279,** 243–248.

66. Lee, N. H., and Fraser, C. M. (1993). Cross-talk between m1 muscarinic acetylcholine and β_2-adrenergic receptors: cAMP and the third intracellular loop of m1 muscarinic receptors confer heterologous regulation. *J. Biol. Chem.* **268,** 7949–7957.

67. Hadcock, J. R., Port, J. D., Gelman, M. S., and Malbon, C. C. (1992). Cross–talk between tyrosine kinase and G–protein–linked receptors: Phosphorylation of β_2–adrenergic receptors in response to insulin. *J. Biol. Chem.* **267,** 26017–26022.

68. Ho, A. K. S., Zhang, Y. J., Duffield, R., and Zheng, G. M. (1991). Evidence for the simultaneous translocation of muscarinic acetylcholine receptor and G protein by carbachol. *Cell. Signal.* **3,** 587–598.

69. Richardson, R. M., Ptasienski, J., and Hosey, M. M. (1992). Functional effects of protein kinase C–mediated phosphorylation of chick heart muscarinic cholinergic receptors. *J. Biol. Chem.* **267**, 10127–10132.
70. Hayes, G., Biden, T. J., Selbie, L. A., and Shine, J. (1992). Structural subtypes of the dopamine D2 receptor are functionally distinct: Expression of the cloned D2$_A$ and D2$_B$ subtypes in a heterologous cell line. *Mol. Endocrinol.* **6**, 920–926.
71. Namba, T., Sugimoto, Y., Negishi, M., Irie, A., Ushikubi, F., Kakizuka, A., Ito, S., Ichikawa, A., and Narumiya, S. (1993). Alternative splicing of C–terminal tail of prostaglandin E receptor subtype EP3 determines G–protein specificity. *Nature (London)* **365**, 166–170.
72. Spengler, D., Waeber, C., Pantaloni, C., Holsboer, F., Bockaert, J., Seeburg, P. H., and Journot, L. (1993). Differential signal transduction by five splice variants of the PACAP receptor. *Nature (London)* **365**, 170–175.
73. Hirata, F., and Axelrod, J. (1980). Phospholipid methylation and biological signal transmission. *Science* **209**, 1082–1090.
74. Jansson, C., Härmälä, A. S., Toivola, D. M., and Slotte, J. P. (1993). Effects of the phospholipid environment in the plasma membrane on receptor interaction with the adenylyl cyclase complex of intact cells. *Biochim. Biophys. Acta* **1145**, 311–319.
75. Jans, D. A. (1992). The mobile receptor hypothesis revisited: A mechanistic role for hormone receptor lateral mobility in signal transduction. *Biochim. Biophys. Acta* **1113**, 271–276.
76. Van Brocklyn, J., Bremer, E. G., and Yates, A. J. (1993). Gangliosides inhibit platelet-derived growth factor-stimulated receptor dimerization in human glioma U-1242MG and Swiss 3T3 cells. *J. Neurochem.* **61**, 371–374.
77. Barrantes, F. J. (1993). Structural-functional correlates of the nicotinic acetylcholine receptor and its lipid microenvironment. *FASEB J.* **7**, 1460–1467.
78. Topper, Y. J., and Freeman, C. S. (1980). Multiple hormone interactions in the developmental biology of the mammary gland. *Physiol. Rev.* **60**, 1049–1106.
79. Holcomb, H. H., Costlow, M. E., Buschow, R. A., and McGuire, W. L. (1976). Prolactin binding in rat mammary gland during pregnancy and lactation. *Biochim. Biophys. Acta* **428**, 104–112.
80. Haslam, S. Z., and Shyamala, G. (1979). Progesterone receptors in normal mammary glands of mice: Characterization and relationship to development. *Endocrinol. (Baltimore)* **105**, 786–795.
81. Muldoon, T. G. (1979). Mouse mammary tissue estrogen receptors: Ontogeny and molecular hetergeneity. *In* "Ontogeny of Receptors and Reproductive Hormone Action" (T. H. Hamilton, J. H. Clark, and W. A. Sadler, eds.), pp. 225–247. Raven Press, New York.
82. Lindenbaum, M., and Chatterton, R. T. (1981). Interaction of steroids with dexamethasone-binding receptor and corticosterone-binding globulin in the mammary gland of the mouse in relation to lactation. *Endocrinol. (Baltimore)* **109**, 363–375.
83. Inagaki, Y., and Kohmoto, K. (1982). Changes in Scatchard plots for insulin binding to mammary epithelial cells from cycling, pregnant, and lactating mice. *Endocrinol. (Baltimore)* **110**, 176–182.
84. Edery, M., Pang, K., Larson, L., Colosi, T., and Nandi, S. (1985). Epidermal growth factor receptor levels in mouse mammary glands in various physiological states. *Endocrinol. (Baltimore)* **117**, 405–411.
85. Lincoln, D. T., Water, M. J., Breipohl, W., Sinowatz, F., and Lobie, P. E. (1990).

Growth hormone receptors expression in the proliferating rat mammary gland. *Acta Histochem.* **40** *[Suppl.]*, 47–49.

86. Lavandero, S., Santibáñez, J. F., Ocaranza, M. P., and Sapag-Hagar, M. (1990). Insulin-like growth factor I receptor levels during the lactogenic cycle in rat mammary gland. *Biochem. Soc. Trans.* **18**, 576–577.

87. Nagasawa, H., Sakai, S., and Banerjee, M. R. (1979). Prolactin receptor. *Life Sci.* **24**, 193–208.

88. Sokka, T., Hämäläinen, T., and Huhtaniemi, I. (1992). Functional LH receptor appears in the neonatal rat ovary after changes in the alternative splicing pattern of the LH receptor mRNA. *Endocrinol. (Baltimore)* **130**, 1738–1740.

89. Migliaccio, A. R., Migliaccio, G., D'Andrea, A., Baiocchi, M., Crotta, S., Nicolis, S., Ottolenghi, S., and Adamson, J. W. (1991). Response to erythropoietin in erythroid subclones of the factor-dependent cell line 32D is determined by translocation of the erythropoietin receptor to the cell surface. *Proc. Natl. Acad. Sci. U. S.A.* **88**, 11086–11090.

PART **3**

Transduction

CHAPTER **8**

G Proteins and Cyclic Nucleotides

CHAPTER OUTLINE

I. Introduction

Because peptide and certain other hormones cannot cross the plasma membrane, they must interact with their receptors on the cell surface. Therefore, if the hormone is to have an effect on cellular processes, a signal must be generated from the other side of the membrane; this signal can then carry out the actions of the hormone. If the hormone itself is considered to be the primary, or first, messenger, then the signal becomes the second messenger.

This part of the book discusses all the second messengers. Chapter 8 begins with a brief discussion of the criteria for these mediators and then presents an overview of the GTP-binding proteins. Finally, the cyclic nucleotides are covered. Chapter 9 describes the role of phospholipids in signal transduction: phosphatidylinositol is involved with the elevation of intracellular calcium and the activation of a protein kinase, whereas phosphatidylcholine may affect membrane fluidity and generate the precursor for the eicosanoids. Arachidonic acid, sphingomyelin, and the lysophospholipids are also mentioned. Chapter 10 describes a number of mediators that are not as well defined as the cyclic nucleotides and calcium; they include the polyamines, oligosaccharides, cellular pH, and the cytoskeleton. Chapter 11 is a general synthesis of the preceding three chapters and has a strong emphasis on protein phosphorylation and how it can directly affect cellular processes.

II. Criteria for Second Messengers

How does one identify a second messenger for a hormone, that is, what characteristics should a molecule have to be called a second messenger? The five basic criteria a compound must satisfy will be discussed using glycogen breakdown as an example: in the liver, glucagon stimulates glycogenolysis via cAMP.

1. The mediator, or its analog, must mimic the action of the hormone. Because cAMP is not very membrane permeable, dibutyryl cAMP is frequently used on intact cells; once inside the cell, the butyryl side chains are removed. Unfortunately, most investigators do not realize that this hydrolysis results in a significant accumulation of butyric acid, which can affect cellular metabolism in its own right (see Chapter 13). Nonetheless, this analog does induce glycogenolysis in liver cells.

2. The hormone must induce elevated levels of the mediator. Glucagon does elevate cAMP levels in liver cells.

3. The hormone must appropriately affect the enzymes of synthesis and/or degradation of the mediator. cAMP is synthesized from ATP by adenylate cyclase and is hydrolytically activated by a cyclic nucleotide phosphodiesterase (PDE) (Fig. 8-1). cAMP concentrations can

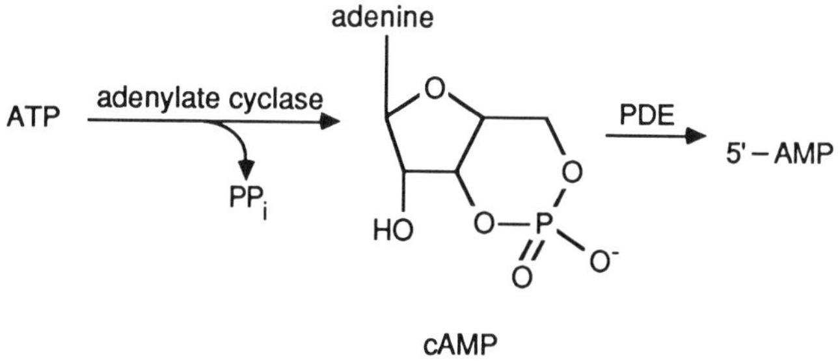

Fig. 8-1. The formation and degradation of cAMP. PDE, Cyclic nucleotide phosphodiesterase.

be elevated by stimulating the adenylate cyclase or inhibiting the PDE. In the liver, glucagon does the former.

4. An appropriate temporal relationship must exist among the hormone, mediator, and hormonal effect. It would be difficult to argue that cAMP is the second messenger of glucagon in the liver if cAMP levels did not rise until *after* glycogenolysis had already started. In fact, the elevation of cAMP concentrations precedes glycogenolysis in this system.

5. Finally, if drugs are available to modulate the endogenous level of the mediator pharmacologically, they should also mimic or inhibit, as appropriate, the effects of the hormone. For example, cAMP levels can be raised by (i) stimulating the adenylate cyclase with either forskolin or aluminum fluoride or (ii) inhibiting the PDE with methylxanthines. Cyclic AMP levels can be lowered by inhibiting the adenylate cyclase with 2′,3′-dideoxyadenosine or 9-(tetrahydro-2-furyl)adenine. Forskolin, aluminum fluoride, and the methylxanthines can stimulate glycogenolysis in liver cells.

Therefore, one can reasonably conclude that cAMP is indeed the second messenger for glucagon in the liver. However, care must be taken not to overinterpret these data. For example, they do not argue that cAMP is the only mediator for glucagon in the liver; in fact, there is evidence that glucagon may activate another transduction system in this organ. Nor do the data state that cAMP will be the mediator for glucagon in all tissues. As far as is known, this statement is true for glucagon; however, the effect of vasopressin is mediated by cAMP in the kidney but by calcium in the liver.

III. G Proteins

A. Components and Cycle

Several major transduction systems use GTP-binding proteins, or simply G proteins, to couple a hormone signal to an effector. Basically, a G protein is a molecular switch with a built-in automatic timer; when bound to GDP, the switch is in the off position, but when bound to GTP, the switch is on. Since the G protein itself is an inefficient GTPase, it will eventually hydrolyze the bound GTP and turn itself off. The G proteins are all homologous at the catalytic site, but can vary considerably elsewhere. Indeed, the size variation alone is tremendous: 20 to 100 kDa.

The GTPase activity of the small G proteins is so low that it requires an accessory factor, the *GTPase-activating protein* (GAP). In addition to augmenting the intrinsic GTPase activity of small G proteins and turning them off, it has been proposed that GAP may also serve as an effector. Finally, GAP can be bound and phosphorylated by RTKs, suggesting that GAP may represent a site of signal input into the system. The possible role of GAP as an effector and signal transducer is discussed further later. Although there is some overlap in G-protein specificity, there appears to be a separate GAP for each small G protein.

External signals can also be fed into the system via a component that triggers the exchange of GDP for GTP, thereby flipping the switch on. The recommended term for this component is the *GDP dissociation stimulator* (GDS), although it has also been called a guanine nucleotide release protein (GNRP), GDP release factor (GRF), and GNP exchange protein (GEP). Recently another method of activation has been proposed: the GDP may be converted to GTP while still bound to the G protein by a nucleoside diphosphate kinase. This probably does not occur under physiological conditions (1), but the close association of this kinase to G_s suggests that it may channel GTP to G proteins (2).

The GDS is opposed by a *GDP dissociation inhibitor* (GDI) that not only inhibits GNP exchange but also represses the intrinsic and GAP-stimulated GTPase activity (3,4). The GDI appears to be preassociated with the small G proteins (5) and probably keeps basal activity at a low level and influences the localization of these molecules. Because the $\beta\gamma$ dimer performs similar functions on the large G proteins, some authorities have suggested that GDI is the small G protein equivalent of the $\beta\gamma$ dimer (6). The system is also dampened by a *GTPase-inhibiting protein* (GIP). It binds the G protein with either GDP or GTP and inhibits GAP.

The general cycle is presented in Fig. 8-2. In response to some stimulus, GDS facilitates the exchange of GDP for GTP and activates the G protein. The G protein by itself or with GAP, which subsequently binds to the G protein, triggers a series of biological effects. Eventually, the GTP is hydrolyzed, GAP dissociates, and the system is inactivated. Both GDI and GIP act to check the cycle. Table 8-1 adds details to this cycle by giving specific examples. The EF-Tu/EF-Ts cycle in translation elongation is probably one of the examples most familar to biology students.

B. Small G Proteins

1. Classification

The first G proteins discovered were involved with the signal tranduction from serpentine receptors; they are heterotrimers whose GTPase subunit

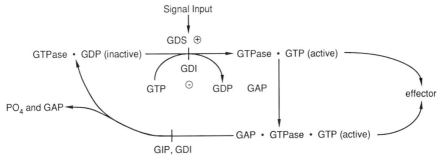

Fig. 8-2. The general cycle for G proteins. GAP, GTPase-activating protein; GDI, GDP dissociation inhibitor; GDS, GDP dissociation stimulator; GIP, GTPase-inhibiting protein.

is about 40 kDa. These molecules are the ones most closely associated with the term G protein, although in this chapter they will be referred to as G protein trimers to clearly distinguish them from the small G proteins. These latter proteins have molecular weights around 20 kDa and exist as either monomers or identical oligomers (7–9). Although their exact function in hormone signal transduction is less clear than that of their larger cousins, there is evidence that they do play an important role.

A classification scheme for these small G proteins is presented in Table 8-2. Most of them are related to Ras both in amino acid sequence and in post-translational modifications. Because some of these modifications are unusual, it would be worthwhile to digress briefly and discuss them (Table 8-3). There are four ways in which lipids can be covalently attached to proteins: the simplest of which involves the attachment of a fatty acid. Myristic acid is coupled to the amino terminus via an amide linkage. This occurs during protein synthesis and the modification is quite stable. Although many myristoylated proteins are membrane associated, others are cytoplasmic. Because myristic acid is so short, it has been proposed that it is not the hydrophobicity of the lipid moiety that is responsible for the membrane binding but that there are membrane receptors that recognize this fatty acid and the adjacent amino acid sequence. Palmitic acid is longer and attached to cysteines by a thioester bond; unlike myristoylation, this modifi-

Table 8-1

Components of the GTPase Cycle for Several Systems

GTPase	GDP dissociation stimulator (GDS)	GTPase activating protein (GAP)	Function
EF-Tu	EF-Ts	Ribosome	Translation proof-reading
Yeast Ras	Cdc25	IRA 1 and 2	Nutrient transduction
Mammalian Ras	RasGDS; Vav	RasGAP	Proliferation
G protein trimer	Hormone receptor	None vs. internal vs. effector	Hormone signal transduction

Table 8-2

Some G Protein Families and Their Functions

Group	Members	Function
Ras superfamily		
Ras family	Ras	Mating and nutrient transduction (yeast); mitogenesis (mammals)
Ras-like family	Ral, Rap	NADPH oxidase activation
Rho family	Rho, Rac	Cytoskeletal organization; activation of NADPH oxidase and PI3K
Rab family	Rab, Ram, SEC4, YPT1	Vesicular trafficking
Ran family	Ran	Chromosomal condensation
ARF family	ARF, CIN4	Golgi–vesicle interactions; stimulation of phospholipase D
G protein trimer	G_s, G_i, G_q, etc.	Hormone signal transduction
Elongation factors	EF-Tu	Translation proofreading
Signal recognition particle	SRP54	Transfer of proteins across the endoplasmic reticulum

cation has a high turnover rate, suggesting a regulatory role. Indeed, palmitic acid turnover is stimulated during serpentine receptor desensitization (Chapter 6) and this modification may determine the accessibility of adjacent serine-rich regions to kinases.

The other two lipid modifications are more complex. Polyprenylation refers to the attachment of a polyprenyl polymer, usually a farnesyl or a geranylgeranyl group (10). The former contains three isopentenyl subunits whereras the latter has four. These polymers are generated by the *polyprenyl* or *isoprenoid pathway*, which also produces sterols; the latter is synthesized from a six-unit precursor that cyclizes to form the phenanthrene nucleus. Proteins targeted for polyprenylation have the sequence C–A–A–X, where A is an aliphatic amino acid and X is any amino acid (Fig. 8-3). If X is leucine, the cysteine receives a geranylgeranyl group; if X is serine, methionine, or asparagine the cysteine will be farnesylated. Initially, the three carboxy-terminal amino acids are removed and the exposed cysteine is methylated. Finally, the polyprenyl group is attached to the cysteine via a thioether linkage. In the small G proteins, there is often an adjacent cysteine that is palmitoylated; although the polyprenylation is not reversible, the methylation and associated palmitoylation do undergo turnover. For example, some small G proteins are maintained in the cytosol as an inactive complex with GDI; hormones that stimulate nucleotide exchange cause the complex to dissociate and the newly exposed carboxy terminus of the G protein is carboxymethylated (11). This modification then favors the association of the G protein with the membrane, where many of its effectors reside.

Table 8-3

Characteristics of the Covalent Lipid Modifications of Proteins

Characteristic	Modification			
	Myristoylation	Palmitoylation	Polyprenylation	Phosphatidyl-inositol glycan
Linkage	N-terminal amide	Thioester to cysteine	Thioether to C-terminal cysteine	C-terminal amide via phospho-ethanolamine
Site of synthesis	Endoplasmic reticulum	Golgi and cytosol	Cytosol[a]	Endoplasmic reticulum[a]
Protein location	Plasmalemma, cytosol	Inner leaflet of plasma membrane	Plasmalemma, cytosol	Outer leaflet of plasma membrane
Turnover	Low	High	None	None except cleavage
Function	N-terminal blocker; membrane–protein association	Membrane anchorage; receptor desensitization	Membrane–protein association	Membrane anchorage (at cell apex)

[a] Location of core modification. Additional modifications occur elsewhere.

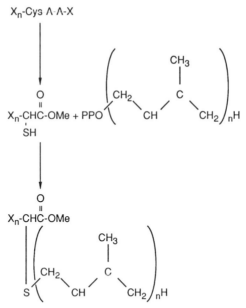

Fig. 8-3. Prenylation pathway. A, Aliphatic amino acid; X, any amino acid.

Like myristoylated proteins, many polyprenylated proteins are membrane associated but the length of the polymer does not always correlate with this property. Therefore, membrane receptors for these proteins have also been postulated to explain their membrane binding.

The last modification, phosphatidylinositol glycan (PI-glycan), is included for completeness; it will be discussed more thoroughly in Chapter 10. Briefly, this is a phospholipid attached to the carboxy terminus of a protein by a phosphoethanolamine–oligosaccharide tether.

Ras is a 21-kDa protein that forms identical dimers and trimers. It is polyprenylated and palmitoylated near the carboxy terminus and myristoylated at the amino terminus. In yeast, Ras activates adenylate cyclase and mediates mating and nutrient transduction; in mammals, it is associated with the stimulation of Raf kinase and mitogenesis (see subsequent discussion). The mammalian RasGAP is 120 kDa: it has the GTPase at the carboxy terminus, a hydrophobic amino terminus, and two SH2 motifs separated by one SH3 motif in the middle (12). It can increase the GTPase activity of Ras 100-fold; however, there is considerable evidence that the mammalian Ras-GAP also has effector functions. For example, RasGAP doubles the activity of Lck, a soluble tyrosine kinase (13), and is required to uncouple the muscarinic receptor from G_K, a G protein trimer that opens the potassium channel (14). These functions reside outside the GTPase domain, since the isolated carboxy terminus of RasGAP has normal GTPase activity but cannot support Ras-induced transcription (15). Candidate structures that might mediate the effector function of GAP include the SH2 and SH3 domains; for example, the SH2–SH3 peptide, in combination with Ras, can stimulate Jun, a transcription factor (16). Furthermore, an excess of SH3 peptide can block oocyte maturation induced by insulin or Ras (17).

NF1, also called *neurofibromin*, is another mammalian GAP; NF1 is defective in the disease neurofibromatosis (18). It is homologous to the yeast RasGAPs IRA1 and IRA2, and although it has a 20-fold higher affinity for Ras than the mammalian RasGAP just described, it is less efficient. In some tumors associated with neurofibromatosis, the total GAP activity is low and the level of Ras–GTP is elevated (19) because the mutant NF1 is unable to inactivate the GTP-bound Ras. Mitogenesis and tumorigenesis result. Unfortunately, the mechanism of NF1 may not be so simple, since other tumors associated with neurofibromatosis have normal Ras–GTP levels (20).

The *Ras-like* family has 50–60% homology to Ras, is polyprenylated and includes Ral and Rap. In neutrophils, Rap is membrane associated under basal conditions. However, after the carboxy terminus is phosphorylated by PKA, Rap dissociates from the membrane, binds RapGDS, and is activated (21). Rap then activates the NADPH oxidase that produces the oxygen radicals used to kill bacteria. Since PKA is regulated by cAMP, a hormone second messenger, there is a possible link between this small G protein and endocrine transduction. Such an association is seen in pancreatic acinar cells, where several gastrointestinal hormones stimulate GNP exchange on Rap, presumably by PKA (22). Rap can also block the actions of Ras by binding to and sequestering RasGAP, a Ras effector.

The *Rho* family is more distantly related to Ras and has 30% homology to Ras. It is also polyprenylated and includes Rho and Rac. This family is involved in cytoskeletal organization: Rho can stimulate actin stress fibers and focal adhesion formation (23), whereas both Rho and Rac are required for growth factor-induced membrane ruffling (24). Rac is also required for NADPH oxidase activation (25).

Like the Rho family, the *Rab* family has a 30% homology to Ras and is polyprenylated. However, its carboxy terminus may vary from the classic C–A–A–X motif; this variation requires a unique set of enzymes for polyprenylation. Both the yeast (YPT1 and SEC4) and mammalian (Rab and Ram) members are involved in vesicular trafficking between cell organelles and the plasmalemma (26,27). Like Rap, Rab can be released from membranes by phosphorylation (28); in this case the kinase is *cell division cycle kinase 2* (Cdc2).

The *Ran* family is unique because it lacks any amino- or carboxy-terminal motifs associated with lipid modification (29). Ran prevents premature chromosomal condensation during mitosis.

The *ARF* family was initially discovered as accessory factors required for ADP–ribosylation by various bacterial toxins; as such, they were called *ADP-ribosylation factors* (ARFs). They do not affect eukaryotic ADP–ribosylating enzymes and do not appear to have any GTPase activity, although GTP can affect their activity (30). They are myristoylated but not polyprenylated and are intermediate in homology between Ras and the G protein trimers. The functions of ARFs are unknown but they are major coat proteins of Golgi stacks. They may play a role in Golgi structure, such as in the budding and uncoating of transfer vesicles (31-33); and they can stimulate phospholipase D (34). They also inhibit the insulin-induced maturation of *Xenopus* oocytes. Since oocyte maturation induced by insulin is mediated by Ras, it has been proposed that ARF may be an inhibitory G protein that opposes Ras, much like G_i opposes G_s.

2. Role in Transduction

As noted earlier, many of the small G proteins are involved in cytoskeletal organization or vesicular trafficking. However, Rap activity can be regulated by PKA and Ras is necessary for the mitogenic activity of many growth factors. The latter data have been obtained from experiments using either microinjected Ras antibodies or dominant inhibitory mutants of Ras; such techniques block specific hormone-induced activities. In general, the activities most strongly affected are DNA synthesis and several proline-directed kinases, such as MAP and Raf kinase (Table 8-4). The latter are closely associated with mitogenesis. Components of the polyphosphatidylinositol pathway and general metabolism are the least affected. Occasionally, there are conflicting reports concerning the involvement of Ras in the action of a particular hormone; most of these disputes arise from the choice of antibodies or mutants. There are, in fact, several forms of Ras and different hormones utilize different types. For example, insulin and IGF-I use H-Ras whereas FGF, EGF, and PDGF act through N-Ras or K-Ras (35).

There are several ways that hormones can couple to Ras and other small G proteins. The first and simplest way would be to act directly on the small G protein. As noted ealier, PKA can phosphorylate Rap and Cdc2 does the same to Rab; the modification releases both from the membrane. Ras is a substrate for PKC, but this phosphorylation does not alter its biological activity.

Second, hormones may act through GDS. NGF, PDGF, FGF, IL-6, EGF, HGF, and insulin stimulate the rate of nucleotide exchange on Ras 2 to 5-fold

Table 8-4
Evidence for a Role for Mammalian Ras in Hormone Signal Transduction

Hormone	DNA synthesis	MAP and Raf kinases	Polyphosphatidyl-inositol pathway[a]
PDGF	Yes	Yes	No
EGF	Yes	Yes	No
CSF-1	Yes		
NGF		Yes	No
Insulin		Yes	No

[a] Includes phospholipase C, protein kinase C, or PI-3 kinase.

(36–40). This activity requires tyrosine kinase activity but not activation of the polyphosphatidylinositide pathway. The most direct pathway would involve the phosphorylation and activation of RasGDS; this is the mechanism in T lymphocytes (41,42). Stimulation of either the T cell receptor–CD4 complex or the IL-2 receptor activates a soluble tyrosine kinase, Lck, which then phosphorylates and activates Vav, a RasGDS (Fig. 8-4). EGF, PDGF, and SCF can also phosphorylate Vav, although this is not a nonspecific effect of all RTKs: for example, neither the IL-3R, GM-CSFR, nor the CSF-1R can modify Vav (43).

Hormones may also activate RasGDS via adaptors. One of the substrates for several RTKs is the protein Shc (44). The tyrosine phosphorylated Shc is then bound by Grb2, an adaptor with one SH2 and two SH3 motifs. Another substrate, IRS-1, performs a similar function after being phosphorylated by the insulin, IGF-I, IL-2, or IL-4 receptor (45-49). Alternatively, autophosphorylated RTKs can directly bind Grb2 (50). The complex between Grb2 and a phosphotyrosine from Shc, IRS-1, or RTK attracts and activates RasGDS (Fig. 8-5; 49,50). This interaction occurs between the amino-terminal SH3 of Grb2 and the proline-rich region of the RasGDS. The system is inactivated by the phosphorylation of RasGDS by an unknown serine–threonine kinase; this modification causes the GDS to dissociate from the membrane and from its substrate, Ras (53,54). In addition, IRS-1 can bind and stimulate a PTP, which may also participate in the inactivation process by removing the phosphates from IRS-1 (55). Note that antibodies against Grb2 block the effects of both Ras and Rac, suggesting that the activation of Rac may also be mediated by this adaptor (56).

Third, the hormones can affect GAP. The receptors for PDGF, EGF, CSF-1, and EPO can bind and phosphorylate RasGAP. However, the importance of this modification is in dispute: (i) the stoichiometry is low (57,58), (ii) the activity of unbound RasGAP is unaffected by phosphorylation (59), and (iii) many hormones can affect GAP activity without phosphorylation (58). Phosphorylation by PKC has also been documented but its effect is equally uncertain (61). It is possible that GAP binding to hormone receptors by itself is sufficient to mediate hormone activity: EGFR-bound RasGAP has half the activity of the unbound form (59). RasGAP may be sequestered in other ways: RasGAP phosphorylation on serine in response to EGF binds to a

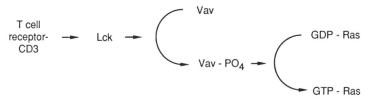

Fig. 8-4. T lymphocyte pathway to activate Ras. The T cell receptor stimulates Lck, which phosphorylates and activates Vav, a Ras GDP dissociation stimulator (RasGDS).

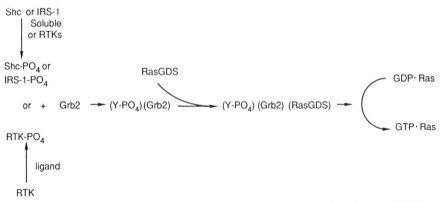

Fig. 8-5. Growth factor pathway to activate Ras. The tyrosine-phosphorylated RTK or adaptor (Shc or IRS-1) stimulates Grb2 to form a ternary complex with the RasGDP dissociation stimulator (RasGDS).

GAP-like protein called p190 (62). This complex has only 25% of the original GAP activity. GAP may be regulated allosterically: phosphatidic acid, arachidonic acid, and phosphoinositols are all known second messengers and all can inhibit GAP activity (63). These compounds can also stimulate RasGIP.

Fourth, hormones may affect GDI. For example, the dissociation of Rac from RhoGDI can be induced by several second messengers, such as arachidonic acid, polyamines, and phosphoinositides (64).

Note that hormones can affect more than one pathway, especially in different cell types (65). Once activated, Ras can bind Raf, a protein kinase that phosphorylates and activates MAP kinase kinase (66-70); MAP kinase, the next substrate in this cascade is a major kinase involved in affecting the activity of transcription factors (see Chapter 12). This pathway also mediates the insulin-induced maturation of *Xenopus* oocytes (71,72).

C. Large G Proteins

The G protein trimers couple the serpentine receptors to their effectors (Chapter 6). The nomenclature for these G proteins is confusing because these proteins were often functionally identified before being purified and sequenced. For example, the G protein stimulating adenylate cyclase is called G_s, whereas that inhibiting this enzyme is G_i; in this case, the structural classification corresponds nicely to the functional classification. However, a G protein that regulates potassium channels, G_K, may actually turn out to be a member of the G_i family. Another G protein, G_p, activates phospholipase $C\beta$ (PLCβ); however, it was subsequently discovered that G_p belonged to the G_q family. To further complicate matters, there is some evidence that there may be another G_p that is not in the G_q group. In this text, the functional classification will only be used when the identity of the G protein is still in doubt.

The G protein is actually a heterotrimer with a subunit structure of $\alpha\beta\gamma$. The α subunit is the GTPase and is primarily responsible for the biological activity of the G protein. As such it can be subjected to the same classification scheme just shown: α_s, α_i, α_q, and so on. α_s is a 45 to 52-kDa protein; the larger variant is a result of alternative splicing of a single mRNA. This may have regulatory significance, since the insert has an additional PKC phosphorylation site. The carboxy terminus binds the hormone receptor and the effector, whereas the amino terminus binds the $\beta\gamma$ dimer (Fig. 8-6). In α_i and α_o, the amino terminus is also myristoylated; this modification enhances membrane-binding (73), increases the affinity of the α subunit for the $\beta\gamma$ dimer (74), and is required for coupling between α_{i2} and adenylate cyclase (75). Although not myristoylated, the α_s subunit is palmitoylated on the third residue and this modification serves the same functions just enumerated for myristoylation (76). α_s also binds aluminum fluoride (an exogenous activator) and is modified by cholera toxin. Cholera toxin removes nicotinamide from NAD^+ and attaches the rest of the molecule to an arginine (Fig. 8-7); this is called mono(ADP–ribosyl)ation. This amino acid is in the catalytic site and its modification inactivates the GTPase. Since the hydrolysis of GTP turns the system off, mono(ADP–ribosyl)ation results in a persistently activated state.

The β subunit is a 35-kDa protein and binds magnesium. The first 30–40 amino acids are involved in binding the α and γ subunits (77). The rest of the molecule is composed of eight repeats of a WD-40 motif. The function of this repeat is unknown but it also occurs in other proteins involved in protein–protein interactions. For example, this motif is present in an activator of phospholipase A_2 (74), that is involved in another transduction pathway (see Chapter 9). The γ subunit is 8.4 kDa, is polyprenylated, and is closest physically to the α subunit (79,80). Initially, researchers thought that there was only a single $\beta\gamma$ dimer for each of the different α subunits and that the dimer was not directly involved with mediating biological activity. However, both assumptions proved incorrect. There are several isoforms for both of these subunits and there appears to be some specificity in their association (78-83); for example, β_1 will bind γ_1 or γ_2; but β_2 will only bind γ_2, and β_3 will bind γ_4. This coupling can also be receptor specific (83,84): the $\alpha_{o1}\beta_3\gamma_4$ mediates the M4R inhibition of voltage-gated calcium channels, whereas $\alpha_{o2}\beta_1\gamma_3$ mediates the SRIF receptor inhibition of these same channels. In addition, certain $\beta\gamma$ isoforms can couple to specific effectors; for example, β_1 selectively couples to PLCβ (85) and β_2 targets β_2AR (86). Other evidence for the biological effects of the $\beta\gamma$ is discussed later.

The α subunit has a much higher intrinsic GTPase activity than the small G proteins. For that reason, investigators assumed that these proteins had no GAP or that a GAP-like domain had been incorporated into the larger α protein. However, several effectors are known to accelerate GTP hydrolysis when they are bound to α. For example, PLCβ increases the GTPase activity of α_q and a cGMP-specific phosphodiesterase will enhance GTP hydrolysis by α_t (87,88). This is not true of all effectors: adenylate cyclase has no GAP

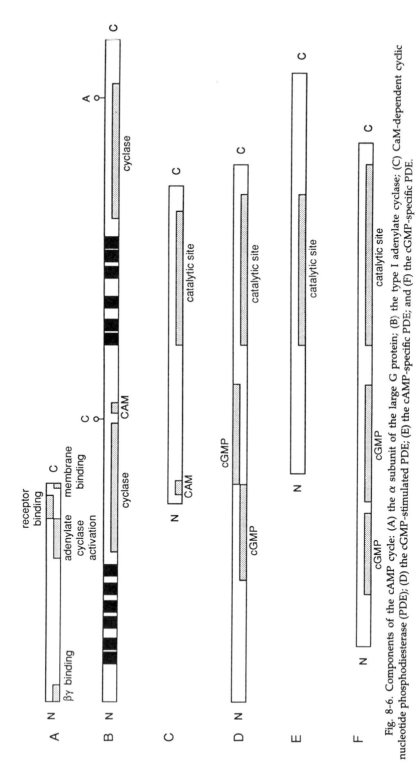

Fig. 8-6. Components of the cAMP cycle: (A) the α subunit of the large G protein; (B) the type I adenylate cyclase; (C) CaM-dependent cyclic nucleotide phosphodiesterase (PDE); (D) the cGMP-stimulated PDE; (E) the cAMP-specific PDE; and (F) the cGMP-specific PDE.

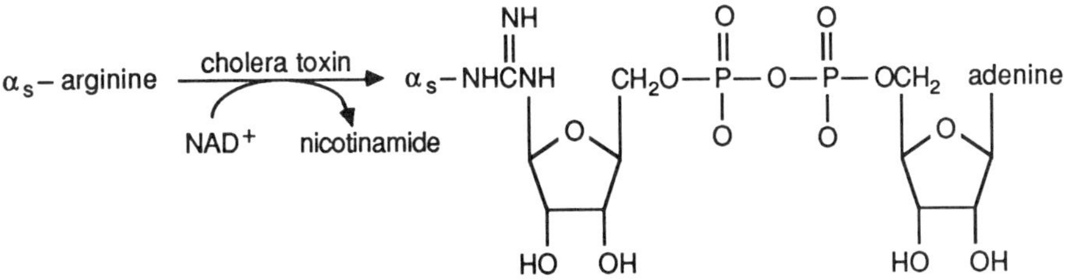

Fig. 8-7. Biochemical mechanism by which cholera toxin activates α_s.

activity. The fact that some effectors of G protein trimers have GAP activity adds further evidence that the GAPs for the small G proteins are also effectors.

There are three or four different α subunit families. The α_s family includes α_s and α_{olf}; the latter forms part of the G protein in the olfactory epithelium and is responsible for the sensory transduction of smell. Both activate adenylate cyclase and α_s can directly open calcium channels, inhibit sodium channels, and stimulate a plasmalemma calcium pump (89). The α_i family includes α_i, α_z, α_o, α_t, and α_g. All of the members of this family except α_z can be mono(ADP-ribosyl)ated by another bacterial toxin, pertussis toxin. The first two inhibit adenylate cyclase and open potassium channels; α_i can also inhibit PLCβ (85). α_o stimulates potassium channels, inhibits adenylate cyclase, and activates PLC (91,92). α_t and α_g transmit sensory signals involved in light and taste perception, respectively; α_t is coupled to a cGMP-specific phosphodiesterase and α_g elevates cAMP in sweet receptors and calcium in bitter receptors (93). The α_q family activates PLCγ and includes α_{11}, α_{14}, α_{15}, and α_{16}. The last group, which includes α_{12} and α_{13}, is sometimes listed separately or incorporated as a subfamily under α_q. γ_{13} has been reported to stimulate a (Na^+, H^+) exchanger, NHE-1 (94).

IV. Cyclic AMP Pathway

A. Components and Cycle

In the cAMP pathway, hormones stimulate or inhibit adenylate cyclase via G_s and G_i, respectively. The G proteins were just discussed. In this section, the enzymes that produce and degrade cAMP will be covered. Six adenylate cyclases have been sequenced; all have the same overall topology (Fig. 8-6). They can be divided into two highly homologous halves: each begins with six transmembrane helices that are followed by the catalytic domain (95). Both catalytic sites are required for activity, although they do not have to be contiguous (96), that is, the molecule can be physically split in half and still be active as long as both halves are present. The cyclases fall into three groups: the first group, which includes the types I and III cyclases, are calmodulin (CaM) dependent. Because type I is also stimulated by α_s but inhibited by $\beta\gamma$, some authorities feel that any G protein input cancels itself out and that calcium–CaM is the major activator of this group. Type III was originally identified in the olfactory epithelium but it has subsequently been found in other tissues (97). Types II and IV form the second group, have shorter carboxy termini, and are stimulated by $\beta\gamma$ in the presence of the α subunit (98); type II can also be activated by phosphorylation by PKC (99). Types V and VI, which constitute the last group, also have shorter carboxy termini but longer amino termini. They are CaM-independent and are inhibited by calcium (94). A PKA site in the carboxy terminus is responsible for heterologous desensitization (95). Some of the cyclases can also be phosphorylated on tyrosine by Src; this modification increases the sensitivity of the cyclase for its agonists by 2 to 3-fold (102). In addition, this last group is the most sensitive to the inhibitory effects of α_i; type II is modestly suppressed and type I is barely affected at all (103,104).

The cyclic nucleotides are degraded by phosphodiesterases (PDEs). There are five classes (Table 8-5), but all have a homologous catalytic domain in the center of the molecule (Fig. 8-6; 105). The regulatory site is usually located in the amino terminus; for example, this is where the CaM and cGMP allosteric sites are found. The function of the carboxy terminus is unknown except in the cGMP-specific PDE, in which it is involved in membrane binding. The calcium–CaM PDE is stimulated by calcium–CaM but inhibited by phosphorylation by either PKA or a CaM-dependent kinase II. The cGMP-stimulated PDE is allosterically activated by cGMP. This represents a rare direct action of cGMP; as noted subsequently, most of the actions of cGMP are mediated by a protein kinase (PKG). The cGMP-inhibited PDE is stimulated by phosphorylation by either PKA or an insulin-activated serine kinase. These three PDEs will utilize either cAMP or cGMP as substrate. The cAMP-specific PDE degrades only cAMP and has no known acute regulators; however, cAMP can induce the transcription of this enzyme. The cGMP-specific PDE uses only cGMP as substrate and was originally thought to be restricted to the retina, where it is activated by transducin (G_t). How-

Table 8-5

Cyclic Nucleotide Phosphodiesterases[a]

Isoform	Substrate	Regulation
Calcium–CaM PDE	cGMP > cAMP	Calcium–CaM (+); PKA (−); CaM-dependent kinase II (+)
cGMP-stimulated PDE	cAMP > cGMP	cGMP (+)
cGMP-inhibited PDE	cAMP > cGMP	PKA (+); insulin-stimulated serine kinase (+)
cAMP-specific PDE	cAMP	PKA (+)[b]
cGMP-specific PDE	cGMP	α_t (+); cGMP allosteric site but no known effect

[a] PDE, Phosphodiesterase; CaM, calmodulin; PKA, protein kinase A.
[b] Via transcription, not direct phosphorylation.

ever, it has recently been found in lungs and platelets. It also has an allosteric cGMP-binding site, although this nucleotide has no observable effect on enzymatic activity.

These components interact in the following manner (Fig. 8-8; 106). Hormones whose actions are mediated by elevated cAMP levels bind to their receptors. The hormone–receptor complex then binds to an inactive G_s; that is, a G_s whose α_s subunit is binding GDP instead of GTP. In some systems, the receptor may be precoupled to G_s; for example, 50% of the βARs are precoupled. This precoupling increases the affinity of the receptor for its ligand. When all three components (hormone, receptor, and G_s) are together, GTP can displace GDP from the α_s subunit. Recent studies have shown that the last 11 amino acids of α_s form a loop that helps bind GDP; when α_s binds the hormone–receptor complex, the loop opens up and the affinity for GDP decreases, thereby facilitating nucleotide exchange (107,108).

The next several steps are controversial: conventional wisdom says that the α_s dissociates from the rest of the complex, although a minority view claims that the dissociation seen under experimental conditions is really an artifact. In addition, it is uncertain whether α_s remains associated with the membrane or whether it diffuses to the adenylate cyclase through the cytoplasm. Regardless of the route, the α_s will now stimulate adenylate cyclase

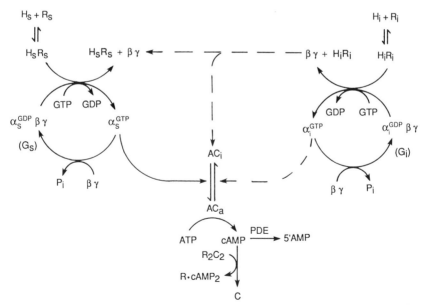

Fig. 8-8. The activation and inhibition of adenylate cyclase. AC_a and AC_i, Active and inactive adenylate cyclase, respectively; C, catalytic subunit of the cAMP-dependent protein kinase; H_i inhibitory hormone (and its receptor, R_i); H_s, stimulatory hormone (and its receptor, R_s); R, regulatory subunit of the cAMP-dependent protein kinase. Other abbreviations are defined in the text and in the legend to Fig. 8-1.

activity, but only as long as the GTP remains intact. Since α_s contains low GTPase activity, the GTP is slowly hydrolyzed to GDP and α_s recombines with the β and γ subunits. Because of this automatic shut-off system, cAMP generation is quickly terminated when hormones are removed. Some analogs of GTP have unusual bonds between the phosphates and cannot be hydrolyzed by GTPases such as α_s. Such analogs permanently activate adenylate cyclase because the system cannot turn itself off. Cholera toxin has a similar effect (see preceding discussion).

Hormones whose actions are mediated by lowering cAMP levels act in a similar manner except that their hormone–receptor complexes bind G_i, which is then activated when GTP displaces the GDP on α_i. However, it is not clear how G_i inhibits adenylate cyclase; by analogy to the G_s system, α_i should directly inhibit adenylate cyclase, but the activity of α_i is very weak. The β subunit is also an effective inhibitor, which has led to the speculation that the released $\beta\gamma$ complex may force α_s to reassociate into G_s, thereby terminating the adenylate cyclase stimulation. In other words, the activation of adenylate cyclase requires that G_s dissociate to liberate α_s:

$$\alpha_s\beta\gamma \rightleftharpoons \alpha_s + \beta\gamma$$

If the concentration of $\beta\gamma$ can be increased from another source such as G_i, the laws of mass action dictate that the equilibrium would shift back to the left. However, the data of one experiment conflict with this hypothesis: the mono(ADP–ribosyl)ation of α_s by cholera toxin not only permanently activates α_s, but also renders α_s unable to reassociate with $\beta\gamma$. Despite this, somatostatin-stimulated G_i is still able to inhibit adenylate cyclase in cholera toxin-treated pituitary cells, suggesting that G_i does not act by promoting the reassociation of G_s (109). Alternatively, $\beta\gamma$ may directly inhibit the adenylate cyclase; in fact, this effect has been shown for type II and IV cyclases.

The α_i also has GTPase activity that is responsible for the termination of its action. Inhibition is also produced by pertussis toxin, which mono(ADP–ribosyl)ates α_i at a carboxy-terminal cysteine. This is a result of two effects: first, the modification inhibits the coupling of G_i to its receptor and, second, it blocks GTP activation in the absence of agonist (104). In most tissues, G_i is present in a 4 to 10-fold excess over G_s. This excess is important in maintaining a low basal activity of adenylate cyclase (111).

B. Outputs

The best known output of this system is the allosteric regulator cAMP, which is generated by adenylate cyclase in response to α_s (Fig. 8-9). This modulator can inhibit a phosphoinositide kinase (112) and a poly(ADP-ribose)glycohydrolase (113); the former enzyme is involved in lipid metabolism (Chapter 9) and the latter reverses a covalent modification of histones (Chapter 13). cAMP can also directly activate several ion channels, such as the cardiac pacemaker channel (114) and the potassium channel in *Drosophila* muscle (115); furthermore, it inhibits the insulin-sensitive glucose carrier in a ki-

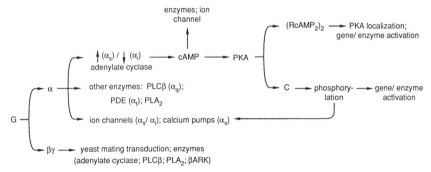

Fig. 8-9. Schematic representation of the various outputs of the cAMP pathway. PLCβ, Phospholipase Cβ; PLA₂, phospholipase A₂; βARK, β-adrenergic receptor kinase. Other abbreviations are defined in the text and in the legend to Fig. 8-8.

nase-independent manner, suggesting another direct effect (116). However, the major target of this molecule is a cAMP-dependent protein kinase or protein kinase A (PKA).

PKA is a heterotetramer (R_2C_2) consisting of two regulatory subunits (R) that inhibit the two catalytic subunits (C). The amino terminus of R contains a dimerization domain as well as a pseudosubstrate site that occupies and inhibits the catalytic site of C (see Fig. 11-1). This region is then followed by two tandem cAMP-binding sites. When cAMP binds the regulatory subunits, the tetramer dissociates and the liberated catalytic subunits become active:

$$R_2C_2 \text{ (inactive)} + 4cAMP \rightleftharpoons (R \cdot cAMP_2)_2 + 2C \text{ (active)}$$

Activation also requires the autophosphorylation of C; the phosphate group forms bonds with basic residues to stabilize the kinase and lower the K_m for ATP and the substrate (117). C is myristoylated; although this modification is not necessary for either the localization or the activation of PKA (118), it does impart greater thermal stability to the kinase (119). There are three isoforms of C, but there are no known functional differences between Cα and Cβ except for their tissue distribution. All three phosphorylate serines or threonines at the following consensus sequence: (+)–(+)–X-S/T, where (+) is a basic amino acid. PKA can phosphorylate an enormous range of substrates. However, Cγ differs slightly in substrate specificity and is less sensitive to a protein kinase inhibitor (120,121). The PKA phosphorylation of receptors has already been discussed in preceding chapters; other substrates include enzymes, cytoskeleton, channels, and transcription factors.

The two major regulatory subunits are RI and RII. RI has a high affinity for cAMP that results in the rapid dissociation of the tetramer and a slow reassociation. It predominates in undifferentiated or embryonic tissues. RII has a lower affinity for cAMP; therefore, dissociation is slow and reassociation is rapid. However, PKA II can autophosphorylate its RII subunit; this modification increases the affinity of RII for cAMP and decreases subunit reassociation. Conversely, Cdc2 can phosphorylate RII in the first cAMP-binding site; this modification decreases the affinity of RII for cAMP and favors the formation of the inactive tetramer. Cdc2 phosphorylation also reduces the affinity of RII for MAP-2, a microtubular accessory protein; therefore, this modification may affect the localization of PKA (122). PKA II is more abundant than PKA I in differentiated tissues.

In addition to structural differences, these two isoenzymes are regulated differently. In rat anterior pituitary cells, PKA I is activated more rapidly and with less GHRH than PKA II (123). In rat liver, a similar phenomenon is seen with glucagon (124,125). These data suggest that PKA I may be involved with acute responses, such as secretion or enzyme activation, whereas PKA II may trigger more prolonged effects, such as gene transcription. Note that this type of regulation may be tissue specific: in normal osteoblasts, PTH activates both PKA I and II with the same time course and concentration dependence (126).

Until recently, protein phosphorylation by the catalytic subunit was thought to be the only action exerted by PKA II, but there is some evidence that RII may have functions independent of the catalytic subunit. For example, RII may help localize PKA to specific parts of the cell, thereby influencing substrate accessibility. RII has a high affinity for the Golgi apparatus and microtubules (127; see also Chapter 10); the latter are substrates for PKA, whose phosphorylation facilitates microtubule assembly. RII also has a high affinity for the nuclear matrix (128). Therefore, RII may be responsible for localizing PKA to certain organelles; this compartmentalization would favor some substrates over others and influence the spectrum of phosphorylation by PKA.

RII has also been reported to inhibit the phosphoprotein phosphatase (129), an enzyme responsible for terminating the glycogenolysis induced by cAMP-stimulated phosphorylation (see Chapter 11). Consequently, RII would complement the kinase by preventing the dephosphorylation of its substrates. More controversial is its possible role in transcription. It is clear from several studies that phosphorylation by PKA is essential for cAMP-induced gene transcription (see Chapter 12), but whether or not RII contributes to this effect is unknown. RII can bind the DNA sequence responsible for cAMP-induced transcription; this binding is cAMP dependent (130). Furthermore, this cAMP response element (CRE) could not activate a reporter gene in mutants lacking RII; responsiveness was restored by RII but not RI (131). However, in other systems, RII does not appear to be necessary.

Heretofore, the discussion has been dominated by PKA; this emphasis is only appropriate, since PKA phosphorylation is an output of major importance. However, the α subunit of G proteins can affect other activities; for example, it can modulate the cGMP-specific PDE (see preceeding discussion) and the phospholipases Cβ (PLCβ) and A$_2$ (PLA$_2$) (see Chapter 9). The α subunit can also directly affect many ion channels, including the calcium and potassium channels (132). Actually, these channels can often be regulated by the same pathway via different mechanisms. In endocrine and smooth muscle cells, the calcium channel is directly modulated by α; in skeletal and cardiac muscle it is phosphorylated by PKA, which can also induce the gene for this channel. Finally, there is some evidence to suggest that G proteins may directly stimulate PI3K (133).

Until recently, all the output for the G proteins was thought to occur through the α subunit, but there is now considerable evidence that the $\beta\gamma$ dimer can also have biological effects (Fig. 8-9) (134). This dimer inhibits adenylate cyclase I and stimulates types II and IV (see preceeding discussion), increases βARK activity (see Chapter 7), and activates both PLCβ and PLA$_2$ (Chapter 9). The latter event occurs in the retina (135). Finally, the $\beta\gamma$ complex mediates both the pheromone induction of the mating response in yeast and the 1-methyladenine stimulation of oocyte meoisis in starfish (136). Some authorities have questioned the significance of these effects because of the high concentrations of $\beta\gamma$ required. In response, those favoring a physiological role for $\beta\gamma$ claim that this dimer can arise from many different G proteins and can, therefore, accumulate to high levels. In addition, it has been argued that the difference in effective concentrations between the α and $\beta\gamma$ subunits is artifactual: many G protein effectors accelerate GTP hydrolysis and shorten the half-life of the active α subunit. However, since α effects are usually measured in the presence of nonhydrolyzable analogs of GTP, the α activity is artificially prolonged, rendering the experimental system more sensitive to α (137). As such, the true effective concentrations of α and $\beta\gamma$ *in vivo* may not be that different.

C. Regulation

The regulation of the adenylate cyclases and PDEs were discussed earlier. In this section, control of the other components of this system will be covered. G proteins can be regulated by (i) compartmentalization, (ii) molecular number, and (iii) covalent modification (138). Early in the history of cyclic nucleotide research, the cell was considered to be a bag of cytoplasm with virtually no internal barriers to diffusion. G proteins were thought to form a common pool for which all receptors could compete. This view turns out to be overly simplistic; first, not all receptors have equal access to all G proteins. G_s activates both the plasmalemma calcium pump and an adenylate cyclase in liver; β-agonists can activate the G_s coupled to the cyclase but not that coupled to the pump (139). Even after a second messenger has been generated, its diffusion is severely restricted: endogenously produced cAMP results in a more restricted pattern of protein phosphorylation than seen with exogenous cAMP analogs (140), presumably because the former is generated at discrete locations and is degraded before it diffuses very far. The strong association of PKA to certain organelles would further limit protein phosphorylation. For example, it has been shown that PKA entry into the nucleus is the rate-limiting event in the hormonal stimulation of transcription (141,142). In addition to affecting G protein access to receptors and effectors during primary stimulation, compartmentalization can also play a role in desensitization. G proteins and receptors are sequestered together; but while internalized they become physically dissociated and recycle at different rates (143).

Feedback regulation of G proteins often occurs by decreasing G protein number. For example, β-agonists, which activate G_s, decrease α_s 25% in lymphoma cells while elevating α_i 3-fold (144); in other words, not only does the α_s pathway get dampened, but its antagonist α_i is stimulated. The muscarinic acetylcholine receptor utilizes G_q in Chinese hamster ovary (CHO) cells and these agonists will down-regulate G_q 40% (143). Heterologous regulation is also usually accomplished by altering G protein number. Many of the symptoms of hyperthyroidism are related to the overactivity of the βARs: rapid heart rate, elevated body temperature, and so on. This relationship is partially a result of the induction of α_s by T_3; conversely, hypothyroidism increases α_i (146). Homologous regulation is often due to changes in G protein half-life whereas heterologous regulation occurs via transcription.

Three types of covalent modification have been described: (i) serine-threonine phosphorylation, (ii) tyrosine phosphorylation, and (iii) mono(ADP–ribosyl)ation. The phosphorylation of α_i by either PKA or PKC impairs its ability to inhibit adenylate cyclase (147–148). There are conflicting reports concerning the phosphorylation of α_s; this problem probably arises from the fact that there are two α_s isoforms. The longer form has an additional short sequence containing a PKC consensus site capable of being phosphorylated (150). α_s, α_i, and α_o can all be tyrosine phosphorylated by Src (151); this modification increases the rate of nucleotide exchange, decreases the α affinity for the $\beta\gamma$ dimer, and stimulates agonist-induced GTPase activity.

As noted already, several bacterial toxins can remove ADP–ribose from NAD^+ and attached it to G proteins. An endogenous enzyme with a similar catalytic activity and protein structure has been isolated (152). Because several of the bacterial toxins modify the G proteins of the cAMP system, it was suggested that the endogenous enzyme might function to modulate this system physiologically. This hypothesis was tested for hCG in a Leydig tumor cell line (153), for LH in Leydig cells (154), and for TSH in a thyroid cell line (153); each stimulates adenylate cyclase in its respective target cells. However, in no system was the stimulation NAD dependent and no mono(ADP–ribosyl)ated G_s could be found. Researchers concluded that none of these hormones acted via mono(ADP–ribosyl)ation.

In other systems, inhibitors of mono(ADP–ribosyl)ation blocked the effects of T_3 on oxidative phosphorylation (155) and histamine on the production of eicosanoids (156). However, no data were given on the effects of T_3 or histamine on actual ADP–ribosylation levels or on enzymes involved in this modification. These crucial data were obtained in platelets, where prostacyclin treatment did result in the mono(ADP–ribosyl)ation of α_s; and this modification was associated with enhanced cAMP production (157). However, mono(ADP–ribosyl)ation does not appear to be the primary mechanism by which receptors activate G proteins; instead, it functions in secondary gain. This conclusion also comes from work in platelets, where thrombin mono(ADP–ribosyl)ates a G protein via PKC, an effector of thrombin that is downstream from the G protein (158). Since the modification requires PKC, one might speculate that the mono(ADP–ribosyl)transferase may be activated by PKC phosphorylation. In rods this transferase can also be stimulated to modify α_s by NO (159,160).

PKA is primarily controlled by cAMP and the type of regulatory subunit (see preceeding discussion). However, there are two other regulatory mechanisms: (i) the protein kinase inhibitor (PKI) and (ii) down-regulation. PKI inhibits PKA by acting as a pseudosubstrate and by sequestering the kinase; its levels can be regulated by several hormones. For example, in the kidney, parathormone, which acts through cAMP, elevates PKI 30–60%; this probably represents negative feedback (161). Conversely, both 1,25-DHCC and calcium lower PKI 90–95% in the kidney. In addition to altering substrate levels, PKI can be tyrosine phosphorylated by the EGFR; this modification impairs PKI activity (162).

cAMP causes RI and RII to dissociate from C. Although this event activates C, it also facilitates the down-regulation of C since the free form is much more susceptible to degradation (163). Long-term exposure to cAMP can also elevate RI and RII; this would drive the equilibrium back to the inactive tetramer.

D. Specificity

One final problem must be addressed: specificity. For simplicity, the presentation just completed implied that there was a unique and clear pathway from hormone receptor to G protein to effector. In truth, there is considerable overlap among these routes (Fig. 8-10; 164). For example, many receptors can activate the same G protein: glucagon, vasopressin, and angiotensin all activate G_p in the liver. Conversely, one receptor can activate many G

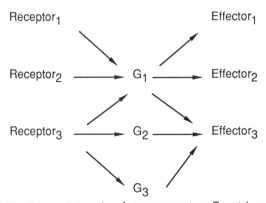

Fig. 8-10. Promiscuous interactions between receptors, G proteins, and effectors.

proteins: LH and PTH activate both G_s and G_p; M2R agonists activate G_p and G_i; and D2R is coupled to calcium channels by α_o and to potassium channels via α_{i3} (165–167). One G protein can induce many effectors: α_s can activate both adenylate cyclase and calcium channels. Finally, an effector can be stimulated by many G proteins: PLCβ can be activated by any member of the G_q family. To further complicate matters, some effectors, such as adenylate cyclase and PLCβ can be affected by the $\beta\gamma$ dimer as well as by the α subunit.

When a receptor is coupled to multiple G proteins, there is often a preferred order: both glucagon and tachykinin couple to both G_s and G_p, but for glucagon the order is $G_s > G_p$ whereas for tachykinin it is the reverse. This ordering introduces the agonist concentration as a critical variable in determining the spectrum of activity of any given receptor. Other factors may also affect the coupling; this is best illustrated by PTH and CT in bone cells, where the two hormones activate the same G proteins (G_s and G_p) but have opposite effects:

1. Cell cycle. CT stimulates the $(Na^+,K^+)ATPase$ in G_2 via cAMP (G_s), but inhibits this same enzyme in S via PKC (G_p) (168). G_s is still present in S and can be activated by other agonists, but it is somehow uncoupled from CT.

2. Hormone concentration. At low concentrations, PTH only stimulates PKC (G_p); at higher concentrations, PKC is unaffected whereas PKA is activated (G_s); at the highest levels, both kinases are stimulated (169).

3. Receptor concentration. The higher the receptor concentration, the more likely that cross-activation of G proteins will occur. For example, at low concentrations M4R inhibits adenylate cyclase via G_i but at higher concentrations it stimulates the cyclase through G_s (170). Whether this phenomenon is unique to transfection systems that yield very high receptor copy numbers or whether it can also occur physiologically is not known.

4. Receptor subcellular localization. In renal cortical cells, PTH receptors located on the basolateral surface are coupled to G_s, but those at the cell apex are not (171).

5. Cell type. PTH induces proliferation in osteoblasts via G_p, but activates bone resorption by osteoclasts via cAMP (G_s). Since osteoblasts and osteoclasts arise from the same lineage, this phenomenon may also represent differential G protein coupling based on the developmental status of the cell or tissue.

6. Other signals. Phosphate depletion depresses PTH-induced calcium responses (G_p) but enhances the elevation of cAMP (G_s); hyperphosphatemia has the reverse effect (172). Furthermore, insulin can suppress the effect of PTH on phosphoinositides (G_p) without having any effect on cAMP (G_s) (173).

7. Temporal patterns. The effects of PKA (G_s) are usually more prolonged than those of PKC (G_p) (174). In a different example, endothelin uses G_{13} for the initial transient contraction of smooth muscle but G_{11-2} for sustained contractions (175).

Obviously this example shows that G protein–receptor coupling can be very flexible and can depend on the agonist concentration, duration of stimulation, accessory signals, and the type, developmental stage, and proliferative state of the tissue. As such, this overlap in specificity allows for considerable integration of signals.

V. Cyclic GMP Pathway

The generation of cGMP has already been covered (see Chapter 6). Briefly, there are two synthetic pathways: one utilizes the membrane-bound guanylate cyclases and the other involves the soluble enzymes. The former cyclases are directly activated by ligand binding, whereas the latter are secondarily stimulated by hormones that elevate calcium levels which, with CaM, trigger the synthesis of nitric oxide. Nitric oxide is the proximate activator of the soluble guanylate cyclases.

There are three major outputs: (i) a PDE, (ii) a protein kinase, and (iii) ion channels (176). The effects of cGMP on several of the PDEs were discussed already (Table 8-4). There are two cGMP-dependent protein kinases or protein kinase Gs (PKGs): a ubiquitous soluble form (PKG I) and a membrane-bound form (PKG II) (177). Because the latter has not been characterized and is very restricted in its tissue distribution, it will not be considered further. The former kinase is very homologous to PKA: there is a dimerization domain in the amino terminus followed by two cGMP-binding sites and finally the catalytic site at the carboxy terminus (see Fig. 11-1). The consensus phosphorylation site for the two kinases is also the same: (+)-(+)-X-S/T. The major difference is that the protein is contiguous rather than being split into R and C subunits as occurs with PKA.

Alternative splicing of the amino terminus gives rise to two forms; PKG Iβ has a reduced affinity for cGMP and may be activated by physiological concentrations of cAMP. Cross-stimulation can also occur after PKG autophosphorylation, which increases affinity of PKG for cAMP. Conversely, high concentrations of cGMP can stimulate PKA (178). Because both PKA and PKG have the identical phosphorylation consensus site and each can be stimulated by either cyclic nucleotide, attempts to elucidate a unique role for PKG have been difficult. PKG is most abundant in the Purkinje cells of the cerebellum and in smooth muscle, where it induces relaxation by lowering intracellular calcium levels. In addition, cGMP, probably through PKG, stimulates cyclic ADP-ribose cyclase (179), which catalyzes the formation of another second messenger (see Chapter 9).

Finally, cGMP can directly interact with several ion channels; the first to be characterized was the cation channel of the photoreceptor (180). The channel is related to the voltage-gated ion channels (see Fig. 6-7); it has six transmembrane helices and a single transmembrane β loop. Presumably, four subunits come together to form an 8-stranded β-barrel pore. There is a single cGMP-binding site in the carboxy terminus. Similar channels have been characterized from other tissues; they differ in their ion specificity and cyclic nucleotide preference.

VI. Cyclic CMP Pathway

Work on other cyclic nucleotides has been less fruitful. Cyclic CMP has been detected in tissues and is elevated in rapidly proliferating tissues; for example, levels in regenerating liver are 130 times those in normal liver (175). Furthermore, dibutyryl cCMP is mitogenic in both leukemic cells (181) and normal mammary epithelium (182). A cytidylate cyclase has also been identified and is similarly elevated in rapidly dividing cells (183). Finally, a very specific cCMP PDE has been partially purified; it does not hydrolyze cAMP or cGMP and is not inhibited by the methylxanthines. Its concentration is low in rapidly proliferating tissues and it can be inhibited by polyamines. Polyamines are associated with rapid growth (see Chapter 10); therefore, their inhibition of this enzyme would allow cCMP, a postulated mitogen, to accumulate and synergize with the polyamines and possibly other growth signals.

VII. Transcellular Signaling

Second messenger signals can be propagated throughout a tissue in the absence of direct hormonal stimulation of each cell. Using autoradiography to detect ^{125}I-labeled hCG binding and cytochemistry to detect activated PKA, receptor–kinase coupling could be studied in granulosa cells (184). Every cell showing hCG binding had activated PKA; every *isolated* cell without hCG binding did not have activated PKA. However, if a cell without hCG binding was in physical contact with one that did, then *both* cells had activated PKA. The hypothesis is that the cAMP generated in cells showing hCG binding is diffusing through gap junctions into the surrounding cells and activating their PKA.

This method of propagation also occurs for the other major transduction system, calcium. For example, in follicular cells angiotensin II initiates calcium waves that are propagated to the adjacent oocyte (185). However, it is not calcium that is actually passing through the gap junctions; instead, the second messenger inositol 1,4,5-trisphosphate diffuses through these pores and opens calcium reservoirs within each cell (186; see also Chapter 9).

VIII. Summary

GTP-binding proteins, or G proteins, are molecular switches with built-in or closely associated automatic timers. They are activated when GTP replaces GDP and inactivated when the intrinsic GTPase activity hydrolyzes GTP. Most of the small G proteins are involved in vesicular trafficking and cytoskeletal organization but Ras has been strongly implicated in the mitogenic signal transduction of several growth factors. There are several postulated mechanisms for how these hormone activate Ras but the most common ones include stimulating guanine nucleotide exchange and sequestering GAP, a protein required to turn the system off. In particular, RTKs can directly stimulate a RasGDS by tyrosine phosphorylation or indirectly stimulate RasGDS via adaptors. The activation of Ras leads to the stimulation of several proline-directed kinases and, eventually, to DNA synthesis.

The large G proteins are trimers. The α subunit is the GTPase and designates which signal pathway will be affected: α_s and α_i alter adenylate cyclase activity and ion channels, whereas α_q activates the phospholipid–calcium pathway (Fig. 8-9). The $\beta\gamma$ dimer can also affect these two pathways, as well as mediate yeast mating transduction. PKA is a major target of cAMP and can have both acute effects by phosphorylating enzymes and ion channels and long-term effects by phosphorylating transcription factors and inducing genes. There is considerable overlap in the coupling of receptors, G proteins, and effectors; the exact biological activity produced is influenced by the agonist concentration, the duration of stimulation, the presence of other signals, and the type, developmental stage, and proliferative state of the tissue.

cGMP is produced by membrane-bound or soluble guanylate cyclases; the former are hormone receptors whereas the latter are second messenger receptors for nitric oxide and carbon monoxide. cGMP can affect PDEs, ion channels, and PKG. cCMP is the newest and least studied member of the cyclic nucleotides. Although associated with proliferation, an unequivocal role in hormone action has not been demonstrated.

Finally, signals can diffuse through gap junctions and spread throughout a tissue without the hormone having to contact each and every cell. This phenomenon has been demonstrated for both cAMP and inositol 1,4,5-trisphosphate, a calcium-releasing second messenger.

References

General References

Boguski, M. S., and McCormick, F. (1993). Proteins regulating Ras and its relatives. *Nature (London)* **366,** 643–654.

Bokoch, G. M. (1993). Biology of the Rap proteins, members of the *ras* superfamily of GTP-binding proteins. *Biochem. J.* **289,** 17–24.

Brown, A. M. (1993). Membrane-delimited cell signaling complexes: Direct ion channel regulation by G proteins. *J. Membr. Biol.* **131,** 93–104.

Casey, P. J. (1992). Biochemistry of protein prenylation. *J. Lipid Res.* **33,** 1731–1740.

Conkin, B. R., and Bourne, H. R. (1993). Structural elements of Gα subunits that interact with Gβγ, receptors, and effectors. *Cell* **73,** 631–641.

Eismann, E., Bönigk, W., and Kaupp, U. B. (1993). Structural features of cyclic nucleotide-gated channels. *Cell. Physiol. Biochem.* **3,** 332–351.

Newman, C. M. H., and Magee, A. I. (1993). Post-translational processing of the ras superfamily of small GTP-binding proteins. *Biochim. Biophys. Acta* **1155,** 79–96.

White, M. F., and Kahn, C. R. (1994). The insulin signaling system. *J. Biol. Chem.* **269,** 1–4.

See also Refs. 6–10, 12, 18, 26, 27, 50, 63, 103, 105, 106, 132, 134, 137, 144, 146, 152, 160, 176, 177, and 181.

Cited References

1. Randazzo, P. A., Northup, J. K., and Kahn, R. A. (1992). Regulatory GTP-binding proteins (ADP-ribosylation factor, G_t, and RAS) are not activated directly by nucleoside diphosphate kinase. *J. Biol. Chem.* **267,** 18182–18189.

2. Bominaar, A. A., Molijn, A. C., Pestel, M., Veron, M., and Van Haastert, P. J. M. (1993). Activation of G-proteins by receptor-stimulated nucleoside diphosphate kinase in *Dictyostelium*. *EMBO J.* **12,** 2275–2279.

3. Hart, M. J., Maru, Y., Leonard, D., Witte, O. N., Evans, T., and Cerione, R. A. (1992). A GDP dissociation inhibitor that serves as a GTPase inhibitor for the Ras-like protein CDC42Hs. *Science* **258,** 812–815.

4. Chuang, T. H., Xu, X., Knaus, U. G., Hart, M. J., and Bokoch, G. M. (1993). GDP dissociation inhibitor prevents intrinsic and GTPase activating protein-stimulated GTP hydrolysis by the Rac GTP-binding protein. *J. Biol. Chem.* **268,** 775–778.

5. Regazzi, R., Kikuchi, A., Takai, Y., and Wollheim, C. B. (1992). The small GTP-binding proteins in the cytosol of insulin-secreting cells are complexed to GDP dissociation inhibitor proteins. *J. Biol. Chem.* **267,** 17512–17519.

6. Bokoch, G. M., and Der, C. J. (1993). Emerging concepts in the *Ras* superfamily of GTP-binding proteins. *FASEB J.* **7,** 750–759.

7. Bourne, H. R., Sanders, D. A., and McCormick, F. (1990). The GTPase superfamily: A conserved switch for diverse cell functions. *Nature (London)* **348,** 125–132.

8. Hall, A. (1990). The cellular functions of small GTP-binding proteins. *Science* **249,** 635–640.

9. Sanders, D. A. (1990). A guide to low molecular weight GTPases. *Cell Growth Diff.* **1,** 251–258.

10. Kleuss, C., Scherübl, H., Hescheler, J., Schultz, G., and Wittig, B. (1993). Selectivity in signal transduction determined by q subunits of heterotrimeric G proteins. *Science* **259,** 832–834.

11. Philips, M. R., Pillinger, M. H., Staud, R., Volker, C., Rosenfeld, M. G., Weissmann, G., and Stock, J. B. (1993). Carboxy methylation of Ras-related proteins during signal transduction in neutrophils. *Science* **259,** 977–980.

12. Grand, R. J. A., and Owen, D. (1991). The biochemistry of ras p21. *Biochem. J.* **279,** 609–631.

13. Amrein, K. E., Flint, N., Panholzer, B., and Burn, P. (1992). Ras GTPase-activating protein: A substrate and a potential binding protein of the protein-tyrosine kinase p56^{lck}. *Proc. Natl. Acad. Sci. U.S.A.* **89**, 3343–3346.
14. Yatani, A., Okabe, K., Polakis, P., Halenbeck, R., McCormick, F., and Brown, A. M. (1990). *ras* p21 and GAP inhibit coupling of muscarinic receptors to atrial K$^+$ channels. *Cell* **61**, 769–776.
15. Schweighoffer, F., Barlat, I., Chevallier-Multon, M. C., and Tocque, B. (1992). Implication of GAP in Ras-dependent transactivation of a polyoma enhancer sequence. *Science* **256**, 825–827.
16. Medema, R. H., de Laat, W. L., Martin, G. A., McCormick, F., and Bos, J. L. (1992). GTPase-activating protein SH2-SH3 domains induce gene expression in a ras-dependent fashion. *Mol. Cell. Biol.* **12**, 3425–3430.
17. Duchesne, M., Schweighoffer, F., Parker, F., Clerc, F., Frobert, Y., Thang, M. N., and Tocqué, B. (1993). Identification of the SH3 domain of GAP as an essential sequence for Ras-GAP-mediated signaling. *Science* **259**, 525–528.
18. Gutmann, D. H., and Collins, F. S. (1993). The neurofibromatosis type 1 gene and its protein product, neurofibromin. *Neuron* **10**, 335–343.
19. DeClue, J. E., Papageorge, A. G., Fletcher, J. A., Diehl, S. R., Ratner, N., Vass, W. C., and Lowy, D. R. (1992). Abnormal regulation of mammalian p21^{ras} contributes to malignant tumor growth in von Recklinghausen (type 1) neurofibromatosis. *Cell* **69**, 265–273.
20. Johnson, M. R., Look, A. T., DeClue, J. E., Valentine, M. B., and Lowy, D. R. (1993). Inactivation of the *NF1* gene in human melanoma and neuroblastoma cell lines without impaired regulation of GTP·Ras. *Proc. Natl. Acad. Sci. U.S.A.* **90**, 5539–5543.
21. Miura, Y., Kaibuchi, K., Itoh, T., Corbin, J. D., Francis, S. H., and Takai, Y. (1992). Phosphorylation of *smg* p21B/*rap*1B p21 by cyclic GMP-dependent protein kinase. *FEBS Lett.* **297**, 171–174.
22. Zimmermann, P., Schnefel, S., Zeuzem, S., Pröfrock, A., Haase, W., and Schulz, I. (1992). Effects of agonists on p21^{ras} and *ras*-related proteins in rat pancreatic acinar cells. *Am. J. Physiol.* **263**, G396–G406.
23. Ridley, A. J., and Hall, A. (1992). The small GTP-binding protein rho regulates the assembly of focal adhesions and actin stress fibers in response to growth factors. *Cell* **70**, 389–399.
24. Ridley, A. J., Paterson, H. F., Johnston, C. L., Diekmann, D., and Hall, A. (1992). The small GTP-binding protein rac regulates growth factor-induced membrane ruffling. *Cell* **70**, 401–410.
25. Abo, A., Pick, E., Hall, A., Totty, N., Teahan, C. G., and Segal, A. W. (1991). Activation of the NADPH oxidase involves the small GTP-binding protein p21^{rac1}. *Nature (London)* **353**, 668–670.
26. Botstein, D., Segev, N., Stearns, T., Hoyt, M. A., Holden, J., and Kahn, R. A. (1988). Diverse biological functions of small GTP-binding proteins in yeast. *Cold Spring Harbor Symp. Quant. Biol.* **53**, 629–636.
27. Balch, W. E. (1989). Biochemistry of interorganelle transport: A new frontier in enzymology emerges from versatile *in vitro* model systems. *J. Biol. Chem.* **264**, 16965–16968.
28. van der Sluijs, P., Hull, M., Huber, L. A., Mâle, P., Goud, B., and Mellman, I. (1992). Reversible phosphorylation–dephosphorylation determines the localization of rab4 during the cell cycle. *EMBO J.* **11**, 4379–4389.

29. Bischoff, F. R., and Ponsting, H. (1991). Catalysis of guanine nucleotide exchange on Ran by the mitotic regulator TCC1. *Nature (London)* **354,** 80–82.
30. Bahnson, T. D., Tsai, S. C., Adamik, R., Moss, J., and Vaughan, M. (1989). Microinjection of a 19-kDa guanine nucleotide-binding protein inhibits maturation of *Xenopus* oocytes. *J. Biol. Chem.* **264,** 14824–14828.
31. Serafini, T., Orci, L., Amherdt, M., Brunner, M., Kahn, R. A., and Rothman, J. E. (1991). ADP-ribosylation factor is a subunit of the coat of Golgi-derived COP-coated vesicles: A novel role for a GTP-binding protein. *Cell* **67,** 239–253.
32. Balch, W. E., Kahn, R. A., and Schwaninger, R. (1992). ADP-ribosylation factor is required for vesicular trafficking between the endoplasmic reticulum and the *cis*-Golgi compartment. *J. Biol. Chem.* **267,** 13053–13061.
33. Kahn, R. A., Randazzo, P., Serafini, T., Weiss, O., Rulka, C., Clark, J., Amherdt, M., Roller, P., Orci, L., and Rothman, J. E. (1992). The amino terminus of ADP-ribosylation (ARF) is a critical determinant of ARF activities and is a potent and specific inhibitor of protein transport. *J. Biol. Chem.* **267,** 13039–13046.
34. Brown, H. A., Gutowski, S., Moomaw, C. R., Slaughter, C., and Sternweis, P. C. (1993). ADP-ribosylation factor, a small GTP-dependent regulatory protein, stimulates phospholipase D activity. *Cell* **75,**1137–1144.
35. Vincent, T. S., Wülfert, E., and Merler, E. (1992). Differences in growth factor signaling pathways determined by p21*ras* specific monoclonal antibodies. *FASEB J.* **6,** A1356.
36. Nakafuku, M., Satoh, T., and Kaziro, Y. (1992). Differentiation factors, including nerve growth factor, fibroblast growth factor, and interleukin-6, induce an accumulation of an active Ras·GTP complex in rat pheochromocytoma PC12 cells. *J. Biol. Chem.* **267,** 19448–19454.
37. Osterop, A. P. R. M., Medema, R. H., Bos, J. L., vanden Zon, G. C. M., Moller, D. E., Flier, J. S., Möller, W., and Maassen, J. A. (1992). Relation between the insulin receptor number in cells, autophosphorylation and insulin-stimulated Ras·GTP formation. *J. Biol. Chem.* **267,** 14647–14653.
38. Zhang, K., Papageorge, A. G., and Lowy, D. R. (1992). Mechanistic aspects of signaling through Ras in NIH 3T3 cells. *Science* **257,** 671–674.
39. Buday, L., and Downward, J. (1993). Epidermal growth factor regulates the exchange rate of guanine nucleotides on p21*ras* in fibroblasts. *Mol. Cell. Biol.* **13,** 1903–1910.
40. Graziani, A., Gramaglia, D., dalla Zonca, P., and Comoglio, P. M. (1993). Hepatocyte growth factor/scatter factor stimulates the Ras-guanine nucleotide exchanger. *J. Biol. Chem.* **268,** 9165–9168.
41. Gulbins, E., Coggeshall, K. M., Baier, G., Katzav, S., Burn, P., and Altman, A. (1993). Tyrosine-stimulated guanine nucleotide exchange activity of Vav in T cell activation. *Science* **260,** 822–825.
42. Evans, G. A., Howard, O. M. Z., Erwin, R., and Farrar, W. L. (1993). Interleukin-2 induces tyrosine phosphorylation of the *vav* proto-oncogene product in human T cells: Lack of requirement for the tyrosine kinase lck. *Biochem. J.* **294,** 339–342.
43. Alai, M., Mui, A. L. F., Cutler, R. L., Bustelo, X. R., Barbacid, M., and Krystal, G. (1992). Steel factor stimulates the tyrosine phosphorylation of the proto-oncogene product, p95*vav*, in human hemopoietic cells. *J. Biol. Chem.* **267,** 18021–18025.
44. Lowenstein, E. J., Daly, R. J., Batzer, A. G., Li, W., Margolis, B., Lammers, R., Ullrich, A., Skolnik, E. Y., Bar-Sagi, D., and Schlessinger, J. (1992). The SH2 and

SH3 domain-containing protein GRB2 links receptor tyrosine kinases to ras signaling. *Cell* **70**, 431–442.

45. Baltensperger, K., Kozma, L. M., Cherniack, A. D., Klarlund, J. K., Chawla, A., Banerjee, U., and Czech, M. P. (1993). Binding of the Ras activator son of sevenless to insulin receptor substrate-1 signaling complexes. *Science* **260**, 1950–1952.

46. Skolnik, E. Y., Batzer, A., Li, N., Lee, C. H., Lowenstein, E., Mohammadi, M., Margolis, B., and Schlessinger, J. (1993). The function of GRB2 in linking the insulin receptor to Ras signaling pathways. *Science* **260**, 1953–1955.

47. Skolnik, E. Y., Lee, C. H., Batzer, A., Vicentini, L. M., Zhou, M., Daly, R., Myers, M. J., Backer, J. M., Ullrich, A., White, M. F., and Schlessinger, J. (1993). The SH2/SH3 domain-containing protein GRB2 interacts with tyrosine-phosphorylated IRS-1 and Shc: implications for insulin control of *ras* signalling. *EMBO J.* **12**, 1929–1936.

48. Tobe, K., Matuoka, K., Tamemoto, H., Ueki, K., Kaburagi, Y., Asai, S., Noguchi, T., Matsuda, M., Tanaka, S., Hattori, S., Fukui, Y., Akanuma, Y., Yazaki, Y., Takenawa, T., and Kadowaki, T. (1993). Insulin stimulates association of insulin receptor substrate-1 with the protein abundant Src homology/growth factor receptor-bound protein 2. *J. Biol. Chem.* **268**, 11167–11171.

49. Burns, L. A., Karnitz, L. M., Sutor, S. L., and Abraham, R. T. (1993). Interleukin-2-induced tyrosine phosphorylation of p52^{shc} in T lymphocytes. *J. Biol. Chem.* **268**, 17659–17661.

50. Downward, J. (1994). The GRB2/Sem-5 adaptor protein. *FEBS Lett.* **338**, 113–117.

51. Olivier, J. P., Raabe, T., Henkemeyer, M., Dickson, B., Mbamalu, G., Margolis, B., Schlessinger, J., Hafen, E., and Pawson, T. (1993). A *Drosophila* SH2-SH3 adaptor protein implicated in coupling the sevenless tyrosine kinase to an activator of Ras guanine nucleotide exchange, Sos. *Cell* **73**, 179–191.

52. Simon, M. A., Dodson, G. S., and Rubin, G. M. (1993). An SH3-SH2-SH3 protein is required for p21^{Ras1} activation and binds to sevenless and Sos proteins *in vitro*. *Cell* **73**, 169–177.

53. Rozakis-Adcock, M., Fernley, R., Wade, J., Pawson, T., and Bowtell, D. (1993). The SH2 and SH3 domains of mammalian Grb2 couple the EGF receptor to the Ras activator mSos1. *Nature (London)* **363**, 83–85.

54. Li, N., Batzer, A., Daly, R., Yajnik, V., Skolnik, E., Chardin, P., Bar-Sagi, D., Margolis, B., and Schlessinger, J. (1993). Guanine-nucleotide-releasing factor hSos1 binds to Grb2 and links receptor tyrosine kinases to Ras signalling. *Nature (London)* **363**, 85–88.

55. Kuhné, M. R., Pawson, T., Lienhard, G. E., and Feng, G. S. (1993). The insulin receptor substrate 1 associates with the SH2-containing phosphotyrosine phosphatase Syp. *J. Biol. Chem.* **268**, 11479–11481.

56. Matuoka, K., Shibasaki, F., Shibata, M., and Takenawa, T. (1993). Ash/Grb-2, a SH2/SH3-containing protein, couples to signaling for mitogenesis and cytoskeletal reorganization by EGF and PDGF. *EMBO J.* **12**, 3467–3473.

57. Molloy, C. J., Bottaro, D. P., Fleming, T. P., Marshall, M. S., Gibbs, J. B., and Aaronson, S. A. (1989). PDGF induction of tyrosine phosphorylation of GTPase activating protein. *Nature (London)* **342**, 711–714.

58. Ellis, C., Moran, M., McCormick, F., and Pawson, T. (1990). Phosphorylation of GAP and GAP-associated proteins by transforming and mitogenic tyrosine kinases. *Nature (London)* **343**, 377–381.

59. Serth, J., Weber, W., Frech, M., Wittinghofer, A., and Pingoud, A. (1992). Binding of the H-ras p21 GTPase activating protein by the activated epidermal growth factor receptor leads to inhibition of the p21 GTPase activity *in vitro*. *Biochemistry* **31**, 6361–6365.

60. Marti, K. B., and Lapetina, E. G. (1992). Epinephrine suppresses rap1B. GAP-activated GTPase activity in human platelets. *Proc. Natl. Acad. Sci. U.S.A.* **89**, 2784–2788.

61. Gschwendt, M., Kittstein, W., and Marks, F. (1993). Protein kinase C forms a complex with and phosphorylates the GTPase activating protein GAP: Phosphorylation by PKC is dependent on tyrosine phosphorylation of GAP and/or a GAP-associated protein. *Biochem. Biophys. Res. Commun.* **194**, 571–576.

62. Moran, M. F., Polakis, P., McCormick, F., Pawson, T., and Ellis, C. (1991). Protein-tyrosine kinases regulate the phosphorylation, protein interactions, subcellular distribution, and activity of p21^{ras} GTPase-activating protein. *Mol. Cell. Biol.* **11**, 1804-1812.

63. Liscovitch, M. (1992). Crosstalk among multiple signal-activated phospholipases. *Trends Biochem. Sci.* **17**, 393-399.

64. Chuang, T. H., Bohl, B. P., and Bokoch, G. M. (1993). Biologically active lipids are regulators of Rac·GDI complexation. *J. Biol. Chem.* **268**, 26206–26211.

65. Satoh, T., Fantl, W. J., Escobedo, J. A., Williams, L. T., and Kaziro, Y. (1993). Platelet-derived growth factor receptor mediates activation of Ras through different signaling pathways in different cell types. *Mol. Cell. Biol.* **13**, 3706–3713.

66. Moodie, S. A., Willumsen, B. M., Weber, M. J., and Wolfman, A. (1993). Complexes of Ras·GTP with Raf-1 and mitogen-activated protein kinase kinase. *Science* **260**, 1658–1661.

67. Van Aelst, L., Barr, M., Marcus, S., Polverino, A., and Wigler, M. (1993). Complex formation between RAS and RAF and other protein kinases. *Proc. Natl. Acad. Sci. U.S.A.* **90**, 6213–6217.

68. Vojtek, A. B., Hollenberg, S. M., and Cooper, J. A. (1993). Mammalian Ras interacts directly with the serine/threonine kinase Raf. *Cell* **74**, 205–214.

69. Warne, P. H., Viciana, P. R., and Downward, J. (1993). Direct interaction of Ras and the amino-terminal region of Raf-1 *in vitro*. *Nature (London)* **364**, 352–355.

70. Zhang, X., Settleman, J., Kyriakis, J. M., Takeuchi-Suzuki, E., Elledge, S. J., Marshall, M. S., Bruder, J. T., Rapp, U. R., and Avruch, J. (1993). Normal and oncogenic p21^{ras} proteins bind to the amino-terminal regulatory domain of c-Raf-1. *Nature (London)* **364**, 308–313.

71. Korn, L. J., Siebel, C. W., McCormick, F., and Roth, R. A. (1987). *Ras* p21 as a potential mediator of insulin action in *Xenopus* oocytes. *Science* **236**, 840–843.

72. Chuang, L. M., Myers, M. G., Seidner, G. A., Birnbaum, M. J., White, M. F., and Kahn, C. R. (1993). Insulin receptor substrate 1 mediates insulin and insulin-like growth factor I-stimulated maturation of *Xenopus* oocytes. *Proc. Natl. Acad. Sci. U.S.A.* **90**, 5172–5175.

73. Jones, T. L. Z., Simonds, W. F., Merendino, J. J., Brann, M. R., and Spiegel, A. M. (1990). Myristoylation of an inhibitory GTP-binding protein α subunit is essential for its membrane attachment. *Proc. Natl. Acad. Sci. U.S.A.* **87**, 568–572.

74. Linder, M. E., Pang, I. H., Duronio, R. J., Gordon, J. I., Sternweis, P. C., and Gilman, A. G. (1991). Lipid modifications of G protein subunits: Myristoylation of $G_{o,\alpha}$ increases its affinity for $\beta\gamma$. *J. Biol. Chem.* **266**, 4654–4659.

75. Gallego, C., Gupta, S. K., Winitz, S., Eisfelder, B. J., and Johnson, G. L. (1992).

Myristoylation of the $G\alpha_{i2}$ polypeptide, a G protein α subunit, is required for its signaling and transformation functions. *Proc. Natl. Acad. Sci. U.S.A.* **89**, 9695–9699.

76. Wedegaertner, P. B., Chu, D. H., Wilson, P. T., Levis, M. J., and Bourne, H. R. (1993). Palmitoylation is required for signaling functions and membrane attachment of $G_q\alpha$ and $G_s\alpha$. *J. Biol. Chem.* **268**, 25001–25008.

77. Lupas, A. N., Lupas, J. M., and Stock, J. B. (1992). Do G protein subunits associate via a three-stranded coiled coil? *FEBS Lett.* **314**, 105–108.

78. Peitsch, M. C., Borner, C., and Tschopp, J. (1993). Sequence similarity of phospholipase A_2 activating protein and the G protein β-subunits: A new concept of effector protein activation in signal transduction. *Trends Biochem. Sci.* **18**, 292–293.

79. Mumby, S. M., Casey, P. J., Gilman, A. G., Gutowski, S., and Sternweis, P. C. (1990). G protein γ subunits contain a 20-carbon isoprenoid. *Proc. Natl. Acad. Sci. U.S.A.* **87**, 5873–5877.

80. Yamane, H. K., Farnsworth, C. C., Xie, H., Howald, W., Fung, B. K. K., Clarke, S., Gelb, M. H., and Glomset, J. A. (1990). Brain G protein γ subunits contain all-*trans*-geranylgeranylcysteine methyl ester at their carboxyl termini. *Proc. Natl. Acad. Sci. U.S.A.* **87**, 5868–5872.

81. Pronin, A. N., and Gautam, N. (1992). Interaction between G-protein β and γ subunit types is selective. *Proc. Natl. Acad. Sci. U.S.A.* **89**, 6220–6224.

82. Schmidt, C. J., Thomas, T. C., Levine, M. A., and Neer, E. J. (1992). Specificity of G protein β and γ subunit interactions. *J. Biol. Chem.* **267**, 13807–13810.

83. Kleuss, C., Scherübl, H., Hescheler, J., Schultz, G., and Wittig, B. (1993). Selectivity in signal transduction determined by γ subunits of heterotrimeric G proteins. *Science* **259**, 832–834.

84. Kleuss, C., Scherübl, H., Hescheler, J., Schultz, G., and Wittig, B. (1992). Different β-subunits determine G-protein interaction with transmembrane receptors. *Nature (London)* **358**, 424–426.

85. Wu, D., and Simon, M. I. (1993). Activation of phospholipase C β_2 by the α and $\beta\gamma$ subunits of trimeric GTP-binding protein. *Proc. Natl. Acad. Sci. U.S.A.* **90**, 5297–5301.

86. Müller, S., Hekman, M., and Lohse, M. J. (1993). Specific enhancement of β-adrenergic receptor kinase activity by defined G-protein β and γ subunits. *Proc. Natl. Acad. Sci. U.S.A.* **90**, 10439–10443.

87. Berstein, G., Blank, J. L., Jhon, D. Y., Exton, J. H., Rhee, S. G., and Ross, E. M. (1992). Phospholipase C–β1 is a GTPase-activating protein for $G_{q/11}$, its physiologic regulator. *Cell* **70**, 411–418.

88. Ross, E. M., and Berstein, G. (1993). Regulation of the M1 muscarinic receptor-G_q-phospholipase C-β pathway by nucleotide exchange and GTP hydrolysis. *Life Sci.* **52**, 413–419.

89. Jouneaux, C., Audigier, Y., Goldsmith, P., Pecker, F., and Lotersztajn, S. (1993). G_s mediates hormonal inhibition of the calcium pump in liver plasma membranes. *J. Biol. Chem.* **268**, 2368–2372.

90. Litsch, I., Sulkholutskaya, I., and Weng, C. (1993). G protein-mediated inhibition of phospholipase C activity in a solubilized membrane preparation. *J. Biol. Chem.* **268**, 8692–8697.

91. Blitzer, R. D., Omri, G., De Vivo, M., Carty, D. J., Premont, R. T., Codina, J., Birnbaumer, L., Cotecchia, S., Caron, M. G., Lefkowitz, R. J., Landau, E. M., and Iyengar, R. (1993). Coupling of the expressed α_{1B}-adrenergic receptor to the

phospholipase C pathway in *Xenopus* oocytes: The role of G_o. *J. Biol. Chem.* **268**, 7532–7537.

92. Carter, B. D., and Medzihradsky, F. (1993). G_o mediates the coupling of the μ opioid receptor to adenylyl cyclase in cloned neural cells and brain. *Proc. Natl. Acad. Sci. U.S.A.* **90**, 4062–4066.

93. McLaughlin, S. K., McKinnon, P. J., and Margolskee, R. F. (1992). Gustducin is a taste-cell-specific G protein closely related to the transducins. *Nature (London)* **357**, 563–569.

94. Voyno-Yasenetskaya, T., Conklin, B. R., Gilbert, R. L., Hooley, R., Bourne, H. R., and Barber, D. L. (1994). $G\alpha13$ stimulates Na-H exchange. *J. Biol. Chem.* **269**, 4721–4724.

95. Krupinski, J., Coussen, F., Bakalyar, H. A., Tang, W. J., Feinstein, P. G., Orth, K., Slaughter, C., Reed, R. R., and Gilman, A. G. (1989). Adenylyl cyclase amino acid sequence: Possible channel- or transporter-like structure. *Science* **244**, 1558–1564.

96. Tang, W. J., Krupinski, J., and Gilman, A. G. (1991). Expression and characterization of calmodulin-activated (type I) adenylylcyclase. *J. Biol. Chem.* **266**, 8595–8603.

97. Xia, Z. G., Choi, E. J., Wang, F., and Storm, D. R. (1992). The type III calcium/ calmodulin-sensitive adenylyl cyclase is not specific to olfactory sensory neurons. *Neurosci. Lett.* **144**, 169–173.

98. Federman, A. D., Conklin, B. R., Schrader, K. A., Reed, R. R., and Bourne, H. R. (1992). Hormonal stimulation of adenylyl cyclase through G_i-protein $\beta\gamma$ subunits. *Nature (London)* **356**, 159–161.

99. Yoshimura, M., and Cooper, D. M. F. (1993). Type-specific stimulation of adenylylcyclase by protein kinase C. *J. Biol. Chem.* **268**, 4604–4607.

100. Ishikawa, Y., Katsushika, S., Chen, L., Halnon, N. J., Kawabe, J., and Homcy, C. J. (1992). Isolation and characterization of a novel cardiac adenylylcyclase cDNA. *J. Biol. Chem.* **267**, 13553–13557.

101. Premont, R. T., Jacobowitz, O., and Iyengar, R. (1992). Lowered responsiveness of the catalyst of adenylyl cyclase to stimulation by G_s in heterologous desensitization: A role for adenosine 3',5'-monophosphate-dependent phosphorylation. *Endocrinol (Baltimore)* **131**, 2774–2784.

102. Luttrell, D. K., Hausdorff, W. P., Moyers, J. E., Gilmer, T. M., Parsons, S. J., Caron, M. G., and Lefkowitz, R. J. (1992). Overexpression of pp60[c-src] is associated with altered regulation of adenylyl cyclase. *Cell. Signal.* **4**, 531–541.

103. Iyengar, R. (1993). Molecular and functional diversity of mammalian G_s-stimulated adenylyl cyclases. *FEBS Lett.* **7**, 768–775.

104. Taussig, R., Iñiguez-Lluhi, J. A., and Gilman, A. G. (1993). Inhibition of adenylyl cyclase by $G_{i\alpha}$. *Science* **261**, 218–221.

105. Conti, M., Jin, S. L. C., Monaco, L., Repaske, D. R., and Swinnen, J. V. (1991). Hormonal regulation of cyclic nucleotide phosphodiesterases. *Endocr. Rev.* **12**, 218–234.

106. Levitzki, A., and Bar-Sinai, A. (1991). The regulation of adenylyl cyclase by receptor-operated G proteins. *Pharmacol. Ther.* **50**, 271–283.

107. Conklin, B. R., Farfel, Z., Lustig, K. D., Julius, D., and Bourne, H. R. (1993). Substitution of three amino acids switches receptor specificity of $G_q\alpha$ to that of $G_i\alpha$. *Nature (London)* **363**, 274–276.

108. Dratz, E. A., Furstenau, J. E., Lambert, C. G., Thireault, D. L., Rarick, H., Schepers, T., Pakhlevaniants, S., and Hamm, H. E. (1993). NMR structure of a receptor-bound G-protein peptide. *Nature (London)* **363**, 276–281.

109. Toro, M. J., Montoya, E., and Birnbaumer, L. (1987). Inhibitory regulation of adenylyl cyclases. Evidence inconsistent with $\beta\gamma$-complexes of G_i proteins mediating hormonal effects by interfering with activation of G_s. *Mol. Endocrinol.* **1**, 669–676.

110. Sunyer, T., Monastirsky, B., Codina, J., and Birnbaumer, L. (1989). Studies on nucleotide and receptor regulation of G_i proteins: Effects of pertussis toxin. *Mol. Endocrinol.* **3**, 1115–1124.

111. Cerione, R. A., Staniszewski, C., Caron, M. G., Lefkowitz, R. J., Codina, J., and Birnbaumer, L. (1985). A role for N_i in the hormonal stimulation of adenylate cyclase. *Nature (London)* **318**, 293–295.

112. O'Shea, J. J., Suárez-Quian, C. A., Swank, R. A., and Klausner, R. D. (1987). The inhibitory effect of cyclic AMP on phosphatidylinositol kinase is not mediated by the cAMP dependent protein kinase. *Biochem. Biophys. Res. Commun.* **146**, 561–567.

113. Tavassoli, M., Tavassoli, M. H., and Shall, S. (1983). Isolation and purification of poly(ADP-ribose) glycohydrolase from pig thymus. *Eur. J. Biochem.* **135**, 449–455.

114. DiFrancesco, D., and Tortora, P. (1991). Direct activation of cardiac pacemaker channels by intracellular cyclic AMP. *Science* **351**, 145–147.

115. Latorre, R., Bacigalupo, J., Delgado, R., and Labarca, P. (1991). Four cases of direct ion channel gating by cyclic nucleotides. *J. Bioenerg. Biomembr.* **23**, 577–597.

116. Piper, R. C., James, D. E., Slot, J. W., Puri, C., and Lawrence, J. C. (1993). GLUT4 phosphorylation and inhibition of glucose transport by dibutyryl cAMP. *J. Biol. Chem.* **268**, 16557–16563.

117. Steinberg, R. A., Cauthron, R. D., Symcox, M. M., and Shuntoh, H. (1993). Autoactivation of catalytic (Cα) subunit of cyclic AMP-dependent protein kinase by phosphorylation of threonine 197. *Mol. Cell. Biol.* **13**, 2332–2341.

118. Clegg, C. H., Ran, W., Uhler, M. D., and McKnight, G. S. (1989). A mutation in the catalytic subunit of protein kinase A prevents myristylation but does not inhibit biological activity. *J. Biol. Chem.* **264**, 20140–20146.

119. Yonemoto, W., McGlone, M. L., and Taylor, S. S. (1993). N-Myristylation of the catalytic subunit of cAMP-dependent protein kinase conveys structural stability. *J. Biol. Chem.* **268**, 2348–2352.

120. Beebe, S. J., Salomonsky, P., Jahnsen, T., and Li, Y. (1992). The Cγ subunit is a unique isozyme of the cAMP-dependent protein kinase. *J. Biol. Chem.* **267**, 25505–25512.

121. Beebe, S. J., Salomonsky, P. M., and Uhler, M. D. (1992). The Cγ- and Cα-subunits of the cAMP-dependent protein kinases have different inhibitor sensitivities. *FASEB J.* **6**, A833.

122. Keryer, G., Luo, Z., Cavadore, J. C., Erlichman, J., and Bornens, M. (1993). Phosphorylation of the regulatory subunit of type IIβ cAMP-dependent protein kinase by cyclin B/p34^{cdc2} kinase impairs its binding to microtubule-associated protein 2. *Proc. Natl. Acad. Sci. U.S.A.* **90**, 5418–5422.

123. Bilezikjian, L. M., Erlichman, J., Fleischer, N., and Vale, W. W. (1987). Differential activation of type I and type II 3',5'-cyclic adenosine monophosphate-dependent protein kinases by growth hormone-releasing factor. *Mol. Endocrinol.* **1**, 137–146.

124. Schwoch, G. (1978). Differential activation of type-I and type-II adenosine 3',5'-cyclic monophosphate-dependent protein kinases in liver of glucagon-treated rats. *Biochem. J.* **170**, 469–477.

125. Byus, C. V., Hayes, J. S., Brendel, K., and Russell, D. H. (1979). Regulation of glycogenolysis in isolated rat hepatocytes by the specific activation of type I cyclic AMP-dependent protein kinase. *Mol. Pharmacol.* **16**, 941–949.

126. Livesey, S. A., Kemp, B. E., Re, C. A., Partridge, N. C., and Martin, T. J. (1982). Selective hormonal activation of cyclic AMP-dependent protein kinase isoenzymes in normal and malignant osteoblasts. *J. Biol. Chem.* **257**, 14983–14987.

127. Lohmann, S. M., DeCamilli, P., Einig, I., and Walter, U. (1984). High-affinity binding of the regulatory subunit (RII) of cAMP-dependent protein kinase to microtubule-associated and other cellular proteins. *Proc. Natl. Acad. Sci. U.S.A.* **81**, 6723–6727.

128. Sikorska, M., Whitfield, J. F., and Walker, P. R. (1988). The regulatory and catalytic subunits of cAMP-dependent protein kinases are associated with transcriptionally active chromatin during changes in gene expression. *J. Biol. Chem.* **263**, 3005–3011.

129. Khatra, B. S., Printz, R., Cobb, C. E., and Corbin, J. D. (1985). Regulatory subunit of cAMP-dependent protein kinase inhibits phosphoprotein phosphatase. *Biochem. Biophys. Res. Commun.* **130**, 567–573.

130. Wu, J. C., and Wang, J. H. (1989). Sequence-selective DNA binding to the regulatory subunit of cAMP-dependent protein kinase. *J. Biol. Chem.* **264**, 9989–9993.

131. Tortora, G., and Cho-Chung, Y. S. (1990). Type II regulatory subunit of protein kinase restores cAMP-dependent transcription in a cAMP-unresponsive cell line. *J. Biol. Chem.* **265**, 18067–18070.

132. Brown, A. M., and Birnbaumer, L. (1990). Ionic channels and their regulation by G protein subunits. *Annu. Rev. Physiol.* **52**, 197–213.

133. Ward, S. G., Reif, K., Ley, S., Fry, M. J., Waterfield, M. D., and Cantrell, D. A. (1992). Regulation of phosphoinositide kinases in T cells: Evidence that phosphatidylinositol 3-kinase is not a substrate for T cell antigen receptor-regulated tyrosine kinases. *J. Biol. Chem.* **267**, 23862–23869.

134. Clapham, D. E., and Neer, E. J. (1993). New roles for G-protein $\beta\gamma$-dimers in transmembrane signalling. *Nature (London)* **365**, 403–406.

135. Jelsema, C. L., and Axelrod, J. (1987). Stimulation of phosphorylation A$_2$ activity in bovine rod outer segments by the $\beta\gamma$ subunits of transducin and its inhibition by the α subunit. *Proc. Natl. Acad. Sci. U.S.A.* **84**, 3623–3627.

136. Jaffe, L. A., Gallo, C. J., Lee, R. H., Ho, Y. K., and Jones, T. L. Z. (1993). Oocytes maturation in starfish is mediated by the $\beta\gamma$-subunit complex of a G-protein. *J. Cell Biol.* **121**, 775–783.

137. Iñiguez-Lluhi, J. A., Kleuss, C., and Gilman, A. G. (1993). The importance of G-protein $\beta\gamma$ subunits. *Trends Cell Biol.* **3**, 230–236.

138. Milligan, G. (1993). Agonist regulation of cellular G protein levels and distribution: Mechanisms and functional implications. *Trends Pharmacol. Sci.* **14**, 413–418.

139. Jouneaux, C., Audigier, Y., Goldsmith, P., Pecker, F., and Lotersztajn, S. (1993). G$_s$ mediates hormonal inhibition of the calcium pump in liver plasma membranes. *J. Biol. Chem.* **268**, 2368–2372.

140. Stocco, D. M., and Chaudhary, L. R. (1990). Evidence for the functional coupling of cyclic AMP in MA-10 mouse Leydig tumour cells. *Cell. Signal.* **2**, 161–170.

141. Bacskai, B. J., Hochner, B., Mahaut-Smith, M., Adams, S. R., Kaang, B. K., Kandel, E. R., and Tsien, R. Y. (1993). Spatially resolved dynamics of cAMP and protein kinase A subunits in *Aplysia* sensory neurons. *Science* **260**, 222–226.

142. Hagiwara, M., Brindle, P., Harootunian, A. T., Armstrong, R., Rivier, J., Vale, W. W., Tsien, R., and Montminy, M. R. (1993). Coupling of hormonal stimulation and transcription via the cyclic AMP-responsive factor CREB is rate limited by nuclear entry of protein kinase A. *Mol. Cell. Biol.* **13,** 4852–4859.

143. Ho, A. K. S., Zhang, Y. J., Duffield, R., and Zheng, G. M. (1991). Evidence for the simultaneous translocation of muscarinic acetylcholine receptor and G protein by carbachol. *Cell. Signal.* **3,** 587–598.

144. Milligan, G., and Green, A. (1991). Agonist control of G-protein levels. *Trends Pharmacol. Sci.* **12,** 207–209.

145. Mullaney, I., Dodd, M. W., Buckley, N., and Milligan, G. (1993). Agonist activation of transfected human M1 muscarinic acetylcholine receptors in CHO cells results in down-regulation of both the receptor and the α subunit of the G-protein G_q. *Biochem. J.* **289,** 125–131.

146. Hadcock, J. R., and Malbon, C. C. (1993). Agonist regulation of gene expression of adrenergic receptors and G proteins. *J. Neurochem.* **60,** 1–9.

147. Pyne, N. J., Murphy, G. J., Milligan, G., and Houslay, M. D. (1989). Treatment of intact hepatocytes with either the phorbol ester TPA or glucagon elicits the phosphorylation and functional inactivation of the inhibitory guanine nucleotide regulatory protein G_i. *FEBS Lett.* **243,** 77–82.

148. Bushfield, M., Murphy, G. J., Lavan, B. E., Parker, P. J., Hruby, V. J., Milligan, G., and Houslay, M. D. (1990). Hormonal regulation of G_i2 α-subunit phosphorylation in intact hepatocytes. *Biochem. J.* **268,** 449–457.

149. Yatomi, Y., Arata, Y., Tada, S., Kume, S., and Ui, M. (1992). Phosphorylation of the inhibitory guanine-nucleotide-binding protein as a possible mechanism of inhibition by protein kinase C of agonist-induced Ca^{2+} mobilization in human platelet. *Eur. J. Biochem.* **205,** 1003–1009.

150. Pyne, N. J., Freissmuth, M., and Palmer, S. (1992). Phosphorylation of the spliced variant forms of the recombinant stimulatory guanine-nucleotide-binding regulatory protein ($G_{s\alpha}$) by protein kinase C. *Biochem. J.* **285,** 333–338.

151. Hausdorff, W. P., Pitcher, J. A., Luttrell, D. K., Linder, M. E., Kurose, H., Parsons, S. J., Caron, M. G., and Lefkowitz, R. J. (1992). Tyrosine phosphorylation of G protein α subunits by pp60[c-src]. *Proc. Natl. Acad. Sci. U.S.A.* **89,** 5720–5724.

152. Vaughan, M., and Moss, J. (1981). Mono(ADP-ribosyl)transferases and their effects on cellular metabolism. *Curr. Top. Cell Regul.* **20,** 205–246.

153. Rebois, R. V., Beckner, S. K., Brady, R. O., and Fishman, P. H. (1983). Mechanism of action of glycopeptide hormones and cholera toxin: What is the role of ADP-ribosylation. *Biochemistry* **80,** 1275–1279.

154. Moger, W. H. (1983). Evidence that ADP-ribosylation is not necessary for luteinizing hormone stimulation of Leydig cell steroidogenesis. *Experientia* **39,** 1407–1408.

155. Thomas, W. E., and Mowbray, J. (1987). Evidence for ADP-ribosylation in the mechanism of rapid thyroid hormone control of mitochondria. *FEBS Lett.* **223,** 279–283.

156. Halldórsson, H., Bödvarsdóttir, T., Kjeld, M., and Thorgeirsson, G. (1992). Role of ADP-ribosylation in endothelial signal transduction and prostacyclin production. *FEBS Lett.* **314,** 322–326.

157. Molina y Vedia, L., Nolan, R. D., and Lapetina, E. G. (1989). The effect of iloprost on the ADP-ribosylation of $G_s\alpha$ (the α-subunit of G_s). *Biochem. J.* **261,** 841–845.

158. Brüne, B., Molina y Vedia, L., and Lapetina, E. G. (1990). Agonist-induced

ADP-ribosylation of a cytosolic protein in human platelets. *Proc. Natl. Acad. Sci. U.S.A.* **87**, 3304–3308.

159. Pozdnyakov, N., Lloyd, A., Reddy, V. N., and Sitaramayya, A. (1993). Nitric oxide-regulated endogenous ADP-ribosylation of rod outer segment proteins. *Biochem. Biophys. Res. Commun.* **192**, 610–615.

160. Brüne, B., Dimmeler, S., Molina y Vedia, L., and Lapetina, E. G. (1994). Nitric oxide: A signal for ADP-ribosylation of proteins. *Life Sci.* **54**, 61–70.

161. Al-Abdaly, F. A., and Henry, H. L. (1989). Hormonal regulation of chick kidney inhibitor of adenosine 3′,5′-monophosphate-dependent protein kinase. *Endocrinol. (Baltimore)* **124**, 2901–2906.

162. Van Patten, S. M., Heisermann, G. J., Cheng, H. C., and Walsh, D. A. (1987). Tyrosine kinase catalyzed phosphorylation and inactivation of the inhibitor protein of the cAMP-dependent protein kinase. *J. Biol. Chem.* **262**, 3398–3403.

163. Richardson, J. M., Howard, P., Massa, J. S., and Maurer, R. A. (1990). Post-transcriptional regulation of cAMP-dependent protein kinase activity by cAMP in GH_3 pituitary tumor cells: Evidence for increased degradation of catalytic subunit in the presence of cAMP. *J. Biol. Chem.* **265**, 13635–13640.

164. Milligan, G. (1993). Mechanisms of multifunctional signalling by G protein-linked receptors. *Trends Pharmacol. Sci.* **14**, 239–244.

165. Abou-Samra, A. B., Jüppner, H., Force, T., Freeman, M. W., Kong, X. F., Schipani, E., Urena, P., Richards, J., Bonventre, J. V., Potts, J. T., Kronenberg, H. M., and Segre, G. V. (1992). Expression cloning of a common receptor for parathyroid hormone and parathyroid hormone-related peptide from rat osteoblast-like cells: A single receptor stimulates intracellular accumulation of both cAMP and inositol trisphosphates and increases intracellular free calcium. *Proc. Natl. Acad. Sci. U.S.A.* **89**, 2732–2736.

166. Baertschi, A. J., Audigier, Y., Lledo, P. M., Israel, J. M., Bockaert, J., and Vincent, J. D. (1992). Dialysis of lactotropes with antisense oligonucleotides assigns guanine nucleotide binding protein subtypes to their channel effectors. *Mol. Endocrinol.* **6**, 2257–2265.

167. Gudermann, T., Birnbaumer, M., and Birnbaumer, L. (1992). Evidence for dual coupling of the murine luteinizing hormone receptor to adenylyl cyclase and phosphoinositide breakdown and Ca^{2+} mobilization: Studies with the cloned murine luteinizing hormone receptor expressed in L cells. *J. Biol. Chem.* **267**, 4479–4488.

168. Chakraborty, M., Chatterjee, D., Kellokumpu, S., Rasmussen, H., and Baron, R. (1991). Cell cycle-dependent coupling of the calcitonin receptor to different G proteins. *Science* **251**, 1078–1082.

169. Jouishomme, H., Whitfield, J. F., Chakravarthy, B., Durkin, J. P., Gagnon, L., Isaacs, R. J., MacLean, S., Neugebauer, W., Willick, G., and Rixon, R. H. (1992). The protein kinase-C activation domain of the parathyroid hormone. *Endocrinol. (Baltimore)* **130**, 53–60.

170. Dittman, A. H., Weber, J. P., Hinds, T. R., Choi, E. J., Migeon, J. C., Nathanson, N. M., and Storm, D. R. (1994). A novel mechanism for coupling of m4 muscarinic acetylcholine receptors to calmodulin-sensitive adenylyl cyclases: Crossover from G protein-coupled inhibition to stimulation. *Biochemistry* **33**,943–951.

171. Kaufmann, M., Muff, R., Stieger, B., Biber, J., Murer, H., and Fischer, J. A. (1994). Apical and basolateral PTH receptors in rat renal cortical membranes. *Endocrinol. (Baltimore)* **134**, 1173–1178.

172. Green, J., Kleeman, C. R., Schotland, S., and Chaimovitz, C. (1991). Acute phosphate depletion dissociates hormonal stimulated second messengers in osteoblast-like cells. *Endocrinol. (Baltimore)* **129**, 848–858.
173. Iida-Klein, A., and Hahn, T. J. (1991). Insulin acutely suppresses parathyroid hormone second messenger generation in UMR-106-01 osteoblast-like cells: Differential effects on phospholipase C and adenylate cyclase activation. *Endocrinol. (Baltimore)* **129**, 1016–1024.
174. Fujimori, A., Cheng, S. L., Avioli, L. V., and Civitelli, R. (1992). Structure–function relationship of parathyroid hormone: Activation of phospholipase-C, protein kinase-A and -C in osteosarcoma cells. *Endocrinol. (Baltimore)* **130**, 29–36.
175. Bitar, K. N., Stein, S., and Omann, G. M. (1992). Specific G proteins mediate endothelin induced contraction. *Life Sci.* **50**, 2119–2124.
176. Lincoln, T. M., and Cornwell, T. L. (1993). Intracellular cyclic GMP receptor proteins. *FASEB J.* **7**, 328–338.
177. Butt, E., Geiger, J., Harchau, T., Lohmann, S. M., and Walter, U. (1993). The cGMP-dependent protein kinase—Gene, protein, and function. *Neurochem. Res.* **18**, 27–42.
178. Jiang, H., Shabb, J. B., and Corbin, J. D. (1993). Cross-activation: Overriding cAMP/cGMP selectivities of protein kinases in tissues. *Biochem. Cell. Biol.* **70**, 1283–1289.
179. Galione, A., White, A., Willmott, N., Turner, M., Potter, B. V. L., and Watson, S. P. (1993). cGMP mobilizes intracellular Ca^{2+} in sea urchin eggs by stimulating cyclic ADP–ribose synthesis. *Nature (London)* **365**, 456–459.
180. Goulding, E. H., Ngai, J., Kramer, R. H., Colicos, S., Axel, R., Siegelbaum, S. A., and Chess, A. (1992). Molecular cloning and single-channel properties of the cyclic nucleotide-gated channel from catfish olfactory neurons. *Neuron* **8**, 45–58.
181. Anderson, T. R. (1982). Cyclic cytidine 3′,5′-monophosphate (cCMP) in cell regulation. *Mol. Cell. Endocrinol.* **28**, 373–385.
182. Sheffield, L. G. (1987). Cyclic cytidine monophosphate stimulates DNA synthesis by bovine mammary tissue *in vitro*. *Cell Biol. Int. Rep.* **11**, 557–562.
183. Newton, R. P., Salvage, B. J., and Hakeem, N. A. (1990). Cytidylate cyclase: Development of assay and determination of kinetic properties of a cytidine 3′,5′-cyclic monophosphate-synthesizing enzyme. *Biochem. J.* **265**, 581–586.
184. Fletcher, W. H., and Greenan, J. R. T. (1985). Receptor mediated action without receptor occupancy. *Endocrinol. (Baltimore)* **116**, 1660–1662.
185. Sandberg, K., Ji, H., Iida, T., and Catt, K. J. (1992). Intercellular communication between follicular angiotensin receptors and *Xenopus laevis* oocytes: Mediation by an inositol 1,4,5-trisphosphate-dependent mechanism. *J. Cell Biol.* **117**, 157–167.
186. Boitano, S., Dirksen, E. R., and Sanderson, M. J. (1992). Intercellular propagation of calcium waves mediated by inositol trisphosphate. *Science* **258**, 292–295.

CHAPTER 9

Calcium, Calmodulin, and Phospholipids

CHAPTER OUTLINE

I. Introduction

The second major transduction system is the polyphosphoinositide (PPI) pathway. Very briefly, phosphoinositide (PI) is phosphorylated on positions 4 and 5 to become PPI (Fig. 9-1); this compound in turn is hydrolyzed by a hormone-dependent phospholipase C (PLC). Two second messengers are produced: a phosphorylated head group (inositol 1,4,5-trisphosphate, IP_3) and diacylglycerol (DG). Inositol 1,4,5-trisphosphate elevates cellular calcium levels and DG stimulates a calcium-activated phospholipid-dependent protein kinase (protein kinase C, PKC). DG can be further hydrolyzed by a diacylglycerol lipase to release a second fatty acid; in this case the fatty acid is predominantly arachidonic acid, a precursor to the eicosanoids (see Chapter 3). This overall scheme is depicted in Fig. 9-2.

II. Criteria for Second Messengers

Satisfying Sutherland's postulates for the PPI pathway is much more difficult than for the cAMP pathway: (i) there are many more mediators generated; (ii) some of these mediators are produced at the end of a long chain of reactions, and (iii) one of these mediators is an ion that is more difficult to manipulate than a small organic molecule. Nonetheless, with care and diligence it can be done for at least some of the second messengers in this pathway, such as calcium:

1. The mediator, or its analog, must mimic the action of the hormone. There are several ways that calcium can be introduced into the cell; the simplest uses the calcium ionophore A23187 (Fig. 9-3). This compound is a hydrophobic calcium chelator; it binds these divalent cations and shuttles

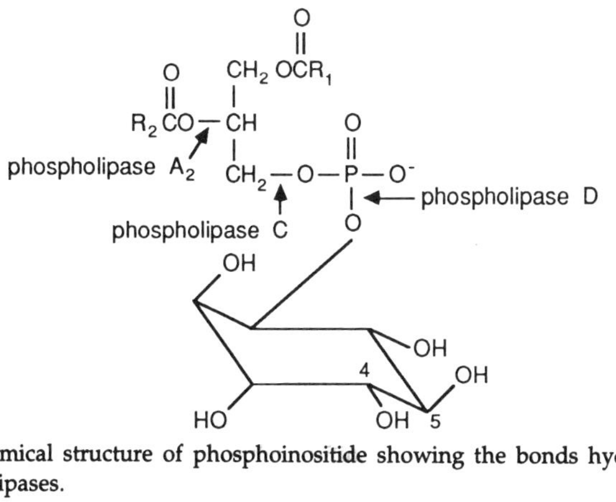

Fig. 9-1. Chemical structure of phosphoinositide showing the bonds hydrolyzed by the different phospholipases.

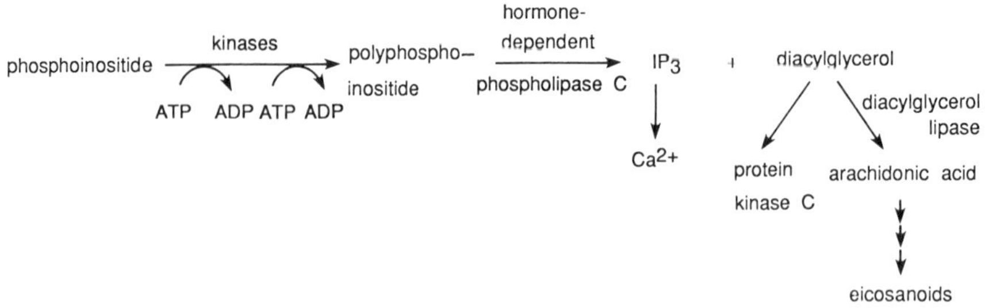

Fig. 9-2. Polyphosphoinositide pathway (general scheme).

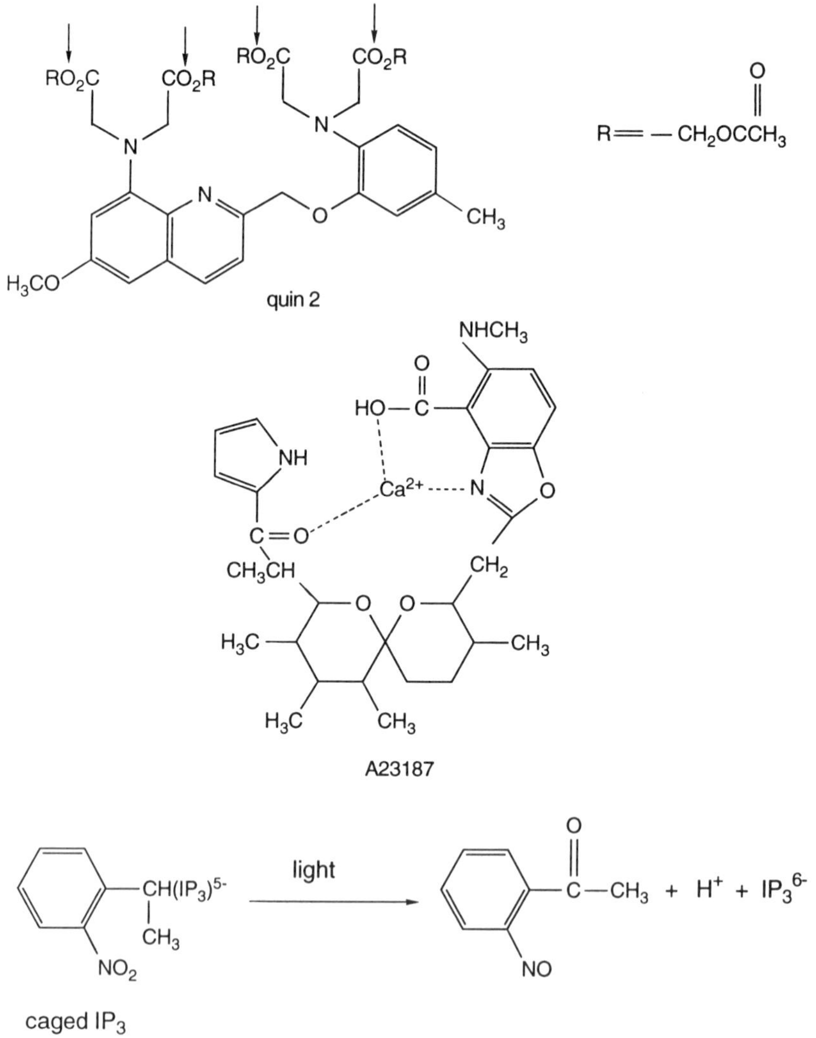

quin 2

A23187

caged IP$_3$

Fig. 9-3. Chemical structures for quin 2, a calcium-triggered fluorescent compound; A23187, a calcium ionophore shown with bound calcium; and caged IP$_3$, which releases IP$_3$ after photolysis. The arrows indicate the quin 2 calcium binding sites, which are exposed after the blocking groups have been removed.

them across the plasmalemma from the medium into the cytosol. If one needs more temporal or spatial control, "caged" calcium can be used. This is another calcium chelator that is sensitive to ultraviolet light. The calcium remains tightly bound to the chelator until it is exposed to UV light, which isomerizes the molecule, thereby disorienting the chelating groups and releasing the calcium. When this compound is used with a laser beam, calcium can be elevated in very discrete locations within the cell. Finally, calcium can be released from internal stores by the natural mediator IP_3. Because of the size and charge of this compound, plasma membranes must be permeabilized with detergents to introduce it into cells. However, it also comes in a hydrophobic caged form that readily passes through the plasmalemma and releases IP_3 by photolysis.

2. The hormone must induce elevated levels of the mediator. There are four methods for measuring calcium levels in response to hormones: (i) calcium-specific electrodes, (ii) fluxes of calcium radioisotopes, (iii) fluorescent calcium-sensitive compounds, and (iv) light-emitting calcium-sensitive proteins (1). Both electrodes and fluxes measure cellular calcium changes indirectly. As discussed later, initial alterations in cellular calcium levels are due to an internal redistribution; exchanges with the extracellular environment, which are detected by the electrodes and fluxes, are secondary events. The other two methods directly determine intracellular calcium concentrations. There are several compounds, such as quin 2, that fluoresce when their acidic groups chelate calcium; the degree of fluorescence is proportional to the calcium concentration. These binding groups are esterified so the compounds can traverse the plasma membrane; once inside, nonspecific esterases remove the blocking groups and the compounds become trapped (Fig. 9-3). The light-producing proteins such as *aequorin* act in a related manner. Aequorin, which is responsible for bioluminescence in certain jellyfish, is a 20-kDa protein containing an organic prosthetic group called *luciferin*. This complex emits light in response to elevated calcium levels; again, the intensity is proportional to the calcium concentration. The disadvantage of this method is that the protein must be microinjected into each cell. This feature can, however, also be an advantage because it allows the calcium fluctuations in a single cell to be followed.

3. The hormone must appropriately affect the enzymes of synthesis and/or degradation of the mediator. Obviously, calcium is an element: it cannot be "synthesized" or "degraded." However, hormones do activate a PLC that releases IP_3; as noted in Chapter 6, the IP_3R is a calcium channel that releases internal stores of this ion. Therefore, PLC activity can be determined. In addition, calcium is removed by ATPase pumps, some of which are hormone regulated.

4. An appropriate temporal relationship must exist among the hormone, mediator, and hormonal effect. The normal course of events is to observe an increase in PLC activity, elevated IP_3, elevated calcium, and then activation of some downstream effector.

5. Finally, if drugs are available to modulate the endogenous level of the mediator pharmacologically, they should also mimic or inhibit, as appropriate, the effects of the hormone. Again, calcium is not synthesized or degraded; rather, it is shifted from one compartment to another via channels and pumps. Therefore, these membrane proteins become the targets for pharmacological manipulations. As noted earlier, calcium ionophores can be used to elevate intracellular calcium levels. On the other hand, calcium levels may be lowered by EGTA, a chelating agent that is relatively specific for calcium. Cellular depletion of calcium is often accelerated by using a combination of both EGTA and an ionophore; because of the EGTA in the medium, the calcium concentration is now reversed and the ionophore will carry calcium out of the cell. Caged chelators that are activated by light are also available for greater temporal and spatial control (2). Finally, one can deplete cells of calcium by blocking the calcium channel. Although there is a single voltage-dependent calcium channel, there are four pharmacological classes of antagonists, each of which binds to one of several sites on the channel (3). The prototypical drugs are verapamil, nifedipine, diltiazem, and lidoflazine; the first drug appears to be the most popular for studies on the PPI pathway.

The enzymes in this pathway can be inhibited by either neomycin or U-7322. The mechanism of neomycin is actually indirect: it binds PPI and prevents PLC access to its substrate. Unfortunately, it also inhibits another phospholipase, PLA_2 (4). U-7322 is a steroid derivative with no reported extraneous effects; however, all drugs have side effects and care should be exercised whenever any of them is used in experiments.

Two enzymes involved in recycling are also targets of drugs. Once the IP_3 is released, it is progressively dephosphorylated before being recycled; lithium salts block the final dephosphorylation, thereby inhibiting the pathway at the recycling step. Unfortunately, lithium also interferes with the binding of GTP to the G proteins (5). Finally, DG kinase phosphorylates DG in preparation for its recycling. It can be inhibited by R 59 949, but it also inhibits PKC, DG lipase, and PLA_2 (6).

Two other mediators have received considerable attention: (i) calmodulin, a calcium-binding protein that can affect the activity of many enzymes, and (ii) PKC. Calmodulin (CaM) presents an additional problem to satisfying Sutherland's postulates: hormones do not acutely change total CaM levels. Rather, hormones elevate calcium that binds to and activates CaM. However, CaM can be covalently tagged by calcium-sensitive fluorescent probes that will emit light only when the calcium-binding sites are occupied and the CaM is active. CaM can be inhibited by compounds that bind to its central hydrophobic helix; these drugs include the phenothiazines and the naphthalene sulfonamides.

PKC can be specifically activated by 12-O-tetradecanoylphorbol-13-acetate (TPA) and other related phorbol esters. However, there are at least seven PKC isoforms (see subsequent discussion) and their sensitivities to TPA differ: PKCϵ is the most sensitive, being stimulated by only 0.01–0.1 n*M* TPA; PKCα, PKCβ, and PKCγ are the least sensitive (10–1000 n*M* TPA); and PKCδ, PKCη, and PKCζ are intermediate in sensitivity (1–10 n*M* TPA) (7). Since prolonged treatment with TPA causes PKC down-regulation, phorbol esters can also be used as specific inhibitors; however, the inhibitory ability of TPA does not always correlate with the sensitivity of the PKC isozymes to TPA stimulation; in addition, the inhibitory effect occasionally shows tissue specificity. For example, in adipocytes PKCα, which is the most resistant to TPA, is down-regulated the most whereas PKCϵ, which is the most sensitive to TPA, is not repressed at all (8). In neuroblastoma cells, PKCα is down-regulated but in leukemia cells it is up-regulated after an 18-hour exposure to TPA (9,10). Finally, TPA can have effects on ion channels and hormone secretion that are not mediated by PKC and appear to be nonspecific actions (11,12). Other protein kinase inhibitors have been postulated to be relatively specific for PKC, but none has withstood the test of time (13). TPA is still the most specific but one must be sure which isoforms are being affected in any given system.

III. The Phosphoinositide Effect

A. Cellular Calcium

Although the free calcium concentration in extracellular fluid is about 1 m*M*, cytoplasmic levels are only 0.01 μ*M* at rest and even during hormonal stimulation only reach 10 μ*M* (14,15). With such a large concentration gradient, calcium is continuously leaking into the cell through calcium channels; however, this low concentration is still maintained by a group of calcium transport ATPases, for example, (Ca^{2+},Mg^{2+})ATPase, (Ca^{2+},Na^{+})ATPase, and (Ca^{2+},H^{+})ATPase (Fig. 9-4). The (Ca^{2+},H^{+})ATPase exchanges two hydrogen ions for one calcium ion for each ATP hydrolyzed (16,17). The pump can be substrate driven: calcium sharply stimulates the pump in the range of

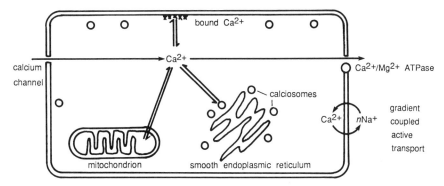

Fig. 9-4. Cellular distribution of calcium and its interchange

0.1–1 μM. CaM activates the pump by increasing its affinity for calcium 30-fold. Finally, the pump is also affected by phosphorylation. PKA increases the V_{max} of the pump without changing K_m or n; PKG has a similar effect, although it does not appear to directly modify the ATPase. The effects of PKC are controversial.

Calcium pumps can also sequester this cation into internal stores. The best characterized pump is the one in the sarcoplasmic reticulum of skeletal muscle. This pump is inhibited by the protein phospholamban; phosphorylation of this inhibitor by PKA or CaMKII causes it to dissociate from the pump (18). CaMKII can also directly modify and activate the pump. In summary, calcium and calcium-regulated processes, such as CaM and CaM-KII, stimulate both plasma membrane and endoplasmic pumps to remove calcium from the cytoplasm.

Calcium enters the cell through ligand- and voltage-gated channels. The ligand-gated calcium channels, such as the glutamate receptors, were covered in Chapter 6. The voltate-gated channels have four repeating motifs containing six transmembrane helices each (see Fig. 6-7). There are three classes: L-type, T-type, and N-type (19). The L-type channel requires a large depolarization (above −10 mV) for activation and produces a large prolonged conductance. Because dihydropyridine (DHP) is a common pharmacological agonist for this channel, it is sometimes known as the DHP receptor. The T-type channel requires very little depolarization (above −70 mV) for stimulation, but it only produces a tiny transient conductance. The N-type channels are so named because they are only found in neurons. They require intermediate degrees of depolarization (above −30 mV) and produce a moderate transient conductance. The α subunits of the L and N channels are homologous, suggesting that these channels are all members of the same family (20).

The skeletal L channel consists of a single subunit of each of the following components: α_1, $\alpha_2-\delta$, β, and γ. The α_1 subunit conforms to the basic motif of the voltage-gated channels and can form a function channel by itself (Fig. 6-7). The α_2 and δ subunits are transcribed from the same gene, are cleaved post-translationally, and remain attached by disulfide bonds. These subunits increase current amplitude and confer valinomycin sensitivity on the channel. The β subunit is a peripheral protein that accelerates the rates of both activation and inactivation. The γ subunit is unique to the skeletal muscle isoform and may be responsible for the high density of this channel in skeletal muscle; it may also determine inactivation properties.

Originally, hormones were thought to elevate intracellular calcium by releasing this cation from internal stores; however, it is now known that in many systems this effect is augmented by calcium influx, for example, through the voltage-gated channels. Hormones can regulate these channels in four ways: (i) G proteins, (ii) phosphorylation, (iii) altering the voltage threshold of the channels, and (iv) altering the membrane voltage. As discussed in Chapter 8, several members of the G_s and G_i families directly affect ion channels. In addition, several second messenger-activated protein kinases can regulate the DHP receptor: PKA activates the skeletal isoform, but not the cardiac or smooth muscle channels (21); conversely, the CaM-dependent protein kinase type II (CaMKII) stimulates the latter two forms but not the former (22–24); PKC increases activity in the skeletal isoform but decreases it in the cardiac type (12,23,25). These kinases have been physiologically linked to hormones in vascular smooth muscle, where PTH activates the L channels via PKA (26).

Hormones can also increase or decrease the threshold at which the channels depolarize. 1,25-DHCC lowers the threshold of L channels so they are activated without depolarization (27). This appears to be a nongenomic effect, since it can be observed within 1 minute. There may be an allosteric site for this sterol on the L channel, like the site for progesterone on the GABA receptor (see Chapter 5). Conversely, ANF, which uses cGMP, inactivates T channels in glomerulosa cells by raising the threshold (28). Finally, hormones can depolarize or hyperpolarize the plasmalemma to stimulate or inhibit the voltage-gated calcium channels. GHRF activates the sodium channel via cAMP; the resulting increase in cytoplasmic sodium depolarizes the pituitary cells and triggers calcium influx (29). This effect is opposed by SRIF, which opens potassium channels and hyperpolarizes the cells. ACTH and angiotensin have similar effects on the adrenal cells (30). The ionic milieu can also be altered metabolically. Aldosterone is secreted from the glomerulosa cells and stimulates sodium–potassium exchange in the kidney. Rising potassium in the extracellular fluid will depolarize the glomerulosa cells enough to activate the T channels and stimulate aldosterone synthesis and secretion; aldosterone will then lower potassium levels by excretion (28). Hypokalemia has the opposite effect.

Intracellular calcium can also be elevated by releasing this cation from internal sources; the major channels here are the IP_3 and ryanodine receptors (see Chapter 6). There is still considerable controversy over exactly where these calcium stores are located. Everyone agrees that one component is a special subcompartment of the smooth endoplasmic reticulum that is found near the plasma membrane and around the nucleus. These vesicles have been reported to contain calcium-binding proteins that facilitate calcium concentration. However, the presence of IP_3Rs on the plasmalemma or on nuclear membranes is still unsettled.

The IP_3R is a ligand-gated calcium channel, but IP_3 is not the only means of regulating this protein. The receptor has an allosteric ATP site whose occupancy increases IP_3-induced calcium fluxes by 50% (31). Alkalinization and CaM can also enhance cation release; the former does so by increasing the affinity of the receptor for IP_3, but the latter does not (32). The role of calcium itself is complex: luminal calcium is required for channel opening but the effects of cytosolic calcium are concentration dependent and are mediated by the accessory protein calmedin. At low cytosolic calcium levels (0.1–0.3 μM), cation flux is augmented; but at 0.3–1 μM calcium ion release is inhibited (33). IP_3R phosphorylation provides another level of control; participating kinases include PKA, PKC, and CaMKII. PKA decreases the amount of calcium released at any given IP_3 concentration, although the IP_3 affinity is not altered (34). On the other hand, PKC increases the rate of release and maximum release of calcium (35); no effects have yet been associated with CaMKII phosphorylation (36). The differential expression of the various isoforms of the IP_3R represents a final regulatory mechanism; there are three major isoforms of the receptor with additional forms generated by alternative splicing (37,38). These forms have different affinities for IP_3 and some lack several of the phosphorylation sites noted earlier (37).

The ryanodine receptor is homologous to the IP_3R and is organized into the same square tetramer (see Chapter 6). This receptor was originally thought to be restricted to muscle cells, where its body was imbedded in the sarcoplasmic reticulum and its large amino terminus formed the foot-like structure that coupled it to the L channel in the T-tubule. However, a second isoform exists in cardiac muscle and a third is widely distributed (39); although it often colocalizes in tissues with IP_3Rs, the two regulate distinctly separate calcium pools (40). The ryanodine receptor is regulated in much the same manner as the IP_3R: it has CaM and ATP allosteric binding sites and the calcium effects are biphasic. However, the calcium concentration curve is shifted to the right: activation occurs at $0.1-1$ μM (vs. $0.1-0.3$ μM for IP_3), whereas inhibition requires $100-1000$ μM (41). The ryanodine receptor can also be activated by CaMKII phosphorylation (42). Finally, although this receptor is unaffected by IP_3, it may have its own endogenous ligand: cyclic ADP–ribose (43–45), which is a metabolite of NAD^+ (Fig. 9-5). Physical binding of cyclic ADP–ribose to the ryanodine receptor has not been demonstrated but this molecule does directly activate cardiac ryanodine receptors in lipid bilayers (46). Its contribution to the elevation of intracellular calcium varies considerably with different systems: it makes a significant contribution to the sperm-induced elevations in *Xenopus* oocytes, but plays no role in the fertilization of hamster oocytes (47).

There are several potential ways that external signals can affect cyclic ADP–ribose (cADP–ribose) levels. First, a cytoplasmic cADP–ribose cyclase

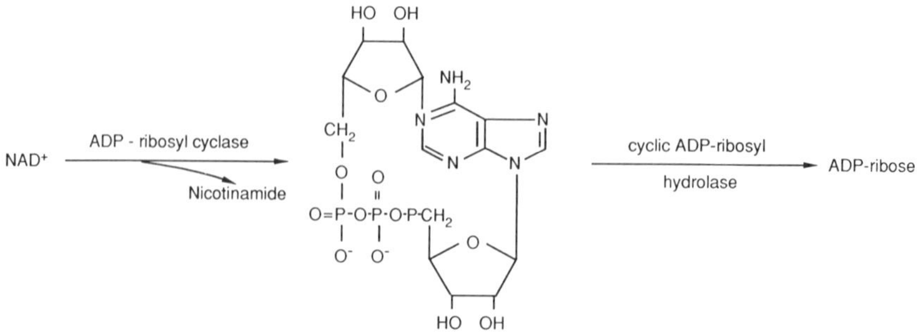

Fig. 9-5. Synthesis and degradation of cyclic ADP–ribose. The most recent data suggest that the ribose is attached at N^1 rather than N^6 (46).

can be stimulated by cGMP, probably through PKG (48). Second, a membrane-bound antigen on lymphocytes, CD38, was recently shown to have cyclase activity (49). Antibody binding stimulated both the enzyme activity and the elevation of intracellular calcium from non-IP$_3$ pools. The existence of hormone receptors homologous to CD38 is certainly a possibility.

Two other calcium stores within the cell are the mitochondria and the cytoplasmic surface of the plasma membrane. Calcium binds to the latter through the negatively charged head groups of the membrane phospholipids. The mitochondria can accumulate large amounts of calcium, but it does not release the cation in response to hormones or second messengers. The mitochondria may simply act as sinks for pathologically elevated calcium, thereby preventing potential cell damage; they may also be involved in long-term calcium homeostasis.

B. Phospholipase C

There are four major groups of phosphatidylinositol-specific PLC: PLCα, PLCβ, PLCγ and PLCδ (50,51). PLCα includes the small PLCs, none of which have been cloned. One attempt at isolating members in this group yielded the Q-2 isozyme of protein disulfide isomerase (52) and another attempt produced a fragment of PLCδ (53). Considering the difficulties in isolating examples from this class, some authorities feel that either this group does not exist or that it consists only of degradation products from the other groups.

In contrast to PLCα, members from the other three classes have been cloned and all share two regions of homology: the X and Y domains (Fig. 9-6). These regions appear to form the catalytic site. In addition, PLCβ has a carboxy-terminal domain involved in binding membranes and G proteins.

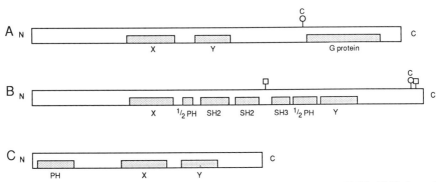

Fig. 9-6. Phosphoinositide-specific phospholipase C isoenzymes: (A) PLCβ, (B) PLCγ, and (C) PLCδ. Phosphorylation sites are represented by circles (serine or threonine) or squares (tyrosine). C, PKC phosphorylation site; PH, pleckstrin homology domain; SH, Src homology domain; X and Y, homologous regions thought to represent the catalytic site.

PLCβ is the major PLC regulated by G proteins (54) and can be activated by either the α or the $\beta\gamma$ subunits. The former usually belongs to the α_q family, which is insensitive to pertussis toxin. Because pertussis toxin could block transduction through this pathway in some tissues, it was postulated that members of the α_i family must also be involved. Indeed, a PLC from *Xenopus* oocytes was subsequently shown to be activated by α_o (55); however, this appears to be a specialized PLC, since these results are not found in most other systems. Rather, it is now known that it was not the α_i that was involved, but the $\beta\gamma$ dimer that can stimulate PLCβ 4- to 8-fold (56). This effect requires high concentrations of $\beta\gamma$ and the amino-terminal two-thirds of PLCβ (57), but since the $\beta\gamma$ dimers can originate from any G protein, they can accumulate from several different pathways to reach the necessary levels. Finally, PLCβ can also be inhibited by G proteins: the inhibition of PLCβ by adenosine and dopamine is mediated, in part, by α_i (58).

PLCβ can be phosphorylated by PKC; although the intrinsic activity does not change, G protein coupling is impaired (59,60). Finally, it is subject to product inhibition by DG (61).

Although PLCβ is most abundant in the brain, PLCγ is more widespread. This group is characterized by two SH2 and an SH3 domain between the catalytic sites; the SH2 domain allows the PLCγ to bind and be activated by the RTKs. Although phosphorylated by many RTKs and soluble tyrosine kinases (62), it is difficult to demonstrate activation *in vitro* because of the high constitutive activity of the purified enzyme. *In vivo*, PLCγ activity may be suppressed by an inhibitor that dissociates after phosphorylation; there is some evidence that this inhibitor is profilin (63; see also Chapter 10). PKC phosphorylation inhibits PLCγ by impairing tyrosine phosphorylation (64); PKA may act in a similar manner (65).

The receptors for EGF, PDGF, and heregulin can also allosterically activate PLCγ; a one-to-one association leads to a 3- to 4-fold stimulation (66). Tyrosine phosphorylation of neither the receptor nor the PLCγ is required; in fact, phosphorylation of PLCγ actually dampens its allosteric activation. The effect appears to be specific, since the insulin receptor is without effect.

In addition to the Src homology domains, PLCγ has a region it shares with several other proteins involved in signal transduction. Because the sequences were identified in the cytoskeletal protein pleckstrin, this region has been christened the pleckstrin homology (PH) domain (67–69). In PLCγ, the PH domain is split and brackets the SH domains. The function of the PH domain remains unknown.

PLCδ is considerably smaller than PLCβ or PLCγ because of a shorter carboxy terminus. This protein is widely distributed in several tissues and can be regulated by many factors, although it is still not clear which ones are physiological. Because some actions of thrombin are mediated by PLCδ (70) and this hormone uses a G protein-coupled receptor, one might assume that G proteins are physiological regulators of this isozyme. However, PLCδ is not controlled by α_q, and the $\beta\gamma$ dimer can only stimulate enzyme activity 2-fold (56). Polyamines increase activity 3-fold (71), whereas both sphingomyelin

(72) and IP_3 (73) inhibit PLCδ. The latter probably represents product inhibition.

C. Phosphoinositide Cycle

In 1953, Hokin and Hokin (74) reported that acetylcholine stimulated the turnover of PI in the pancreas; this phenomenon became known as the PI effect. In 1975, Mitchell (75) published several other important observations:

1. Hormones that stimulate PI breakdown also stimulate calcium influx.

2. Phosphoinositide hydrolysis precedes calcium influx.

3. Phosphoinositide turnover does not require elevated calcium levels.

4. Calcium ionophores could mimic the overall effect of the hormones but did not stimulate PI breakdown.

It is now known that this latter finding is not true in all systems (see subsequent discussion). However, the data were sufficient for Mitchell to propose that these hormones acted by stimulating the breakdown of PI, which then evoked calcium fluxes. Finally, it has been shown that PPI is the actual substrate being hydrolyzed; increased PI turnover in most systems is secondary to the recycling of the PPI breakdown products (see Fig. 9-7).

The hormone–receptor complexes are primarily coupled to PPI hydrolysis in two ways (see preceeding discussion): G proteins and tyrosine phosphorylation. The RTKs and the soluble tyrosine kinases that are coupled to cytokine receptors phosphorylate and activate the PLCγ. On the other hand, the serpentine receptors use G proteins to activate PLCβ. These PLCs may also be secondarily stimulated by other second messengers: both PLCβ and PLCγ can be phosphorylated by second messenger-activated kinases and PLCδ can be stimulated by polyamines (see Chapter 10).

Initially, the source of calcium for elevating cytosolic concentrations was believed to be internal because removal of this cation from the medium did not acutely block cytoplasmic fluctuations. However, repeated stimulations did lead to successively smaller fluctuations in the absence of external calcium, suggesting that external calcium is necessary to replenish internal stores. Cell fractionation studies show that hormone stimulation depletes calcium stores in the microsomes but not in the mitochondria or elsewhere. The major component of the microsomes was the smooth endoplasmic reticulum, which is known to sequester calcium in muscle cells. However, there is some controversy over whether the pool is a simple subcompartment of the smooth endoplasmic reticulum or whether it is a more highly specialized structure. Although these internal vesicles are the sole source of calcium in many systems, it is now known that other systems also take advantage of high external calcium concentrations by activating calcium plasmalemma channels to augment the fluxes from internal stores. Calcium release from internal stores is mediated by the IP_3R whereas fluxes across the plasma

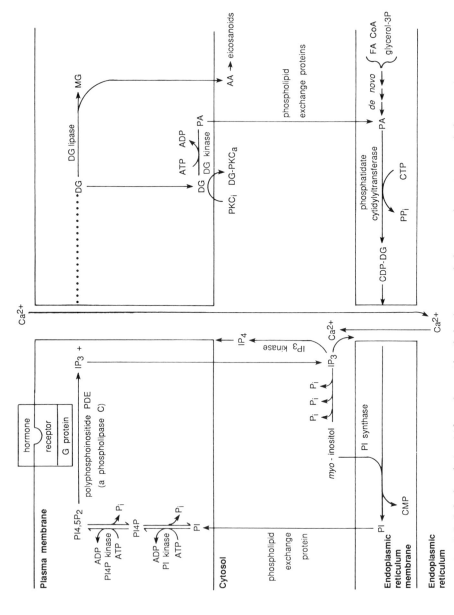

Fig. 9-7. Polyphosphoinositide pathway (detailed scheme, including recycling). AA, Arachidonic acid; FA CoA, fatty acyl coenzyme A; MG, monoacylglycerol; PA, phosphatidic acid. Other abbreviations are defined in the text.

membrane utilize the voltage-gated channels. In addition, there is evidence that there are ligand-gated channels at the cell surface; some of these channels are activated by PPI metabolites and are involved in calcium replenishment (see subsequent discussion).

Initial studies with quin 2 showed that agonists evoked a rise in cytoplasmic calcium levels that were smooth and static as long as the agonists were present. However, studies using aequorin in single cells revealed that calcium is released in pulses 7 seconds in duration and 20–100 seconds apart (76). The latency, frequency, and amplitude can be dependent on the agonist concentration; at high concentrations, the pulses fuse to form a bona fide plateau. The earlier studies using quin 2 were monitoring entire cell populations; these individual pulses were lost in the resulting statistical summation. These pulses are initiated from the subplasmalemma vesicles immediately underneath the stimulus and spread outward in waves (77). These waves are generated by IP_3; local calcium is released as the IP_3 diffuses throughout the cell (78). Calcium itself is too quickly buffered or sequestered to diffuse very far.

These pulses are not secondary to fluctuations in IP_3 generation, since exogenously administered IP_3 evokes this same pattern (79), nor are they a property of the IP_3R (80). Two models have been proposed to explain this pattern of calcium release. In the *two pool model*, calcium is stored in an IP_3-sensitive pool and an IP_3-insensitive pool (81); the latter is regulated by calcium and may correspond to the ryanodine-sensitive pool. Calcium released by IP_3 in turn releases more calcium from the IP_3-insensitive pool; the emptying of these two sources is responsible for the rapid rise and then decline in cytosolic calcium. The pools must be replenished before the next pulse can occur. In the *calcium agonist model*, the pulses are explained in terms of the biphasic effects of calcium on the IP_3R (82). IP_3 releases calcium, which synergizes with IP_3 to accelerate cation release. However, as calcium levels rise, it eventually becomes inhibitory and further release is attenuated.

In addition to these global fluctuations, changes in calcium concentrations can be much more restricted. For example, in exocrine cells, high affinity IP_3Rs exists on the luminal surface; IP_3, generated at the basal surface in response to secretagogues, diffuses to and specifically activates these high-affinity IP_3Rs (83,84). The resulting spikes are local and do not spread but are sufficient to induce secretion. Such an arrangement would not only be energetically efficient but would also be less likely to disrupt the rest of the cellular machinery. If fact, some investigators have suggested that this mechanism, by which high-affinity IP_3Rs are located only where they are needed, may represent the physiological situation and that the global changes described earlier only occur in response to pharmacological stimulation.

As noted already, many systems activate plasma membrane channels to allow extracellular calcium to supplement the internal release. This calcium influx is not pulsed, although it does increase the frequency and velocity of the IP_3-induced waves (85). Therefore, extracellular calcium does not overwhelm the endogenously produced calcium waves that are so important for frequency signaling.

There are several advantages to coding information in patterns rather than simple amplitude. First, the system has greater fidelity, especially at low hormone concentrations. Brief pulses of calcium also prevent calcium overload and toxicity, conserve energy, and prevent desensitization. Finally, patterns can increase the repertoire of responses of a single hormone. For example, during the follicular phase, GnRH levels are low and induce calcium oscillations that stimulate LH transcription in pituitary cells but inhibits LH release (86). At ovulation, high GnRH levels produce calcium pulses or a plateau that inhibit LH transcription but release the pool of LH that has accumulated during the follicular phase.

Once the calcium stores have been emptied, they must be replenished: three mechanisms have been postulated. In the simplest, the same mediator that activated calcium release also activates plasma membrane channels to start refilling the internal pools. There is evidence that IP_3 does just that in hepatocytes and T lymphocytes (87,88). However, this mechanism would not allow for the differential regulation of calcium release and replenishment. This control could be accomplished if the plasma membrane channels were activated by a distinct mediator; the most likely candidate is a metabolite of IP_3, inositol 1,3,4,5-tetrakisphosphate (IP_4). This mechanism appears to be active in endothelial cells (89). cGMP has also been proposed as a signaling molecule for calcium replenishment (90). In pancreatic acinar cells, the calcium influx is blocked by inhibitors of guanylate cyclase and this inhibition is reversed by cGMP analogs. A third postulated mediator has been partially characterized from lymphocytes and oocytes (91,92). It is a small (< 0.5 kDa), phosphorylated molecule with vicinal hydroxy groups but no aldehyde or ketone groups; it is not IP_3 or IP_4.

A final mechanism is highly speculative but intuitively appealing; it is based on the interaction between the L channel and the ryanodine receptor in skeletal muscle. The action potential in the T-tubule is sensed by the L channel, which conveys this information to the ryanodine receptor in the lateral sacs of the sarcoplasmic reticulum. This information is transmitted through the long amino terminus that forms a foot-like process connecting the T-tubule and lateral sacs (see Chapter 6). Could the IP_3R or nonmuscle ryanodine receptor contact a plasma membrane channel and inform it of the status of internal calcium stores? This physical association would also guarantee that calcium influx would occur very close to internal calcium pools, so replenishment could occur without significantly affecting cytoplasmic calcium concentrations. The IP_3-insensitive pools appear to be filled first and then the calcium is transferred to IP_3-sensitive stores.

The final pathway is presented in Fig. 9-6 (93). The phosphorylation of PI, hydrolysis of PPI, and effects of IP_3 have already been discussed. The recycling has only been mentioned briefly. The synthesis of PI can only occur in the endoplasmic reticulum and involves four processes: the translocation of the phospholipids between the two membrane systems, the activation of

DG, the dephosphorylation of IP_3, and the recoupling of the two components. The translocation is accomplished by various phospholipid exchange proteins. These exchange proteins are important, since PI is limiting and long-term stimulation cannot be sustained without them (94). The activation of DG involves its phosphorylation to phosphatidic acid and conjugation to CTP. Inositol 1,4,5-trisphosphate is sequentially dephosphorylated by phosphatases, the last of which is inhibited by lithium; experimentally, lithium is used to block recycling. Phosphoinositide synthase is then responsible for joining the inositol and CDP–DG. Studies examining the turnover of PI measure the incorporation of radioactive phosphate into PI. Since this occurs before hydrolysis, radioactive incorporation is really a reflection of recycling. In fact, increased incorporation could be seen in the complete absence of PPI hydrolysis if the hormone simply stimulated a total increase in PI content through the *de novo* pathway.

D. Output

1. Calcium and Calmodulin

Calcium is a major output of this transduction system and there are several enzymes whose activities are affected by concentrations of this cation; examples include the calcium activation of glyceraldehyde phosphate dehydrogenase, pyruvate dehydrogenase, and α-ketoglutarate dehydrogenase. More frequently, however, calcium acts in concert with calcium-binding peptides such as calmodulin (CaM).

CaM is a 148-amino-acid peptide (16.7 kDa); it is heat stable, ubiquitous, both histologically and phylogenetically, and highly conserved evolutionarily. The peptide structurally resembles a dumbbell: it has two globular ends separated by a 7-turn helix (Fig. 9-8A; 95). Each globular end contains two calcium-binding sites that have a helix–loop–helix configuration wrapped around the cation; the innermost site in each end uses the long connecting helix as one of the sides. The two binding sites in the carboxy-terminal half have a slightly higher affinity than those in the amino-terminal half, but the difference is within an order of magnitude: most of the dissociation constants reported for these sites range between 10^{-5} and 10^{-6} M. Each globular end also has a hydrophobic groove.

The amino-terminal half of the long helix is hydrophobic whereas the carboxy-terminal half is acidic; this helix is one of the sites of interaction between CaM and the enzymes it activates (96). This fact has been determined in two ways: affinity labeling and amino acid derivatization. CaM activity can be blocked by several hydrophobic aromatic compounds, such as the phenothiazines and the napthalene sulfonamides. The phenothiazines can be altered so they will covalently attach to CaM; such a stable bond allows the chemist to identify the attachment site that turns out to be the hydrophobic region of the long helix. Furthermore, this same region has several methionines that can be selectively derivatized; these modifications also destroy CaM activity. Finally, the target sites in many CaM-binding

A

B

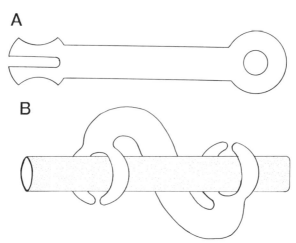

Fig. 9-8. Schematic representation of the calmodulin (CaM) molecule and its interactions with substrates. (A) Each globular domain has two calcium-binding sites and a groove. The two globular domains are turned 90° with respect to each other and are separated by a 7-turn α helix. (B) α-Helical substrates bind to CaM in the grooves of the globular domains.

proteins are complementary to this long helix, that is, they are half hydrophobic and half basic.

The globular ends are also involved in binding some target proteins. The first calcium domain is required to activate the myosin light chain kinase, the second domain enhances calcineurin activity, and one of the carboxy-terminal domains stimulates the membrane-bound guanylate cyclase in *Tetrahymena* (97). X-Ray crystallographic data of CaM bound to target proteins demonstrate that CaM is not a rigid dumbell (98,99). The target site is a short α helix that is grabbed at either end by the hydrophobic groove in the globular termini of CaM. The intervening α helix is quite flexible and allows the globular ends to properly position themselves (Fig. 9-8B). The function of calcium in activating CaM is not clear; in general, it probably stabilizes the overall conformation. However, non-calcium-binding mutants of CaM are still viable in yeast (100), suggesting that calcium may not be essential for all the functions of CaM.

The major mechanism by which hormones control CaM activity is by altering the cytoplasmic calcium concentration. Calmodulin itself does not appear to be acutely regulated by hormones, that is, the peptide is synthesized constitutively. This conclusion was reached after an extensive survey failed to reveal any hormonally regulated system in which CaM levels fluctuated (101,102). However, hormones may still be important in the maintenance of basal levels of CaM or in long-term regulation (103). CaM levels decline in the fat pads of diabetic rats (104) and in the myometrium of ovariectomized rabbits (105); levels are restored by insulin and estrogen replacement therapy, respectively. Furthermore, the CaM content of rat mammary glands rises 2- to 3-fold during pregnancy (106,107). Hormones can also regulate the cellular localization of CaM (103); usually CaM is associated with the plasma membrane and hormones can release CaM into the cytosol and nucleus, where it then effects cellular processes. This liberation may be secondary to the cytoskeletal remodeling that often accompanies hormone stimulation (see Chapter 10).

Finally, CaM can be covalently modified. Casein kinase II can phosphorylate CaM and inhibit its activity (108). Tyrosine phosphorylation by the insulin and PDGF receptors is still controversial because of its unusual requirement for basic peptides. This modification increases the affinity of CaM for calcium and enhances the CaM stimulation of PDE (108). Finally, one of the lysines in CaM is constitutively methylated; this does not affect biological activity, but does prevent the ubiquitination and rapid degradation of CaM.

Many enzymes are regulated by CaM but only some of the more important or better understood ones will be discussed. Some enzymes, such as the cyclic nucleotide phosphodiesterase and adenylate cyclase, have already been covered (see Chapter 8), whereas others, such as the myosin light chain kinase, are discussed later (see Chapter 11). In these examples, CaM binds to the enzyme as a transient extrinsic subunit. However, in phosphorylase kinase, CaM is actually a permanent part of the enzyme complex (109); this enzyme is critical in glycogenolysis, in which it phosphorylates, thereby activating, the glycogen phosphorylase (see Chapter 11). The phosphorylase kinase has the following quaternary structure: $(\alpha\beta\gamma\delta)_4$. The γ subunit contains the catalytic site and the δ subunit is CaM. The α and β subunits are additional regulatory components; their phosphorylation increases the affinity of the enzyme for calcium, thereby making activation easier.

Because phosphorylation is such a common mechanism to control cellular processes, it is not surprising that CaM can activate more general protein kinases as well. The *CaM-dependent protein kinase, type II* (CaMKII) is very large (600–650 kDa) and is composed of identical subunits arranged in a two-layered oligomer (110). The kinase contains several homologous subunits: α, β and β' are the most common. All the subunits are catalytic, bind CaM, and can be phosphorylated. In the α subunits, the amino-terminal kinase and CaM-binding domains are located peripherally and are connected to the centrally aggregated carboxy termini via thin strands; there are five subunits in each tier. The β subunits create a similar flower-like structure, except that a two-tiered octamer, not a decamer, results. The regulatory site binds the ATP-binding site and inhibits kinase activity (see Fig. 11-1); CaM activates the kinase by binding to the regulatory domain and freeing the ATP site (111). Autophosphorylation within this same regulatory region also prevents it from occupying the ATP site. This modification has two effects: first, it increases the affinity of the regulatory domain for CaM 1000-fold and, second, it can preserve 40% of the kinase activity even in the absence of CaM. The higher CaM affinity maintains CaM binding to the kinase long after calcium levels have begun to fall. This phenomenon enables CaMKII to act as a calcium sensor: if the calcium pulses are occurring fast enough, the CaMKII will remain fully active despite the fluctuating ion levels.

The existence of CaMKII implies the existence of CaMKI; indeed, there are four CaM-dependent protein kinases. However, only CaMKII has a broad enough specificity to have widespread effects. The effects of the others are too specific to be of general interest.

Another CaM-regulated enzyme, *calcineurin* or protein phosphatase 2B (PP-2B), reverses phosphorylation (see Chapter 11), it is a widespread, multifunctional phosphatase (112). This enzyme is composed of two subunits, α and β. The α subunit is 61 kDa and binds both zinc and ferric ions; it also contains the catalytic and CaM-binding sites. Interestingly, the β subunit (19 kDa) is another member of the CaM family and has four calcium-binding sites. Therefore, this phosphatase is controlled by *two* calcium-binding peptides—CaM and the β subunit.

2. Protein Kinase C

The other major second messenger produced by the PPI pathway is DG, which activates another protein kinase, PKC (113–115). This kinase is divided into four conserved (C) regions and the intervening variable (V) regions (see Fig. 11-1). C1 contains the TPA-DG-binding site. It is subdivided into two cysteine-rich domains, each of which forms a half-site that binds TPA with low affinity; together they form a single high-affinity binding site. C2 contains four zinc ions and binds calcium. C2 does not conform to any calcium-binding motif and so the binding may be indirect via phosphatidylserines. C2 also binds to *r*eceptors for *a*ctivated *C k*inase (RACKs), which are responsible for localizing PKC to certain sites (116). The sequence of one RACK is known and is homologous to the G_β family (117). Since members of this family are also known to bring the βAR kinase and the G_α to the plasmalemma to bind membrane proteins, G_β may have a general role in macromolecular assembly. C3 and C4 are the ATP-binding and catalytic sites, respectively. V1 is at the extreme amino terminus and contains a pseudosubstrate site that inhibits kinase activity; it is thought that the binding of calcium and phospholipids alters the conformation of PKC in such a way that this region is displaced from the catalytic site. There are also several autophosphorylation sites; although the unmodified PKC can bind substrate and cofactors, it is not active until it has been autophosphorylated (118).

There are three major PKC families. Group A is also called the classical or conventional PKCs and includes the PKC isoforms α, β, and γ. They possess the C2 domain and are calcium dependent. They can be activated by lysopholipids (119) and have good activity toward the classical kinase substrates such as histones, myelin basic protein, and protamine (120). Group B, or the new PKCs, includes PKC isoenzymes δ, ϵ, η, and θ. They do not have a C2 domain and are calcium independent, although they still require DG and phosphatidylserine. They are not activated by lysophospholipids and do not phosphorylate the classical kinase substrates well. Group C, or the atypical PKCs, includes PKCζ, PKCι, PKCμ, and PKCλ; they lack both the C2 and half of the C1 domains. They are calcium and DG independent but still require phosphatidylserine. Many of these isoforms also differ in the signaling pathways they affect. For example, only PKCα and PKCϵ phosphorylate and inhibit PLCγ (121); PKCα, PKCβ, and PKCϵ activate the transcription factor AP-1, but PKCγ does not (122); PKCα and PKCδ induce myeloid differentiation, but PKCβ, PKCϵ, PKCη, and PKCζ do not (123); the conventional PKCs phosphorylate the insulin receptor, but the new PKCs do not (124). Most isoforms are cytoplasmic; on activation, PKC is translocated to the plasmalemma where binding to phospholipids occurs. However, PKCμ has a putative transmembrane domain (125) and PKCη is located exclusively in the nuclei of several tissues such as epithelium (126). Tissue distribution also differs among the isoforms: PKCα, PKCδ, PKCϵ, and PKCζ are ubiquitous whereas other isozymes have a more restricted tissue distribution. For example, PKCβ is abundant in the brain and spleen, PKCη is mostly located in skin and lungs, and PKCθ is found predominantly in skeletal muscle and hematopoietic stem cells (120). Finally, the different isoforms also vary in their length of activation: PKCα is transiently stimulated whereas PKCβ retains its activity longer.

There are several mechanisms to regulate PKC. Calcium is a major activator for the Group A PKCs and phospholipids affect all PKCs. The most important phospholipids are DG and phosphatidylserine; the latter appears to coordinate calcium binding with the C2 region. However, other lipids can also affect PKC activity: both phosphatidylinositol 4,5-bisphosphate (PIP$_2$) and lipoxygenase metabolites can stimulate PKC, whereas sphingolipids are inhibitors. Arachidonic acid is an activator of PKCγ. Covalent modifications have also been reported: PKCδ can be phosphorylated and activated by several tyrosine kinases (127). PKC can be activated by cleavage in V3 by the protease calpain. Removal of the regulatory amino terminus renders PKC permanently active, even in the absence of calcium and phospholipids. In addition to being constitutively active, the clipped PKC, also called PKM, would no longer be bound to the membrane; the resolubilized PKC could have greater access to its substrates or even be able to phosphorylate a different spectrum of substrates (128). However, there is conflicting evidence on whether or not this type of cleavage actually occurs in intact cells (129,130). Finally, PKC can be inhibited by the 14-3-3 protein, an acidic 60-kDa protein; 14-3-3 probably acts as a PKC pseudosubstrate as PKI is for PKA (131).

Numerous substrates for PKC have been identified, but how many of them are physiological is still not clear. These substrates include (i) membrane receptors and transport systems, (ii) kinases, (iii) contractile and cytoskeletal proteins, (iv) proteins involved in gene expression and protein synthesis, and (v) metabolic enzymes, especially the rate-limiting enzymes in central metabolic pathways.

3. PI 3' Kinase

As noted at the beginning of this chapter, the central phospholipid in the PPI pathway is phosphatidylinositol 4,5-bisphosphate (PIP_2), which is hydrolyzed to yield IP_3 and DG. However, other isomers also exist; for example, PI-3' kinase (PI3K) generates phosphatidylinositol 1,3,5-trisphosphate ($PI,3,5-P_2$). PI3K is activated by several mitogens and the resulting phospholipid has been closely associated with mitogenesis (132–134). The kinase has an 85-kDa regulatory subunit (p85) and a 110-kDa catalytic subunit (p110). The regulatory subunit has two SH2 domains and one SH3 domain and becomes associated with activated RTKs. Many of these RTKs will phosphorylate p85 on tyrosines concomitant with enzyme activation; however, it now appears that this phosphorylation is a fortuitous event that is unrelated to kinase activity. For example, insulin can stimulate PI3K by phosphorylating an adaptor, IRS-1 or p185, that then activates PI3K without the phosphorylation of p85 (135,136). The binding of the SH2 groups of p85 to the phosphotyrosine of the RTKs or to their adaptors is sufficient to effect a conformational change and kinase activation (137). PI3K may also be activated by small G proteins such as Rho (138).

The question remaining is, "What role does its product $PI3,5-P_2$ play?" It may generate a second messenger like PIP_2, but there are no known PLCs that will hydrolyze this phospholipid. Instead, it is believed that the intact $PI3,5-P_2$ is the mediator. Since it is a phospholipid, it may affect PKC activity; indeed, it can activate PKCζ (139). It is also a critical link between some RTKs and Ras activation (140). For the insulin receptor, this linkage may be mediated by IRS-1, which can bind Grb2 and stimulate a RasGDS. Finally, it may also play a role in RTK endocytosis (141). In yeast, VPS34 is homologous to p110 and has PI3K activity; another protein, VPS15, is a kinase that targets VPS34 to the membranes where the two proteins are involved in vacuole sorting and morphogenesis. In a similar fashion, it is postulated that p85 may target p110 to active RTKs. The resulting synthesis of $PI3,5-P_2$ may alter the physical properties of the plasmalemma and encourage endocytosis. For example, this phospholipid may induce plasma membrane curvature or bind to other proteins involved in endocytosis. The hypothesis is supported by the finding that the PI3K binding site in the PDGFR is necessary and sufficient for internalization of the receptor (142). Another yeast protein homologous to PI3K is Tor2, which is necessary for cell cycle progression past G_1 (143); this activity in yeast supports the association between PI3K and mitosis seen in mammalian systems.

4. Calpain

Calpain is an acronym for *cal*cium-activated, *pa*pain-like protease (144). There are two isozymes that have homologous catalytic subunits and identical regulatory subunits; both subunits bind calcium. The regulatory subunit also has a phospholipid-binding site that is responsible for membrane association. The catalytic subunit prefers to cleave at interfaces between hydrophobic and hydrophilic domains; such sites exist in many CaM-binding proteins (see preceding discussion). Several of these proteins become CaM independent after cleavage; they include phosphorylase kinase, calcium ATPase, PDE, and calcineurin. Although not CaM dependent, PKC is also cleaved by calpain and rendered independent of calcium and DG. It is not clear if this activation is physiological, since many of these enzymes have very short half-lives once they are cleaved. Another substrate is a phospho-tyrosine phosphatase whose hydrophobic carboxy terminus localizes the enzyme to the plasma membrane (145). After calpain removes this domain, the phosphatase shifts to the cytosol and doubles its activity. Finally, many cytoskeletal components are calpain substrates. It has been postulated that this cleavage may loosen the actin–cytoskeleton meshwork to allow endo- or exocytosis; both processes are calcium regulated.

Calpain is regulated by three modulators: calcium, phospholipids, and calpastatin. Calcium activates both isozymes, but the concentration requirement differs; calpain I only needs micromolar amounts of calcium, whereas calpain II requires millimolar concentrations. However, phospholipids can reduce this requirement. Finally, calpain can be inhibited by calpastatin, a protein composed of four internal repeats. Each domain can bind and inhibit one calpain molecule. In addition to these allosteric modulators, calpain can also be phosphorylated by CaMKII; this modification doubles the protease activity (146).

5. Other Outputs

There are several other potential outputs. First, PPI and/or DG may be subject to further hydrolysis to release arachidonic acid, which can be active by itself as well as being a precursor to the eicosanoids. These compounds are covered in more detail later in this chapter. PIP_2 has activity independent of its hydrolysis products; in particular, it binds to many cytoskeletal elements to regulate actin polymerization (147; see also Chapter 10). It can also activate PKC, although it is not as efficient as other phospholipids (148). IP_3 and its metabolites have been shown to affect the activity of several enzymes. IP_2 stimulates phosphofructokinase (149), DNA polymerase (150), and a calcium ATPase (151). IP_3 induces a calcium ATPase (152) and protein phosphatase 1 (153) while inhibiting protein tyrosine phosphatase IA (154), aldolase (155), and the (Na^+,Ca^{2+}) exchanger (152). IP_4 stimulates both the AMP deaminase and protein phosphatase 1 (153) but inhibits the calcium ATPase (152).

E. Regulation

1. Interrelationships of the Branches

The calcium and PKC branches of the PPI pathway can interact in four different ways: (i) synergistically, (ii) antagonistically, (iii) independently, and (iv) temporally. In most systems, the two branches reinforce each other (115). For example, in platelets, thrombin-induced protein phosphorylation is only partially mimicked by PKC activators or calcium ionophores alone, but is fully mimicked by a combination of the two. Examples of antagonism are much rarer: in neuronal cells, calcium elicits hyperpolarization by increasing potassium currents whereas PKC activators depolarize the cells by decreasing potassium currents (156). In lymphocytes, the two branches act independently: TPA stimulates mitosis without any apparent changes in intracellular calcium concentrations (157). Finally, the two branches can interact temporally (14): IP_3 and calcium trigger the acute responses whereas PKC and its phosphorylated substrates have more prolonged effects. Glucose-provoked insulin secretion from the pancreas is biphasic: the initial peak is mimicked by A23187 whereas the later sustained release is mimicked by TPA. A similar phenomenon occurs with aldosterone production in adrenal glomerulosa cells.

Such an array of interactions may, at first seem contradictory: how can two branches antagonize, or be independent of, one another when they are both part of the same pathway? Recent studies suggest that these two branches may, in fact, be independently regulated. For example, hormones can stimulate a phosphatidylcholine-specific phospholipase C that hydrolyzes phosphatidylcholine (PC) into DG and phosphocholine (see subsequent discussion). The phosphocholine does not effect intracellular calcium levels but the DG can still activate those PKC isozymes that are calcium independent. Conversely, calcium levels can be regulated independently of PKC activation; for example, calcium can be recruited from IP_3-independent pools or from the external medium through plasma membrane channels. In these cases, no DG is produced and PKC is not activated. Differential tissue distribution results in another form of independent control. In brain, IP_3 receptors and PKC are not always localized in the same regions (158). Although both are present in the molecular layer of the cerebellum, hippocampus, corpus striatum, and cerebral cortex, IP_3 receptors are unmeasurable in the external plexiform layer of the olfactory bulb and in the substantia gelatinosa, even though PKC can still be detected in concentrations comparable to those in other brain regions. Therefore, there are mechanisms of regulating these outputs separately.

2. Homologous Regulation

Homologous regulation consists primarily of negative feedback by one of the two major products of this pathway: calcium or PKC (Fig. 9-9). Negative feedback mediated by PKC takes three forms: (i) inhibition of phospholipase C, (ii) removal of active products of the pathway, and (iii) decreasing the hormonal sensitivity of the cell to subsequent stimulation. First, PKC phosphorylates both PLCβ and PLCγ and impairs their activation (59,60,64). PKC also phosphorylates DG kinase, which converts DG to phosphatidic acid (159). Although this modification does not directly affect enzyme activity, it does stabilize the kinase. Calcium is removed by stimulation of the calcium transport ATPases, which pump the cation out of the cell (64): the sarcoplasmic calcium ATPase is phosphorylated by PKC, whereas the (Ca^{2+}, H^+); ATPase is activated by calcium and CaM. Finally, PKC can reduce its own

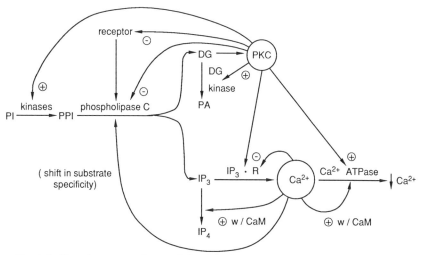

Fig. 9-9. Homologous regulation of the polyphosphoinositide pathway. The major feedback control is effected by the principal outputs, PKC and IP_3 (circled). DG, Diacylglycerol; PA, phosphatidic acid.

levels (down-regulate itself); however, these reports must be cautiously interpreted. Whenever TPA is used to activate PKC, down-regulation is inevitable and rapid (160); this appears to be a result of enzyme degradation. However, when PKC is naturally stimulated, its activity persists. As a result, PKC down-regulation as induced by TPA may be an artifact or an exaggerated response due to the great potency of TPA or to its long half-life. Because DG is metabolized within minutes of its formation, the natural control of PKC may be through levels of its DG activator rather than through down-regulation. A similar situation occurs with progesterone receptors: progesterone agonists down-regulate the receptor, whereas the natural steroid does not (161). The reason is that progesterone has such a short half-life that it does not occupy the receptor long enough to down-regulate it; the agonists all have much longer half-lives. The final mechanism by which PKC exerts negative feedback is by phosphorylation of the hormone receptors. For example, this modification of the EGFR lowers its affinity for EGF and reduces the responsiveness of the cell to further stimulation by EGF (162).

Calcium is the other major product and also contributes to this negative feedback. First, elevated calcium levels in combination with calcimedin interfere with the binding of IP_3 to its receptor, thereby decreasing further calcium release (33). The IP_4 receptor is much less sensitive to the inhibitory effect of high calcium (163); this differential regulation would allow elevated calcium levels to block further release of calcium into the cytoplasm without interfering with the replenishment of internal stores. In fact, calcium and CaM actually stimulate the IP_3 3-phosphokinase so IP_4 can be formed and the regeneration process can begin (164). A second way that calcium is involved in negative feedback is through altering the substrate specificity of the phospholipase C. At low concentrations the enzyme prefers the fully phosphorylated PPI and IP_3 is liberated; however, at higher concentrations, the phospholipase switches to phosphatidylinositol 4,5-bisphosphate and IP_2 is freed. Because IP_2 does not bind to the IP_3 receptor, the internal calcium release ceases; however, DG is still generated and can continue to activate PKC.

Positive feedback is less common but does occur. For example, PKC stimulates the kinases that synthesize PPI (165). The effect presumably occurs via phosphorylation and would enhance the response of the system to subsequent stimulation.

2. Heterologous Regulation

The relationship between the PPI and cAMP pathways can be synergistic or antagonistic (Fig. 9-10); the former occurs during glycogenolysis in the liver (166; see also Chapter 11), whereas the latter occurs in platelets. The PPI pathway can antagonize the cAMP system at several levels. For example, PKC can phosphorylate the β-adrenergic and hCG receptors (see Chapter 7). Unlike the phosphorylation of the EGFR, the modification of these receptors does not change their affinities but uncouples them from the adenylate cyclase. Another possible mechanism is suggested by the fact that both systems use G proteins. Activation of the PPI pathway should liberate $\beta\gamma$ subunits, which could then tie up the α_s subunit of the cAMP pathway. This mechanism would be analogous to the one postulated for G_i (see Chapter 8). Finally, the calcium generated by the PPI pathway can bind to CaM to stimulate the phosphodiesterase that hydrolyzes cAMP, thereby destroying its biological activity. Conversely, cAMP can inhibit both the PI kinases and the phospholipase C; the former does not require phosphorylation but appears to be a direct effect of cAMP (167).

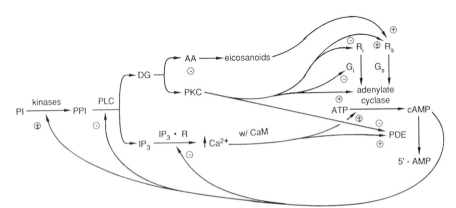

Fig. 9-10. Heterologous regulation of the polyphosphoinositide pathway. AA, Arachidonic acid; DG, diacylglycerol; PLC, phospholipase C. Other abbreviations are defined in the legend to Fig. 8-8.

In other systems, the two pathways complement one another. Indeed, glucagon and ACTH activate both pathways (168,169). Synergism can occur in several ways. First, PKC can enhance cAMP production and reduce its elimination. For example, PKC can phosphorylate and inhibit R_i, G_i, and PDE while stimulating several adenylate cyclase isozymes (see Chapter 8). Second, many of the eicosanoids produced by the PPI pathway have receptors that stimulate adenylate cyclase, resulting in a signal amplification. Conversely, PKA can phosphorylate IP_3R and increase its affinity for IP_3 (170).

The effect of calcium–CaM on adenylate cyclase activity is biphasic (171,172). The catalytic subunit of the cyclase binds CaM and both basal and hormone-stimulated activity require calcium concentrations of $0.01-0.1 \ \mu M$; higher levels ($\geq 1 \ \mu M$) inhibit the enzyme. Therefore, although basal levels of calcium are required for cyclase activity, the elevated concentrations observed during activation of the PPI pathway would both inhibit the cyclase and stimulate the phosphodiesterase, resulting in lower cAMP levels.

IV. Other Phospholipids

A. Phosphatidylcholine

1. Hydrolysis

As work on the PPI pathway became more sophisticated and quantitative, certain discrepancies began to arise. In particular, the data showed that far more DG was produced than PIP_2 was hydrolyzed. For example, in hepatocytes, vasopressin hydrolyzed 9 ng PIP_2/mg tissue but generated 400 ng DG/mg (173). Furthermore, the discrepancies were greatest at later time points. By tagging phospholipids with different fatty acids, it was determined that PIP_2 supplied the DG acutely, but that PC was the source of DG after the first few minutes of stimulation (115). There are two ways that PC can release DG: (i) a PC-specific PLC (PC–PLC) can hydrolyze PC in a manner analogous to the PPI pathway or (ii) PC can be acted on by a PC-specific phospholipase D (PC–PLD). The latter reaction would actually produce phosphatidic acid (PA) and choline (Fig. 9-1); the former would have to be degraded further by a PA phosphohydrolase to produce DG. Both pathways exist; the contribution by each will vary depending on the specific system (174,175).

The PC–PLD can be regulated in two ways: (i) it can be directly activated by Rho (176), ARF (177), and possibly other G proteins and (ii) it can be secondarily activated by PKC and calcium. In the latter case, the PPI pathway is the first to be stimulated; then the PKC will phosphorylate and inhibit PLC while activating the PLD. Essentially, PKC switches the transduction system from PIP_2 to PC. The net effect is the continued production of DG for PKC activation, while IP_3 and calcium are reduced.

PC–PLC in *Xenopus* oocytes can be activated by Ras (178). The effects of this enzyme can also be potentiated by factors that interfere with PC recycling (179). CTP:phosphocholine cytidylyltransferase is involved in the reutilization of DG and can be regulated by hormone mediators. For example, CCK, α-adrenergic agonists, and bombesin inhibit this enzyme in the pancreas by elevating calcium and activating CaM. When cytidylyltransferase activity is suppressed, DG recycling is delayed and DG accumulates.

The other product of PC–PLC is phosphocholine which, until recently, was not thought to act as a second messenger. The first suggestion that this metabolite might have transducive functions came from studies showing that PC hydrolysis activated the transcription factor NF-κB but that this effect was independent of DG and PKC (180). Since phosphocholine was the only other product of this reaction, it was a prime candidate to activate NF-κB. Subsequently, phosphocholine was demonstrated to be mitogenic by itself and to mediate the mitogenic effects of several growth factors (181). Therefore, PC–PLC generates two second messengers: DG which can activate PKC and phosphocholine which can stimulate cell division.

2. Synthesis

In addition to being an alternative source for DG, the accumulation of PC can alter membrane properties in a way that enhances cAMP production. PC can be synthesized from phosphatidylserine via a decarboxylation to phosphatidylethanolamine followed by successive methylations (Fig. 9-11; 182). Although two different phospholipid methyltransferases were originally postulated, later data suggest that there may be only one. Because phosphatidylserine is predominantly located on the cytoplasmic face of the plasmalemma and PC is usually on the extracellular side, this conversion to PC is accompanied by a transverse migration across the membrane. The source of the methyl groups is S-adenosylmethionine, which is converted to S-adenosylhomocysteine (SAH). The methyltransferase is subject to product inhibition by SAH, and several drugs have been developed to take advantage of this fact. For example, 3-deazaadenosine and its structural variants are, or can be, metabolized to SAH analogs and are potent inhibitors of the methyltransferase.

Phospholipid methylation has been closely associated with cAMP production in several systems. In fibroblasts, bradykinin stimulates phospholipid methylation before cAMP content rises; in most systems, an elevation in cAMP concentrations is the most common response to PC synthesis (183). However, in *Xenopus* oocytes, progesterone stimulation of phospholipid methylation is associated with a decline in cAMP levels (185). In both systems, the methylation peaks at 15 seconds, although the changes in cAMP content require 2–5 minutes, suggesting a cause-and-effect relationship. This is supported by the use of methyltransferase inhibitors, which also inhibit the changes in cAMP concentrations. Finally, cholera toxin and fluoride can stimulate the adenylate cyclase through G$_s$ without affecting the PC levels; this finding, along with the time courses, would eliminate the possibility that the changes in PC metabolism are secondary events.

How might phospholipid methylation influence cAMP production? One

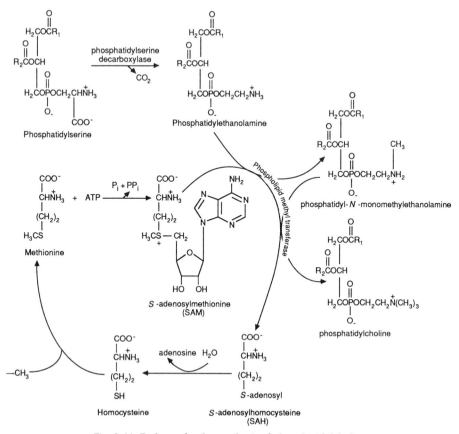

Fig. 9-11. Pathway for the synthesis of phosphatidylcholine.

argument is that it decreases membrane fluidity, thereby facilitating the coupling of receptor, G proteins, and adenylate cyclase (182). The ability of isoproterenol, a β-adrenergic agonist, to stimulate adenylate cyclase in turkey erythrocytes is influenced by membrane fluidity; loading the membranes with cholesterol decreases membrane fluidity and dampens isoproterenol-induced cyclase activity. Conversely, loading the membranes with vaccenic acid increases fluidity and enhances cyclase activity. Finally, increasing the PC content of these membranes also increases their fluidity and coupling efficiency.

Second, phospholipid methylation may act through calcium (182,183). Calcium influxes are stimulated after phospholipid methylation but before changes in cAMP content are observed; these fluxes usually occur in 0.5 to 2 minutes depending on the system. Furthermore, methylation inhibitors also inhibit these fluxes, suggesting that they were evoked by the methylation. Since bradykinin has been shown to stimulate the PPI pathway (185), it is possible that the changes in membrane fluidity induced by changes in PC metabolism could also have facilitated PPI hydrolysis, which then led to the calcium fluxes. Regardless of the exact mechanism, the resulting calcium fluctuations would alter adenylate cyclase activity (see preceding discussion).

Third, the increase in PC may stimulate a PC-specific phospholipase A_2 (PC–PLA_2) that would release arachidonic acid for eicosanoid synthesis (182,183); many receptors for the eicosanoids are coupled to adenylate cyclase. Methyltransferase inhibitors block the release of arachidonic acid and cAMP elevation; mepacrine (also called quinacrine) is an inhibitor of PLA_2 and has the same effect. Alternatively, the active agent may not be arachidonic acid or its metabolites but the other hydrolytic product, lysophosphatidylcholine. Lysophospholipids, which lack a fatty acid in the second position, are strong detergents and, in sufficiently large concentrations, can lyse cells (see subsequent discussion). Indeed, the active ingredient in several snake toxins is a PLA_2 and the toxicity of the venom can be directly attributed to this lytic effect. In smaller amounts, lysophosphatidylcholine might act as a membrane fusogen and aid in secretion; phospholipid methylation has been implicated in a number of secretory systems. Lysophospholipids have also been implicated in the regulation of the (Na^+,H^+) antiport system that influences cellular pH (186). A summary of some of these mechanisms is shown in Fig. 9-12.

This scheme is not without its critics; there are, in fact, three basic problems with this hypothesis (187). First, in many systems the elevation in cAMP precedes phospholipid methylation and the methylation can be induced by cAMP. These systems include glucagon in the liver, ACTH in adipocytes, and hCG in Leydig cells. This is in contrast to the findings in turkey erythrocytes and *Xenopus* oocytes just noted.

Second, the various inhibitors used all have side effects: the methyl-

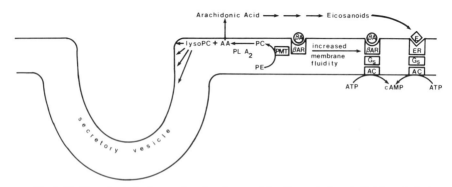

Fig. 9-12. Hypothetical scheme showing the possible effects of phospholipid methylation. AA, Arachidonic acid; AC, adenylate cyclase; βA, β-agonist; βAR, β-adrenergic receptor; E, eicosanoids; ER, eicosanoid receptor; lysoPC, lysophosphatidylcholine; PE, phosphatidylethanolamine; PLA_2, phospholipase A_2; PMT, phospholipid methyltransferase. Other abbreviations are described in the text.

transferase inhibitors can also inhibit other types of methylation reactions; mepacrine can bind to chromatin, and can inhibit both oxidative phosphorylation and the mitochondrial ATPase. Furthermore, the effects of these drugs can be inconsistent: some methyltransferase inhibitors will block the actions of certain hormones in a particular system whereas other inhibitors cannot, although both effectively suppress methyltransferase activity.

Third, methyltransferase activity does not necessarily correspond to PC content. PC can be synthesized by two separate pathways: the methylation pathway (Fig. 9-11) and the salvage pathway. The latter pathway activates phosphocholine with CTP to form CDP-choline, which is then coupled to DG to form PC. In the liver, the two pathways are reciprocally controlled to maintain a constant PC content. For example, glucagon, β-agonists, and vasopressin stimulate the methyltransferase but inhibit the salvage pathway; 3-deazaadenosine inhibits the methyltransferase but stimulates the salvage pathway. Similarly, exogenous choline activates the salvage pathway and suppresses methylation; choline deficiency has the opposite effect. If this type of control operated in all tissues, PC content would remain constant regardless of the methyltransferase activity and membrane fluidity would not be altered. However, PC could still be a significant source of arachidonic acid, DG, and lysophosphatidylcholine, even if total PC content and membrane fluidity did not fluctuate.

B. Arachidonic Acid

As noted earlier, arachidonic acid (AA) commonly occupies the second position of many phospholipids. After release by PLA_2, this acid can act as a precursor to the eicosanoids (see Chapter 3) or arachidonylethanolamide, a ligand for the cannabinoid receptor (188). However, AA can exert several activities by itself (189): it activates PKCγ, Ras and Rac, sphingomyelinase, and the soluble guanylate cyclase. It also directly stimulates potassium and calcium channels and potentiates the glutamate (NMDA) channels. On the other hand, it inhibits CaMKII, the myosin light chain phosphatase, and estradiol binding to its receptor. The immediate source of the AA is phosphatidylethanolamine (PE), which is located in the inner leaflet of the plasmalemma and has a high content of this fatty acid (190,191). However, PC indirectly makes a major contribution by transferring its arachidonic acid to the lysophosphatidylethanolamine to regenerate PE. PI is also rich in AA and may be responsible for as much as one-third of the liberated AA in some systems (183). AA can be released from intact PI by PLA_2 or from DG by DG lipase after PLC hydrolysis; for example, the latter pathway provides 12–15% of the AA released in platelets (192).

There are two forms of PLA_2: extracellular and cytosolic (193). The extracellular form is regulated by the small peptide inhibitors lipocortin I and II (194,195). The lipocortins are activated by calcium, which translocates the inhibitors to the plasma membrane, and are inhibited by PKC and RTKs via phosphorylation. The cytosolic PLA_2 is affected by several hormone mediators: it is activated by $\beta\gamma$ in the retina and by α_{i2} or α_{i3} elsewhere (196), by micromolar amounts of calcium (197), by alkalinization (198), by ATP (199), by phosphatidic acid (200), and by DG independent of PKC (201). The effects of phosphorylation are controversial. In a system using purified recombinant components, PLA_2 could be phosphorylated and activated by MAPK; PKA and PKC could also phosphorylate PLA_2 but no change in activity was observed (202). Since PKA (203) and PKC (204) stimulate PLA_2 in neural and renal tissues, respectively, an indirect role for these kinases cannot be ruled out. CaMKII inhibits PLA_2 in neurons (203) but has not yet been tested in a purified system. The effect of calcium is much simpler: it brings the PLA_2 to the membrane where the substrates are located (205).

C. Sphingolipids

Sphingolipids are membrane lipids with a structure similar to phospholipids: a backbone containing two fatty acids and a head group. However, the backbone is serine instead of glycerol. In sphingosine, the carboxylic acid of serine is attached to palmitic acid by a carbon–carbon bond rather than by the ester bond seen in phospholipids. When the second fatty acid is coupled via an amide bond, the molecule becomes ceramide. The head group defines three different classes of sphingolipids: the cerebrosides contain a single sugar; gangliosides contain complex sugars; and sphingomyelin contains phosphocholine.

The sphingosines have several biological activities (206–209): they inhibit PKC and CaMKII but stimulate casein kinase II and tyrosine kinases. They enhance PLD activity, induce the dephosphorylation of an anti-onco-gene, activate platelets, and release calcium from IP_3-like pools. However, they can inhibit melanoma cell motility and phagocytosis, and reduce muscarinic receptor affinity for its agonist. Ceramide appears to mediate the TNFα-induced activation of MAP kinase (210) and of a transcription factor (211); it can also activate a unique, but still unidentified, protein kinase and phosphatase (212). It is a competitive inhibitor of DG kinase; this effect would block the recycling of DG and allow this second messenger to accumulate (213). Gangliosides and cerebrosides can stimulate CaMKII (214); they can either stimulate or inhibit RTKs, calcium fluctuations, and the calcium–CaM PDE, depending on the particular sphingolipid being tested.

Regulation appears to involve sphingomyelinase, which hydrolyzes sphingomyelin into ceramide and phosphocholine; sphingosine can be derived from the further breakdown of ceramide. Glucocorticoids, 1,25-DHCC, DG, IFNγ, IL-1, and TNFα have all been shown to stimulate sphingomyelinase. The strongest evidence for a physiological role for sphingolipids in hormone action is in the TNFα system: activation occurs within 1 minute at physiological concentrations of TNFα and the effect is specific for sphingolipids (206). Furthermore, ceramide has been shown to mediate the TNFα activation of a transcription factor (211). Another product of this pathway, sphingosine-1-phosphate, may mediate the mitogenic effects of PDGF (215).

D. Lysophospholipids

Lysophospholipids were briefly discussed earlier as possible mediators of endo- or exocytosis. However, other biological activities have also been associated with them (216). Nanomolar concentrations can elevate calcium and lower cAMP levels (217); in micromolar amounts, these molecules are mitogenic in fibroblasts. Lysophospholipids can also activate MAP kinase (218) and are involved with chemotaxis and smooth muscle relaxation (115). Lysophospholipids are the product of PLA_2 hydrolysis; lysosphingolipids have similar biological activities and arise from the breakdown of sphingolipids (219).

There are three possible mechanisms of action of lysophospholipids: first, they may act through plasma membrane receptors. This hypothesis is supported by the fact that these lipids are active extracellularly, where their effects are cell specific. Recently, they have been photoaffinity labeled to a 38- to 40-kDa membrane protein (220). The receptor appears to be coupled to G_i (217).

Alternatively, these lipids may serve as precursors to the platelet-activating factor (PAF): an alkylether PC can be converted to PAF by PLA_2 and lyso-PAF:acetyl CoA acetyltransferase (221–223). Both these enzymes can be activated by PKA, PKC, or CaMKII, depending on the system. PAF is degraded by PAF–acetylhydrolase; this enzyme can be regulated by steroids. Serum levels of the hydrolase are induced by progesterone and glucocorticoids and are repressed by estradiol (224). The elevation occurs via gene induction, since protein synthesis is required (225). The PAF would then be secreted and would act in an autocrine/paracrine fashion (see Chapter 3).

Finally, lysopholipids can activate the conventional PKCs (226), as well as a different, but still unidentified, protein kinase (227). The latter can be further stimulated by calcium but other phospholipids are without effect.

E. Lipoxygenase Pathway

The role of several lipoxygenase products in hormone action has been investigated. In many systems, lipoxygenase inhibitors specifically block the action of the hormone. This inhibition can be overcome by a particular product of this pathway. Finally, the hormone can elevate the levels of these molecules. These systems include ACTH and EGF in steroidogenesis (228,229), dopamine and GnRH in SRIF and LH release, respectively (230,231), and angiotensin in aldosterone synthesis (232) and the inhibition of renin release (Table 9-1; 233). The coupling between the hormone and the pathway is still unknown for most of these hormones. In an epithelial cell line, EGF appears to induce the gene for 12-lipoxygenase, since the elevation in enzyme activity requires protein synthesis and a 10-hour lag (234); a similar mechanism has been shown for angiotensin (235).

The mechanism of action of these molecules is also uncertain. Their inhibition of CaMKII (236) and the direct regulation of potassium channels (237) suggest that these products can act as allosteric molecules. However,

Hormone	Activity	Presumed mediator
Angiotensin	Inhibit renin release; steroidogenesis	12-Hydroxy-6,8,11,14-eicosatetraenoic acid (12-HETE)
Dopamine	SRIF release	8,9-Epoxyeicosatrienoic acid
GnRH	LH release	Leukotriene C_4
ACTH	Steroidogenesis	5-Hydroperoxy-6,8,11,14-eicosatetraenoic acid (5-HPETE)
EGF	Steroidogenesis	12-HETE

plasma membrane receptors for lipoxygenase products have been identified on mast cells (238) and their effect on sodium conductance appears to be mediated by G_{i3} (239), which would be characteristic of membrane receptors. The stimulation of leukocytes by 5-HETE also appears to involve G proteins (240). Finally, their effects on endothelial and melanoma cell morphology are mediated by PKC (241,242), whereas their mediation of EGF-induced actin polymerization involves the MAP kinase activation of PLA_2 (243). However, whether these effects are direct or mediated through a receptor is not clear.

V. Summary

Hormones can utilize several phospholipid metabolites as second messengers (Fig. 9-13). Hormones can activate PI-specific PLCβ via G_q or PLCγ via tyrosine phosphorylation. The head group, IP_3, triggers the release of calcium from internal stores. The influx of calcium from the external medium can also be induced, but it is not clear whether this is a direct result of IP_3 or of one of its metabolites, such as IP_4. The calcium is released in pulses whose frequency contains information about the intensity of the signal. Although calcium can modulate some enzymes, this cation usually acts in combination with CaM. Calcium–CaM binds many target proteins but the greatest effects are seen with a multifunctional protein kinase, CaMKII, and a protein phosphatase, calcineurin.

DG is an allosteric activator of another kinase, PKC, which actually represents a large family of kinases, some of which also require calcium and phospholipids. The hydrolysis of PC will generate DG for PKC stimulation without elevating calcium, since the phosphocholine head group does not affect calcium levels. This pathway appears to be more important at later time periods after hormone stimulation. PC hydrolysis can be accomplished by a PC–PLC or by a combination of PC–PLD and PA phosphohydrolase. PC–PLC can be activated by Ras and PLD by G proteins.

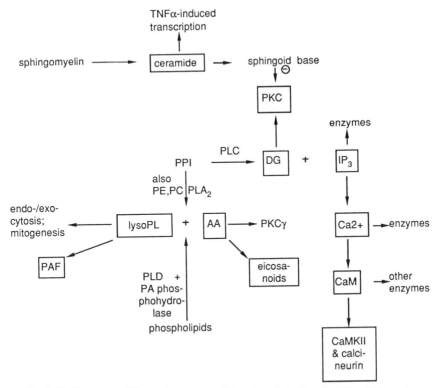

Fig. 9-13. Summary of the major outputs of the phospholipid and sphingolipid pathways. The principal effectors are boxed. AA, Arachidonic acid; CaM, calmodulin; DG, diacylglycerol; lysoPL, lysophospholipid; PA, phosphatidic acid; PAF, platelet-activating factor; PC, phosphatidylcholine; PE, phosphatidylethanolamine; PLC, phospholipase C; PLD, phospholipase D.

Another phospholipase, PLA_2, produces arachidonic acid, which can directly affect protein kinases and ion channels or be converted to various eicosanoids. PLA_2 releases AA primarily from PE and PC and can be hormonally regulated via G proteins, calcium, and phosphorylation. A small amount of AA may come from DG via DG lipase. PLA_2 also generates a lysophospholipid as the other product; this metabolite may affect endo- and exocytosis, mitogenesis, cAMP synthesis, and calcium release. Finally, sphingomyelinase can initiate the breakdown of sphingomyelin into ceramide and sphingosine. The former mediates the effect of TNFα on transcription whereas the latter can modulate the activity of many kinases.

Homologous regulation of the PPI pathway revolves around feedback inhibition by the two major products, PKC and calcium. They stimulate the removal of their activators and suppress further PPI hydrolysis. Heterologous regulation by cAMP can be synergistic or antagonistic, depending on the system being studied.

References

General References

Berridge, M. J. (1993). Inositol trisphosphate and calcium signalling. *Nature (London)* **361,** 315–325.

Billah, M. M. (1993). Phospholipase D and cell signaling. *Curr. Opin. Immunol.* **5,** 114–123.

Divecha, N., Banfić, H., and Irvine, R. F. (1993). Inositides and the nucleus and inositides in the nucleus. *Cell* **74,** 405–407.

Fewtrell, C. (1993). Ca^{2+} oscillations in non-excitable cells. *Annu. Rev. Physiol.* **55,** 427–454.

Galione, A. (1994). Cyclic ADP-ribose, the ADP-ribosyl cyclase pathway and calcium signalling. *Mol. Cell. Endocrinol.* **98,** 125–131.

Lu, K. P., and Means, A. R. (1993). Regulation of the cell cycle by calcium and calmodulin. *Endocr. Rev.* **14,** 40–58.

Menniti, F. S., Oliver, K. G., Putney, J. W., and Shears, S. B. (1993). Inositol phosphates and cell signaling: New views of $InsP_5$ and $InsP_6$. *Trends Biochem. Sci.* **18,** 53–56.

Sanderson, M. J., Charles, A. C., Boitano, S., and Dirksen, E. R. (1994). Mechanisms and function of intercellular calcium signaling. *Mol. Cell. Endocrinol.* **98,** 173–187.

Sando, J. J., Maurer, M. C., Bolen, E. J., and Grisham, C. M. (1992). Role of cofactors in protein kinase C activation. *Cell. Signal.* **4,** 595–609.

Schulman, H., and Hanson, P. I. (1993). Multifunctional Ca^{2+}/calmodulin-dependent protein kinase. *Neurochem. Res.* **18,** 65–77.

Sumida, C., Graber, R., and Nunez, E. (1993). Role of fatty acids in signal transduction: Modulators and messengers. *Prostaglandins Leukotrienes Essent. Fatty Acids* **48,** 117–122.

Zeisel, S. H. (1993). Choline phospholipids: Signal transduction and carcinogenesis. *FASEB J.* **7,** 551–557.

See also Refs. 1, 2, 13–17, 19, 22–24, 37, 39, 41, 50, 51, 77, 80, 92, 103, 111–115, 120, 132–134, 144, 147, 150, 153, 168, 171, 172, 174, 175, 180, 187, 189, 191–195, 206–209, 214, 216, 221, and 223.

Cited References

1. Cobbold, P. H., and Rink, T. J. (1987). Fluorescence and bioluminescence measurement of cytoplasmic free calcium. *Biochem. J.* **248,** 313–328.
2. Adams, S. R., and Tsien, R. Y. (1993). Controlling cell chemistry with caged compounds. *Annu. Rev. Physiol.* **55,** 755–784.
3. Murphy, K. M. M., Gould, R. J., Largent, B. L., and Snyder, S. H. (1983). A unitary mechanism of calcium antagonist drug action. *Proc. Natl. Acad. Sci. U.S.A.* **80,** 860–864.
4. Nakashima, S., Tohmatsu, T., Shirato, L., Takenake, A., and Nozawa, Y. (1987). Neomycin is a potent agent for arachidonic acid release in human platelets. *Biochem. Biophys. Res. Commun.* **146,** 820–826.
5. Peters, D. J. M., Snaar-Jagalska, B. E., van Haastert, P. J. M., and Schaap, P. (1992). Lithium, an inhibitor of cAMP-induced inositol 1,4,5-trisphosphate accumulation in *Dictyostelium discoideum,* inhibits activation of guanine-nucleo-

tide-binding regulatory proteins, reduces activation of adenylylcyclase, but potentiates activation of guanylyl cyclase by cAMP. *Eur. J. Biochem.* **209**, 299–304.

6. Joseph, S., and Krishnamurthi, S. (1989). Pharmacological manipulation of diacylglycerol-dependent protein kinase C. *Trends Pharmacol. Sci.* **10**, 396.

7. Marquez, C., Martinez-A., C., Kroemer, G., and Bosca, L. (1992). Protein kinase C isoenzymes display differential affinity for phorbol esters: Analysis of phorbol ester receptors in B cell differentiation. *J. Immunol.* **149**, 2560–2568.

8. Standaert, M. L., Cooper, D. R., Hernandez, H., Arnold, T. P., and Farese, R. V. (1993). Differential down-regulation of insulin-sensitive protein kinase-C isoforms by 12-*O*-tetradecanoylphorbol-13-acetate in rat adipocytes and BC3H-1 myocytes. *Endocrinol. (Baltimore)* **132**, 689–692.

9. Edashige, K., Sato, E. F., Akimaru, K., Kasai, M., and Utsumi, K. (1992). Differentiation of HL-60 cells by phorbol ester is correlated with up-regulation of protein kinase C-α. *Arch. Biochem. Biophys.* **299**, 200–205.

10. Leli, U., Shea, T. B., Cataldo, A., Hauser, G., Grynspan, F., Beermann, M. L., Liepkalns, V. A., Nixon, R. A., and Parker, P. J. (1993). Differential expression and subcellular localization of protein kinase C α, β, γ, δ, and ε isoforms in SH-SY5Y neuroblastoma cells: Modifications during differentiation. *J. Neurochem.* **60**, 289–298.

11. Kelleher, D., Pandol, S. J., and Kagnoff, M. F. (1988). Phorbol myristate acetate induces IL-2 secretion by HUT 78 cells by a mechanism independent of protein kinase C translocation. *Immunology* **65**, 351–355.

12. Hockberger, P., Toselli, M., Swandulla, D., and Lux, H. D. (1989). A diacylglycerol analogue reduces neuronal calcium currents independently of protein kinase C activation. *Nature (London)* **338**, 340–342.

13. Casnellie, J. E. (1991). Protein kinase inhibitors: Probes for the functions of protein phosphorylation. *Adv. Pharmacol.* **22**, 167–205.

14. Rasmussen, H., and Barrett, P. Q. (1984). Calcium messenger system: An integrated view. *Physiol. Rev.* **64**, 938–984.

15. Reinhart, P. H., Taylor, W. M., and Bygrave, F. L. (1984). The role of calcium ions in the mechanism of action of α-adrenergic agonists in rat liver. *Biochem. J.* **223**, 1–13.

16. Strehler, E. E. (1991). Recent advances in the molecular characterization of plasma membrane Ca^{2+} pumps. *J. Membr. Biol.* **120**, 1–15.

17. Carafoli, E. (1992). The Ca^{2+} pump of the plasma membrane. *J. Biol. Chem.* **267**, 2115–2118.

18. Xu, A., Hawkins, C., and Narayanan, N. (1993). Phosphorylation and activation of the Ca^{2+}-pumping ATPase of cardiac sarcoplasmic reticulum by Ca^{2+}/calmodulin-dependent protein kinase. *J. Biol. Chem.* **268**, 8394–8397.

19. Miller, R. J. (1992). Voltage-sensitive Ca^{2+} channels. *J. Biol. Chem.* **267**, 1403–1406.

20. Fujita, Y., Mynlieff, M., Dirksen, R. T., Kim, M. S., Niidome, T., Nakai, J., Friedrich, T., Iwabe, N., Miyata, T., Furuichi, T., Furutama, D., Mikoshiba, K., Mori, Y., and Beam, K. G. (1993). Primary structure and functional expression of the ω-conotoxin-sensitive N-type calcium channel from rabbit brain. *Neuron* **10**, 585–598.

21. Rotman, E. I., De Jongh, K. S., Florio, V., Lai, Y., and Catterall, W. A. (1992). Specific phosphorylation of a COOH-terminal site on the full-length form of the α1 subunit of the skeletal muscle calcium channel by cAMP-dependent protein kinase. *J. Biol. Chem.* **267**, 16100–16105.

22. Chang, C. F., Gutierrez, L. M., Mundina-Weilenmann, C., and Hosey, M. M. (1991). Dihydropyridine-sensitive calcium channels from skeletal muscle. II. Functional effects of differential phosphorylation of channel subunits. *J. Biol. Chem.* **266**, 16395–16400.

23. Witcher, D. R., Kovacs, R. J., Schulman, H., Cefali, D. C., and Jones, L. R. (1991). Unique phosphorylation site on the cardiac ryanodine receptor regulates calcium channel activity. *J. Biol. Chem.* **266**, 11144–11152.

24. McCarron, J. G., McGeown, J. G., Reardon, S., Ikebe, M., Fay, F. S., and Walsh, J. V. (1992). Calcium-dependent enhancement of calcium current in smooth muscle by calmodulin-dependent protein kinase II. *Nature (London)* **357**, 74–77.

25. Satoh, H. (1992). Inhibition in L-type Ca^{2+} channel by stimulation of protein kinase C in isolated guinea pig ventricular cardiomyocytes. *Gen. Pharmacol.* **23**, 1097–1102.

26. Wang, R., Wu, L., Karpinski, E., and Pang, P. K. T. (1991). The effects of parathyroid hormone on L-type voltage-dependent calcium channel currents in vascular smooth muscle cells and ventricular myocytes are mediated by a cyclic AMP dependent mechanism. *FEBS Lett.* **282**, 331–334.

27. Caffrey, J. M., and Farach-Carson, M. C. (1989). Vitamin D_3 metabolites modulate dihydropyridine-sensitive calcium currents in clonal rat osteosarcoma cells. *J. Biol. Chem.* **264**, 20265–20274.

28. Barrett, P. Q., Bollag, W. B., Isales, C. M., McCarthy, R. T., and Rasmussen, H. (1989). Role of calcium in angiotensin II-mediated aldosterone secretion. *Endocr. Rev.* **10**, 496–518.

29. Lussier, B. T., French, M. B., Moor, B. C., and Kraicer, J. (1991). Free intracellular Ca^{2+} concentration and growth hormone (GH) release from purified rat somatotrophs. III. Mechanism of action of GH-releasing factor and somatostatin. *Endocrinol. (Baltimore)* **128**, 592–603.

30. Enyeart, J. J., Mlinar, B., and Enyeart, J. A. (1993). T-type Ca^{2+} channels are required for adrenocorticotropin-stimulated cortisol production by bovine adrenal zona fasciculata cells. *Mol. Endocrinol.* **7**, 1031–1040.

31. Ferris, C. D., Huganir, R. L., and Snyder, S. H. (1990). Calcium flux mediated by purified inositol 1,4,5-trisphosphate receptor in reconstituted lipid vesicles is allosterically regulated by adenine nucleotides. *Proc. Natl. Acad. Sci. U.S.A.* **87**, 2147–2151.

32. Boynton, A. L., Dean, N. M., and Hill, T. D. (1990). Inositol 1,3,4,5-tetrakisphosphate and regulation of intracellular calcium. *Biochem. Pharmacol.* **40**, 1933–1939.

33. Bezprozvanny, I., Watras, J., and Ehrlich, B. E. (1991). Bell-shaped calcium-response curves of Ins(1,4,5)P$_3$- and calcium-gated channels from endoplasmic reticulum of cerebellum. *Nature (London)* **351**, 751–754.

34. Quinton, T. M., and Dean, W. L. (1992). Cyclic AMP-dependent phosphorylation of the inositol-1,4,5-trisphosphate receptor inhibits Ca^{2+} release from platelet membranes. *Biochem. Biophys. Res. Commun.* **184**, 893–899.

35. Matter, N., Ritz, M. F., Freyermuth, S., Rogue, P., and Malviya, A. N. (1993). Stimulation of protein kinase C leads to phosphorylation of nuclear inositol 1,4,5-trisphosphate receptor and accelerated calcium release by inositol 1,4,5-trisphosphate from isolated rat liver nuclei. *J. Biol. Chem.* **268**, 732–736.

36. Ferris, C. D., Huganir, R. L., Bredt, D. S., Cameron, A. M., and Snyder, S. H. (1991). Inositol trisphosphate receptor: Phosphorylation by protein kinase C

and calcium calmodulin-dependent protein kinases in reconstituted lipid vesicles. *Proc. Natl. Acad. Sci. U.S.A.* **88**, 2232–2235.

37. Mikoshiba, K. (1993). Inositol 1,4,5-trisphosphate receptor. *Trends Pharmacol. Sci.* **14**, 86–89.

38. Magnusson, A., Haug, L. S., Walaas, S. I., and Østvold, A. C. (1993). Calcium-induced degradation of the inositol (1,4,5)-trisphosphate receptor/Ca^{2+}-channel. *FEBS Lett.* **323**, 229–232.

39. Sorrentino, V., and Volpe, P. (1993). Ryanodine receptors: How many, where and why? *Trends Pharmacol. Sci.* **14**, 98–103.

40. Marks, A. R., Tempst, P., Chadwick, C. C., Riviere, L., Fleicher, S., and Nadal-Ginard, B. (1990). Smooth muscle and brain inositol 1,4,5-trisphosphate receptors are structurally and functionally similar. *J. Biol. Chem.* **265**, 20719–20722.

41. Tepikin, A. V., and Petersen, O. H. (1992). Mechanism of cellular oscillations in secretory cells. *Biochim. Biophys. Acta* **1137**, 197–207.

42. Hohengger, M., and Suko, J. (1993). Phosphorylation of the purified cardiac ryanodine receptor by exogenous and endogenous protein kinases. *Biochem. J.* **296**, 303–308.

43. Takasawa, S., Nata, K., Yonekura, H., and Okamoto, H. (1993). Cyclic ADP-ribose in insulin secretion from pancreatic β cells. *Science* **259**, 370–373.

44. White, A. M., Watson, S. P., and Galione, A. (1993). Cyclic ADP-ribose-induced Ca^{2+} release from rat brain microsomes. *FEBS Lett.* **318**, 259–263.

45. Kim, H., Jacobson, E. L., and Jacobson, M. K. (1993). Position of cyclization in cyclic ADP-ribose. *Biochim. Biophys. Res. Commun.* **194**, 1143–1147.

46. Mészáros, L. G., Bak, J., and Chu, A. (1993). Cyclic ADP-ribose as an endogenous regulator of the non-skeletal type ryanodine receptor Ca^{2+} channel. *Nature (London)* **364**, 76–79.

47. Lee, C. H., Aarhus, R., and Walseth, T. F. (1993). Calcium mobilization by dual receptors during fertilization of sea urchin eggs. *Science* **261**, 352–355.

48. Galione, A., White, A., Willmott, N., Turner, M., Potter, B. V. L., and Watson, S. P. (1993). cGMP mobilizes intracellular Ca^{2+} in sea urchin eggs by stimulating cyclic ADP-ribose synthesis. *Nature (London)* **365**, 456–459.

49. Howard, M., Grimaldi, J. C., Bazan, J. F., Lund, F. E., Santos-Argumedo, L., Parkhouse, R. M. E., Walseth, T. F., and Lee, H. C. (1993). Formation and hydrolysis of cyclic ADP-ribose catalyzed by lymphocyte antigen CD38. *Science* **262**, 1056–1059.

50. Rhee, S. G., Kim, H., Suh, P. G., and Choi, W. C. (1991). Multiple forms of phosphoinositide-specific phospholipase C and different modes of activation. *Biochem. Soc. Trans.* **19**, 337–341.

51. Guillon, G., Mouillac, B., and Savage, A. L. (1992). Modulation of hormone-sensitive phospholipase C. *Cell. Signal.* **4**, 11–23.

52. Srivastava, S. P., Fuchs, J. A., and Holtzman, J. L. (1993). The reported cDNA sequence for phospholipase Cα encodes protein disulfide isomerase, isozyme Q-2 and not phospholipase-C. *Biochem. Biophys. Res. Commun.* **193**, 971–978.

53. Taylor, G. D., Fee, J. A., Silbert, D. F., and Hofmann, S. L. (1992). PI-specific phospholipase C "α" from sheep seminal vesicles is a proteolytic fragment of PI-PLC δ. *Biochem. Biophys. Res. Commun.* **188**, 1176–1183.

54. Berstein, G., Blank, J. L., Smrcka, A. V., Higashijima, T., Sternweis, P. C., Exton, J. H., and Ross, E. M. (1992). Reconstitution of agonist-stimulated phosphatidylinositol 4,5-bisphosphate hydrolysis using purified m1 muscarinic receptor, $G_{q/11}$, and phospholipase C-β1. *J. Biol. Chem.* **267**, 8081–8088.

55. Blitzer, R. D., Omri, G., De Vivo, M., Carty, D. J., Premont, R. T., Codina, J., Birnbaumer, L., Cotecchia, S., Caron, M. G., Lefkowitz, R. J., Landau, E. M., and Iyengar, R. (1993). Coupling of the expressed α_{1B}-adrenergic receptor to the phospholipase C pathway in *Xenopus* oocytes: The role of G_o. *J. Biol. Chem.* **268**, 7532–7537.

56. Park, D., Jhon, D. Y., Lee, C. W., Lee, K. H., and Rhee, S. G. (1993). Activation of phospholipase C isozymes by G proteins $\beta\gamma$ subunits. *J. Biol. Chem.* **268**, 4573–4576.

57. Wu, D., and Simon, M. I. (1993). Activation of phospholipase C β_2 by the α and $\beta\gamma$ subunits of trimeric GTP-binding protein. *Proc. Natl. Acad. Sci. U.S.A.* **90**, 5297–5301.

58. Litsch, I., Sulkholutskaya, I., and Weng, C. (1993). G protein-mediated inhibition of phospholipase C activity in a solubilized membrane preparation. *J. Biol. Chem.* **268**, 8692–8697.

59. Ryu, S. H., Kim, U. H., Wahl, M. I., Brown, A. B., Carpenter, G., Huang, K. P., and Rhee, S. G. (1990). Feedback regulation of phospholipase C-β by protein kinase C. *J. Biol. Chem.* **265**, 17941–17945.

60. Pachter, J. A., Pai, J. K., Mayer-Ezell, R., Petrin, J. M., Dobek, E., and Bishop, W. R. (1992). Differential regulation of phosphoinositide and phosphatidylcholine hydrolysis by protein kinase C-β1 overexpression: Effects on stimulation by α-thrombin, guanosine 5'-O-(thiotriphosphate), and calcium. *J. Biol. Chem.* **267**, 9826–9830.

61. Haeffner, E. W., and Wittmann, U. (1992). Ca^{2+} and partly GTPγS-dependent particulate phospholipase C hydrolyzing phosphatidylinositol 4-phosphate and phosphatidylinositol 4,5-bisphosphate is inhibited by diacyl(acyl-acetyl)glycerols. *J. Lipid Mediators* **5**, 237–248.

62. Liao, F., Shin, H. S., and Rhee, S. G. (1993). *In vitro* tyrosine phosphorylation of PLC-γ1 and PLC-γ2 by src-family protein tyrosine kinases. *Biochem. Biophys. Res. Commun.* **191**, 1028–1033.

63. Machesky, L. M., and Pollard, T. D. (1993). Profilin as a potential mediator of membrane-cytoskeleton communication. *Trends Cell Biol.* **3**, 381–385.

64. Park, D. J., Min, H. K., and Rhee, S. G. (1992). Inhibition of CD3-linked phospholipase C by phorbol ester and by cAMP is associated with decreased phosphotyrosine and increased phosphoserine contents of PLC-γ1. *J. Biol. Chem.* **267**, 1496–1501.

65. Alava, M. A., DeBell, K. E., Conti, A., Hoffman, T., and Bonvini, E. (1992). Increased intracellular cyclic AMP inhibits inositol phospholipid hydrolysis induced by perturbation of the T cell receptor/CD3 complex but not by G-protein stimulation: Association with protein kinase A-mediated phosphorylation of phospholipase C-γ1. *Biochem. J.* **284**, 189–199.

66. Hernández-Sotomayor, S. M. T., and Carpenter, G. (1993). Non-catalytic activation of phospholipase C-γ1 *in vitro* by epidermal growth factor receptor. *Biochem. J.* **293**, 507–511.

67. Shaw, G. (1993). Identification of novel pleckstrin homology (PH) domains provides a hypothesis for PH domain function. *Biochem. Biophys. Res. Commun.* **195**, 1145–1151.

68. Musacchio, A., Gibson, T., Rice, P., Thompson, J., and Saraste, M. (1993). The PH domain: A common piece in the structural patchwork of signalling proteins. *Trends Biochem. Sci.* **18**, 343–348.

69. Touhara, K., Inglese, J., Pitcher, J. A., Shaw, G., and Lefkowitz, R. J. (1994).

Binding of G protein $\beta\gamma$-subunits to pleckstrin homology domains. *J. Biol. Chem.* **269**, 10217–10220.

70. Cho, Y. S., Han, M. K., Chae, S. W., Park, C. U., and Kim, U. H. (1993). Selectivity of phospholipase C isozymes in growth factor signaling. *FEBS Lett.* **334**, 257–260.

71. Haber, M. T., Fukui, T., Lebowitz, M. S., and Lowenstein, J. M. (1991). Activation of phosphoinositide-specific phospholipase Cδ from rat liver by polyamines and basic proteins. *Arch. Biochem. Biophys.* **288**, 243–249.

72. Pawelczyk, T., and Lowenstein, J. M. (1992). Regulation of phospholipase Cδ activity by sphingomyelin and sphingosine. *Arch. Biochem. Biophys.* **297**, 328–333.

73. Kanematsu, T., Takeya, H., Watanabe, Y., Ozaki, S., Yoshida, M., Koga, T., Iwanaga, S., and Hirata, M. (1992). Putative inositol 1,4,5-trisphosphate binding proteins in rat brain cytosol. *J. Biol. Chem.* **267**, 6518–6525.

74. Hokin, M. R., and Hokin, L. E. (1953). Enzyme secretion and the incorporation of P^{32} into phospholipides of pancreas slices. *J. Biol. Chem.* **203**, 966–997.

75. Michell, R. H. (1975). Inositol phospholipids and cell surface receptor function. *Biochim. Biophys. Acta* **415**, 81–147.

76. Woods, N. M., Cuthbertson, K. S. R., and Cobbold, P. H. (1986). Repetitive transient rises in cytoplasmic free calcium in hormone-stimulated hepatocytes. *Nature (London)* **319**, 600–602.

77. Cheek, T. R. (1989). Spatial aspects of calcium signalling. *J. Cell Sci.* **93**, 211–216.

78. Allbritton, N. L., Meyer, T., and Stryer, L. (1992). Range of messenger action of calcium ion and inositol 1,4,5-trisphosphate. *Science* **258**, 1812–1815.

79. Wakui, M., Potter, B. V. L., and Petersen, O. H. (1989). Pulsatile intracellular calcium release does not depend on fluctuations in inositol trisphosphate concentration. *Nature (London)* **339**, 317–320.

80. Jacob, R. (1990). Calcium oscillations in electrically non-excitable cells. *Biochim. Biophys. Acta* **1052**, 427–438.

81. Berridge, M. J. (1990). Calcium oscillations. *J. Biol. Chem.* **265**, 9583–9586.

82. Finch, E. A., Turner, T. J., and Goldin, S. M. (1991). Calcium as a coagonist of inositol 1,4,5-trisphosphate-induced calcium release. *Science* **252**, 443–446.

83. Thorn, P., Lawrie, A. M., Smith, P. M., Gallacher, D. V., and Petersen, O. H. (1993). Local and global cytosolic Ca^{2+} oscillations in exocrine cells evoked by agonists and inositol trisphosphate. *Cell* **74**, 661–668.

84. Kasai, H., Li, Y. X., and Miyashita, Y. (1993). Subcellular distribution of Ca^{2+} release channels underlying Ca^{2+} waves and oscillations in exocrine pancreas. *Cell* **74**, 669–677.

85. Girard, S., and Clapham, D. (1993). Acceleration of intracellular calcium waves in *Xenopus* oocytes by calcium influx. *Science* **260**, 229–232.

86. Leong, D. A., and Thorner, M. O. (1991). A potential code of luteinizing hormone-releasing hormone-induced calcium ion responses in the regulation of luteinizing hormone secretion among individual gonadotropes. *J. Biol. Chem.* **266**, 9016–9022.

87. Hansen, C. A., Yang, L., and Williamson, J. R. (1991). Mechanisms of receptor-mediated Ca^{2+} signaling in rat hepatocytes. *J. Biol. Chem.* **266**, 18573–18579.

88. Khan, A. A., Steiner, J. P., Klein, M. G., Schneider, M. F., and Snyder, S. H. (1992). IP_3 receptor: Localization to plasma membrane of T cells and cocapping with the T cell receptor. *Science* **257**, 815–818.

89. Lückhoff, A., and Clapham, D. E. (1992). Inositol 1,3,4,5-tetrakisphosphate activates an endothelial Ca^{2+}-permeable channel. *Nature (London)* **355**, 356–358.

90. Bahnson, T. D., Pandol, S. J., and Dionne, V. E. (1993). Cyclic GMP modulates depletion-activated Ca^{2+} entry in pancreatic acinar cells. *J. Biol. Chem.* **268**, 10808–10812.

91. Randriamampita, C., and Tsien, R. Y. (1993). Emptying of intracellular Ca^{2+} stores releases a novel small messenger that stimulates Ca^{2+} influx. *Nature (London)* **364**, 809–814.

92. Parekh, A. B., Terlau, H., and Stühmer, W. (1993). Depletion of $InsP_3$ stores activates a Ca^{2+} and K^+ current by means of a phosphatase and a diffusible messenger. *Nature (London)* **364**, 814–818.

93. Putney, J. W., and Bird, G. St. J. (1993). The inositol phosphate-calcium signaling system in nonexcitable cells. *Endocr. Rev.* **14**, 610–631.

94. Thomas, G. M. H., Cunningham, E., Fensome, A., Ball, A., Totty, N. F., Truong, O., Hsuan, J. J., and Cockcroft, S. (1993). An essential role for phosphatidylinositol transfer protein in phospholipase C-mediated inositol lipid signaling. *Cell* **74**, 919–928.

95. Babu, Y. S., Sack, J. S., Greenhough, T. J., Bugg, C. E., Means, A. R., and Cook, W. J. (1985). Three-dimensional structure of calmodulin. *Nature (London)* **315**, 37–40.

96. Johnson, J. D., and Mills, J. S. (1986). Calmodulin. *Med. Res. Rev.* **6**, 341–363.

97. VanBerkum, M. F. A., and Means, A. R. (1991). Three amino acid substitutions in domain I of calmodulin prevent the activation of chicken smooth muscle myosin light chain kinase. *J. Biol. Chem.* **266**, 21488–21495.

98. Meador, W. E., Means, A. R., and Quiocho, F. A. (1992). Target enzyme recognition by calmodulin: 2.4 Å structure of a calmodulin-peptide complex. *Science* **257**, 1251–1255.

99. Rao, U., Teeter, M. M., Erickson-Viitanen, S., and DeGrado, W. F. (1992). Calmodulin binding to α_1-purothionin: Solution binding and modeling of the complex. *Proteins Struct. Funct. Genet.* **14**, 127–138.

100. Geiser, J. R., van Tuinen, D., Brockerhoff, S. E., Neff, M. M., and Davis, T. N. (1991). Can calmodulin function without binding calcium? *Cell* **65**, 949–959.

101. Chafouleas, J. G., Pardu, R. L., Brinkley, B. R., Dedman, J. R., and Means, A. R. (1980). Effect of viral transformation on the intracellular regulation of calmodulin and tubulin. *In* "Calcium-Binding Proteins Structure and Function" (F. L. Siegel, E. Carafoli, R. H. Kretsinger, D. H. MacLennan, and R. H. Wasserman, eds.), pp. 189–196. Elsevier/North-Holland Biomedical Press, Amsterdam.

102. Bolander, F. F. (1985). Possible roles of calcium and calmodulin in mammary gland differentiation *in vitro*. *J. Endocrinol.* **104**, 29–34.

103. Gnegy, M. E. (1993). Calmodulin in neurotransmitter and hormone action. *Annu. Rev. Pharmacol. Toxicol.* **32**, 45–70.

104. Solomon, S. S., Palazzolo, M. R., Green, S., and Raghow, R. (1990). Expression of calmodulin gene is down-regulated in diabetic BB rats. *Biochem. Biophys. Res. Commun.* **168**, 1007–1012.

105. Matsui, K., Higashi, K., Fukunaga, K., Miyazaki, K., Maeyama, M., and Miyamoto, E. (1983). Hormone treatments and pregnancy alter myosin light chain kinase and calmodulin levels in rabbit myometrium. *J. Endocrinol.* **97**, 11–19.

106. Pizarro, M., Puente, J., and Hagar, M. S. (1981). Calmodulin and cyclic nucleotide-phosphodiesterase activities in rat mammary gland during the lactogenic cycle. *FEBS Lett.* **136**, 127–130.

107. Riss, T. L., Bechtel, P. J., and Baumrucker, C. R. (1984). Calmodulin content of rat mammary tissue and isolated cells during pregnancy and lactation. *Biochem. J.* **219**, 927–934.
108. Sacks, D. B., Davis, H. W., Williams, J. P., Sheehan, E. L., Garcia, J. G. N., and McDonald, J. M. (1992). Phosphorylation by casein kinase II alters the biological activity of calmodulin. *Biochem. J.* **283**, 21–24.
109. Cohen, P., Cohen, P. T., Shenolikar, S., Nairn, A., and Victor, P. S. (1979). The role of calmodulin in the structure and regulation of phosphorylase kinase from rabbit skeletal muscle. *Eur. J. Biochem.* **100**, 329–337.
110. Kanaseki, T., Ikeuchi, Y., Sugiura, H., and Yamauchi, T. (1991). Structural features of Ca^{2+}/calmodulin-dependent protein kinase II revealed by electron microscopy. *J. Cell Biol.* **115**, 1049–1060.
111. Hanson, P. I., and Schulman, H. (1992). Neuronal Ca^{2+}/calmodulin-dependent protein kinases. *Annu. Rev. Biochem.* **61**, 559–601.
112. Pallen, C. J., and Wang, J. H. (1985). A multifunctional calmodulin-stimulated phosphatase. *Arch. Biochem. Biophys.* **237**, 281–291.
113. Stabel, S., and Parker, P. J. (1991). Protein kinase C. *Phamacol. Ther.* **51**, 71–95.
114. Azzi, A., Boscoboinik, D., and Hensey, C. (1992). The protein kinase C family. *Eur. J. Biochem.* **208**, 547–557.
115. Nishizuka, Y. (1992). Intracellular signaling by hydrolysis of phospholipids and activation of protein kinase C. *Science* **258**, 607–614.
116. Mochly-Rosen, D., Miller, K. G., Scheller, R. H., Khaner, H., Lopez, J., and Smith, B. L. (1992). p65 fragments, homologous to the C2 region of protein kinase C, bind to the intracellular receptors for protein kinase C. *Biochemistry* **31**, 8120–8124.
117. Ron, D., Chen, C. H., Caldwell, J., Jamieson, L., Orr, E., and Mochly-Rosen, D. (1994). Cloning of an intracellular receptor for protein kinase C: A homolog of the β subunit of G proteins. *Proc. Natl. Acad. Sci. U.S.A.* **91**, 839–843.
118. Filipuzzi, I., Fabbro, D., and Imber, R. (1993). Unphosphorylated α-PKC exhibits phorbol ester binding but lacks protein kinase activity in vitro. *J. Cell. Biochem.* **52**, 78–83.
119. Sasaki, Y., Asaoka, Y., and Nishizuka, Y. (1993). Potentiation of diacylglycerol-induced activation of protein kinase C by lysophospholipids: Subspecies difference. *FEBS Lett.* **320**, 47–51.
120. Hug, H., and Sarre, T. F. (1993). Protein kinase C isoenzymes: Divergence in signal transduction? *Biochem. J.* **291**, 329–343.
121. Ozawa, K., Yamada, K., Kazanietz, M. G., Blumberg, P. M., and Beaven, M. A. (1993). Different isozymes of protein kinase C mediate feedback inhibition of phospholipase C and stimulatory signals for exocytosis in rat RBL-2H3 cells. *J. Biol. Chem.* **268**, 2280–2283.
122. Hata, A., Akita, Y., Suzuki, K., and Ohno, S. (1993). Functional divergence of protein kinase C (PKC) family members: PKCγ difers from PKCα and -βII and nPKCε in its competence to mediate-12-O-tetradecanoyl phorbol 13-acetate (TPA)-response transcriptional activation through a TPA-response element. *J. Biol. Chem.* **268**, 9122–9129.
123. Mischak, H., Pierce, J. H., Goodnight, J., Kazanietz, M. G., Blumberg, P. M., and Mushinski, J. F. (1993). Phorbol ester-induced myeloid differentiation is mediated by protein kinase C-α and -δ and not by protein kinase C-βII, -ε, -ζ, and -η. *J. Biol. Chem.* **268**, 20110–20115.
124. Chin, J. E., Dickens, M., Tavare, J. M., and Roth, R. A. (1993). Overexpression of

protein kinase C isoenzymes α, βI, γ, and ϵ in cells overexpressing the insulin receptor: Effects on receptor phosphorylation and signaling. *J. Biol. Chem.* **268**, 6338–6347.

125. Johannes, F. J., Prestle, J., Eis, S., Oberhagemann, P., and Pfizenmaier, K. (1994). PKCμ is a novel, atypical member of the protein kinase C family. *J. Biol Chem.* **269**, 6140–6148.

126. Greif, H., Ben-Chaim, J., Shimon, T., Bechor, E., Eldar, H., and Livneh, E. (1992). The protein kinase C-related PKC-L(η) gene product is localized in the cell nucleus. *Mol. Cell. Biol.* **12**, 1304–1311.

127. Li, W., Mischak, H., Yu, J. C., Wang, L. M., Mushinski, J. F., Heidaran, M. A., and Pierce, J. H. (1994). Tyrosine phosphorylation of protein kinase C-δ in response to its activation. *J. Biol. Chem.* **269**, 2349–2352.

128. Tusupov, O. K., Severin, S. E., and Shvets, V. I. (1991). Proteolytic fragment of protein kinase C (kinase M) phosphorylates *in vitro* phosphatidylinositol-4-phosphate. *Biochem. Biophys. Res. Commun.* **176**, 1007–1013.

129. Buday, L., Seprödi, J., Farkas, G., Mészáros, G., Romhányi, T., Bánhegyi, G., Mandl, J., Antoni, F., and Farago, A. (1987). Proteolytic activation of protein kinase C in the extracts of cells treated for a short time with phorbol ester. *FEBS Lett.* **223**, 15–19.

130. Pontremoli, S., Melloni, E., Damiani, G., Salamino, F., Sparatore, B., Michetti, M., and Horecker, B. L. (1988). Effects of a monoclonal anti-calpain antibody on responses of stimulated human neutrophils: Evidence for a role for proteolytically modified protein kinase C. *J. Biol. Chem.* **263**, 1915–1919.

131. Aitken, A., Collinge, D. B., van Heusden, B. P. H., Isobe, T., Rosebloom, P. H., Rosenfeld, G., and Soll, J. (1992). 14-3-3 proteins: A highly conserved, widespread family of eukaryotic proteins. *Trends Biochem. Sci.* **17**, 498–501.

132. Downes, C. P., and Carter, A. N. (1991). Phosphoinositide 3-kinase: A new effector in signal transduction. *Cell. Signal.* **3**, 501–513.

133. Parker, P. J., and Waterfield, M. D. (1992). phosphatidylinositol 3-kinase: A novel effector. *Cell Growth Diff.* **3**, 747–752.

134. Stephens, L. R., Jackson, T. R., and Hawkins, P. T. (1993). Agonist-stimulated synthesis of phosphatidylinositol-(3,4,5)-triphosphate: A new intracellular signalling system? *Biochim. Biophys. Acta* **1179**, 27–75.

135. Myers, M. G., Backer, J. M., Sun, X. J., Shoelson, S., Hu, P., Schlessinger, J., Yoakim, M., Schaffhausen, B., and White, M. F. (1992). IRS-1 activates phosphatidylinositol 3′-kinase by associating with *src* homology 2 domains of p85. *Proc. Natl. Acad. Sci. U.S.A.* **89**, 10350–10354.

136. Yonezawa, K., Ueda, H., Hara, K., Nishida, K., Ando, A., Chavanieu, A., Matsuba, H., Shii, K., Yokono, K., Fukui, Y., Calas, B., Grigorescu, F., Dhand, R., Gout, I., Otsu, M., Waterfield, M. D., and Kasuga, M. (1992). Insulin-dependent formation of a complex containing an 85-kDa subunit of phosphatidylinositol 3-kinase and tyrosine-phosphorylated insulin receptor substrate 1. *J. Biol. Chem.* **267**, 25958–25966.

137. Shoelson, S. E., Sivaraja, M., Williams, K. P., Hu, P., Schlessinger, J., and Weiss, M. A. (1993). Specific phosphopeptide binding regulates a conformational change in the PI 3-kinase SH2 domain associated with enzyme activation. *EMBO J.* **12**, 795–802.

138. Zhang, J., King, W. G., Dillon, S., Hall, A., Feig, L., and Rittenhouse, S. E. (1993). Activation of platelet phosphatidylinositide 3-kinase requires the small GTP-binding protein Rho. *J. Biol. Chem.* **268**, 22251–22254.

139. Nakanishi, H., Brewer, K. A., and Exton, J. H. (1993). Activation of the ζ isozyme of protein kinase C by phosphatidylinositol 3,4,5-trisphosphate. *J. Biol. Chem.* **268**, 13–16.
140. Yamauchi, K., Holt, K., and Pessin, J. E. (1993). Phosphatidylinositol 3-kinase functions upstream of Ras and Raf in mediating insulin stimulation of c-*fos* transcription. *J. Biol. Chem.* **268**, 14597–14600.
141. Herman, P. K., Stack, J. H., and Emr, S. D. (1992). An essential role for a protein and lipid kinase complex in secretory protein sorting. *Trends Cell Biol.* **2**, 363–368.
142. Joly, M., Kazlauskas, A., Fay, F. S., and Corvera, S. (1994). Disruption of PDGF receptor trafficking by mutation of its PI-3 kinase binding sites. *Science* **263**, 684–687.
143. Kunz, J., Henriquez, R., Schneider, U., Deuter-Reinhard, M., Movva, N. R., and Hall, M. N. (1993). Target of rapamycin in yeast, TOR2, is an essential phosphatidylinositol kinase homolog required for G_1 progression. *Cell* **73**, 585–596.
144. Croall, D. E., and Demartino, G. N. (1991). Calcium-activated neutral protease (calpain) system: Structure, function, and regulation. *Physiol. Rev.* **71**, 813–847.
145. Frangioni, J. V., Oda, A., Smith, M., Salzman, E. W., and Neel, B. G. (1993). Calpain-catalyzed cleavage and subcellular relocation of protein phosphotyrosine phosphatase 1B (PTP-1B) in human platelets. *EMBO J.* **12**, 4843–4856.
146. McClelland, P., Adam, L. P., and Hathaway, D. R. (1994). Identification of a latent Ca^{2+}/calmodulin dependent protein kinase II phosphorylation site in vascular calpain II. *J. Biochem. (Tokyo)* **115**, 41–46.
147. Pike, L. J. (1992). Phosphatidylinositol 4-kinases and the role of polyphosphoinositides in cellular regulation. *Endocr. Rev.* **13**, 692–706.
148. Chauhan, A., Brockerhoff, H., Wisniewski, H. M., and Chauhan, V. P. S. (1991). Interaction of protein kinase C with phosphoinositides. *Arch. Biochem. Phys.* **287**, 283–287.
149. Mayr, G. W. (1989). Inositol 1,4-bisphosphate is an allosteric activator of muscle-type 6-phosphofructo-1-kinase. *Biochem. J.* **259**, 463–470.
150. Rana, R. S., and Hokin, L. E. (1990). Role of phosphoinositides in transmembrane signaling. *Physiol. Rev.* **70**, 115–164.
151. Memon, A. R., Chen, Q., and Boss, W. F. (1989). Inositol phospholipids activate plasma membrane ATPase in plants. *Biochem. Biophys. Res. Commun.* **162**, 1295–1301.
152. Fraser, C. L., and Sarnacki, P. (1992). Regulation of plasma membrane-bound Ca^{2+}-ATPase pump by inositol phosphates in rat brain. *Am. J. Physiol.* **262**, F411–F416.
153. Joseph, S. K., and Williamson, J. R. (1989). Inositol polyphosphates and intracellular calcium release. *Arch. Biochem. Biophys.* **273**, 1–15.
154. Stader, C., and Hofer, H. W. (1992). A major lienal phosphotyrosine phosphatase is inhibited by phospholipids and inositol trisphosphate. *Biochem. Biophys. Res. Commun.* **189**, 1404–1409.
155. Thieleczek, R., Mayr, G. W., and Brandt, N. R. (1989). Inositol polyphosphate-mediated repartitioning of aldolase in skeletal muscle triads and myofibrils. *J. Biol. Chem.* **264**, 7349–7356.
156. Higashida, H., and Brown, D. A. (1986). Two polyphosphatidylinositide metabolites control two K^+ currents in a neuronal cell. *Nature (London)* **323**, 333–335.
157. Gelfand, E. W., Cheung, R. K., Mills, G. B., and Grinstein, S. (1985). Mitogens

trigger a calcium-independent signal for proliferation in phorbol-ester-treated lymphocytes. *Nature (London)* **315**, 419–420.

158. Worley, P. F., Baraban, J. M., Colvin, J. S., and Snyder, S. H. (1987). Inositol trisphosphate receptor localization in brain: Variable stoichiometry with protein kinase C. *Nature (London)* **325**, 159–161.

159. Kanoh, H., Yamada, K., Sakane, F., and Imaizumi, T. (1989). Phosphorylation of diacylglycerol kinase *in vitro* by protein kinase C. *Biochem. J.* **258**, 455–462.

160. Issandou, M., and Rozengurt, E. (1989). Diacylglycerols, unlike phorbol esters, do not induce homologous desensitization or down-regulation of protein kinase C in Swiss 3T3 cells. *Biochem. Biophys. Res. Commun.* **163**, 201–208.

161. Wei, L. L., Krett, N. L., Francis, M. D., Gordon, D. F., Wood, W. M., O'Malley, B. W., and Horwitz, K. B. (1988). Multiple human progesterone receptor messenger ribonucleic acids and their autoregulation by progestin agonists and antagonists in breast cancer cells. *Mol. Endocrinol.* **2**, 62–72.

162. Fearn, J. C., and King, A. C. (1985). EGF receptor affinity is regulated by intracellular calcium and protein kinase C. *Cell* **40**, 991–1000.

163. Theibert, A. B., Supattapone, S., Worley, P. F., Baraban, J. M., Meek, J. L., and Snyder, S. H. (1987). Demonstration of inositol 1,3,4,5-tetrakisphosphate receptor binding. *Biochem. Biophys. Res. Commun.* **148**, 1283–1289.

164. Erneux, C., Moreau, C., Vandermeers, A., and Takazawa, K. (1993). Interaction of calmodulin with a putative calmodulin-binding domain of inositol 1,4,5-triphosphate 3-kinase: Effects of synthetic peptides and site-directed mutagenesis of Trp165. *Eur. J. Biochem.* **214**, 497–501.

165. Nozawa, Y., Nakashima, S., and Nagata, K. (1991). Phospholipid-mediated signaling in receptor activation of human platelets. *Biochim. Biophys. Acta* **1082**, 219–238.

166. Bygrave, F. L., and Benedetti, A. (1993). Calcium: Its modulation in liver by cross-talk between the actions of glucagon and calcium-mobilizing agonists. *Biochem. J.* **296**, 1–14.

167. O'Shea, J. J., Suárez-Quian, C. A., Swank, R. A., and Klausner, R. D. (1987). The inhibitory effect of cyclic AMP on phosphatidylinositol kinase is not mediated by the cAMP dependent protein kinase. *Biochem. Biophys. Res. Commun.* **146**, 561–567.

168. Rasmussen, H. (1986). The calcium messenger system. *N. Engl. J. Med.* **314**, 1094–1101 and 1164–1170.

169. Wakelam, M. J. O., Murphy, G. J., Hruby, V. J., and Houslay, M. D. (1986). Activation of two-signal transduction systems in hepatocytes by glucagon. *Nature (London)* **323**, 68–71.

170. Hajnóczky, G., Gao, E., Nomura, T., Hoek, J. B., and Thomas, A. P. (1993). Multiple mechanisms by which protein kinase A potentiates inositol 1,4,5-trisphosphate-induced Ca^{2+} mobilization in permeabilized hepatocytes. *Biochem. J.* **293**, 413–422.

171. Tomlinson, S., Mac Neil, S., and Brown, B. L. (1985). Calcium, cyclic AMP and hormone action. *Clin. Endocrinol. (Oxford)* **23**, 595–610.

172. MacNeil, S., Lakey, T., and Tomlinson, S. (1985). Calmodulin regulation of adenylate cyclase activity. *Cell Calcium* **6**, 213–226.

173. Augert, G., Blackmore, P. F., and Exton, J. H. (1989). Changes in the concentration and fatty acid composition of phosphoinositides induced by hormones in hepatocytes. *J. Biol. Chem.* **264**, 2574–2580.

174. Liscovitch, M., Ben-Av, P., Danin, M., Faiman, G., Eldar, H., and Livneh, E.

(1993). Phospholipase D-mediated hydrolysis of phosphatidylcholine: Role in cell signalling. *J. Lipid Mediators* **8,** 177–182.

175. Boarder, M. R. (1994). A role for phospholipase D in control of mitogenesis. *Trends Pharmacol. Sci.* **15,** 57–62.

176. Bowman, E. P., Uhlinger, D. J., and Lambeth, J. D. (1993). Neutrophil phospholipase D is activated by a membrane-associated Rho family small molecular weight GTP-binding protein. *J. Biol. Chem.* **268,** 21509–21512.

177. Brown, H. A., Gutowski, S., Moomaw, C. R., Slaughter, C., and Sternweis, P. C. (1993). ADP-ribosylation factor, a small GTP-dependent regulatory protein, stimulates phospholipase D activity. *Cell* **75,** 1137–1144.

178. Dominguez, I., Marshall, M. S., Gibbs, J. B., García de Herreros, A., Cornet, M. E., Graziani, G., Diaz-Meco, M. T., Johansen, T., McCormick, F., and Moscat, J. (1991). Role of GTPase activating protein in mitogenic signalling through phosphatidylcholine-hydrolysing phospholipase C. *EMBO J.* **10,** 3215–3220.

179. Matozaki, T., Sakamoto, C., Nishisaki, H., Suzuki, T., Wada, K., Matsuda, K., Nakano, O., Konda, Y., Nagao, M., and Kasuga, M. (1991). Cholecystokinin inhibits phosphatidylcholine synthesis via a Ca^{2+}-calmodulin-dependent pathway in isolated rat pancreatic acini: A possible mechanism for diacylglycerol accumulation. *J. Biol. Chem.* **266,** 22246–22253.

180. Arenzana-Seisdedos, F., Fernandez, B., Dominguez, I., Jacqué, J. M., Thomas, D., Diaz-Meco, M. T., Moscat, J., and Virelizier, J. L. (1993). Phosphatidylcholine hydrolysis activates NF-κB and increases human immunodeficiency virus replication in human monocytes and T lymphocytes. *J. Virol.* **67,** 6596–6604.

181. Cuadrado, A., Carnero, A., Dolfi, F., Jiménez, B., and Lacal, J. C. (1993). Phosphorylcholine: A novel second second messenger essential for mitogenic activity of growth factors. *Oncogene* **8,** 2959–2968.

182. Hirata, F., and Axelrod, J. (1980). Phospholipid methylation and biological signal transmission. *Science* **209,** 1082–1090.

183. Bareis, D. L., Manganiello, V. C., Hirata, F., Vaughan, M., and Axelrod, J. (1983). Bradykinin stimulates phospholipid methylation, calcium influx, prostaglandin formation, and cAMP accumulation in human fibroblasts. *Proc. Natl. Acad. Sci. U.S.A.* **80,** 2514–2518.

184. Godeau, F., Ishizaka, T., and Koide, S. S. (1985). Early stimulation of phospholipid methylation in *Xenopus* oocytes by progesterone. *Cell Differ.* **16,** 35–41.

185. Jackson, T. R., Hallam, T. J., Downes, C. P., and Hanley, M. R. (1987). Receptor coupled events in bradykinin action: Rapid production of inositol phosphates and regulation of cytosolic free Ca^{2+} in a neural cell line. *EMBO J.* **6,** 49–54.

186. Baran, D. T., and Kelly, A. M. (1988). Lysophosphatidylinositol: A potential mediator of 1,25-dihydroxyvitamin D-induced increments in hepatocyte cytosolic calcium. *Endocrinol. (Baltimore)* **122,** 930–934.

187. Mato, J. M., and Alemany, S. (1983). What is the function of phospholipid N-methylation? *Biochem. J.* **213,** 1–10.

188. Felder, C. C., Briley, E. M., Axelrod, J., Simpson, J. T., Mackie, K., and Devane, W. A. (1993). Anandamide, an endogenous cannabimimetic eicosanoid, binds to the cloned human cannabinoid receptor and stimulates receptor-mediated signal transduction. *Proc. Natl. Acad. Sci. U.S.A.* **90,** 7656–7660.

189. Sumida, C., Graber, R., and Nunez, E. (1993). Role of fatty acids in signal transduction: Modulators and messengers. *Prostaglandins Leukotrienes Essent. Fatty Acids* **48,** 117–122.

190. Colard, O., Breton, M., Pepin, D., Chevy, F., Bereziat, G., and Polonovski, J.

(1989). Arachidonate cannot be released directly from diacyl-*sn*-glycero-3-phosphocholine in thrombin-stimulated platelets. *Biochem. J.* **259**, 333–339.

191. Smith, W. L. (1989). The eicosanoids and their biochemical mechanisms of action. *Biochem. J.* **259**, 315–324.

192. Nozawa, Y., Nakashima, S., and Nagata, K. (1991). Phospholipid-mediated signaling in receptor activation of human platelets. *Biochim. Biophys. Acta* **1082**, 219–238.

193. Kudo, I., Murakami, M., Hara, S., and Inoue, K. (1993). Mammalian non-pancreatic phospholipases A_2. *Biochim. Biophys. Acta* **1170**, 217–231.

194. Flower, R. J. (1988). Lipocortin and the mechanism of action of the glucocorticoids. *Br. J. Pharmacol.* **94**, 987–1015.

195. Crompton, M. R., Moss, S. E., and Crumpton, M. J. (1988). Diversity in the lipocortin/calpactin family. *Cell* **55**, 1–3.

196. Cantiello, H. F., Patenaude, C. R., Codina, J., Birnbaumer, L., and Ausiello, D. A. (1990). $G_{\alpha i-3}$ regulates epithelial Na^+ channels by activation of phospholipase A_2 and lipoxygenase pathways. *J. Biol. Chem.* **265**, 21624–21628.

197. Brooks, R. C., McCarthy, K., Lapetina, E. G., and Morell, P. (1989). Receptor-stimulated phospholipase A_2 activation is coupled to influx of external calcium and not to mobilization of intracellular calcium in C62B glioma cells. *J. Biol. Chem.* **264**, 20147–20153.

198. Sweat, J. D., Connolly, T. M., Cragoe, E. J., and Limbird, L. E. (1986). Evidence that Na^+/H^+ exchange regulates receptor-mediated phospholipase A_2 activation in human platelets. *J. Biol. Chem.* **261**, 8667–8673.

199. Hazen, S. L., and Gross, R. W. (1991). ATP-dependent regulation of rabbit myocardial cytosolic calcium-independent phospholipase A_2. *J. Biol. Chem.* **266**, 14526–14534.

200. Sato, T., Ishimoto, T., Akiba, S., and Fujii, T. (1993). Enhancement of phospholipase A_2 activation by phosphatidic acid endogenously formed through phospholipase D action in rat peritoneal mast cell. *FEBS Lett.* **323**, 23–26.

201. Burch, R. M. (1988). Diacylglycerol stimulates phospholipase A_2 from Swiss 3T3 fibroblasts. *FEBS Lett.* **234**, 283–286.

202. Nemenoff, R. A., Winitz, S., Qian, N. X., Van Putten, V., Johnson, G. L., and Heasley, L. E. (1993). Phosphorylation and activation of a high molecular weight form of phospholipase A_2 by p42 microtubule-associated protein 2 kinase and protein kinase C. *J. Biol. Chem.* **268**, 1960–1964.

203. Piomelli, D., and Greengard, P. (1991). Bidirectional control of phospholipase A_2 activity by Ca^{2+}/calmodulin-dependent protein kinase II, cAMP-dependent protein kinase, and casein kinase II. *Proc. Natl. Acad. Sci. U.S.A.* **88**, 6770–6774.

204. Parker, J., Daniel, L. W., and Waite, M. (1987). Evidence of protein kinase C involvement in phorbol diester-stimulated arachidonic acid release and prostaglandin synthesis. *J. Biol. Chem.* **262**, 5385–5393.

205. Glaser, K. B., Mobilio, D., Chang, J. Y., and Senko, N. (1993). Phospholipase A_2 enzymes: Regulation and inhibition. *Trends Pharmacol. Sci.* **14**, 92–98.

206. Kolesnick, R. N. (1991). Sphingomyelin and derivatives as cellular signals. *Prog. Lipid Res.* **30**, 1–38.

207. Zeller, C. B., and Marchase, R. B. (1992). Gangliosides as modulators of cell function. *Am. J. Physiol.* **262**, C1341–C1355.

208. Kolesnick, R. (1992). Ceramide: A novel second messenger. *Trends Cell Biol.* **2**, 232–236.

209. Hannun, Y. A. (1994). The sphingomyelin cycle and the second messenger function of ceramide. *J. Biol. Chem.* **269,** 3125–3128.
210. Raines, M. A., Kolesnick, R. N., and Golde, D. W. (1993). Sphingomyelinase and ceramide activate mitogen-activated protein kinase in myeloid HL-60 cells. *J. Biol. Chem.* **268,** 14572–14575.
211. Schütze, S., Potthoff, K., Machleidt, T., Berkovic, D., Wiegmann, K., and Krönke, M. (1992). TNF activates NF-κB by phosphatidylcholine-specific phospholipase C-induced "acidic" sphingomyelin breakdown. *Cell* **267,** 765–776.
212. Dobrowsky, R. T., Kamibayashi, C., Mumby, M. C., and Hannun, Y. A. (1993). Ceramide activates heterotrimeric protein phosphatase 2A. *J. Biol. Chem.* **268,** 15523–15530.
213. Younes, A., Kahn, D. W., Besterman, J. M., Bittman, R., Byun, H. S., and Kolesnick, R. N. (1992). Ceramide is a competitive inhibitor of diacylglycerol kinase *in vitro* and in intact human leukemia (HL-60) cells. *J. Biol. Chem.* **267,** 842–847.
214. Merrill, A. H. (1991). Cell regulation by sphingosine and more complex sphingolipids. *J. Bioenerg. Biomembr.* **23,** 83–104.
215. Olivera, A., and Spiegel, S. (1993). Sphingosine-1-phosphate as second messenger in cell proliferation induced by PDGF and FCS mitogens. *Nature (London)* **365,** 557–560.
216. Durieux, M. E., and Lynch, K. R. (1993). Signalling properties of lysophosphatidic acid. *Trends Pharmacol. Sci.* **14,** 249–254.
217. Jalink, K., van Corven, E. J., and Moolenaar, W. H. (1990). Lysophosphatidic acid, but not phosphatidic acid, is a potent Ca^{2+}-mobilizing stimulus for fibroblasts: Evidence for an extracellular site of action. *J. Biol. Chem.* **265,** 12232–12239.
218. Kumagai, N., Morii, N., Fujisawa, K., Yoshimasa, T., Nakao, K., and Narumiya, S. (1993). Lysophosphatidic acid induces tyrosine phosphorylation and activation of MAP-kinase and focal adhesion kinase in cultured Swiss 3T3 cells. *FEBS Lett.* **329,** 273–276.
219. Desai, N. N., Carlson, R. O., Mattie, M. E., Olivera, A., Buckley, N. E., Seki, T., Brooker, G., and Spiegel, S. (1993). Signaling pathways for sphingosylphosphorylcholine-mediated mitogenesis in Swiss 3T3 fibroblasts. *J. Cell Biol.* **121,** 1385–1395.
220. van der Bend, R. L., Brunner, J., Jalink, K., van Corven, E. J., Moolenaar, W. H., and van Blitterswijk, W. J. (1992). Identification of a putative membrane receptor for the bioactive phospholipid, lysophosphatidic acid. *EMBO J.* **11,** 2495–2501.
221. Chilton, F. H., Cluzel, M., and Triggiani, M. (1991). Recent advances in our understanding of the biochemical interactions between platelet-activating factor and arachidonic acid. *Lipids* **26,** 1021–1027.
222. Hayashi, M., Imai, Y., and Oh-ishi, S. (1991). Phorbol ester stimulates PAF synthesis *via* the activation of protein kinase C in rat leukocytes. *Lipids* **26,** 1054–1059.
223. Ninio, E., and Joly, F. (1991). Transmembrane signalling and paf-acether biosynthesis. *Lipids* **26,** 1034–1037.
224. Yasuda, K., and Johnston, J. M. (1992). The hormonal regulation of platelet-activating factor-acetylhydrolase in the rat. *Endocrinol. (Baltimore)* **130,** 708–716.
225. Narahara, H., Frenkel, R. A., and Johnston, J. M. (1993). Secretion of platelet-

activating factor acetylhydrolase following phorbol ester-stimulated differentiation of HL-60 cells. *Arch. Biochem. Biophys.* **301,** 275–281.

226. Sasaki, Y., Asaoka, Y., and Nishizuka, Y. (1993). Potentiation of diacylglycerol-induced activation of protein kinase C by lysophospholipids: Subspecies difference. *FEBS Lett.* **320,** 47–51.

227. Martiny-Baron, G., and Scherer, G. F. E. (1989). Phospholipid-stimulated protein kinase in plants. *J. Biol. Chem.* **264,** 18052–18059.

228. Majercik, M. H., and Puett, D. (1990). Arachidonic acid modulates steroidogenesis in cultured Leydig tumor cells via lipoxygenase metabolite(s). *Progr. Abstr. 72nd Annu. Meet. Endocr. Soc.,* 402.

229. Mikami, K., Omura, M., and Tamura, Y. (1990). Possible site of action of 5-hydroperoxyeicosatetraenoic acid in ACTH-stimulated steroidogenesis in rat adrenal glands. *Progr. Abstr. 72nd Annu. Meet. Endocr. Soc.,* 284.

230. Junier, M. P., Dray, F., Blair, I., Capdevila, J., Dishman, E., Falck, J. R., and Ojeda, S. R. (1990). Epoxygenase products of arachidonic acid are endogenous constituents of the hypothalamus involved in D_2 receptor-mediated, dopamine-induced release of somatostatin. *Endocrinol. (Baltimore)* **126,** 1534–1540.

231. Dan-Cohen, H., Sofer, Y., Schwartzman, M. L., Natarajan, R. D., Nadler, J. L., and Naor, Z. (1992). Gonadotropin releasing hormone activates the lipoxygenase pathway in cultured pituitary cells: Role in gonadotropin secretion and evidence for a novel autocrine/paracrine loop. *Biochemistry* **31,** 5442–5448.

232. Stern, N., Yanagawa, N., Saito, F., Hori, M., Natarajan, R., Nadler, J., and Tuck, M. (1993). Potential role of 12 hydroxyeicosatetraenoic acid in angiotensin II-induced calcium signal in rat glomerulosa cells. *Endocrinol. (Baltimore)* **133,** 843–847.

233. Antonipillai, I., Horton, R., Natarajan, R., and Nadler, J. (1989). A 12-lipoxygenase product of arachidonate metabolism is involved in angiotensin action on renin release. *Endocrinol. (Baltimore)* **125,** 2028–2034.

234. Chang, W. C., Ning, C. C., Lin, M. T., and Huang, J. D. (1992). Epidermal growth factor enhances a microsomal 12-lipoxygenase activity in A431 cells. *J. Biol. Chem.* **267,** 3657–3666.

235. Gu, J. L., Natarajan, R., Ben-Ezra, J., Valente, G., Scott, S., Yoshimoto, T., Yamamoto, S., Rossi, J. J., and Nadler, J. L. (1994). Evidence that a leukocyte type of 12-lipoxygenase is expressed and regulated by angiotensin II in human adrenal glomerulosa cells. *Endocrinol. (Baltimore)* **134,** 70–77.

236. Piomelli, D., Wang, J. K. T., Sihra, T. S., Nairn, A. C., Czernik, A. J., and Greengard, P. (1989). Inhibition of Ca^{2+}/calmodulin-dependent protein kinase II by arachidonic acid and its metabolites. *Proc. Natl. Acad. Sci. U.S.A.* **86,** 8550–8554.

237. Piomelli, D., and Greengard, P. (1990). Lipoxygenase metabolites of arachidonic acid in neuronal transmembrane signalling. *Trends Pharmacol. Sci.* **11,** 367–373.

238. Vonakis, B. M., and Vanderhoek, J. Y. (1992). 15-Hydroxyeicosatetraenoic acid (15-HETE) receptors: Involvement in the 15-HETE-induced stimulation of the cryptic 5-lipoxygenase in PT-18 mast/basophil cells. *J. Biol. Chem.* **267,** 23625–23631.

239. Cantiello, H. F., Patenaude, C. R., Codina, J., Birnbaumer, L., and Ausiello, D. A. (1990). $G_{\alpha i-3}$ regulates epithelial Na^+ channels by activation of phospholipase A_2 and lipoxygenase pathways. *J. Biol. Chem.* **265,** 21624–21628.

240. O'Flaherty, J. T., and Rossi, A. G. (1993). 5-Hydroxyicosatetraenoate stimulates

neutrophils by a stereospecific, G protein-linked mechanism. *J. Biol. Chem.* **268**, 14708–14714.

241. Tang, D. G., Chen, Y. Q., Diglio, C. A., and Honn, K. V. (1993). Protein kinase C-dependent effects of 12(S)-HETE on endothelial cell vitronectin receptor and fibronectin receptor. *J. Cell Biol.* **121**, 689–704.

242. Timar, J., Tang, D., Bazaz, R., Haddad, M. M., Kimler, V. A., Taylor, J. D., and Honn, K. V. (1993). PKC mediates 12(S)-HETE-induced cytoskeletal rearrangement in B16a melanoma cells. *Cell Motil. Cytoskel.* **26**, 49–65.

243. Peppelenbosch, M. P., Tertoolen, L. G. J., Hage, W. J., and de Laat, S. W. (1993). Epidermal growth factor-induced actin remodeling is regulated by 5-lipoxygenase and cycloxygenase products. *Cell* **74**, 565–575.

CHAPTER 10

Miscellaneous
Second
Messengers

CHAPTER OUTLINE

I. Polyamines

Inevitably concomitant with growth and differentiation in almost any system is the increase in *polyamines* (1,2). These small molecules are straight-chain organic compounds with two or more amino groups. They are very positively charged and are required for DNA synthesis, transcription, and translation. Therefore, it is not surprising that they have been implicated in hormone action.

A. Polyamine Synthesis and Degradation

In eukaryotes, polyamine synthesis begins with ornithine, a product of the urea cycle (Fig. 10-1). Its decarboxylation by ornithine decarboxylase (ODC) is the committed step and leads to the first polyamine, *putrescine*. *Spermidine* and *spermine* are then synthesized by the sequential addition of aminopropyl groups to each end of the putrescine. The donor is S-adenosylmethionine (SAM); the attachment of the adenosine to the sulfur renders the thioether bonds labile. Normally the methyl group is donated in biosynthetic pathways; however, in polyamine synthesis, SAM is decarboxylated and the other side chain, the aminopropyl group, is transferred to putrescine to form spermidine. A second transfer to the other end of spermidine yields spermine. The regulation of ODC occurs primarily through altering enzyme

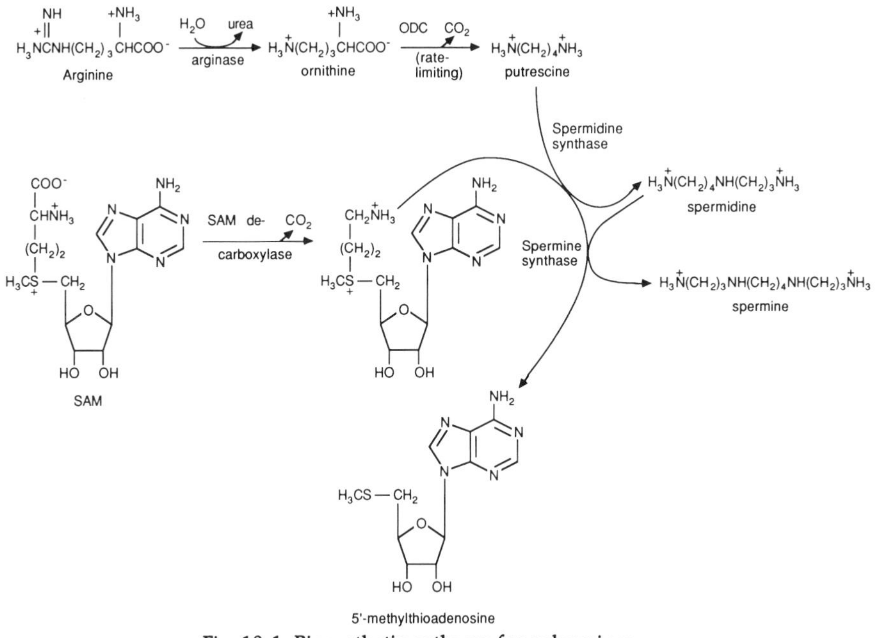

Fig. 10-1. Biosynthetic pathway for polyamines.

levels, although some investigators have suggested that it may also be regulated by G proteins (2). Putrescine, the initial product of this pathway, feeds back to inhibit the translation of ODC mRNA, decreases the half-life of the enzyme, and induces an enzyme inhibitor, the ODC-antizyme. The enzyme can be stimulated via these same mechanisms: for example, protein kinase C (PKC) increases ODC transcription (3), whereas prolactin (PRL) decreases the antizyme. ODC activity can also be increased by cAMP and IP_3, but these effects are probably not mediated by direct phosphorylation or allosterism but by changing enzyme and/or antizyme levels.

There are several useful inhibitors for this pathway. ODC can be inhibited by the substrate analogs HAVA (α-hydrazino-δ-amino-valeric acid) and DFMO (α-difluoromethylornithine). The former is a competitive inhibitor but the latter is a suicidal inhibitor, which irreversibly reacts with the enzyme. S-Adenosylmethionine decarboxylase can be inhibited by MGBG [methylglyoxal bis(guanylhydrazone)], a polyamine analog, which binds to an allosteric site on the enzyme. S-Adenosylmethionine decarboxylase has an absolute requirement for putrescine; this ensures that SAM will not be decarboxylated unless there is putrescine available to accept the aminopropyl group. A second allosteric site binds spermine and inhibits the enzyme; this represents simple negative feedback. MGBG is either a putrescine antagonist or a spermine agonist; in either case, enzyme activity is suppressed.

Polyamines are inactivated by acetylation (4). This modification has three major effects: first, it blocks the cationic site; second, it accelerates their excretion, because the polyamine uptake system in the kidneys does not recognize the acetylated form; finally, they are substrates for polyamine oxidase, whose product can either be recycled or further degraded by diamine oxidase. The N^1-acetyltransferase is regulated by many hormones, growth factors, and second messengers, including cAMP and PKC.

B. Model Systems

1. Mammary Gland

Mammary gland differentiation is one system in which polyamines may mediate hormone actions (5,6). Insulin, cortisol, and PRL are all required for mammary gland differentiation *in vitro*. Cortisol and PRL also elevate polyamine levels and stimulate the enzymes in the biosynthetic pathway: PRL stimulates arginase and ODC, whereas cortisol stimulates SAM decarboxylase and spermidine synthase. Furthermore, PRL can also elevate intracellular polyamine levels by increasing their transport. Because of their charge, polyamines do not readily cross membranes but require a transport system. The V_{max} for this system is stimulated 2.5-fold by PRL; the K_m does not change. In addition, stimulation during the first 12 hours does not depend on transcription or translation, suggesting that this effect is an early event in PRL action. This transport could be very important in altering intracellular polyamine concentrations, because polyamine levels in the blood increase 3-fold during pregnancy.

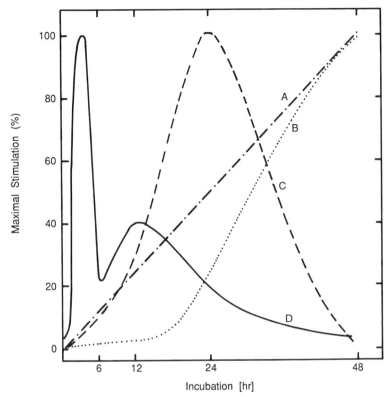

Fig. 10-2. Time course of differentiation and the activation of polyamine synthesis in mouse mammary gland explants cultured with insulin, cortisol, and prolactin. (A) Spermidine levels and the enzymatic activities of argininase, SAM decarboxylase, and spermidine synthase all rise linearly. The other lines represent (B) casein and α-lactalbumin accumulation, (C) DNA synthesis, and (D) ornithine decarboxylase activity. Hormones were present throughout the culture period.

Figure 10-2 shows the time course of DNA synthesis, differentiation (that is, casein and α-lactalbumin accumulation), spermidine, and the enzyme activities for polyamine synthesis; this time course study was performed in mouse mammary gland explants cultured with insulin, cortisol, and PRL. Clearly, increases in ODC activity and spermidine levels precede differentiation. Furthermore, although the activities of SAM decarboxylase, spermidine synthase, and the second ODC peak require transcription and translation, the first ODC peak does not, again suggesting that this initial stimulation is a primary event.

Additional support for the role of polyamines in hormone-induced mammary differentiation comes from inhibitor studies. MGBG inhibits DNA synthesis, elevations in spermidine levels, and the production of milk proteins. This is not a nonspecific inhibition, since it can be reversed by exogenous spermidine. However, the true test for any postulated second messenger is whether or not the putative mediator can replace the hormone: in the mouse mammary gland, spermidine can replace cortisol but not PRL, and it cannot replace any of the hormones in rat or rabbit mammary glands. In summary, polyamines appear to be involved in the hormonal induction of milk proteins, but they cannot be the sole mediators of hormone action in this system.

2. Kidney

Another system in which polyamines may mediate hormone effects is the kidney (7,8). In brief, administration of testosterone *in vivo* stimulates ODC activity within 30 seconds, the levels of all polyamines within 2 minutes, and both endocytosis and the uptake of amino acid and glucose analogs within 5 minutes. All these effects are blocked by DFMO and reversed by exogenous putrescine. Finally, putrescine alone can mimic all the actions of testosterone. Similar results are obtained with β-agonists. Unfortunately, the supraphysiological dose of testosterone and the use of intact animals complicate the interpretation of these data; furthermore, at least one group has not been able to duplicate the result with testosterone (9). However, if the original results are eventually validated and shown to be physiologically relevant, it would characterize a hormone system in which polyamines have satisfied all the criteria for a second messenger.

C. Output

1. Casein Kinase II

Given that polyamines are at least involved in hormone action, how do they affect cellular functions? As mentioned earlier, they are required for DNA synthesis, transcription, and translation but their mechanism of action in these processes is unknown. In part, this requirement may be due to their ability to stabilize nucleic acid structure and neutralize the negative charges; they accomplish this function by lying in the minor groove of the helix and coordinating the phosphates with their amino groups. They appear to have a binding preference for TATA sequences and it has been suggested that polyamines may keep the promoter available for binding transcription factors while suppressing spurious transcription in the absence of these factors (10).

Other major effects are mediated by a polyamine-dependent protein kinase, also called *casein kinase II* (CKII) (11,12). This ubiquitous protein kinase can use either ATP or GTP, although it has higher affinity for the former. It is a heterotetramer and has two 38-kDa α and two 27-kDa β subunits. The α subunit possesses the catalytic site, but the β subunit is still required for full enzymatic activity. The α subunit also has the binding site for heparin, which inactivates the kinase.

The β subunit is the regulatory subunit. It can be autophosphorylated at the extreme amino terminus, which is highly conserved. Autophosphorylation has no effect on tetramer formation or response to polyamines, but it does affect the rate of catalysis (13,14). This subunit also contains the binding site for polyamines. CKII is activated by spermidine in a two-step process: initially, the positively charged polyamines bind to the negatively charged heparin or other proteoglycan inhibitor and cause it to dissociate from the kinase; polyamines then directly bind to the β subunit. Spermidine increases the V_{max} of the kinase 5-fold but does not affect the K_m. Some authorities have questioned the physiological role of polyamines in the regulation of CKII; however, inhibitors of polyamine synthesis inhibit this kinase, and CKII activity is correlated with endogenous polyamine levels (15). Other polybasic molecules can also activate CKII; indeed, the phosphorylation of some substrates, such as calmodulin (CaM) and ODC, requires basic peptides instead of polyamines (16). In these instances, polyamines can actually be inhibitory, presumably by competing with the basic peptides for CKII binding.

The β subunit can be modified by several kinases. PKC can phosphorylate CKII but this only stimulates the kinase 50% (17). Cdc2, a proline-directed kinase associated with the cell cycle (see Chapter 11), phosphorylates CKII at the carboxy terminus near the site of tetramer formation (18,19), but the effects are controversial. Some researchers claim that this modification results in as much as a 5-fold stimulation in kinase activity (20), whereas others report that deleting this site has no effect on activity or tetramer formation (13,21). Epidermal growth factor (EGF), insulin-like growth factor-I (IGF-I), and insulin can also increase phosphorylation and activity of CKII. However, CKII cannot be directly modified by receptor tyrosine kinases (RTKs) since phosphorylation occurs exclusively on serines and threonines (22). Recently, some authorities have questioned the role of growth factors in regulating CKII; they claim that CKII activity remains relatively constant. However, other groups have shown that CKII activity is elevated 2- to 3-fold during cell growth (23). Furthermore, there is a shift of this kinase into the nucleus, where CKII is brought closer to many of its substrates (24).

Several substrates for this kinase have been identified, but the effects of phosphorylation are not always clear because CKII is involved in a number of "silent phosphorylations." Silent phosphorylations are those that have no direct effect on a substrate, but are required for subsequent phosphorylation by other kinases. For example, CKII modifies glycogen synthase; although this change has no immediate effect on synthase activity, the phosphorylation facilitates the subsequent modification of this synthase by glycogen synthase kinase 3. Phosphorylation by this latter kinase does inhibit the synthase. The converse is also possible; the modification of acetyl coenzyme A carboxylase by CKII facilitates the dephosphorylation of this enzyme at the protein kinase A (PKA) site.

CKII is a major nuclear kinase and many of its substrates interact with nucleic acids. CKII phosphorylation increases the activities of DNA ligase (25), topoisomerase II (26), and several transcription factors (see Chapter 12). The translation initiation factor eIF-2 is also phosphorylated. This factor is responsible for bringing the first amino acid to the ribosome. Phosphorylation results in a slight increase in affinity for Met–tRNA^{Met_i}, but the significance of this event is unknown. Finally, CKII can phosphorylate the 20 S protease complex (27); IRS-1, a major mediator of insulin action (28); and other kinases such as Cdc2 (29). The effects of these modifications are unknown.

2. Other Outputs

Polyamines also affect enzymes. Polyamines can stimulate DNA and RNA polymerases, DNA gyrases, DNA methylases, and topoisomerases I and II (1). The effects of polyamines on acetyltransferase, deacetylase, and poly(ADP-ribosyl)synthetase are discussed in Chapter 13. However, in many of these enzymes, divalent cations can substitute for the polyamines, suggesting that the effects of polyamines in these systems is nonspecific and due simply to their charges.

Another way that polyamines can affect enzyme activity is by binding to substrates. For example, the ability of polyamines to stimulate phosphoinositide (PI) kinases has been attributed to its binding to negative phospholipids and making them better substrates. In a similar manner, polyamines inhibit phospholipase C (PLC), phospholipase A_2 (PLA$_2$), and diacylglycerol (DG) kinase; in this case, polyamine binding protects the substrates (30–32).

Polyamines can also bind enzyme modulators. The central helix in CaM is partially acidic and can bind polyamines; this binding blocks the activation of calcineurin and the calcium–CaM-dependent phosphodiesterase (PDE) (33). Finally, the polyamine pathway can affect enzymes by competing for limiting precursors. For example, in plants both the polyamine and the ethylene pathways utilize SAM. Because this metabolite is limiting, the levels of polyamines and ethylene vary in a reciprocal manner (32).

In addition to enzymes, polyamines can affect hormone receptors. They enhance the binding of growth hormone (GH), follicle stimulating hormone (FSH), and insulin to their membrane receptors; promote the binding of glycine to the N-methyl-D-aspartate (NMDA) glutamate receptor (34); increase the stability of the estrogen receptor (1); promote the conversion of the progesterone and vitamin D receptor complexes to the dimers; and facilitate the binding of these dimers to DNA (35,36).

Finally, polyamines themselves may be used to modify proteins (37). A translation initiation factor, eIF-5A (formerly called eIF-4D), contains the unusual amino acid *hypusine*:

$$\overset{\displaystyle NH_2}{\underset{\displaystyle \,}{|}}\qquad\qquad \overset{\displaystyle OH}{\underset{\displaystyle \,}{|}}$$
$$HOOCCH(CH_2)_4NHCH_2CHCH_2CH_2NH_2$$

which is formed when the butylamine group from spermidine is transferred to lysine; the resulting deoxyhypusine is then hydroxylated (38). The precise function of this modification is unknown, but it is required for activity of eIF-5A (39). Another type of protein modification is the attachment of polyamines to glutamines via transglutamination; because polyamines are bifunctional, cross-linking has also been observed. For example, it has been shown that transglutamyl linkage of IL-2 dimers is essential for its cytotoxic effects on oligodendrocytes (40). However, the general significance of this alteration is still unknown.

II. Oligosaccharides

The second messenger for insulin is still unknown; although the insulin receptor contains tyrosine kinase activity, it appears as though this activity cannot account for all the actions of insulin. In an attempt to identify another mediator, insulin was incubated with liver plasma membranes, which contain insulin receptors, and the supernatant was examined for insulin-like activity (41,42). Indeed, the supernatant stimulated mitochondrial pyruvate dehydrogenase, the cAMP PDE, acetyl coenzyme A carboxylase, steroidogenesis, and the phosphatases in glycogen metabolism; it also inhibited adenylate cyclase, PKA, and pyruvate kinase. The supernatant from untreated membranes was inactive. The activity has not been definitively identified, but preliminary characterization suggests that it is a 1- to 2-kDa oligosaccharide.

The source of this carbohydrate appears to be a PI-glycan: that is, a phosphoinositide in which additional sugars are attached to the inositol. Several lines of evidence support this hypothesis. First, such a PI-glycan has been purified from membranes and its polar head group can be removed by a PLC specific for this glycolipid. This head group has all the activity of the insulin mediator. Second, its sugar composition is similar to that for the natural messenger; this composition includes a non-N-acetylated glucosamine, which is unusual in eukaryotic systems. Finally, this PI-glycan can be labeled in intact cells and, following insulin stimulation, this label appears in the putative mediator.

A. Synthesis

This PI-glycan is strikingly similar to one that anchors proteins in membranes (43,44). There are many ways in which fatty acids can be attached to proteins (see Chapter 8). The PI-glycan anchor involves the coupling of phosphoinositide to the carboxy terminus of a protein via an oligosaccharide–phosphoethanolamine (PE) bridge (Fig. 10-3). The PI-glycan is synthesized first; the sugars are added sequentially followed by the PE. The glucosamine is actually added as N-acetylglucosamine, which is then deacetylated. The inositol is initially acylated, but this fatty acid may be removed or reattached as the structure undergoes remodeling. This modification is important, since the presence of a fatty acid on inositol inhibits the activity of PLCs. The fatty acids attached to the glycerol backbone of the PI can also be exchanged during this period.

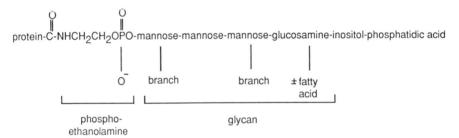

Fig. 10-3. Structure of a protein–glycolipid complex. The structure of PI-glycan would be similar except there would be no protein or phosphoethanolamine.

All proteins that will be coupled to this anchor have a hydrophobic carboxy terminus preceded by a triplet of small amino acids. In the endoplasmic reticulum, this extension is cleaved and the preformed PI-glycan is attached via a pseudopeptidation reaction. In the Golgi, the oligosaccharide branches are added. The core sugar sequence shown in Fig. 10-3 is identical for all known PI-glycan anchors, but the sequence of the branches can vary considerably. In addition, there are other documented variations: for example, there can be additional PEs or phosphoceramide can replace the phosphatidic acid (45).

B. Function

This modification can have several functions. First, it targets certain proteins to the apical surface. Second, it can increase the lateral mobility of membrane proteins. Most integral membrane proteins have diffusion rates slower than those of lipids, but proteins with PI-glycan anchors are only held in the plasmalemma by a phospholipid; therefore, their lateral diffusion rate approaches that of lipids (46). Third, it allows for the quick release of the intact protein from the cell surface via a phospholipase. Several hormones can trigger this release; for example, insulin stimulates the release of alkaline phosphatase, heparin, and lipoprotein lipase (47). However, it is not clear if this liberation is part of the biological action of insulin or simply represents protein turnover. Fourth, the PI-glycan may allow the protein to couple with other transducers; several antigenic markers in immune cells are anchored by PI-glycan and are coupled to the soluble tyrosine kinase Lck (48). This is a specific interaction, since replacement of the PI-glycan with a transmembrane helix uncouples these markers from Lck.

However, the most controversial aspect of this modification is its proposed role in signal transduction. Two potential mediators are generated by the breakdown of the PI-glycan. The first is DG, which can activate PKC. However, note that the fatty acids in the PI-glycan are usually saturated and therefore differ from those in polyphosphoinositide (PPI). Since the fatty acid composition of DG has been shown to influence its ability to activate the different isozymes of PKC, the effects of the PI-glycan-generated DG may differ from its PPI-generated counterpart.

The other product is the oligosaccharide, or glycan. As noted earlier, insulin stimulates the appearance of an oligosaccharide that is capable of acutely affecting the activities of several enzymes. These effects are presumably mediated by allosteric mechanisms. However, the glycan can also influence gene induction: it can elevate α_2-microglobulin mRNA and suppress phosphoenolpyruvate carboxykinase mRNA (49). The glycan cannot mimic the action of insulin on glucose transport, S6 kinase activity, amino acid uptake, or tyrosine aminotransferase activity. Other hormones known to release oligosaccharides include thyroid-stimulating hormone (TSH) (50), interleukin-2 (IL-2) (51), nerve growth factor (NGF) (52–54), transforming growth factor-β (TGF-β) (55), and prolactin (56).

However, there are problems with this scheme, not the least of which is the fact that PI-glycan anchors are located in the outer leaflet of plasma membranes (57,58). Extracellular oligosaccharides or PI-glycan-specific PLCs are active, suggesting that the glycan is either taken up into the cells or binds to an external receptor. In addition, if the oligosaccharide originates from a membrane-anchored protein, two bonds must be hydrolyzed: the one between inositol and glycerol and the one between the glycan and the protein. The first bond can be hydrolyzed by a PI-glycan PLC or PLD, whereas the latter would require a protease. Alternatively, the substrate may be the PI-glycan precursor in the endoplasmic reticulum. In this case, only one bond must be broken; however, the insulin receptor in the plasma membrane must somehow be coupled to the PI-glycan in the endoplasmic reticulum via some other mediator. This link could be provided by G_o or G_i, which have been shown to mediate the insulin-induced release of PI-glycan (59).

III. Cellular pH

All mitogens increase the cytoplasmic pH by 0.1–0.3 units by activating a (Na^+,H^+) antiporter (60–62). Antiporter mutants or inhibitors will block growth; this effect can be reversed if cellular alkalinization is achieved by adding bicarbonate to the medium. These experiments suggest that the elevation of cellular pH is obligatory for mitogenesis; however, alkalinization by itself will not induce growth. There are several forms of the antiporter: NHE-1 is ubiquitous and is the one most closely associated with growth factors, whereas NaH-2 is restricted to certain epithelial cells. NHE-1 is a typical transporter with 10 transmembrane helices; it also has a long carboxy terminus containing several potential phosphorylating sites that are important for growth factor regulation.

NHE-1 can be regulated in several ways. First, it can be substrate driven by mitogens that elevate calcium levels: one of the ways in which calcium concentrations are returned to basal levels is by using the (Ca^{2+},H^+)ATPase, which elevates cytosolic H^+ as calcium is extruded (63,64). The acid then activates the NHE-1. Cortisol, aldosterone, and triiodothyronine (T_3) elevate NHE-1 activity by inducing the gene for this antiporter (65). NHE-1 can also be acutely modulated by phosphorylation: PKC stimulates NHE-1 by increasing the H^+ affinity of the antiporter (66). The effects of PKA are confusing: β-adrenergic agonists, prostaglandin E_1 (PGE_1), and parathormone all increase NHE-1 activity, but somatotropin release-inhibiting factor (SRIF) and dopamine receptor (D_2) agonists inhibit the antiporter (67). All these hormones elevate cAMP levels; however, the effects are independent of cAMP concentrations and G proteins. Either cAMP is acting indirectly or these hormones are utilizing other second messengers. For example, parathormone can stimulate PLC whereas D_2 agonists inhibit this enzyme; these actions could, respectively, stimulate and inhibit PKC, which requires the DG generated by PLC. As such, these hormones may actually be acting through PKC and not PKA. Finally, NHE-1 can be activated by the G protein, α_{13} (68), calmodulin, and cGMP.

The function of cellular alkalinization is unknown. Certainly all enzymes have pH optima, but it has not been demonstrated that enzymes involved in mitogenesis have higher pH optima than those involved in other activities. Alternatively, pH may have effects on transcription or the cytoskeleton (see subsequent discussion).

IV. Cytoskeleton

Cell shape often reflects the metabolic and developmental activities of the cell; for example, the change from squamous to columnar epithelium when secretory processes are stimulated. Cell morphology, in turn, is determined by elements of the cytoskeleton: microtubules, microfilaments, and intermediate filaments. First these components are discussed individually; then their roles in hormone action are examined.

A. Components

Microtubules are hollow tubes, 20–30 nm in diameter and 4.5–7.0 nm thick (69). They are composed of two nearly identical globular proteins: α and β tubulin. These subunits are 50–60 kDa in size and alternate as they spiral along the length of the tube like a collapsed spring. Each subunit has a GTP-binding site; this nucleotide is hydrolyzed during the noncovalent polymerization process:

$$n(\text{tubulin}-\text{GTP}) \longrightarrow (\text{tubulin}-\text{GDP})_n + nP_i$$

Colchicine, vinblastine, and *vincristine* disrupt microtubules by binding to the GTP site and preventing assembly. As a consequence, these compounds are very useful in studying the role of microtubules in various cellular processes; unfortunately, they also have several side effects. For example, colchicine can (i) bind to cell membranes and inhibit fluid and nucleoside transport, (ii) suppress protein synthesis and secretion, (iii) alter intermediate filament organization, and (iv) affect cell shape at concentrations that do not disrupt microtubules.

In contrast to these drugs, *toxol* promotes microtubule formation. In particular, it (i) stabilizes microtubules against the disruptive actions of low temperatures and calcium, (ii) lowers the critical tubulin concentration required for polymerization, and (iii) decreases the lag time for assembly. Unfortunately, the microtubules formed under the influence of toxol are randomly located and disorganized.

In addition to α and β tubulin, several other proteins are involved with the formation and structure of microtubules (70). The microtubule-associated proteins 1 and 2 (MAP 1 and 2) are 270- to 300-kDa proteins that form knobs along the length of the microtubules. Their axial periodicity of 32 nm corresponds to about one MAP molecule per nine tubulin dimers. MAP 1 and 2 cross-link microtubules with themselves and other cytoskeletal elements, act as anchorage sites for PKA and CaM, and can generate force. The latter effect is analogous to the action of dynein in cilia and flagella. The τ proteins constitute another group of cytoskeletal proteins that range in size from 58 to 65 kDa. They are homologous to MAP in the carboxy terminus and serve a similar function: they cross-link microtubules.

Microfilaments are structurally identical to the thin filaments of muscle; indeed, their subunits, both called *actin*, are homologous. Actin is a 42-kDa globular protein that binds ATP; the ATP is hydrolyzed when the subunits noncovalently polymerize:

$$n(\text{actin}-\text{ATP}) \longrightarrow (\text{actin}-\text{ADP})_{n \cdot} + nP_i$$

The actin forms two rows that twist so a complete turn occurs every 13–14 monomers; the resulting filament is 6–7 nm in diameter. As in microtubules, microfilament assembly can be affected by drugs, the most useful of which is *cytochalasin B*, which disrupts microfilaments. Like all drugs, it has side effects, including (i) binding to cell membranes and inhibiting both hexose transport and, in plant cells, photopolarization; (ii) suppressing protein synthesis and secretion; (iii) inducing nuclear extrusion; (iv) inhibiting cell movement and phagocytosis; and (v) blocking cytokinesis in concentrations that do not disrupt microfilaments. Cytochalasin D does not inhibit hexose transport but does have many of the other undesirable effects. Therefore, all experiments using any of these compounds should check for these effects and, if appropriate, controls should be established for them.

Like microtubules, microfilaments have many accessory proteins. These are primarily concerned with organizing the actin filaments, controlling their polymerization, or facilitating their interaction with membrane proteins. Some of the more common ones are list in Table 10-1.

Both microtubules and microfilaments are involved in cell motility and structure. The microtubules form the mitotic spindle, cilia, and flagella, whereas microfilaments are essential for pinocytosis and phagocytosis. Both have structural functions as well: microtubules form the marginal band in

Table 10-1

Actin Accessory Proteins

Protein	Function
Bundling and cross-linking proteins	
Actin-binding protein	Organizes actin into orthogonal nets
α-Actinin	Organizes actin into loose parallel bundles
Fimbrin	Organizes actin into tight parallel bundles
Filamin	Cross-links actin
Actin disruption proteins	
Cap100	Blocks barbed end but does not sever actin
Depactin	Nibbles at actin
Fragmin	Blocks barbed end
Gelsolin/villin	Severs actin; caps barbed end; however, fragments may act as polymer nuclei
Profilin	Binds and sequesters monomer; catalyzes ADP–ATP exchange to promote polymerization and stabilization
Scinderin	Severs actin
Thymosin β4	Inhibits ADP–ATP exchange
Membrane interfacing proteins	
MARCKS	Binds actin to membrane
Talin	Binds vinculin to membrane (for example, via fibronectin receptor)
Vinculin	Binds actin to talin
Actin filament stabilizers	
Caldesmon	Prevents actin reorganization
Nebulin	Promotes actin nucleation and stabilizes the filament in skeletal muscle
Tropomyosin	Stabilizes actin

erythrocytes, whereas microfilaments form the terminal web beneath the plasma membrane and within the microvilli.

After the discovery of microtubules and microfilaments, another group of filaments was found. Because their sizes (8–10 nm in diameter) were between those of the other two, they were called *intermediate filaments* (69,71,72). The molecules have a central α helix; the helices from two molecules align themselves in a parallel fashion and twist around each other in a coiled coil motif. Two such dimers then associate in a staggered, antiparallel arrangement to form a tetramer. This aggregation continues until the intermediate filament is complete. Discussing these filaments in much detail is beyond the scope of this chapter; however, the basic properties of some of the major groups are summarized in Table 10-2. Intermediate filaments can be disrupted by the drug *acrylamide*.

B. Model Systems

The cytoskeleton is not involved in the actions of all hormones. For example, in rat adipocytes, neither colchicine, vinblastine, nor vincristine has any

Table 10-2

Basic Properties of Some of the More Common Intermediate Filaments

Property	Keratin filaments (tonofilaments)	Desmin filaments	Vimentin filaments	Neurofilaments	Lamins	Nestin
Source	Epithelium	Skeletal, cardiac, and smooth muscle	Mesenchyme and derivatives	Neurons (central and peripheral nervous systems)	Nucleated cells	Neuroepithelial stem cells
Subunits and organization	Acidic and basic keratins (40–65 kDa); dimers containing one of each	Desmin (50 kDa)	Vimentin (52 kDa)	Core (68 kDa) and two peripheral proteins (150 and 200 kDa)	Lamins (60–70 kDa)	Nestin
Location	Junctional complexes (desmosomes)	Z and M lines; intercalating discs	Perinuclear	Cellular appendages	Between heterochromatin and inner nuclear membrane	Like vimentin, but does not extend as far into cytoplasm
Possible functions	Cell adhesion	Framework for myofibrils; align Z lines; biogenesis of T–SR system	Framework for nuclear membrane; role in nuclear transport	Tensile strength for axon	Forms nuclear lamina	Early neural differentiation

effect on insulin-induced glucose oxidation (73). Cytochalasin B has no effect on insulin-induced proteins or on insulin inhibition of lipolysis, but at high concentrations it does suppress glucose oxidation. This suppression is not observed with cytochalasin D, indicating that it is secondary to the inhibition of glucose transport. Therefore, neither microtubules nor microfilaments play any role in the action of insulin in adipocytes. Similar results have been reported for melanocyte-stimulating hormone (MSH) action in melanoma cells (74).

Steroidogenesis, however, does involve the cytoskeleton (75). In rat luteal cells, cytochalasin B inhibits the progesterone synthesis induced by either human chorionic gonadotropin (hCG) or cAMP. The drug does not suppress protein synthesis, lower hCG receptor number or affinity, or affect cAMP production. Furthermore, the inhibition of steroid synthesis could not be reversed by adding glucose to the medium or using cytochalasin D, indicating that glucose transport is not a problem. Finally, colchicine has no effect at all.

Similar effects are observed in adrenal tumor cells (76). Again, cytochalasin B suppresses the stimulation of side-chain cleavage by adrenocorticotropic hormone (ACTH) and cAMP. However, it does not inhibit protein synthesis, cholesterol transport into the cell, or ATP levels. Furthermore, it has no effect on cleavage either in isolated mitochondria or by the purified enzyme. These data suggest that microfilaments may be involved in the hormonal stimulation of cholesterol transport from the plasma membrane to the mitochondria, where cleavage takes place. This effect appears to be related to cell shape. If adrenal tumor cells are cultured on plastic treated with poly(2-hydroxyethyl methacrylate), they will round up and respond to ACTH with respect to steroidogenesis. However, if the cells are cultured on plastic coated with polylysine, they assume a flatter appearance and fail to respond to ACTH (77).

There also appears to be a role for intermediate filaments in steroidogenesis: some cholesterol in the adrenal gland is stored as droplets attached to vimentin (78). Acrylamide stimulates steroid synthesis by disrupting the intermediate filaments and liberating the cholesterol for transport to the mitochondria (79). Therefore, both microfilaments and intermediate filaments have been implicated in steroidogenesis: the latter is involved in cholesterol storage and the former transports this sterol to the mitochondria.

The mammary gland represents another example of a system in which the cytoskeleton and substratum influence hormone action (80,81). In the rabbit, PRL converts the squamous cuboidal epithelium to a cuboidal columnar epithelium; it also increases the number and length of microvilli and develops the Golgi and rough endoplasmic reticulum. Finally, PRL induces milk protein synthesis. Are the changes in the cytoarchitecture and gene induction linked or are they independent events? This question can be answered by isolating the epithelial cells and culturing them in petri dishes coated with a collagen gel. The cells will form a flat monolayer; because the substratum is fixed and the cells form junctional complexes, the cells are forced to maintain a squamous configuration. In the presence of PRL, the cellular morphology does not change and there is no stimulation of milk proteins or their mRNAs. However, if the collagen gel is loosened from the petri dish, it will float and shrink, allowing the cells to change shape. Now PRL induces both the previously described morphological changes and milk protein synthesis. Similar results have been reported for the mouse mammary epithelium, although the effect is less complete (81). In attached cells, some casein mRNA does accumulate in the presence of hormones, but it is only 40% of that accumulated in floating gels. Furthermore, casein phosphorylation and secretion are impaired on attached gels. These data suggest that epithelial cell–substratum interactions may be more important than cell shape: if basement membrane components are provided, the cell does not have to be in a secretory conformation. However, if the cell must make its own basement membrane, cell shape plays a greater role (82). How the substratum influences gene expression is discussed later.

C. Regulation

The interactions between the cytoskeleton and its modulators are depicted in Fig. 10-4. The cytoskeleton can be affected by hormones, substratum, and mechanical forces; the altered cytoskeleton then generates a biological effect. There are several possible mechanisms behind these interactions.

Hormones can alter the cytoskeleton by direct interactions, by covalent modification, or by allosterism via second messengers. Both the EGF receptor (83) and human EGF-like receptor 2 (HER2) (84) are associated with the cytoskeleton. This association is mediated by the intracellular domain, although neither the carboxy-terminal autophosphorylation sites nor kinase activity is required. Association does require the high-affinity receptor dimer. Such an association may directly affect cytoskeletal organization or membrane attachment. The PDGF receptor also binds to the cytoskeleton but its effects are mediated by tyrosine phosphorylation (85). In skeletal muscle, the PDGFR is localized to the myotendinous junction where it phosphorylates talin; the subsequent dissociation of talin from vinculin allows the cytoskeleton to reorganize.

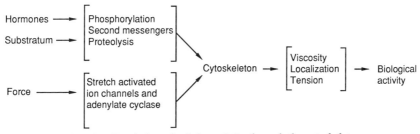

Fig. 10-4. Regulation of cellular activity through the cytoskeleton.

Serine–threonine phosphorylation is the major form of covalent modification. In general, phosphorylation disrupts the cytoskeleton: it decreases polymerization and impairs the binding of the cytoskeleton to other components and to the plasmalemma (86–88). This result is independent of the type of kinase. Recently, the soluble tyrosine kinase FAK (focal adhesion kinase) has been found to phosphorylate paxillin and tensin, although the effects of this modification are unknown (89). FAK is phosphorylated and activated by integrins, which are cellular receptors for elements of the substratum. Therefore, the integrin–FAK pathway is a means for the extracellular matrix to affect the cytoskeleton. Several hormones can also activate FAK.

Deimination is another type of covalent modification that refers to the conversion of arginine within a protein to citrulline. This modification leads to the disassembly of vimentin, desmin, and glial fibrillary acidic protein (GFAP) in the presence of micromolar calcium (90). Mono(ADP-ribosyl)ation of desmin also leads to depolymerization (91). Finally, the cytoskeleton can be degraded by calpain; talin, filamin, and fodrin are particularly susceptible to this calcium-regulated protease (92). Fodrin is the nonerythrocyte isoform of spectrin, a long rod-like protein that forms a cytoskeletal network with actin just underneath the plasma membrane. Many of these effects are interrelated; for example, the dephosphorylation of neurofilaments renders them more susceptible to proteolysis by calpain (93).

Several second messengers can bind components of the cytoskeleton. Calcium can act through PKC, calmodulin-dependent protein kinase II (CaMKII), calpain (see preceding discussion), or CaM (see subsequent discussion). However, it can also act alone. In the presence of calcium, gelsolin fragments actin and caps the barbed ends but, as calcium falls, gelsolin loses the ability to sever actin and the fragments can then act as nucleation sites (94). In combination with CaM, it also regulates caldesmin. Caldesmin suppresses the actin-activated ATPase of smooth muscle myosin; this prevents muscle relaxation and maintains muscle tension. Calcium–CaM binds at the carboxy terminus of caldesmin and removes this inhibition (95). Phosphorylation by PKC at the carboxy terminus or by CaMKII or CKII at the amino terminus also eliminates the inhibition (96–98). MARCKS (*m*yristoylated *a*lanine-*r*ich *C* *k*inase *s*ubstrate) is another target of CaM. MARCKS cross-links actin and binds it to the plasma membrane. CaM binding to MARCKS impairs actin cross-linking but not membrane binding; as such, CaM increases the plasticity of the network without disrupting its membrane attachment. On the other hand, PKC phosphorylation of MARCKS impairs both actin cross-linking and membrane binding, resulting in the solubilization of the actin (99).

Phospholipids are other mediators that affect the cytoskeleton. Phosphoinositol 4.5-biphosphate (PIP_2) binds to gelsolin, profilin, scinderin, and Cap100 and prevents these elements from disrupting actin (100). When hormones activate PLC, PIP_2 is hydrolyzed and gelsolin is free to sever actin and cap the barbed ends while profilin sequesters the monomers: as a result, actin depolymerizes. When the signal is terminated, PIP_2 is regenerated and binds gelsolin and profilin; actin rapidly repolymerizes from primed fragments. In this way, hormones can affect actin remodeling.

One final allosteric modulator is pH. As noted already, scinderin is an actin-severing protein that is inhibited by binding to PIP_2. Calcium and alkalinization shift scinderin from PIP_2 to actin near the plasma membrane; PIP_2 and actin compete for the same site on scinderin. Scinderin then severs actin in the vicinity of the plasmalemma. This local disruption is thought to play a role in exocytosis.

The substratum acts in a manner similar to that of hormones: various components in the extracellular matrix bind to plasma membrane receptors to generate second messengers that can then affect the cytoskeleton. The best characterized cellular receptor for the substratum is integrin (101,102), which is associated with tyrosine kinases, calpain activation, and changes in the cellular pH and cAMP levels (103,104). It can also stimulate the synthesis of PIP_2, thereby potentiating the effect of hormones that hydrolyze this substrate (105). The mechanism by which mechanical force alters the cytoskeleton is even less well characterized; however, stretch-activated ion channels (106) and adenylate cyclase (107,108) have been reported. Therefore, it appears that force also affects the cytoskeleton via the generation of second messengers.

How are these changes in the cytoskeleton converted into biological activity? First, the depolymerization or proteolysis of components of the cytoskeleton can decrease cytosol viscosity and facilitate exo- and endocytosis. Second, the cytoskeleton is involved in compartmentalization; for example, its role in the transport of cholesterol from its stores into the mitochondria has already been mentioned. The cytoskeleton can also influence the cellular localization of proteins that bind to it: its binding to RII of PKA may affect substrate availability and its binding to glucocorticoid receptors may regulate its nuclear transport. mRNAs are other cellular components that the cytoskeleton can partition. The cytoskeleton binds ribosomes and *ribonucleoprotein* (RNP) particles; RNPs sequester certain mRNAs and render them translationally inactive. The degree of translation is determined by a balance between the mRNA in the two pools. This redistribution may also affect the half-life of mRNA. For example, laminin, another component of the extracellular matrix with a cellular receptor, increases the casein mRNA half-life in mammary cells from 10 to 41 hour whereas the half-life of total mRNA is only slightly altered (109). This stabilization is blocked by either cytochalasin D or colchicine. Finally, it has been proposed that the tension generated by changes in cell shape can be transmitted along the components of the cytoskeleton all the way to the nuclear matrix, where these forces can affect gene induction (110). This transduction from physical to chemical information is postulated to occur through changes in thermodynamic variables. For example, tension could alter free energy to promote the unraveling of chromatin; this change in chromatin structure might then facilitate transcription (see Chapter 13).

V. Summary

In addition to the cyclic nucleotides and phospholipids, several other systems can mediate or affect signal transduction across the plasmalemma. These include polyamines, oligosaccharides, pH, and the cytoskeleton. Polyamines are essential for DNA replication, transcription, and translation; they also affect the activity of many enzymes, including the multifunctional protein kinase CKII. Both the synthesis of polyamines and the activity of this kinase are under hormonal control. The oligosaccharides are released from a PI-glycan by a specific PLC, which liberates the polysaccharide moiety; the sugar residues, in turn, affect enzyme activity and gene expression, whereas the DG may activate certain isozymes of PKC. Alkalinization is an inevitable consequence of mitogenesis, but is not sufficient by itself to induce cell division. Mitogens raise the pH by activating the (Na^+, H^+)antiporter via PKC phosphorylation.

The cytoskeleton is also involved in hormone action: for example, microfilaments are required to transport cholesterol into the mitochondria for the hCG- or ACTH-induced side-chain cleavage. In addition to cytoplasmic transport, the cytoskeleton is important in mediating hormone-induced changes in cell morphology required for specific functions. Hormones can affect the cytoskeleton by covalent modifications such as phosphorylation or proteolysis, or by allosteric effects by second messengers. The altered cytoskeleton, in turn, can affect biological activity by decreasing the cytoplasmic viscosity, by transporting materials within the cell, or by affecting translation via the ribosomes and RNP particles that are attached to it.

References

General References

Blackshear, P. J. (1993). The MARCKS family of cellular protein kinase C substrates. *J. Biol. Chem.* **268**, 1501–1504.

Considine, R. V., and Caro, J. F. (1993). Protein kinase C: Mediator or inhibitor of insulin action? *J. Cell. Biochem.* **52**, 8–13.

Dym, M. (1994). Basement membrane regulation of Sertoli cells. *Endocr. Rev.* **15**, 102–115.

Juliano, R. L., and Haskill, S. (1993). Signal transduction from the extracellular matrix. *J. Cell Biol.* **120**, 577–585.

McConville, M. J., and Ferguson, M. A. J. (1993). The structure, biosynthesis and function of glycosylated phosphatidylinositols in the parasitic protozoa and higher eukaryotes. *Biochem. J.* **294**, 305–324.

Schafer, W. R., and Rine, J. (1992). Protein prenylation: Genes, enzymes, targets, and functions. *Annu. Rev. Genet.* **26**, 209–237.

See also Refs. 1, 2, 4, 6, 11, 12, 32, 34, 37, 41–44, 47, 48, 59, 60, 66, 70–72, 86–88, 92, 94, 99–102, 104, 106, and 108.

Cited References

1. Scalabrino, G., Lorenzini, E. C., and Ferioli, M. E. (1991). Polyamines and mammalian hormones. Part I: Biosynthesis, interconversion and hormone effects. *Mol. Cell. Endocrinol.* **77**, 1–35.
2. Scalabrino, G., and Lorenzini, E. C. (1991). Polyamines and mammalian hormones. Part II: Paracrine signals and intracellular regulators. *Mol. Cell. Endocrinol.* **77**, 37–56.
3. Butler, A. P., Mar, P. K., McDonald, F. F., and Ramsay, R. L. (1991). Involvement of protein kinase C in the regulation of ornithine decarboxylase mRNA by phorbol esters in rat hepatoma cells. *Exp. Cell Res.* **194**, 56–61.
4. Casero, R. A., and Pegg, A. E. (1993). Spermidine/spermine N^1-acetyltransferase—The turning point in polyamine metabolism. *FASEB J.* **7**, 653–661.
5. Oka, T., Sakai, T., Lundgren, D. W., and Perry, J. W. (1978). Polyamines in growth and development of mammary gland. *In* "Hormones, Receptors, and Breast Cancer" (W. L. McGuire, ed.), pp. 301–323. Raven Press, New York.
6. Oka, T., Perry, J. W., Takemoto, T., Sakai, T., Terada, N., and Inoue, H. (1981). The multiple regulatory roles of polyamines in the hormonal induction of mammary gland development. *Adv. Polyamine Res.* **3**, 309–320.
7. Koenig, H., Goldstone, A., and Lu, C. Y. (1983). Polyamines regulate calcium fluxes in a rapid plasma membrane response. *Nature (London)* **305**, 530–534.
8. Koenig, H., Goldstone, A. D., and Lu, C. Y. (1983). β-Adrenergic stimulation of Ca^{2+} fluxes, endocytosis, hexose transport, and amino acid transport in mouse kidney cortex is mediated by polyamine synthesis. *Proc. Natl. Acad. Sci. U.S.A.* **80**, 7210–7214.
9. Berger, F. G., and Porter, C. W. (1986). Putrescine does not mediate the androgen-response in mouse kidney. *Biochem. Biophys. Res. Commun.* **138**, 771–777.
10. Matthews, H. R. (1993). Polyamines, chromatin structure and transcription. *Bioessays* **15**, 561–566.
11. Issinger, O. G. (1993). Casein kinases: Pleiotropic mediators of cellular regulation. *Pharmacol. Ther.* **59**, 1–30.
12. Litchfield, D. W., and Lüscher, B. (1993). Casein kinase II in signal transduction and cell cycle regulation. *Mol. Cell. Biochem.* **127/128**, 187–199.
13. Boldyreff, B., Meggio, F., Pinna, L. A., and Issinger, O. G. (1992). Casein kinase-2 structure-function relationship: Creation of a set of mutants of the β subunit that variably surrogate the wild type β subunit function. *Biochem. Biophys. Res. Commun.* **188**, 228–234.
14. Lin, W. J., Sheu, G. T., and Traugh, J. A. (1993). Autophosphorylation affects activity of casein kinase II: Evidence from mutations in the β subunit. *FASEB J.* **7**, A1160.
15. Filhol, O., Loue-Mackenbach, P., Cochet, C., and Chambaz, E. M. (1991). Casein kinase II and polyamines may interact in the response of adrenocortical cells to their trophic hormone. *Biochem. Biophys. Res. Commun.* **180**, 623–630.
16. Sarno, S., Marin, O., Meggio, F., and Pinna, L. A. (1993). Polyamines as negative regulators of casein kinase-2: The phosphorylation of calmodulin triggered by polylysine and by the α[66-86] peptide is prevented by spermine. *Biochem. Biophys. Res. Commun.* **194**, 83–90.
17. Sanghera, J. S., Charlton, L. A., Paddon, H. B., and Pelech, S. L. (1992).

Purification and characterization of echinoderm casein kinase II: Regulation by protein kinase C. *Biochem. J.* **283**, 829–837.

18. Litchfield, D. W., Lozeman, F. J., Cicirelli, M. F., Harrylock, M., Ericsson, L. H., Piening, C. J., and Krebs, E. G. (1991). Phosphorylation of the β subunit of casein kinase II in human A431 cells: Identification of the autophosphorylation site and a site phosphorylated by p34*cdc2*. *J. Biol. Chem.* **266**, 20380–20389.

19. Marin, O., Meggio, F., Draetta, G., and Pinna, L. A. (1992). The consensus sequences for cdc2 kinase and for casein kinase-2 are mutually incompatible: A study with peptides from the β-subunit of casein kinase-2. *FEBS Lett.* **301**, 111–114.

20. Mulner-Lorillon, O., Cormier, P., Labbé, J. C., Dorée, M., Poulhe, R., Osborne, H., and Bellé, R. (1990). M-Phase-specific cdc2 protein kinase phosphorylates the β subunit of casein kinase II and increases casein kinase II activity. *Eur. J. Biochem.* **193**, 529–534.

21. Meggio, F., Boldyreff, B., Issinger, O. G., and Pinna, L. A. (1993). The autophosphorylation and p34*cdc2* phosphorylation sites of casein kinase-2 β-subunit are not essential for reconstituting the fully-active heterotetrameric holoenzyme. *Biochim. Biophys. Acta* **1164**, 223–225.

22. Ackerman, P., Glover, C. V. C., and Osheroff, N. (1990). Stimulation of casein kinase II by epidermal growth factor: Relationship between the physiological activity of the kinase and the phosphorylation state of its β subunit. *Proc. Natl. Acad. Sci. U.S.A.* **87**, 821–825.

23. Lorenz, P., Pepperkok, R., Ansorge, W., and Pyerin, W. (1993). Cell biological studies with monoclonal and polyclonal antibodies against human casein kinase II subunit β demonstrate participation of the kinase in mitogenic signaling. *J. Biol. Chem.* **268**, 2733–2739.

24. Ahmed, K., Yenice, S., Davis, A., and Goueli, S. A. (1993). Association of casein kinase 2 with nuclear chromatin in relation to androgenic regulation of rat prostate. *Proc. Natl. Acad. Sci. U.S.A.* **90**, 4426–4430.

25. Prigent, C., Lasko, D. D., Kodama, K., Woodgett, J. R., and Lindahl, T. (1992). Activation of mammalian DNA ligase I through phosphorylation by casein kinase II. *EMBO J.* **11**, 2925–2933.

26. Corbett, A. H., De Vore, R. F., and Osheroff, N. (1992). Effect of casein kinase II-mediated phosphorylation on the catalytic cycle of topoisomerase II: Regulation of enzyme activity by enhancement of ATP hydrolysis. *J. Biol. Chem.* **267**, 20513–20518.

27. Ludemann, R., Lerea, K. M., and Etlinger, J. D. (1993). Copurification of casein kinase II with 20 S proteasomes and phosphorylation of a 30-kDa proteasome subunit. *J. Biol. Chem.* **268**, 17413–17417.

28. Tanasijevic, M. J., Myers, M. G., Thoma, R. S., Crimmins, D. L., White, M. F., and Sacks, D. B. (1993). Phosphorylation of the insulin receptor substrate IRS-1 by casein kinase II. *J. Biol. Chem.* **268**, 18157–18166.

29. Russo, G. L., Vandenberg, M. T., Yu, I. J., Bae, Y. S., Franza, B. R., and Marshak, D. R. (1992). Casein kinase II phosphorylates p34*cdc2* kinase in G_1 phase of the HeLa cell division cycle. *J. Biol. Chem.* **267**, 20317–20325.

30. Smith, C. D., and Snyderman, R. (1988). Modulation of inositol phospholipid metabolism by polyamines. *Biochem. J.* **256**, 125–130.

31. Wojcikiewicz, R. J. H., and Fain, J. N. (1988). Polyamines inhibit phospholipase C-catalysed polyphosphoinositide hydrolysis: Studies with permeabilized GH₃ cells. *Biochem. J.* **255**, 1015–1021.

32. Schuber, F. (1989). Influence of polyamines on membrane functions. *Biochem. J.* **260**, 1–10.
33. Walters, J. D., and Johnson, J. D. (1988). Inhibition of cyclic nucleotide phosphodiesterase and calcineurin by spermine, a calcium-independent calmodulin antagonist. *Biochim. Biophys. Acta* **957**, 138–142.
34. Scott, R. H., Sutton, K. G., and Dolphin, A. C. (1993). Interactions of polyamines with neuronal ion channels. *Trends Neurosci.* **16**, 153–160.
35. Thomas, T., and Kiang, D. T. (1988). Modulation of the binding of progesterone receptor to DNA by polyamines. *Cancer Res.* **48**, 1217–1222.
36. Morishima, Y., Inaba, M., Nishizawa, Y., Morii, H., Hasuma, T., Matsui-Yuasa, I., and Otani, S. (1994). The involvement of polyamines in the activation of vitamin D receptor from porcine intestinal mucosa. *Eur. J Biochem.* **219**, 349–356.
37. Pegg, A. E. (1986). Recent advances in the biochemistry of polyamines in eukaryotes. *Biochem. J.* **234**, 249–262.
38. Murphey, R. J., and Gerner, E. W. (1987). Hypusine formation in protein by a two-step process in cell lysates. *J. Biol. Chem.* **262**, 15033–15036.
39. Park, M. H. (1989). The essential role of hypusine in eukaryotic translation initiation factor 4D (eIF-4D): Purification of eIF-4D and its precursors and comparison of their activities. *J. Biol. Chem.* **264**, 18531–18535.
40. Eitan, S., and Schwartz, M. (1993). A tranglutaminase that converts interleukin-2 into a factor cytotoxic to oligodendrocytes. *Science* **261**, 106–108.
41. Saltiel, A. R. (1991). The role of glycosyl-phosphoinositides in hormone action. *J. Bioenerg. Biomembr.* **23**, 29–41.
42. Romero, G. (1991). Inositolglycans and cellular signalling. *Cell Biol. Int. Rep.* **15**, 827–852.
43. Menon, A. K. (1991). Biosynthesis of glycosyl-phosphatidylinositol. *Cell Biol. Int. Rep.* **15**, 1007–1021.
44. McConville, M. J., and Ferguson, M. A. J. (1993). The structure, biosynthesis and function of glycosylated phosphatidylinositols in the parasitic protozoa and higher eukaryotes. *Biochem. J.* **294**, 305–324.
45. Conzelmann, A., Puoti, A., Lester, R. L., and Desponds, C. (1992). Two different types of lipid moieties are present in glycophosphoinositol-anchored membrane proteins of *Saccharomyces cerevisiae*. *EMBO J.* **11**, 457–466.
46. Cross, G. A. M. (1990). Glycolipid anchoring of plasma membrane proteins. *Annu. Rev. Biol.* **6**, 1–39.
47. Saltiel, A. R., Osterman, D. G., Darnell, J. C., Chan, B. L., and Sorbara-Cazan, L. R. (1989). The role of glycosylphosphoinositides in signal transduction. *Recent Prog. Horm. Res.* **45**, 353–379.
48. Stefanová, I., Horejsí, V., Ansotegui, I. J., Knapp, W., and Stockinger, H. (1991). GPI-anchored cell-surface molecules complexed to protein tyrosine kinases. *Science* **254**, 1016–1019.
49. Alvarez, L., Avila, M. A., Mato, J. M., Castaño, J. G., and Varela-Nieto, I. (1991). Insulin-like effects of inositol phosphate-glycan on messenger RNA expression in rat hepatocytes. *Mol. Endocrinol.* **5**, 1062–1068.
50. Martiny, L., Antonicelli, F., Thuilliez, B., Lambert, B., Jacquemin, C., and Haye, B. (1990). Control by thyrotropin of the production by thyroid cells of an inositol phosphate-glycan. *Cell. Signal.* **2**, 21–27.
51. Eardley, D. D., and Koshland, M. E. (1991). Glycosylphosphatidylinositol: A candidate system for interleukin-2 signal transduction. *Science* **251**, 78–81.

52. Chan, B. L., Chao, M. V., and Saltiel, A. R. (1989). Nerve growth factor stimulates the hydrolysis of glycosylphosphatidylinositol in PC-12 cells: A mechanism of protein kinase C regulation. *Proc. Natl. Acad. Sci. U.S.A.* **86,** 1756–1760.
53. Represa, J., Avila, M. A., Miner, C., Giraldez, F., Romero, G., Clemente, R., Mato, J. M., and Varela-Nieto, I. (1991). Glycosyl-phosphatidyl-inositol/inositol phosphoglycan: A signaling system for the low-affinity nerve growth factor receptor. *Proc. Natl. Acad. Sci. U.S.A.* **88,** 8016–8019.
54. Varela-Nieto, I., Represa, J., Avila, M. A., Miner, C., Mato, J. M., and Giraldez, F. (1991). Inositol phospho-oligosaccharide stimulates cell proliferation in the early developing inner ear. *Dev. Biol.* **143,** 432–435.
55. Vivien, D., Petitfrère, E., Martiny, L., Sartelet, H., Galéra, P., Haye, B., and Pujol, J. P. (1993). IPG (inositolphosphate glycan) as a cellular signal for TGF-β1 modulation of chondrocyte cell cycle. *J. Cell. Physiol.* **155,** 437–444.
56. Fanjul, L. F., Marrero, I., González, J., Quintana, J., Santana, P., Estévez, F., Mato, J. M., and Ruiz de Galarreta, C. M. (1993). Does oligosaccharide-phosphatidylinositol (glycosyl-phosphatidylinositol) hydrolysis mediate prolactin signal transduction in granulosa cells? *Eur. J. Biochem.* **216,** 747–755.
57. Saltiel, A. R., and Cuatrecasas, P. (1988). In search of a second messenger for insulin. *Am. J. Physiol.* **255,** C1–C11.
58. Varela, I., Alvarez, J. F., Clemente, R., Ruiz-Albusac, J. M., and Mato, J. M. (1990). Asymmetric distribution of the phosphatidylinositol-linked phospho-oligosaccharide that mimics insulin action in the plasma membrane. *Eur. J. Biochem.* **188,** 213–218.
59. Kilgour, E. (1993). A role for inositol-glycan mediators and G-proteins in insulin action. *Cell. Signal.* **5,** 97–105.
60. Barber, D. L. (1991). Mechanisms of receptor-mediated regulation of Na-H exchange. *Cell. Signal.* **3,** 387–397.
61. Fliegel, L., and Fröhlich, O. (1993). The Na^+/H^+ exchanger: An update on structure, regulation and cardiac physiology. *Biochem. J.* **296,** 273–285.
62. Tse, M., Levine, S., Yun, C., Brant, S., Counillon, L. T., Pouyssegur, J., and Donowitz, M. (1993). Structure/function studies of the epithelial isoforms of the mammalian Na^+/H^+ exchanger gene family. *J. Membr. Biol.* **135,** 93–108.
63. Conlin, P. R., Cirillo, M., Zerbini, G., Williams, G. H., and Canessa, M. L. (1993). Calcium-mediated intracellular acidification and activation of Na^+-H^+ exchange in adrenal glomerulosa cells stimulated with potassium. *Endocrinol. (Baltimore)* **132,** 1345–1352.
64. Wöll, E., Ritter, M., Scholz, W., Häussinger, D., and Lang, F. (1993). The role of calcium in cell shrinkage and intracellular alkalinization by bradykinin in Ha-*ras* oncogene expressing cells. *FEBS Lett.* **322,** 261–265.
65. Sacktor, B., and Kinsella, J. L. (1986). Hormonal regulation of renal Na^+-H^+ exchange activity. *Curr. Top. Membr. Transp.* **26,** 223–244.
66. Moolenaar, W. H., Defize, L. H. K., van der Saag, P. T., and de Laat, S. W. (1986). The generation of ionic signals by growth factors. *Curr. Top. Membr. Transp.* **26,** 137–156.
67. Ganz, M. B., Pachter, J. A., and Barber, D. L. (1990). Multiple receptors coupled to adenylate cyclase regulate Na-H exchange independent of cAMP. *J. Biol. Chem.* **265,** 8989–8992.
68. Voyno-Yasenetskaya, T., Conklin, B. R., Gilbert, R. L., Hooley, R., Bourne, H. R., and Barber, D. L. (1994). Gα13 stimulates Na-H exchange. *J. Biol. Chem.* **269,** 4721–4724.

69. Alberts, B., Bray, D., Lewis, J., Raff, M., Roberts, K., and Watson, J. D. (1994). "Molecular Biology of the Cell," 3rd Ed. Garland, New York.

70. MacRae, T. H. (1992). Microtubule organization by cross-linking and bundling proteins. *Biochim. Biophys. Acta* **1160**, 145–155.

71. Bloemendal, H., and Pieper, F. R. (1989). Intermediate filaments: Known structure, unknown function. *Biochim. Biophys. Acta* **1007**, 245–253.

72. van de Klundert, F. A. J. M., Raats, J. M. H., and Bloemendal, H. (1993). Intermediate filaments: Regulation of gene expression and assembly. *Eur. J. Biochem.* **214**, 351–366.

73. Jarett, L., and Smith, R. M. (1979). Effect of cytochalasin B and D on groups of insulin receptors and on insulin action in rat adipocytes. Possible evidence for a structural relationship of the insulin receptor to the glucose transport system. *J. Clin. Invest.* **63**, 571–579.

74. DiPasquale, A., and McGuire, J. (1976). MSH stimulates adenylate cyclase and tyrosinase in cultivated melanoma cells in the presence of cytochalasin B. *Exp. Cell Res.* **102**, 264–268.

75. Azhar, S., and Menon, K. M. J. (1981). Receptor-mediated gonadotropin action in the ovary. Action of cytoskeletal element-disrupting agents on gonadotropin-induced steroidogenesis in rat luteal cells. *Biochem. J.* **194**, 19–27.

76. Mrotek, J. J., and Hall, P. F. (1977). Response of adrenal tumor cells to adrenocorticotropin: Site of inhibition by cytochalasin B. *Biochemistry* **16**, 3177–3181.

77. Betz, G., and Hall, P. F. (1987). Steroidogenesis in adrenal tumor cells: Influence of cell shape. *Endocrinol. (Baltimore)* **120**, 2547–2554.

78. Almahbobi, G., and Hall, P. F. (1990). The role of intermediate filaments in adrenal steroidogenesis. *J. Cell Sci.* **97**, 679–687.

79. Shiver, T. M., Sackett, D. L., Knipling, L., and Wolff, J. (1992). Intermediate filaments and steroidogenesis in adrenal Y-1 cells: Acrylamide stimulation of steroid production. *Endocrinol. (Baltimore)* **131**, 201–207.

80. Suard, Y. M. L., Haeuptile, S. T., and Kraehenbuhl, J. P. (1983). Cell proliferation and milk protein gene expression in rabbit mammary cell cultures. *J. Cell Biol.* **96**, 1435–1442.

81. Lee, E. Y. P., Lee, W., Kaetzel, C. S., Parry, G., and Bissell, M. J. (1985). Interaction of mouse mammary epithelial cells with collagen substrata: Regulation of casein gene expression and secretion. *Proc. Natl. Acad. Sci. U.S.A.* **82**, 1419–1423.

82. Howlett, A. P., and Bissell, M. J. (1990). Regulation of mammary epithelial cell function: A role for stromal and basement membrane matrices. *Protoplasma* **159**, 85–95.

83. van Belzen, N., Spaargaren, M., Verkleij, A. J., and Boonstra, J. (1990). Interaction of epidermal growth factor receptors with the cytoskeleton is related to receptor clustering. *J. Cell. Physiol.* **145**, 365–375.

84. Carraway, C. A. C., Carvajal, M. E., Li, Y., and Carraway, K. L. (1993). Association of p185^{neu} with microfilaments via a large glycoprotein complex in mammary carcinoma microvilli: Evidence for a microfilament-associated signal transduction particle. *J. Biol. Chem.* **268**, 5582–5587.

85. Tidball, J. G., and Spencer, M. J. (1993). PDGF stimulation induces phosphorylation of talin and cytoskeletal reorganization in skeletal muscle. *J. Cell Biol.* **123**, 627–635.

86. Wiche, G. (1989). High-M_r microtubule-associated proteins: Properties and functions. *Biochem. J.* **259**, 1–12.

87. Klymkowsky, M. W., Bachant, J. B., and Domingo, A. (1989). Functions of intermediate filaments. *Cell Motil. Cytoskel.* **14**, 309–331.
88. Luna, E. J., and Hitt, A. L. (1992). Cytoskeleton-plasma membrane interactions. *Science* **258**, 955–964.
89. Schaller, M. D., and Parsons, J. T. (1993). Focal adhesion kinase: An integrin-linked protein tyrosine kinase. *Trends Cell Biol.* **3**, 258–262.
90. Inagaki, M., Takahara, H., Nishi, Y., Sugawara, K., and Sato, C. (1989). Ca^{2+}-dependent deimination-induced disassembly of intermediate filaments involves specific modification of the amino-terminal head domain. *J. Biol. Chem.* **264**, 18119–18127.
91. Huang, H. Y., Graves, D. J., Robson, R. M., and Huiatt, T. W. (1993). ADP-ribosylation of the intermediate filament protein desmin and inhibition of desmin assembly *in vitro* by muscle ADP-ribosyltransferase. *Biochem. Biophys. Res. Commun.* **197**, 570–577.
92. Croall, D. E., and Demartino, G. N. (1991). Calcium-activated neutral protease (calpain) system: Structure, function, and regulation. *Physiol. Rev.* **71**, 813–847.
93. Greenwood, J. A., Troncoso, J. C., Costello, A. C., and Johnson, G. V. W. (1993). Phosphorylation modulates calpain-mediated proteolysis and calmodulin binding of the 200-kDa and 160-kDa neurofilament proteins. *J. Neurochem.* **61**, 191–199.
94. Forscher, P. (1989). Calcium and polyphosphoinositide control of cytoskeletal dynamics. *Trends Neurosci.* **12**, 468–474.
95. Evans, R. M. (1988). Cyclic AMP-dependent protein kinase-induced vimentin filament disassembly involves modification of the N-terminal domain of intermediate filament subunits. *FEBS Lett.* **234**, 73–78.
96. Ikebe, M., and Hornick, T. (1991). Determination of the phosphorylation sites of smooth nuscle caldesmon by protein kinase C. *Arch. Biochem. Biophys.* **288**, 538–542.
97. Sobue, K., and Sellers, J. R. (1991). Caldesmon, a novel regulatory protein in smooth muscle and nonmuscle actomyosin systems. *J. Biol. Chem.* **266**, 12115–12118.
98. Bogatcheva, N. V., Vorotnikov, A. V., Birukov, K. G., Shirinsky, V. P., and Gusev, N. B. (1993). Phosphorylation by casein kinase II affects the interaction of caldesmon with smooth muscle myosin and tropomyosin. *Biochem. J.* **290**, 437–442.
99. Aderem, A. (1992). Signal transduction and the actin cytoskeleton: The roles of MARCKS and profilin. *Trends Biochem. Sci.* **17**, 438–443.
100. Pike, L. J. (1992). Phosphatidylinositol 4-kinases and the role of polyphosphoinositides in cellular regulation. *Endocr. Rev.* **13**, 692–706.
101. Schwartz, M. A. (1992). Transmembrane signalling by integrins. *Trends Cell Biol.* **2**, 304–308.
102. Juliano, R. L., and Haskill, S. (1993). Signal transduction from the extracellular matrix. *J. Cell Biol.* **120**, 577–585.
103. Fox, J. E. B., Taylor, R. G., Taffarel, M., Boyles, J. K., and Goll, D. E. (1993). Evidence that activation of platelet calpain is induced as a consequence of binding of adhesive ligand to the integrin, glycoprotein IIb-IIIa. *J. Cell Biol.* **120**, 1501–1507.
104. Adams, J. C., and Watt, F. M. (1993). Regulation of development and differentiation by the extracellular matrix. *Development* **117**, 1183–1198.
105. McNamee, H. P., Ingber, D. E., and Schwartz, M. A. (1993). Adhesion to

fibronectin stimulates inositol lipid synthesis and enhances PDGF-induced inositol lipid breakdown. *J. Cell Biol.* **121,** 673–678.

106. Sachs, F. (1991). Mechanical transduction by membrane ion channels: A mini review. *Mol. Cell. Biochem.* **104,** 57–60.

107. Watson, P. A. (1990). Direct stimulation of adenylate cyclase by mechanical forces in S49 mouse lymphoma cells during hyposmotic swelling. *J. Biol. Chem.* **265,** 6569–6575.

108. Watson, P. A. (1991). Function follows form: Generation of intracellular signals by cell deformation. *FASEB J.* **5,** 2013–2019.

109. Zeigler, M. E., and Wicha, M. S. (1992). Posttranscriptional regulation of α-casein mRNA accumulation by laminin. *Exp. Cell Res.* **200,** 481–489.

110. Ingber, D. E., and Jamieson, J. D. (1984). Cells as tensegrity structures: Architectural regulation of histodifferentiation by physical forces transduced over basement membrane. *In* "Gene Expression during Normal and Malignant Differentiation" (L. C. Anderson, C. G. Gahmberg, and P. Ekblou, eds.), pp. 13–32. Academic Press, New York.

CHAPTER 11

Phosphorylation and Other Nontranscriptional Effects of Hormones

I. Introduction

The rise of molecular biology has resulted in an undue emphasis on gene regulation. Certainly transcriptional control is a major mechanism by which hormones affect cellular processes and it is discussed Part 4. However, other mechanisms do not involve gene regulation but are no less important. The major portion of this chapter will discuss the regulation of phosphorylation by protein kinases and phosphatases and their effects on certain model systems. The chapter ends with an examination of hormonal control of transport.

II. Phosphorylation

A. General

Perhaps the major transcriptional mechanism for cellular regulation is the covalent modification of cellular constituents; phosphorylation is at the forefront of these modifications (1–3). A number of serine–threonine protein kinases have already been discussed in previous chapters; their structure and control are summarized in Table 11-1. Protein kinases A and C (PKA, PKC) have been studied most extensively. The roles of the other protein kinases are less well characterized because many of their major substrates are still unidentified.

Such identification is complicated by the question of physiological relevance: almost any protein can be phosphorylated by any given kinase under the appropriate *in vitro* conditions. Therefore, how does one determine if a particular modification is a genuine regulatory mechanism? Krebs and Beavo (4) proposed four criteria that should be satisfied before a phosphorylation reaction can be deemed physiologically relevant.

1. The substrate should be phosphorylated *in vitro* at a reasonable rate and in a stoichiometric manner.

2. This phosphorylation should appropriately alter the function of the substrate. For example, if the substrate is an enzyme, its activity should be modulated.

3. The phosphorylation and dephosphorylation should occur in intact cells or tissues and should be correlated with the functional changes in the substrate.

4. Finally, the mediators controlling the responsible kinases and/or phosphatases should fluctuate in a manner correlated with the degree of phosphorylation. The levels of the kinases rarely change: therefore, the correlation must be made between the kinase effector and the modification. For example, if a particular phosphorylation is catalyzed by PKA, then cAMP levels should rise as the degree of phosphorylation increases.

Table 11-1
Summary of Multipurpose Serine–Threonine Protein Kinases Involved with Hormone Action

Kinase	Subunits	Regulation	Substrate specificity
PKA	R_2C_2	cAMP (removal of inhibitor)	$(+)-(+)-X-S/T^a$
PKG	Homodimer	cGMP (direct activation)	$(+)_{2-3}-X-S/T^b$
PKC	Monomer	Ca^{2+} and/or phospholipid (direct activation)	$(+)_{1-3}-X_{1-2}-S/T-X_{1-2}-(+)_{1-3}^b$
CaMKII	Homodecamer (α); homooctamer (β)	Ca^{2+} and CaM (direct activation); autophosphorylation	$R-X-X-S/T^c$
CKII	$\alpha\beta$ dimer	Polyamines; S–T phosphorylation	$S/T-X/(-)-X/(-)-(-)$
MAP kinase	Monomer	T and Y phosphorylation by MAP kinase kinase	$P-X_{1-2}-S/T-P$
Proline-directed kinase	Cdc2 + cyclin A	T and Y phosphorylation on cyclin	$S/T-P$ or $P-L-S/T-P$
H1 kinase	Cdc2 + cyclin B + Suc1	T and Y phosphorylation on cyclin	$S/T-P-X-(+)$
Raf kinase	Monomer	S and Y(?) phosphorylation	$\Phi-\Phi-X-S/T-\Phi-\Phi^d$
S6KI	Monomer	S–T phosphorylation by insulin, etc.	$R-(R)-R-X-X-S$
S6KII	Monomer	Phosphorylation by MAP kinase	$R-(R)-R-X-X-S$
DNA-PK	Trimer	Requires DNA binding	$(-)-S/T-Q$ or $Q-S/T-Q$

[a] Arginine is the preferred basic amino acid.
[b] Either arginine or lysine may be the basic amino acid.
[c] Valine often follows S–T.
[d] Φ is a hydrophobic amino acid, especially aliphatic ones.

Both glycogenolysis and smooth muscle contraction, which will be described in this chapter, meet these criteria, but the data for many other systems are still incomplete.

In addition to the multipurpose kinases listed in Table 11-1, there are also a number of more specific serine–threonine kinases (Table 11-2), some of which are affected by the former kinases. This type of serial activation is quite common and is probably related to the way in which these kinases are regulated (5). As noted earlier, kinase levels are usually constant and activation rarely increases enzyme activity more than 20-fold. Therefore, to increase the gain of this system, several kinases are arranged in a cascade that can greatly amplify the initial response. This cascade can also increase the range of substrates phosphorylated and can introduce regulatory sites for better integration of the response.

Table 11-2
Summary of Specific, Hormone-Related, Serine–Threonine Protein Kinases

Protein kinase	Regulator	Effect of stimulation
Glycogen metabolism		
Phosphorylase kinase	PKA; calcium	Glycogenolysis
Glycogen synthase kinase 3 (GSK-3)	PKC; MAPK-activated protein kinase	Glycogenolysis; transcription inhibition
Smooth muscle contraction		
Myosin light chain kinase (MLCK)	Calcium, CaM	Smooth muscle contraction
Translation		
Double-stranded RNA-dependent kinase	Interferon	Inhibits translation
CaMKIII	Calcium, CaM	Inhibits translation
Other		
β-Adrenergic receptor kinase	Receptor occupancy	Desensitization
Hydroxymethylglutaryl coenzyme A (HMG CoA) reductase kinase	Phosphorylation by another kinase	Inhibits steroid synthesis

Another common characteristic of protein phosphorylation is its hierarchical nature (6,7). Hierarchy refers to the phenomenon in which phosphorylation at one site influences phosphorylation at subsequent sites. Usually, the first modification is regulated by second messengers, although this phosphorylation by itself is without effect. Its only purpose is to facilitate or inhibit the subsequent modifications. Such an arrangement permits graded or threshold effects and allows for regulatory integration.

There are several examples of hierarchical phosphorylation; in glycogen synthase, there are four pairs of sites where the modification of the first is required for phosphorylation of the second. At the amino terminus, PKA phosphorylation must precede that by casein kinase I (CKI). At the carboxy terminus, there are two additional sites where CKI is the secondary kinase; at one either PKA or PKC must act first, whereas at the other site initial phosphorylation must occur by PKA or calmoldulin dependent protein kinase II (CaMKII). Finally, in the middle of glycogen synthase, there is a site that must be modified by CKII before glycogen synthase kinase-3 (GSK-3) can phosphorylate it.

There are also examples in which the first phosphorylation inhibits the second. The hormone-sensitive lipase can be phosphorylated at either S-563 or S-565, but not both. Normally, PKA would phosphorylate the former and activate the lipase, but prior modification at the latter site will block PKA action.

Finally, many second messengers like calcium are released in pulses, whose frequency can be sensed by kinases (8,9). For example, CaMKII is initially activated by calcium–CaM, but subsequent autophosphorylation renders the kinase partially active in the absence of calcium–CaM. This modification allows CaMKII to remain partially active for several seconds after calcium levels decline. Depending on the pulse frequency, CaMKII may still be active when the next calcium elevation occurs, allowing the signals to be summed. The greater the frequency, the greater the summation. This phenomenon converts the signal frequency into a graded response by the kinase.

B. Protein Kinases

The four major kinase families (10) are (i) PKA-related kinases, (ii) CaM kinase, (iii) casein kinase-related kinases, and (iv) tyrosine kinases. The PKA family prefers basic residues at the amino terminus of the phosphorylation site (Table 11-1) and includes PKA, PKG, PKC, β-adrenergic receptor kinase (βARK), and S6 kinase (S6K). The CaM kinase family has a similar sequence

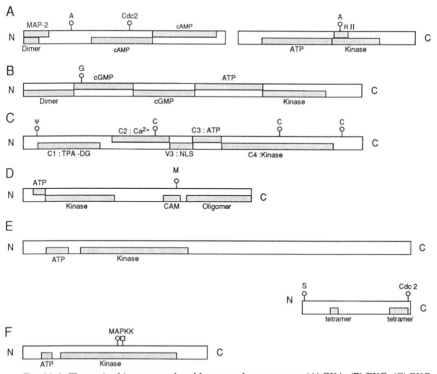

Fig. 11-1. The major kinases regulated by second messengers: (A) PKA, (B) PKG, (C) PKC, (D) CaMKII, (E) CKII (α and β subunits), and (F) MAPK. Phosphorylation sites are designated by circles and the responsible kinase by the following letters: A, PKA; C, PKC; G, PKG; M, CaMKII; P, GSK-3; ψ, pseudosubstrate site. Other abbreviations are defined in the text.

preference and is structurally closely related to the PKA family. The casein kinase family includes both the casein kinases and the proline-directed kinases (PDKs); the former prefer acidic residues near the site of modification, whereas the latter require proline. The PDKs include mitogen-activated protein (MAP) kinase, cell division cycle kinase 2 (Cdc2), and GSK-3 kinase. The tyrosine kinases obviously contain those kinases that phosphorylate tyrosine; however, the tyrosine and serine–threonine kinases are homologous and there is some mixing of the two groups. For example, the double-stranded RNA (dsRNA)-activated protein kinase is a serine–threonine kinase but belongs in this family. The Raf and Mos kinases may be other such examples.

Many of these kinases have already been discussed in previous chapters: βARK (Chapter 7); PKA and PKG (Chapter 8); PKC and CaMKII (Chapter 9); and CKII (Chapter 10). All these kinases have similar structures: a homologous kinase domain, a regulatory domain, and a (pseudo)autophosphorylation site (Fig. 11-1). The latter two elements tonically inhibit the kinase in the absence of a positive modulator. The proline-directed kinases and several other miscellaneous kinases will be discussed in this chapter.

1. Proline-Directed Protein Kinases

One of the first kinases in this class was initially discovered as a kinase that phosphorylated the *microtubule-associated protein-2* (MAP-2); it became known as the MAP-2 kinase or, more simply, MAPK (11–13). Later, it was discovered to have more widespread effects and be stimulated by growth factors. Not wanting to change an entrenched acronym, the scientific community merely redefined MAPK to mean *mitogen-activated protein kinase*, although some have argued for a new term: *extracellular-signal regulated kinase* (ERK). This text will use the older MAPK.

MAPK exists in several isoforms and must be phosphorylated on both threonine and tyrosine for activation (14). This finding was initially exciting, since it suggested a direct link between serine–threonine kinases and the receptor tyrosine kinases (RTKs). However, RTKs do not phosphorylate MAPK; rather, a MAPK kinase that can modify MAPK on both amino acids and activate it has recently been isolated (15). This MAPK kinase is phosphorylated and activated by yet another kinase, a MAPK kinase kinase (Fig. 11-2). Several other kinases are also capable of activating MAPK kinase, including Raf and Mos (see subsequent text), but at the present time the physiological significance of each of these MAPK kinase kinases is still uncertain (16,17).

The MAPK can be activated by many growth factors, including insulin, insulin-like growth factor-II (IGF-II), epidermal growth factor (EGF), nerve growth factor (NGF), platelet-derived growth factor (PDGF), stem cell factor (SCF), and thrombin. The activation mechanism is still incompletely known; as noted earlier, the RTKs do not directly phosphorylate any known member of the cascade. However, both they and some of their tyrosine phosphorylated adaptors, such as Shc and IRS-1, can bind Grb2 (see Chapter 8); Grb2, in turn, binds and activates Ras GDP dissociation stimulator (RasGDS).

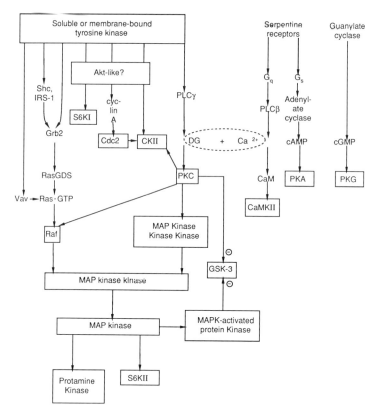

Fig. 11-2. Flowchart of some hormonally regulated protein kinases. Kinases are boxed.

Ras–GTP then activates Raf, a protein kinase in the MAPK cascade (Fig. 11-2). Alternatively, MAPK can be activated through the polyphosphoinositide (PPI) pathway, which involves PKC and a MAPK kinase kinase. These pathways are not totally independent; for example, PKC can phosphorylate and activate Raf (18). MAPK can also be activated by autophosphorylation. Normally, this is such a slow process that it was not originally considered to be physiologically relevant. However, there may be modulators that can significantly accelerate the rate of this reaction; for example, Elk-1 can increase the rate of MAPK autophosphorylation as much as 100-fold depending on conditions (19).

This pathway can also be inhibited by several kinases. Cdc2 (discussed below) phosphorylates and inhibits the MAPK kinase (20). Several studies have documented the inhibitory effects of PKA but the exact site is in dispute. Most data suggest that PKA blocks MAPK activation at or very near the Raf step (21,22).

Finally, MAPK activation can be prolonged by the inhibition of MAPK phosphatases. Both NGF and EGF inhibit the protein tyrosine phosphatase that acts on MAPK, although they differ in their effects on serine–threonine phosphatases (23). This difference may explain why the NGF stimulation of MAPK has a longer duration than that of EGF and can induce the transloca-tion of MAPK into the nucleus (24). The substrates of MAPK run the gamut of cellular proteins: elements of the cytoskeleton (MAP-2), hormone recep-tors (EGFR), transcription factors (Myc, Jun, and SRF), and enzymes (tyrosine hydroxylase and acetyl coenzyme A carboxylase), including other kinases (S6KII and Lck).

GSK-3 was first discovered as a component of glycogen metabolism (25). It is activated by tyrosine phosphorylation by a still unidentified kinase (26) and acts as a general inhibitor (27). Its phosphorylation inhibits glycogen synthase, the transcription factor Jun, and the product of the *engrailed* gene (28). The latter is required for pattern formation in *Drosophila*. GSK-3β activity can be reduced by phosphorylation by the conventional PKCs (29) or by a MAPK-activated protein kinase (30); for example, both kinases indi-rectly activate Jun by suppressing the inhibiting activity of GSK-3.

The cell cycle kinases have had several acronyms: MPF for *m*aturation *p*romoting *f*actor or *M* phase *p*romoting *f*actor and Cdc2 for *c*ell-*d*ivision-*cy*-cle kinase (31–33). The former label (MPF) refers to the kinase activity, whereas the latter term (Cdc2) designates a specific gene product; the dis-tinction is important, since Cdc2 is inactive alone. Complexed with cyclin A, Cdc2 is a multipurpose proline-directed protein kinase (PDPK) that is active on many substrates during interphase. It can be stimulated by EGF and NGF by tyrosine phosphorylation on the cyclin subunit (34). Complexed with cyclin B and Suc1, Cdc2 is active only during mitosis. The presence of Suc1 shifts the substrate specificity of the complex to proteins involved with cell division; for example, Cdc2 will phosphorylate (i) histone H1 that is involved with chromosomal condensation, (ii) lamins that result in nuclear envelope breakdown, (iii) single-stranded DNA-binding proteins that are required for the initiation and elongation in DNA synthesis, and (iv) the retinoblastoma gene product, which inhibits DNA synthesis in its underphosphorylated form (see Chapter 16). Because of the foremost effect, this complex is also called the H1 kinase.

The cell cycle begins when cyclin B is induced. Initially, the protein loosely associates with Cdc2, but the binding becomes tighter after T-161 of Cdc2 is phosphorylated. This modification is very quickly followed by phos-phorylation at T-14 and Y-15; these amino acids are in the ATP-binding site and inhibit the kinase. When DNA synthesis is complete, the latter two site are dephosphorylated by Cdc25, a threonine–tyrosine phosphatase, and the now-activated Cdc2 initiates mitosis. At the end of mitosis, cyclin B is de-graded and Cdc2 once again becomes inactive.

2. Other Protein Kinases

Like MAPK, Raf kinase is stimulated by several growth factors, including insulin, PDGF, fibroblast growth factor (FGF), EGF, NGF, colony-stimulating factor-1 (CSF-1), interleukin-2 (IL-2), IL-3, and granulocyte–macrophage-

CSF (GM-CSF) (35,36). Also, like MAPK, Raf kinase can be activated by phosphorylation on serines, threonines, and tyrosines, although the latter site is still controversial. The best data on tyrosine phosphorylation comes from the study of cytokines: IL-2, IL-3, and GM-CSF all lead to the stoichiometric phosphorylation and activation of Raf (36). The cytokine receptors are thought to bind and activate soluble tyrosine kinases such as Lck and Src (see Chapter 6), and Raf can be phosphorylated by Lck (37) and activated by Src (38). On the other hand, activation via the RTKs is associated with phosphorylation on serine and threonine, not tyrosine. Raf can be phosphorylated and activated by the conventional PKCs (39); it can also be modified by MAPK, but this event is not associated with any change in kinase activity (40). Finally, Raf can be activated by Ras; this appears to occur through direct binding between the two proteins (41–43).

The MAPK cascade presented in Fig. 11-2 is highly speculative; the uncertainity arises from two major factors. First, there are several feedback loops that allow a particular kinase to act at more than one site. For example, tyrosine kinases can activate PKC by stimulating phospholipase Cγ (PLCγ) and the PPI pathway; PKC, in turn, can phosphorylate several tyrosine kinases and affect their activity. Second, there is some tissue and species specificity with respect to the particular sequence. The major known substrates for MAPK include other kinases and transcription factors, such as the serum response factor.

The S6Ks, also known as the ribosomal S6 kinases (RSKs), were first identified as kinases that phosphorylated ribosomal protein S6 in response to mitogens (44). Two major groups of S6Ks have been isolated and characterized. S6KI was purified from rat liver, has a single kinase domain, and has a molecular mass of 70 kDa. It is activated by insulin, EGF, FGF, and PDGF via serine–threonine phosphorylation; however, the responsible kinase has not yet been identified. It is slower acting that the S6KII; its activity is maximal 5–20 minutes after stimulation, whereas S6KII is fully activated in only 2–5 minutes (45,46). S6KII was purified from frog oocytes, contains two kinase domains, and has a larger molecular mass of 90 kDa. The amino-terminal kinase sequence is most similar to that of the PKA family and to S6KI; for this reason, the S6K activity is thought to reside in this domain. The carboxy-terminal kinase sequence most closely resembles phosphorylase kinase, although phosphorylase b is not a substrate for S6KII. It is activated by several mitogens, including EGF, FGF, PDGF, and bombesin; this stimulation is achieved through phosphorylation by MAPK (Fig. 11-2; 47,48). It is also activated by several cytokines in the IL-6 family and it mediates the effects of these hormones on gene transcription (49). In addition, to ribosomal protein S6, S6KII modifies several transcription factors including the serum response factor, Fos, and the retinoic acid X receptor (RXR).

Several other kinases are of potential interest. Akt is a PKC-related kinase that possesses an SH2 domain (50); as such, it may represent the long-sought-after interface between the RTKs and the serine–threonine kinases. The DNA-activated protein kinase (DNA-PK) must bind DNA for activity (51,52). It has not yet been sequenced, but it has a unique consensus phosphorylation site: it requires glutamine adjacent to the serine or threonine. It modifies many nuclear proteins including nuclear receptors, transcription factors, DNA topoisomerases, and RNA polymerase II. The dsRNA-activated protein kinase is another nucleic acid-binding protein kinase (53). The amino terminus binds dsRNA, which is required for activity; this need can be eliminated by autophosphorylation. The kinase is induced by interferon and modifies a component of the translation machinery; translation is inhibited and viral replication is blocked (see Chapter 14).

C. Protein Phosphatases

1. Serine–Threonine Phosphatases

If phosphorylation is important, so must dephosphorylation be (54,55). The major serine–threonine phosphatases are listed in Table 11-3. Many of them show the same variety of regulation by second messengers exhibited by the protein kinases. Protein phosphatase-1 (PP-1), the central phosphatase in reversing glycogenolysis (see subsequent text), is a dimer consisting of a catalytic and a localization subunit (56). The latter differs depending on the location of the enzyme; for example, the G subunit attaches PP-1 to glycogen particles. Control of the phosphatase activity occurs by regulating the interaction between PP-1 and its two inhibitory proteins, Inhibitor-1 and Inhibitor-2, which are thought to act like pseudosubstrates. Phosphorylation of the G subunit by PKA causes PP-1 to dissociate from glycogen; the free form is much more likely to bind and be inhibited by Inhibitor-1 (57). This binding also requires the phosphorylation of Inhibitor-1 by PKA. PP-1 is stimulated by insulin-induced S6KII phosphorylation of the G subunit (58) and by phosphorylation of Inhibitor-2 by Cdc2 or GSK-3. Both these proline-directed kinases modify the same site and lead to the dissociation of Inhibitor-2 from PP-1. A nuclear-localizing subunit is also subject to phosphorylation. This subunit inhibits PP-1 activity; but after PKA or CKII phosphorylation, it dissociates from PP-1 (59).

Calcineurin (PP-2B) is also a dimer consisting of a catalytic and a regulatory subunit. The latter is a member of the CaM family and binds calcium; this binding activates PP-2B activity. PP-2B can be further stimulated by the binding of exogenous calcium–CaM or phospholipids (60). It can be inhibited by CaMKII and PKC phosphorylation of the CaM-binding domain (61). However, the most intriguing regulation is by the immunosuppressants, cyclosporin A and FK506 (62,63). These drugs are used clinically to suppress tissue rejection. The mechanism of action of these drugs involves the inhibition of PP-2B after complexing with endogenous proteins: cyclosporin A binds cyclophilin and FK506 binds the FK506-binding protein (FKBP). Apparently, activation of T lymphocytes requires the dephosphorylation of a transcription factor by PP-2B for factor to enter the nucleus and bind DNA

Table 11-3

Summary of Several Widespread Multifunctional Phosphatases

Phosphatase	Location	Function	Structure	Regulation
PP-1	Glycogen particle; microsomes; ribosomes; myofibrils	Glycogen metabolism; cholesterol and protein synthesis; smooth muscle relaxation	Dimer: catalytic (37 kDa) and organelle-binding (103 kDa) subunits; different binding subunits for each organelle	Inhibited by PKA phosphorylation of glycogen-binding subunit, G (catalytic subunit dissociates and binds Inhibitor-1); stimulated by insulin-induced S6KII phosphorylation of G; stimulated by Cdc2 and GSK-1 phosphorylation and inactivation of Inhibitor-2; stimulated by phosphorylation of nuclear subunit by PKA and CKII
PP-2A	Cytosol	Glycolysis; gluconeogenesis; fatty acid synthesis; amino acid catabolism	Trimer: catalytic (36 kDa) and two regulatory (60 and 54–55 kDa) subunits	Inhibited by regulatory subunits; stimulated by polycations (for example, spermine), ceramide, and insulin-induced S–T kinase; activated by PKG phosphorylation
PP-2B (calcineurin)	Cytosol	Dephosphorylation of RII (PKA), Inhibitor-1, CaM-dependent PDE, and microtubules	Dimer: catalytic (61 kDa) and regulatory (19 kDa) subunit; latter is a member of CaM family and binds calcium	Stimulated by calcium alone and in combination with CaM and by phospholipid binding to regulatory subunit; inhibited by CaMKII and PKC phosphorylation; inhibited by immunosuppressants
PP-1C	Cytosol	Cholesterol synthesis	Monomer of 45 kDa	Unknown

(64,65); this activation is blocked by the immunosuppressants. It is suspected that cyclophilin and FKBP may have endogenous ligands that are involved in the physiological regulation of PP-2B.

Protein phosphatase-2A (PP-2A) is a dual phosphatase that can be converted to a tyrosine phosphatase by ATP. PP-2A is also known as the polycation-stimulated phosphatase because it can be activated *in vitro* by polycations such as spermine, but the physiological role of polyamines in the regulation of this phosphatase remains to be determined. PP-2A can be stoichiometrically phosphorylated on tyrosine by the insulin and EGF receptors (66); this modification inhibits the phosphatase. These hormones can also phosphorylate and inhibit PP-2A indirectly through a protamine kinase kinase (67). Finally, there is some indirect evidence that atrial natriuretic factor (ANF) can stimulate PP-2A by PKG-induced phosphorylation (68). In addition to phosphorylation, PP-2A can be carboxymethylated in a cAMP-dependent manner (69). Although the mechanism is unknown, cAMP-induced phosphorylation and activation of the responsible carboxymethylase would represent the simplest explanation. This modification does not alter PP-2A activity but it does change its substrate specificity. Lastly, PP-2A may have allosteric regulators; for example, ceramide, a putative second messenger (see Chapter 9), has been reported to stimulate PP-2A (70).

PP-1, PP-2A, and PP-2B are all homologous; the last serine–threonine phosphatase is phosphatase-2C (PP-2C), a monomer with a unique sequence. Almost nothing is known about its regulation or role in dephosphorylation.

2. Phosphotyrosine Phosphatases

The other major group of phosphatases, the phosphotyrosine phosphatases (PTPs), removes phosphate from phosphotyrosine (71,72). The PTPs are divided into three classes: soluble (class I) and membrane-bound (classes II and III). The former are structurally quite simple: they all have a homologous catalytic domain of about 250 amino acids and either an amino- or a carboxy-terminal extension possessing some regulatory domain (Fig. 11-3). The latter is involved in localization, ligand binding, or protein stability. For example, PTP-IA has a very hydrophobic carboxy terminus that associates with the endoplasmic reticulum; PTP-S has a carboxy terminus that binds DNA (73); and the amino terminus of PTP-IB is homologous to protein 4.1, which is known to interact with the cytoskeleton. Some of these PTPs can be hormonally regulated; for example, PTP-IA can be cleaved by calpain resulting in a change in cellular location and an enhanced activity (74). However, the most interesting PTPs from an endocrine point of view are the SH-PTPs; each has two SH2 domains and binds to a variety of RTKs (75–77). This association activates the SH-PTP 5- to 10-fold (78). In addition to direct stimulation, the binding of SH-PTP to an RTK may also function in translocating the PTP to the membrane where some of its substrates or activators may reside. This possibility is supported by the fact that PTP activity is markedly activated toward some substrates by negative phospholipids (79).

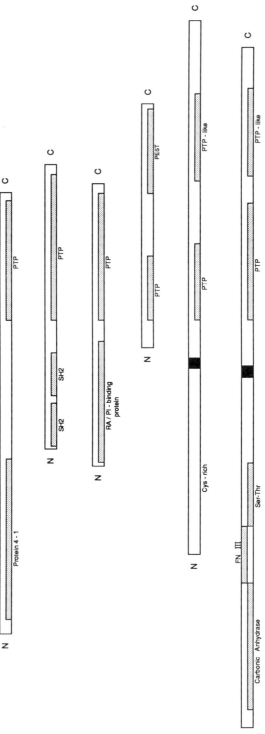

Fig. 11-3. Several phosphotyrosine phosphatases. The top four are soluble PTPs (class I) each having a different type of regulatory site. The bottom two PTPs are membrane-bound (class III). The black area represents the transmembrane domain. FN III, Fibronectin type III domain. Other abbreviations are defined in the text.

Indeed, the RTK itself may be a substrate, although RTKs differ widely in their susceptibility to PTPs (80,81). Finally, SH-PTPs may act as adaptors for RTKs; for example, Grb2 does not bind directly to the PDGFR but to an SH-PTP that is already bound to the receptor (82).

Allosteric activation of SH-PTPs by other phosphotyrosine-containing proteins also occurs; IRS-1, an insulin substrate, can bind and activate these PTPs (83). Allosteric stimulation by other ligands is more controversial; PTP-IA is inhibited by micromolar amounts of inositol 1,4,5-trisphosphate (IP_3) (84), but the physiological significance of this effect is uncertain. Another PTP has an amino terminus that is homologous to retinaldehyde-binding protein and PI transfer protein. Both these proteins bind small molecules that are active in signal transduction, and the homology with this PTP suggests that the PTP may also bind and be regulated by retinoids or IP_3 (85). The last group in this class has PEST sequences. PEST is an acronym using the single letter designations for the amino acids proline, glutamic acid, serine, and threonine. These sequences are recognized by the catabolic machinery of the cell; as such, any protein containing them has a short half-life. Phosphorylation is another potential regulatory mechanism for these enzymes; PTP-IA is phosphorylated in the carboxy terminus by Cdc2, PKC, and during mitosis, but this modification does not result in any change in activity (86,87).

The membrane-bound PTPs have either one (class II) or two (class III) cytoplasmic catalytic domains. The former is represented by a single example, which possesses fibronectin type III domains; the latter can be divided into several families, depending on the structure of the extracellular domain. Type I has a cysteine-rich structure that is most compatible with ligand binding, although no soluble ligands of this family have been identified. Two other groups have fibronectin type III modules either with (type III) or without immunoglobulin-like domains (type II). These two groups have been implicated in cell-matrix interactions and are much more widely distributed than the first family. Type IV has an amino terminus so short that it is difficult to imagine it can bind anything. Finally, type V has a very complex extracellular structure composed of several modules: the extreme amino terminus is homologous to carbonic anhydrase (88,89). This module is followed by a fibronectin type III region, a serine–threonine-rich region, and lastly a hydrophilic domain (Fig. 11-3). Although the amino terminus does not have carbonic anhydrase activity, its altered sequence is not predicted to disrupt the three-dimensional structure of the enzyme. As such, this domain should form a deep hydrophobic pocket that could accommodate a ligand.

As noted earlier, the class III PTPs have two enzyme-like domains. It is universally agreed that the membrane proximal domain is active (88,90), but the status of the distal domain is uncertain. Some authorities claim it is also active but is not routinely detected in phosphatase assays because it has a unique substrate specificity (91). Others claim that the distal domain is required for activation of the proximal one, although the proximal site is active when cloned alone (92). As such, the distal site would represent a regulatory domain. Another possible regulatory mechanism is phosphorylation; many of these PTPs have phosphorylation sites, but their effects have yet to be characterized. Finally, dimerization of the class III PTP occurs and inhibits the phosphatase activity (93).

Two other PTP groups will also be briefly mentioned. First, the cysteine phosphatases are 18-kDa proteins with no homology to the just-discussed PTPs (94). One of their distinguishing characteristics is their activation by purines, especially cGMP. Second, there are several mixed-function phosphatases that are capable of removing phosphates from serines, threonines, and tyrosines. PP-2A is one such enzyme; its phosphotyrosine phosphatase activity is differentially enhanced by ATP and by the small t and middle T antigens from various viruses (see Chapter 16). Cdc25, which dephosphorylates and activates Cdc2, is another. Finally, MAPK phosphatase 1 specifically removes phosphates from both threonines and tyrosines in MAPK (95); this phosphatase is the mammalian homolog of the vaccinia virus phosphatase.

Several functions have been attributed to PTPs. First and most obvious is their regulatory role in tyrosine phosphorylation. They can oppose the actions of tyrosine kinases by dephosphorylating their substrates. In addition, they can have more direct effects on RTKs; these kinases are activated by autophosphorylation and can be inactivated by dephosphorylation. For example, the insulin receptor has been shown to be a substrate for the class III PTPs (96). PTPs can also inhibit guanylate cyclase (97). This cyclase is inhibited by a kinase-like domain between the membrane and cyclase site; the inhibitory region can be inactivated by tyrosine phosphorylation. PTPs remove the phosphate and allow the regulatory domain to once again suppress cyclase activity. However, PTPs can stimulate tyrosine kinases as well. Many soluble tyrosine kinases are inhibited by autophosphorylation sites and can be stimulated by their dephosphorylation. For example, the PTP CD45 can dephosphorylate and activate Lck (98); Cdc25 can do the same for Cdc2. Finally, PTPs have postulated roles in exocytosis (99) and protein turnover (100), although their roles in these functions are not as well delineated as those in the control of general phosphorylation.

D. Model Systems

1. Glycogen Metabolism

Glycogen metabolism is an excellent example of how phosphorylation can regulate cellular processes (Fig. 11-4; 1). Three separate hormones will be considered: cAMP-dependent hormones (glucagon in liver and epinephrine in muscle); vasopressin, which acts through the PPI pathway; and insulin, whose second messengers are unknown but may involve oligosaccharides. For accuracy, note that in the liver glucagon has been shown to activate both adenylate cyclase and the PPI pathway; this is not surprising, since the two mediators reinforce one another in this system. However, for simplicity the pathways will be considered separately.

LIVER   MUSCLE

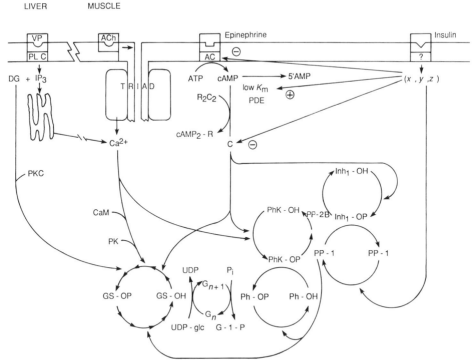

Fig. 11-4. Hormonal regulation of glycogen metabolism in the liver and muscle. AC, Adenylate cyclase; GS, glycogen synthase; G_n, glycogen; G-1-P, glucose 1-phosphate; Inh_1, inhibitor-1; Ph, glycogen phosphorylase; PhK, glycogen phosphorylase kinase; PK, CaM-dependent protein kinase; PLC, phospholipase C; R_2C_2, PKA tetramer; UDP-glc, UDP-glucose; x, y, z, unknown mediators of insulin action. Other abbreviations are defined in the text and in Table 11-3.

Glucagon and epinephrine inhibit glycogen synthesis and stimulate glycogenolysis; all these effects are mediated by phosphorylation by PKA. Glycogen synthase in muscle has a substrate binding site for UDP–glucose and allosteric sites for ADP and glucose 6-phosphate. The former inhibits the enzyme (if ADP is high, then energy levels are low and the cell should not be storing glucose but burning it) and the latter stimulates it (if glucose 6-phosphate levels are high, it should be stored). The enzyme has seven phosphorylation sites. Phosphorylation at five of these sites results in an increased K_m for UDP–glucose, an increased K_a for glucose 6-phosphate, and a decreased K_i for ADP, that is, it binds to its inhibitor more efficiently but binds to its substrate and activator less efficiently. Essentially, the enzyme is inhibited. These phosphorylation sites are modified by different protein kinases and the phosphorylations are additive. As a result, glycogen synthase is not regulated in a strictly on–off fashion but is controlled by a mechanism that is more like a rheostat. This enzyme is inhibited by PKA-mediated phosphorylation.

Glycogen breakdown is accomplished by glycogen phosphorylase, which exists in two forms: phosphorylase *b* is a dimer that is subject to allosteric control, but phosphorylase *a* is a tetramer that is fully active and insensitive to allosteric modulators. The conversion from phosphorylase *b* to phosphorylase *a* is a result of phosphorylation by phosphorylase kinase. This kinase has a subunit composition of $(\alpha\beta\gamma\delta)_4$: γ contains the catalytic site, δ is CaM, and α and β are regulatory subunits that are both phosphorylated. This phosphorylation, which is also performed by PKA, leads to a 15- to 20-fold increase in activity; it also decreases the K_a of the δ subunit for calcium, another activator.

Finally, the previously described phosphorylations can be reversed by PP-1. Therefore, to maintain glycogenolysis, this enzyme must be inactivated. Once again, this is done by PKA, which phosphorylates the G subunit of PP-1. This modification causes PP-1 to dissociate from the glycogen particle and bind Inhibitor-1. This binding also requires that Inhibitor-1 be phosphorylated by PKA.

Vasopressin can also stimulate glycogenolysis; this effect is mediated by the PPI pathway. The free calcium binds to the δ subunit (CaM) of phosphorylase kinase, resulting in further activation. The phosphorylation of the glycogen phosphorylase will then stimulate the enzyme to break down glycogen. Calcium can also bind free CaM to activate a CaM-dependent protein kinase; both this kinase and PKC, another output of the PPI pathway, can phosphorylate and further inactivate glycogen synthase.

Insulin inhibits glycogenolysis by generating one or more small mediators (see Chapter 10). First, phosphorylation by PKA is stopped by (i) suppressing adenylate cyclase to lower cAMP levels, (ii) stimulating the phosphodiesterase to lower cAMP levels further, and (iii) directly inhibiting the kinase. Second, insulin reverses the phosphorylation of glycogen synthase, glycogen phosphorylase, and phosphorylase kinase; that is, the synthase is reactivated and the phosphorylase returns to tight allosteric control. Insulin accomplishes this dephosphorylation by inducing S6KII to phosphorylate and activate PP-1 (51).

2. Smooth Muscle Contraction

Contraction occurs when the thick filaments (primarily *myosin*) and thin filaments (actin) in muscle slide past one another. This requires the stimulation of an actin-activated $Mg^{2+}-ATPase$ that resides in the head region of the heavy chain of myosin. Also associated with the head are two light chains. Contraction is initiated when intracellular calcium levels rise (Fig. 11-5); because the sarcoplasmic reticulum in smooth muscle is not as well developed as it is in skeletal muscle, the calcium is thought to originate from both intra- and extracellular sources. Calcium and CaM activate CaMKII, which in turn phosphorylates and activates a kinase that modifies one of the myosin light chains (101). This myosin light chain kinase (MLCK) phosphorylates the

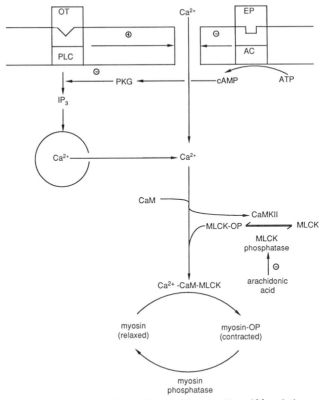

Fig. 11-5. Hormonal regulation of smooth muscle contraction. Abbreviations are defined in the text and in Fig. 11-4. EP, Epinephrine; MLCK, myosin light chain; OT, oxytocin.

P-light chain, which then stimulates the Mg^{2+}-ATPase and triggers contraction. This effect is augmented by arachidonic acid, another product of phospholipases. Arachidonic acid inhibits the MLCK phosphatase that reverses the phosphorylation of CaMKII (102). Relaxation occurs when intracellular calcium levels return to basal levels.

This system is also regulated by β-agonists; however, in smooth muscle contraction, calcium and cAMP antagonize each other. The β-agonists elevate cAMP to such high levels that it can cross-activate PKG. PKG presumably phosphorylates some component of the PPI pathway and interferes with the production of IP_3.

III. Glucose Transport

In addition to metabolism and contraction, transport systems can also be directly regulated by hormones and their mediators. In its simplest form, the transporter may be incorporated into the receptor; an example would be the nicotinic acetylcholine receptor (nAChR), which contains an ion channel. Glucose transport represents a more complex system (103–105).

In most cells, glucose transport is by facilitated diffusion, that is, it is transported by a carrier down its concentration gradient and no energy input is required. The transporter is symmetrical in that glucose can travel in either direction with equal ease. However, glucose transport does require that the hexose be properly oriented: the reducing end always points toward the cytoplasm. The carrier is 55 kDa, contains 15% carbohydrate, and binds cytochalasin B stoichiometrically (106,107). It crosses the plasma membrane 12 times, although only the last 6 transmembrane helices are believed to be directly involved in glucose transport. The transport of glucose by its carrier is analogous to an enzymatic reaction:

$$\text{glucose}_{\text{out}} + \text{carrier} \rightleftharpoons \text{glucose} - \text{carrier} \rightarrow \text{glucose}_{\text{in}} + \text{carrier}$$

Such an analysis yields values for K_m and V_{max}; although they are not exactly equivalent to the enzymatic parameters, they do convey similar information. Insulin stimulates glucose transport by increasing both the V_{max} (transport capacity) and the K_m (transport affinity).

Initial studies used cytochalasin B to assay glucose carriers in the plasma membrane and in the low-density microsomal fraction. Researchers found that insulin increases the content of transporters in the plasma membrane, although it decreases the content in microsomes; this result correlates with the observed stimulation of glucose transport. One can also assay for the carrier by measuring transport activity in the different cellular fractions, and the same results are obtained. Therefore, insulin increases V_{max} by inducing the migration of glucose carriers from the microsomes to the plasma membrane (Fig. 11-6).

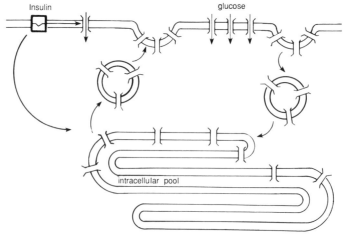

Fig. 11-6. Schematic representation of the two postulated mechanisms for the regulation of glucose transport by insulin.

However, other data have not supported this migration hypothesis as the sole mechanism for insulin-induced glucose uptake (108–110). First, *cycloheximide*, an inhibitor of protein synthesis, also blocks the translocation of the glucose transporter from the microsomes to the plasma membrane but does not inhibit insulin-stimulated glucose uptake. Second, there is a quantitative discrepancy between transporter migration and glucose transport: the former only increases 2.6-fold whereas the latter is stimulated 11-fold. Finally, there is a temporal discrepancy: the carrier reaches the cell surface several minutes before glucose uptake is increased, suggesting the existence of an activation step.

The mechanism for these effects on transporter migration and activation is still unknown. It is known that neither MAPK (111) nor the postulated oligosaccharide mediator of insulin is involved (112) but that IRS-1 and PI3K are required (113,114). After being phosphorylated by the insulin receptor, IRS-1 binds and activates PI3K. The latter appears to be involved in vesicular trafficking (see Chapter 9) and may facilitate the translocation of membrane vesicles laden with glucose transporters to the cell surface. In addition to IRS-1 and PI3K, some authorities propose a role for PKC but this is still controversial. The proponents of the PKC mechanism argue that insulin can activate PLC and PKC and that PKC inhibitors and antisense RNA can block insulin-induced glucose transport (115). However, the stimulation of PKC requires pharmacological concentrations of insulin (116) and the effects of PKC inhibitors are additive, suggesting that they are interfering with different pathways or producing nonspecific effects (117). It is possible that PKC is involved in only part of the transport process. For example, it has been argued that PKC may be responsible for the transporter migration but not its activation (118). In those tissues where translocation is the dominant mechanism of stimulation, the importance of PKC will be obvious. However, in systems where the activation is preeminent, PKC may not appear to play any role.

Although insulin is the major hormone regulating glucose transport, other hormones can influence this action of insulin. The simplest mechanism would be to alter carrier levels; for example, T_3 stimulates the mRNA for the glucose transporter 3-fold in rat skeletal muscle (119). Other hormones can have more acute effects; for example, G_s agonists oppose, and G_i agonists enhance, the actions of insulin on glucose transport. The effects of these compounds in isolated plasma membranes are blocked by cholera and pertussis toxins, respectively, and are not correlated with cAMP levels (120). These data suggest that the G proteins are acting directly on the transporter. A role for phosphorylation by PKA has also been postulated; PKA can phosphorylate the carboxy terminus of the carrier (121,122). However, others point out that only the internal transporters are modified; the plasma membrane carriers are not phosphorylated (123). Furthermore, the degree of modification is quite small and adenosine can block the effect of β-agonists on glucose transport without affecting phosphorylation of the transporter. Recently, it has been proposed that the inhibitory effect of cAMP is independent of PKA, that is, cAMP may directly bind the carboxy terminus of the glucose transporter (124). If confirmed, this mechanism would explain why PKA phosphorylation is so low and sometimes unrelated to carrier activity.

IV. Summary

Two major ways that hormones can directly affect cellular metabolism are by phosphorylation and membrane transport. The activities of many enzymes are influenced by phosphorylation, and the responsible kinases are frequently under the control of hormone mediators: PKA by cAMP, PKG by cGMP, PKC by calcium and phospholipids, CaM-dependent protein kinase by CaM, and casein kinase II by polyamines. In addition, many other kinases may not be directly regulated by second messengers but form part of protein kinase cascades initiated by hormones. These cascades amplify the signal and introduce additional sites for regulation.

The serine–threonine phosphatases, which regulate the reverse process, are subject to similar controls: PP-1 by PKA and insulin-induced S6KII; PP-2A by polyamines and PKG; and PP-2B by calcium, CaM, CaMKII, and PKC. The soluble phosphotyrosine phosphatases have domains that affect localization, ligand binding, and protein stability. Of particular note is one group that has SH2 domains, binds RTKs, and is phosphorylated and activated by RTKs. The membrane-bound PTPs may mediate hormone or cell-matrix transduction.

Transport may be affected in several ways. First, hormone receptors may form part of the transporter, as in the case of the nAChR and the sodium channel. Second, transporters may be regulated by hormone mediators, such as the G proteins of β-agonists, which increase glucose transport. Finally, transporter numbers may be altered by gene induction, for example, by T_3, or by cellular redistribution, as postulated for the insulin regulation of glucose transport.

References

General References

Baldwin, S. A. (1993). Mammalian passive glucose transporters: Members of an ubiquitous family of active and passive transport proteins. *Biochim. Biophys. Acta* **1154**, 17–49.

Blenis, J. (1993). Signal transduction via the MAP kinases: Proceed at your own RSK. *Proc. Natl. Acad. Sci. U.S.A.* **90**, 5889–5892.

Considine, R. V., and Caro, J. F. (1993). Protein kinase C: Mediator or inhibitor of insulin action? *J. Cell. Biochem.* **52**, 8–13.

Davis, R. J. (1993). The mitogen-activated protein kinase signal transduction pathway. *J. Biol. Chem.* **268**, 14553–14556.

Goldstein, B. J. (1993). Regulation of insulin receptor signaling by protein-tyrosine dephosphorylation. *Receptor* **3**, 1–15.

Hubbard, M. J., and Cohen, P. (1993). On target with a new mechanism for the regulation of protein phosphorylation. *Trends Biochem. Sci.* **18**, 172–177.

Nishida, E., and Gotoh, Y. (1993). The MAP kinase cascade is essential for diverse signal transduction pathways. *Trends Biochem. Sci.* **18**, 128–131.

Samuel, C. E. (1993). The eIF-2α protein kinases, regulators of translation in eukaryotes from yeasts to humans. *J. Biol. Chem.* **268**, 7603–7606.

Walton, K. M., and Dixon, J. E. (1993). Protein tyrosine phosphatases. *Annu. Rev. Biochem.* **62**, 101–120.

See also Refs. 1–7, 10–13, 22, 27, 31–33, 35, 36, 44, 51–56, 71, 72, 98, 101, 103–105, 115, and 116.

Cited References

1. Blackshear, P. J., Nairn, A. C., and Kuo, J. F. (1988). Protein kinases 1988: A current perspective. *FASEB J.* **2**, 2957–2969.

2. Cohen, P. (1988). Protein phosphorylation and hormone action. *Proc. R. Soc. London B* **234**, 115–144.

3. Shenolikar, S. (1988). Protein phosphorylation: Hormones, drugs, and bioregulation. *FASEB J.* **2**, 2753–2764.

4. Krebs, E. B., and Beavo, J. A. (1979). Phosphorylation–dephosphorylation of enzymes. *Annu. Rev. Biochem.* **48**, 923-959.

5. Shacter, E., Stadtman, E. R., Jurgensen, S. R., and Chock, P. B. (1988). Role of cAMP in cyclic cascade regulation. *Meth. Enzymol.* **159**, 3–19.

6. Roach, P. J. (1990). Control of glycogen synthase by hierarchal protein phosphorylation. *FASEB J.* **4**, 2961–2968.

7. Roach, P. J. (1991). Multisite and hierarchal protein phosphorylation. *J. Biol. Chem.* **266**, 14139–14142.

8. Dupont, G., and Goldbeter, A. (1992). Protein phosphorylation driven by intracellular calcium oscillations: A kinetics analysis. *Biophys. Chem.* **42**, 257–270.

9. Meyer, T., Hanson, P. I., Stryer, L., and Schulman, H. (1992). Calmodulin trapping by calcium-calmodulin-dependent protein kinase. *Science* **256**, 1199–1202.

10. Hanks, S. K., Quinn, A. M., and Hunter, T. (1988). The protein kinase family: Conserved features and deduced phylogeny of the catalytic domains. *Science* **241**, 42–52.

11. Cobb, M. H., Boulton, T. G., and Robbins, D. J. (1991). Extracellular signal-regulated kinases: ERKs in progress. *Cell Regul.* **2**, 965–978.

12. Anderson, N. G. (1992). MAP kinases—Ubiquitous signal transducers and potentially important components of the cell cycling machinery in eukaryotes. *Cell. Signal.* **4**, 239–246.

13. Pelech, S. L., and Sanghera, J. S. (1992). Mitogen-activated protein kinases: Versatile transducers for cell signaling. *Trends Biochem. Sci.* **17**, 233–238.

14. Anderson, N. G., Maller, J. L., Tonks, N. K., and Sturgill, T. W. (1990). Requirement for integration of signals from two distinct phosphorylation pathways for activation of MAP kinase. *Nature (London)* **343**, 651–653.

15. Crews, C. M., Alessandrini, A., and Erikson, R. L. (1992). The primary structure

of MEK, a protein kinase that phosphorylates the *ERK* gene product. *Science* **258**, 478–480.

16. Tsuda, L., Inoue, Y. H., Yoo, M. A., Mizuno, M., Hata, M., Lim, Y. M., Adachi-Yamada, T., Ryo, H., Masamune, Y., and Nishida, Y. (1993). A protein kinase similar to MAP kinase activator acts downstream to the Raf kinase in *Drosophila. Cell* **72**, 407–414.

17. Posada, J., Yew, N., Ahn, N. G., Vande Woude, G. F., and Cooper, J. A. (1993). Mos stimulates MAP kinase in *Xenopus* oocytes and activates a MAP kinase kinase *in vitro. Mol. Cell. Biol.* **13**, 2546–2553.

18. Kolch, W., Heldecker, G., Kochs, G., Hummel, R., Vahidl, H., Mischak, H., Finkenzeller, G., Marmé, D., and Rapp, U. R. (1993). Protein kinase Cα activates RAF-1 by direct phosphorylation. *Nature (London)* **364**, 249–252.

19. Rao, V. N., and Reddy, E. S. P. (1993). Elk-1 proteins are phosphoproteins and activators of mitogen-activated protein kinase. *Cancer Res.* **53**, 3449–3454.

20. Rossomando, A. J., Dent, P., Sturgill, T. W., and Marshak, D. R. (1994). Mitogen-activated protein kinase kinase 1 (MKK1) is negatively regulated by threonine phosphorylation. *Mol. Cell. Biol.* **14**, 1594–1602.

21. Wu, J., Dent, P., Jelinek, T., Wolfman, A., Weber, M. J., and Sturgill, T. W. (1993). Inhibition of the EGF-activated MAP kinase signaling pathway by adenosine 3′,5′-monophosphate. *Science* **262**, 1065–1069.

22. Cook, S. J., and McCormick, F. (1993). Inhibition by cAMP of Ras-dependent activation of Raf. *Science* **262**, 1069–1074.

23. Peraldi, P., Scimeca, J. C., Filloux, C., and Van Obberghen, E. (1993). Regulation of extracellular signal-regulated protein kinase-1 (ERK-1; pp44/mitogen-activated protein kinase) by epidermal growth factor and nerve growth factor in PC12 cells: Implication of ERK1 inhibitory activities. *Endocrinol. (Baltimore)* **132**, 2578–2585.

24. Nguyen, T. T., Scimeca, J. C., Filloux, C., Peraldi, P., Carpentier, J. L., and Van Obberghen, E. (1993). Co-regulation of the mitogen-activated protein kinase, extracellular signal-regulated kinase 1, and the 90-kDa ribosomal S6 kinase in PC12 cells: Distinct effects of the neurotrophic factor, nerve growth factor, and the mitogenic factor, epidermal growth factor. *J. Biol. Chem.* **268**, 9803–9810.

25. Plyte, S. E., Hughes, K., Nikolakaki, E., Pulverer, B. J., and Woodgett, J. R. (1992). Glycogen synthase kinase-3: Functions in oncogenesis and development. *Biochim. Biophys. Acta* **1114**, 147-162.

26. Hughes, K., Nikolakaki, E., Plyte, S. E., Totty, N. F., and Woodgett, J. R. (1993). Modulation of the glycogen kinase-3 family by tyrosine phosphorylation. *EMBO J.* **12**, 803–808.

27. Woodgett, J. R., Plyte, S. E., Pulverer, B. J., Mitchell, J. P., and Hughs, K. (1993). Roles of glycogen synthase kinase-3 in signal transduction. *Biochem. Soc. Trans.* **21**, 905–907.

28. Siegfried, E., Chou, T. B., and Perrimon, N. (1992). *wingless* signaling acts through *zeste-white 3*, a *Drosophila* homolog of *glycogen synthase kinase-3*, to regulate *engrailed* and establish cell fate. *Cell* **71**, 1167–1179.

29. Goode, N., Hughes, K., Woodgett, J. R., and Parker, P. J. (1992). Differential regulation of glycogen synthase kinase-3β by protein kinase C isotypes. *J. Biol. Chem.* **267**, 16878–16882.

30. Sutherland, C., Leighton, I. A., and Cohen, P. (1993). Inactivation of glycogen synthase kinase-3β by phosphorylation: new kinase connections in insulin and growth-factor signalling. *Biochem. J.* **296**, 15–19.

31. Wang, J. Y. J. (1992). Oncoprotein phosphorylation and cell cycle control. *Biochim. Biophys. Acta* **1114**, 179–192.
32. Müller, R., Mumberg, D., and Lucibello, F. C. (1993). Signals and genes in the control of cell-cycle progression. *Biochem. Biophys. Acta* **1155**, 151–179.
33. Nigg, E. A. (1993). Cellular substrates of p34^{cdc2} and its companion cyclin-dependent kinases. *Trends Cell Biol.* **3**, 296–301.
34. Ostergaard, H. L., and Trowbridge, I. S. (1991). Negative regulation of CD45 protein tyrosine phosphatase activity by ionomycin in T cells. *Science* **253**, 1423–1425.
35. Li, P., Wood, K., Mamon, H., Haser, W., and Roberts, T. (1991). Raf-1: A kinase currently without a cause but not lacking in effects. *Cell* **64**, 479–482.
36. Rapp, U. R. (1991). Role of *Raf-1* serine/threonine protein kinase in growth factor signal transduction. *Oncogene* **6**, 495–500.
37. Thompson, P. A., Ledbetter, J. A., Rapp, U. R., and Bolen, J. B. (1991). The Raf-1 serine-threonine kinase is a substrate for the p56^{lck} protein tyrosine kinase in human T-cells. *Cell Growth Diff.* **2**, 609–617.
38. Williams, N. G., Roberts, T. M., and Li, P. (1992). Both p21^{ras} and pp60^{v-src} are required, but neither alone is sufficient, to activate the Raf-1 kinase. *Proc. Natl. Acad. Sci. U.S.A.* **89**, 2922–2926.
39. Sozeri, O., Vollmer, K., Liyanage, M., Frith, D., Kour, G., Mark, G. E., and Stabel, S. (1992). Activation of the c-Raf protein kinase by protein kinase C phosphorylation. *Oncogene* **7**, 2259–2262.
40. Mori, A., Aizawa, H., Saido, T. C., Kawasaki, H., Mizuno, K., Murofushi, H., Suzuki, K., and Sakai, H. (1991). Site-specific phosphorylation by protein kinase C inhibits assembly-promoting activity of microtubule-associated protein 4. *Biochemistry* **30**, 9341–9346.
41. Moodie, S. A., Willumsen, B. M., Weber, M. J., and Wolfman, A. (1993). Complexes of Ras·GTP with Raf-1 and mitogen-activated protein kinase kinase. *Science* **260**, 1658–1661.
42. Van Aelst, L., Barr, M., Marcus, S., Polverino, A., and Wigler, M. (1993). Complex formation between RAS and RAF and other protein kinases. *Proc. Natl. Acad. Sci. U.S.A.* **90**, 6213–6217.
43. Vojtek, A. B., Hollenberg, S. M., and Cooper, J. A. (1993). Mammalian Ras interacts directly with the serine/threonine kinase Raf. *Cell* **74**, 205–214.
44. Kozma, S. C., Ferrari, S., and Thomas, G. (1993). Unmasking a growth factor/oncogene-activated S6 phosphorylation cascade. *Cell. Signal.* **1**, 219–225.
45. Chen, R. H., Chung, J., and Blenis, J. (1991). Regulation of pp90^{rsk} phosphorylation and S6 phosphotransferase activity in Swiss 3T3 cells by growth factor-, phorbol ester-, and cyclic AMP-mediated signal transduction. *Mol. Cell. Biol.* **11**, 1861–1867.
46. Chung, J., Chen, R. H., and Blenis, J. (1991). Coordinate regulation of pp90^{rsk} and a distinct protein-serine/threonine kinase activity that phosphorylates recombinant pp90^{rsk} in vitro. *Mol. Cell. Biol.* **11**, 1868–1874.
47. Sturgill, T. W., Ray, L. B., Erikson, E., and Maller, J. L. (1988). Insulin-stimulated MAP-2 kinase phosphorylates and activates ribosomal protein S6 kinase II. *Nature (London)* **334**, 715–718.
48. Susa, M., Olivier, A. R., Fabbro, D., and Thomas, G. (1989). EGF induces biphasic S6 kinase activation: Late phase is protein kinase C-dependent and contributes to mitogenicity. *Cell* **57**, 817–824.
49. Yin, T., and Yang, Y. C. (1994). Mitogen-activated protein kinases and ribo-

somal S6 protein kinases are involved in signaling pathways shared by interleukin-11, interleukin-6, leukemia inhibitory factor, and oncostatin M in mouse 3T3-L1 cells. *J. Biol. Chem.* **269**, 3731–3738.

50. Bellacosa, A., Testa, J. R., Staal, S. P., and Tsichlis, P. N. (1991). A retroviral oncogene, *akt*, encoding a serine-threonine kinase containing an SH2-like region. *Science* **254**, 274–277.

51. Lees-Miller, S. P., and Anderson, C. W. (1992). The DNA-activated protein kinase, DNA-PK: A potential coordinator of nuclear events. *Cancer Cells* **3**, 341–346.

52. Finnie, N., Gottlieb, T., Hartley, K., and Jackson, S. P. (1993). Transcription factor phosphorylation by the DNA-dependent protein kinase. *Biochem. Soc. Trans.* **21**, 930–935.

53. Meurs, E., Chong, K., Galabru, J., Thomas, N. S. B., Kerr, I. M., Williams, B. R. G., and Hovanessian, A. G. (1990). Molecular cloning and characterization of the human double-stranded RNA-activated protein kinase induced by interferon. *Cell* **62**, 379–390.

54. Cohen, P. T. W., Brewis, N. D., Hughes, V., and Mann, D. J. (1990). Protein serine/threonine phosphatases: An expanding family. *FEBS Lett.* **268**, 355–359.

55. Mumby, M. C., and Walter, G. (1993). Protein serine/threonine phosphatases: Structure, regulation, and functions in cell growth. *Physiol. Rev.* **73**, 673–699.

56. Bollen, M., and Stalmans, W. (1992). The structure, role, and regulation of type 1 protein phosphatases. *Crit. Rev. Biochem. Mol. Biol.* **27**, 227–281.

57. Villa-Moruzzi, E. (1992). Activation of type-1 protein phosphatase by cdc2 kinase. *FEBS Lett.* **304**, 211–215.

58. Sutherland, C., Campbell, D. G., and Cohen, P. (1993). Identification of insulin-stimulated protein kinase-1 as the rabbit equivalent of rsk^{mo}-2: Identification of two threonines phosphorylated during activation by mitogen-activated protein kinase. *Eur. J. Biochem.* **212**, 581–588.

59. Van Eynde, A., Beullens, M., Stalmans, W., and Bollen, M. (1994). Full activation of a nuclear species of protein phosphatase-1 by phosphorylation with protein kinase A and casein kinase-2. *Biochem. J.* **297**, 447–449.

60. Politino, M., and King, M. M. (1990). Calcineurin-phospholipid interactions: Identification of the phospholipid-binding subunit and analyses of a two-stage binding process. *J. Biol. Chem.* **265**, 7619–7622.

61. Hashimoto, Y., and Soderling, T. R. (1989). Regulation of calcineurin by phosphorylation: Identification of the regulatory site phosphorylated by Ca^{2+}/calmodulin-dependent protein kinase II and protein kinase C. *J. Biol. Chem.* **264**, 16524–16529.

62. Schreiber, S. L. (1992). Immunophilin-sensitive protein phosphatase action in cell signaling pathways. *Cell* **70**, 365–368.

63. Walsh, C. T., Zydowsky, L. D., and McKeon, F. D. (1992). Cyclosporin A, the cyclophilin class of peptidylprolyl isomerases, and blockade of T cell signal transduction. *J. Biol. Chem.* **267**, 13115–13118.

64. Heitman, J., Movva, N. R., and Hall, M. N. (1992). Proline isomerases at the crossroads of protein folding, signal transduction, and immunosuppression. *New Biol.* **4**, 448–460.

65. McCaffrey, P. G., Perrino, B. A., Siderling, T. R., and Rao, A. (1993). NF-AT$_{p}$, a T lymphocyte DNA-binding protein that is a target for calcineurin and immunosuppressive drugs. *J. Biol. Chem.* **268**, 3747–3752.

66. Chen, J., Martin, B. L., and Brautigan, D. L. (1992). Regulation of protein

serine–threonine phosphatase type-2A by tyrosine phosphorylation. *Science* **257**, 1261–1264.

67. Guo, H., and Damuni, Z. (1993). Autophosphorylation-activated protein kinase phosphorylates and inactivates protein phosphatase 2A. *Proc. Natl. Acad. Sci. U.S.A.* **90**, 2500–2504.

68. White, R. E., Lee, A. B., Shcherbatko, A. D., Lincoln, T. M., Schonbrunn, A., and Armstrong, D. L. (1993). Potassium channel stimulation by natriuretic peptides through cGMP-dependent dephosphorylation. *Nature (London)* **361**, 263–266.

69. Floer, M., and Stock, J. (1994). Carboxy methylation of protein phosphatase 2A from *Xenopus* eggs is stimulated by cAMP and inhibited by okadaic acid. *Biochem. Biophys. Res. Commun.* **198**, 372–379.

70. Dobrowsky, R. T., Kamibayashi, C., Mumby, M. C., and Hannun, Y. A. (1993). Ceramide activates heterotrimeric protein phosphatase 2A. *J. Biol. Chem.* **268**, 15523–15530.

71. Fischer, E. H., Charbonneau, H., and Tonks, N. K. (1991). Protein tyrosine phosphatases: A diverse family of intracellular and transmembrane enzymes. *Science* **253**, 401–406.

72. Brautigan, D. L. (1992). Great expectations: Protein tyrosine phosphatases in cell regulation. *Biochim. Biophys. Acta* **1114**, 63–77.

73. Radha, V., Kamatkar, S., and Swarup, G. (1993). Binding of a protein-tyrosine phosphatase to DNA through its carboxy-terminal noncatalytic domain. *Biochemistry* **32**, 2194–2201.

74. Frangioni, J. V., Oda, A., Smith, M., Salzman, E. W., and Neel, B. G. (1993). Calpain-catalyzed cleavage and subcellular relocation of protein phosphotyrosine phosphatase 1B (PTP-B) in human platelets. *EMBO J.* **12**, 4843–4856.

75. Feng, G. S., Hui, C. C., and Pawson, T. (1993). SH2-Containing phosphotyrosine phosphatase as a target of protein-tyrosine kinases. *Science* **259**, 1607–1611.

76. Vogel, W., Lammers, R., Huang, J., and Ullrich, A. (1993). Activation of a phosphotyrosine phosphatase by tyrosine phosphorylation. *Science* **259**, 1611–1614.

77. Maegawa, H., Ugi, S., Ishibashi, O., Tachikawa-Ide, R., Takahara, N., Tanaka, Y., Takagi, Y., Kikkawa, R., Shigeta, Y., and Kashiwagi, A. (1993). Src homology 2 domains of protein tyrosine phosphatase are phosphorylated by insulin receptor kinase and bind to the COOH-terminus of insulin receptors *in vitro*. *Biochem. Biophys. Res. Commun.* **194**, 208–214.

78. Lechleider, R. J., Sugimoto, S., Bennett, A. M., Kashishian, A. S., Cooper, J. A., Shoelson, S. E., Walsh, C. T., and Neel, B. G. (1993). Activation of the SH2-containing phosphotyrosine phosphatase SH-PTP2 by its binding site, phosphotyrosine 1009, on the human platelet-derived growth factor receptor β. *J. Biol. Chem.* **268**, 21478–21481.

79. Zhao, Z., Shen, S. H., and Fischer, E. H. (1993). Stimulation by phospholipids of a protein-tyrosine-phosphatase containing two *src* homology 2 domains. *Proc. Natl. Acad. Sci. U.S.A.* **90**, 4251–4255.

80. Yi, T., and Ihle, J. N. (1993). Association of hematopoietic cell phosphatase with c-Kit after stimulation with c-Kit ligand. *Mol. Cell. Biol.* **13**, 3350–3358.

81. Yi, T., Mui, A. L. F., Krystal, G., and Ihle, J. N. (1993). Hematopoietic cell phosphatase associates with the interleukin-3 (IL-3) receptor β chain and down-regulates IL-3-induced tyrosine phosphorylation and mitogenesis. *Mol. Cell. Biol.* **13**, 7577–7586.

82. Li, W., Nishimura, R., Kashishian, A., Batzer, A. G., Kim, W. J. H., Cooper, J. A., and Schlessinger, J. (1994). A new function for a phosphotyrosine phosphatase: Linking GRB2-Sos to a receptor tyrosine kinase. *Mol. Cell. Biol.* **14,** 509–517.

83. Kuhné, M. R., Pawson, T., Lienhard, G. E., and Feng, G. S. (1993). The insulin receptor substrate 1 associates with the SH2-containing phosphotyrosine phosphatase Syp. *J. Biol. Chem.* **268,** 11479–11481.

84. Stader, C., and Hofer, H. W. (1992). A major lienal phosphotyrosine phosphatase is inhibited by phospholipids and inositol trisphosphate. *Biochem. Biophys. Res. Commun.* **189,** 1404–1409.

85. Gu, M., Warshawsky, I., and Majerus, P. W. (1992). Cloning and expression of a cytosolic megakaryocyte protein-tyrosine-phosphatase with sequence homology to retinaldehyde-binding protein and yeast SEC14p. *Proc. Natl. Acad. Sci. U.S.A.* **89,** 2980–2984.

86. Schievella, A. R., Paige, L. A., Johnson, K. A., Hill, D. E., and Erikson, R. L. (1993). Protein tyrosine phosphatase-1B undergoes mitosis-specific phosphorylation on serine. *Cell Growth Diff.* **4,** 239–246.

87. Flint, A. J., Gebbink, M. F. G. B., Franza, B. R., Hill, D. E., and Tonks, N. K. (1993). Multi-site phosphorylation of the protein tyrosine phosphatase, PTP1B: Identification of cell cycle regulated and phorbol ester stimulated sites of phosphorylation. *EMBO J.* **12,** 1937–1946.

88. Krueger, N. X., and Saito, H. (1992). A human transmembrane protein-tyrosine-phosphatase, PTPζ, is expressed in brain and has an N-terminal receptor domain homologous to carbonic anhydrases. *Proc. Natl. Acad. Sci. U.S.A.* **89,** 7417–7421.

89. Barnea, G., Silvennoinen, O., Shaanan, B., Honegger, A. M., Canoll, P. D., D'Eustachio, P., Morse, B., Levy, J. B., LaForgia, S., Huebner, K., Musacchio, J. M., Sap, J., and Schlessinger, J. (1993). Identification of a carbonic anhydrase-like domain in the extracellular region of RPTPγ defines a new subfamily of receptor tyrosine phosphatases. *Mol. Cell. Biol.* **13,** 1497–1506.

90. Itoh, M., Streuli, M., Krueger, N. X., and Saito, H. (1992). Purification and characterization of the catalytic domains of the human receptor-linked protein tyrosine phosphatases HPTPβ, leukocyte common antigen (LCA), and leukocyte common antigen-related molecule (LAR). *J. Biol. Chem.* **267,** 12356–12363.

91. Wang, Y., and Pallen, C. J. (1991). The receptor-like protein tyrosine phosphatase HPTPα has two active catalytic domains with distinct substrate specificies. *EMBO J.* **10,** 3231–3237.

92. Tan, X., Stover, D. R., and Walsh, K. A. (1993). Demonstration of protein tyrosine phosphatase activity in the second of two homologous domains of CD45. *J. Biol. Chem.* **268,** 6835–6838.

93. Desai, D. M., Sap, J., Schlessinger, J., and Weiss, A. (1993). Ligand-mediated negative regulation of a chimeric transmembrane receptor tyrosine phosphatase. *Cell* **73,** 541–554.

94. Manao, G., Pazzagli, L., Cirri, P., Caselli, A., Camici, G., Cappugi, G., Saeed, A., and Ramponi, G. (1992). Rat liver low M_r phosphotyrosine protein phosphatase isoenzymes: Purification and amino acid sequences. *J. Protein Chem.* **11,** 333–345.

95. Alessi, D. R., Smythe, C., and Keyse, S. M. (1993). The human CL100 gene encodes a Tyr/Thr-protein phosphatase which potently and specifically inactivates MAP kinase and suppresses its activation by oncogenic Ras in *Xenopus* oocyte extracts. *Oncogene* **8,** 2015–2020.

96. Hashimoto, N., Feener, E. P., Zhang, W. R., and Goldstein, B. J. (1992). Insulin receptor protein-tyrosine phosphatases: Leukocyte common antigen-related phosphatase rapidly deactivates the insulin receptor kinase by preferential dephosphorylation of the receptor regulatory domain. *J. Biol. Chem.* **267**, 13811–13814.

97. Bottari, S. P., King, I. N., Reichlin, S., Dahlstroem, I., Lydon, N., and de Gasparo, M. (1992). The angiotensin AT_2 receptor stimulates protein tyrosine phosphatase activity and mediates inhibition of particulate guanylate cyclase. *Biochem. Biophys. Res. Commun.* **183**, 206–211.

98. Tonks, N. K., and Charbonneau, H. (1989). Protein tyrosine dephosphorylation and signal transduction. *Trends Biochem. Sci.* **14**, 497–500.

99. Jena, B. P., Padfield, P. J., Ingebritsen, T. S., and Jamieson, J. D. (1991). Protein tyrosine phosphatase stimulates Ca^{2+}-dependent amylase secretion from pancreatic acini. *J. Biol. Chem.* **266**, 17744–17746.

100. Seger, R., Ahn, N. G., Posada, J., Munar, E. S., Jensen, A. M., Cooper, J. A., Cobb, M. H., and Krebs, E. G. (1992). Purification and characterization of mitogen-activated protein kinase activator(s) from epidermal growth factor-stimulated A431 cells. *J. Biol. Chem.* **267**, 14373–14381.

101. Abdel-Latif, A. A. (1991). Biochemical and functional interactions between the inositol 1,4,5-trisphosphate-Ca^{2+} and cyclic AMP signalling systems in smooth muscle. *Cell. Signal.* **3**, 371–385.

102. Gong, M. C., Fuglsang, A., Alessi, D., Kobayashi, S., Cohen, P., Somlyo, A. V., and Somlyo, A. P. (1992). Arachidonic acid inhibits myosin light chain phosphatase and sensitizes smooth muscle to calcium. *J. Biol. Chem.* **267**, 21492–21498.

103. Simpson, I. A., and Cushman, S. W. (1986). Hormonal regulation of mammalian glucose transport. *Annu. Rev. Biochem.* **55**, 1059–1089.

104. Ismail-Beigi, F. (1993). Metabolic regulation of glucose transport. *J. Membr. Biol.* **135**, 1–10.

105. Klip, A., Ramlal, T., Bilan, P. J., Marette, A., Liu, Z., and Mitsumoto, Y. (1993). What signals are involved in the stimulation of glucose transport by insulin in muscle cells? *Cell. Signal.* **5**, 519–529.

106. Bell, G. I., Burant, C. F., Takeda, J., and Gould, G. W. (1993). Structure and function of mammalian facilitative sugar transporters. *J. Biol. Chem.* **268**, 19161–19164.

107. Gould, G., W., and Holman, G. D. (1993). The glucose transporter family: Structure, function and tissue-specific expression. *Biochem. J.* **295**, 329–341.

108. Baly, D. L., and Horuk, R. (1987). Dissociation of insulin-stimulated glucose transport from the translocation of glucose carriers in rat adipose cells. *J. Biol. Chem.* **262**, 21–24.

109. Calderhead, D. M., and Lienhard, G. E. (1988). Labeling of glucose transporters at the cell surface in 3T3-L1 adipocytes: Evidence for both translocation and a second mechanism in the insulin stimulation of transport. *J. Biol. Chem.* **263**, 12171–12174.

110. Gibbs, E. M., Lienhard, G. E., and Gould, G. W. (1988). Insulin-induced translocation of glucose transporters to the plasma membrane precedes full stimulation of hexose transport. *Biochemistry* **27**, 6681–6685.

111. Fingar, D. C., and Birnbaum, M. J. (1994). Characterization of the mitogen-activated protein kinase/90-kilodalton ribosomal protein S6 kinase signaling pathway in 3T3-L1 adipocytes and its role in insulin-stimulated glucose transport. *Endocrinol. (Baltimore)* **134**, 728–735.

112. Kelly, K. L., Mato, J. M., Merida, I., and Jarett, L. (1987). Glucose transport and antilipolysis are differentially regulated by the polar head group of an insulin-sensitive glycophospholipid. *Proc. Natl. Acad. Sci. U.S.A.* **84**, 6404–6407.

113. Rice, K. M., and Garner, C. W. (1994). Correlation of the insulin receptor substrate-1 with insulin-responsive deoxyglucose transport in 3T3-L1 adipocytes. *Biochem. Biophys. Res. Commun.* **198**, 523–530.

114. Okada, T., Kawano, Y., Sakakibara, T., Hazeki, O., and Ui, M. (1994). Essential role of phosphatidylinositol 3-kinase in insulin-induced glucose transport and antilipolysis in rat adipocytes: Studies with a selective inhibitor wortmannin. *J. Biol. Chem.* **269**, 3568–3573.

115. Farese, R. V. (1990). Lipid-derived mediators in insulin action. *Proc. Soc. Exp. Biol. Med.* **195**, 312–324.

116. Blackshear, P. J., Haupt, D. M., and Stumpo, D. J. (1991). Insulin activation of protein kinase C: A reassessment. *J. Biol. Chem.* **266**, 10946–10952.

117. Guma, A., Munoz, P., Camps, M., Testar, X., Palacin, M., and Zorzano, A. (1992). Inhibitors such as staurosporine, H-7 or polymyxin B cannot be used in skeletal muscle to prove the role of protein kinase C on insulin action. *Biosci. Rep.* **12**, 413–424.

118. Cooper, D. R., Watson, J. E., Hernandez, H., Yu, B., Standaert, M. L., Ways, D. K., Arnold, T. T., Ishizuka, T., and Farese, R. V. (1992). Direct evidence for protein kinase C involvement in insulin-stimulated hexose uptake. *Biochem. Biophys. Res. Commun.* **188**, 142–148.

119. Weinstein, S. P., Watts, J., and Haber, R. S. (1991). Thyroid hormone increases muscle/fat glucose transporter gene expression in rat skeletal muscle. *Endocrinol. (Baltimore)* **129**, 455–464.

120. Honnor, R. C., Naghshineh, S., Cushman, S. W., Wolff, J., Simpson, I. A., and Londos, C. (1992). Cholera and pertussis toxins modify regulation of glucose transport activity in rat adipose cells: Evidence for mediation of a cAMP-independent process by G-proteins. *Cell. Signal.* **4**, 87–98.

121. James, D. E., Hiken, J., and Lawrence, J. C. (1989). Isoproterenol stimulates phosphorylation of the insulin-regulatable glucose transporter in rat adipocytes. *Proc. Natl. Acad. Sci. U.S.A.* **86**, 8368–8372.

122. Lawrence, J. C., Hiken, J. F., and James, D. E. (1990). Phosphorylation of the glucose transporter in rat adipocytes: Identification of the intracellular domain at the carboxyl terminus as a target for phosphorylation in intact cells and *in vitro*. *J. Biol. Chem.* **265**, 2324–2332.

123. Nishimura, H., Saltis, J., Habberfield, A. D., Garty, N. B., Greenberg, A. S., Cushman, S. W., Londos, C., and Simpson, I. A. (1991). Phosphorylation state of the GLUT4 isoform of the glucose transporter in subfractions of the rat adipose cell: Effects of insulin, adenosine, and isoproterenol. *Proc. Natl. Acad. Sci. U.S.A.* **88**, 11500–11504.

124. Piper, R. C., James, D. E., Slot, J. W., Puri, C., and Lawrence, J. C. (1993). GLUT4 phosphorylation and inhibition of glucose transport by dibutyryl cAMP. *J. Biol. Chem.* **268**, 16557–16563.

PART **4**

Gene Regulation
by Hormones

CHAPTER **12**

Hormonally Regulated Transcription Factors

CHAPTER OUTLINE

I. Introduction

In Part 3, mechanisms by which hormones and their second messengers directly affect cellular processes were discussed. This part of the book describes mechanisms by which these molecules affect gene expression. Chapter 12 discusses the hormonal control of transcription factors and their mechanisms of action. Chapter 13 then examines the role of DNA organization and conformation on transcription; in particular, nucleosomes and their covalent modification, DNA methylation, and DNA conformation will be discussed. Finally, the hormonal control of various post-transcriptional events is summarized; such events include RNA stability, processing, transport, and translation, as well as the post-translational modification of proteins.

II. Transcription Factors: General

For completeness, this section will at least briefly cover each major structural class of transcription factors (1–4). This discussion will then be followed by a more detailed examination of those groups that are hormonally regulated (see Table 12-1). In reviewing the known factors, it is important to keep in mind several basic principles (1). First, the α-helix is the most common secondary structure used to bind DNA; presumably this frequency is a result of the greater versatility or stability of the α helix versus the β structure. All hormone response element (HRE) recognition helices in eukaryotic transcription factors have the same basic structure: an amino-terminal half that binds the DNA bases and a carboxy-terminal half that interacts with the deoxyribose–phosphate backbone (5). Second, the factors primarily bind in the major groove because the nucleotides are more accessible, especially to an α helix. Minor groove contacts are usually made by an isolated peptide strand, which augments the major contacts in the wider groove. Third, the DNA backbone constitutes about half of all the contacts. Although these contacts are to the deoxyribose–phosphate backbone, they are not necessarily nonspecific since the base sequence can produce local alterations in the DNA structure that are sufficient to add to the overall specificity of binding. Finally, there is no unique correspondence between amino acids and the bases they contact; that is, there is no simple code for determining to what nucleotide sequence a given protein sequence will bind.

A. DNA-Binding and Dimerization Motifs

1. Helix–Turn–Helix (HTH)

One of the simplest and evolutionarily earliest DNA-binding motifs is the *HTH*. The bacterial prototype consists of two α helices separated by a β turn (Fig. 12-1A). The second, or carboxy-terminal, helix is the recognition helix and lies in the major groove to make specific contacts with the bases.

Table 12-1
Transcription Factors Mediating Hormone Action

Transcription factor	Activating hormone or second messenger
Zinc twist	
Nuclear receptors	Steroids, sterols, retinoids, T_3
Peroxisome proliferator activated receptor (PPAR)	Fatty acids
Leucine zippers (bZIP)	
Jun-Fos (AP-1)	PKC > PKA
CREB	PKA > PKC
C/EBPβ (NF-IL6)	CaM, IL-6 (via MAPK)
Helix–loop–helix (bHLH)	
Aromatic hydrocarbon (Ah) receptor	Aromatic hydrocarbons
MyoD	Inhibited by PKC
bHLH-ZIP	
Myc-Max	CKII, MAPK
Fos interacting protein (FIP)	PKC > PKA
Helix–span–helix	
AP-2	PKC > PKA
POU family	
Pit-1 and Oct-1	TRH (via calcium)
Unknown Class	
Serum response factor (SRF)	Various growth factors (via CKII and MAPK)
NF-κB	PKC and reactive O_2 intermediates > PKA
IFN stimulated gene factor	IFN and other growth factors (via tyrosine phosphorylation)
CTF/NF1	TGFβ

The first helix lies on top of the second at a right angle and makes nonspecific contacts with the backbone. The amino-terminal tail also binds in an adjacent major groove. Transcription factors with HTH motifs bind as dimers to DNA sequences with dyad symmetry.

Higher organisms have a variation on this structure called the *homeodomain* (Fig. 12-1B). This family has three helices; as in the HTH proteins, the carboxy-terminal helix lies in the major groove to make specific contacts. To make this contact, the bases at the ends of the recognition sequence are tilted to slightly bend around the third helix. The first two helices lie on top. Because of the additional helix, the amino-terminal tail is displaced and lies in the 5' minor groove. Although the binding is weak ($K_d \sim 10^{-7}$ M), it adds to the overall DNA affinity of this family. Alone, the third helix has a K_d of $\sim 1-2 \times 10^{-9}$ M. Examples of this family include the homeotic proteins of *Drosophila*, the MAT factors in yeast, and a transcription factor for the somatropin release-inhibiting factor (SRIF) gene in the gastrointestinal tract of mammals (6,7).

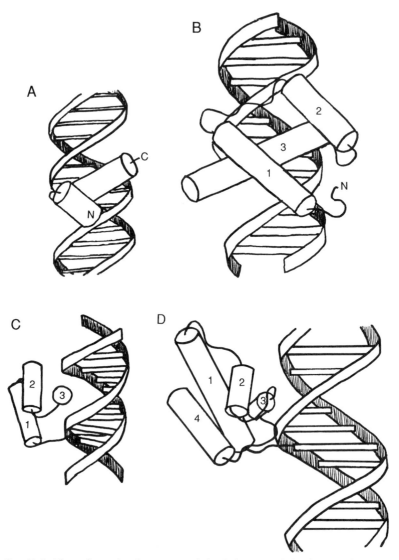

Fig. 12-1. Three-dimensional structure of the helix–turn–helix family of transcription factors. (A) helix–turn–helix, (B) homeodomain (viewed from above), (C) homeodomain (viewed from the side), (D) POU_S domain.

The *POU* family represents a variation of the homeodomain (8). The name is an acronym derived from the first three groups of transcription factors in which the motif was recognized: Pit-1, the Oct subfamily, and Unc-86. This motif contains a standard homeodomain, called POU_H, preceded by a conserved 75- to 82-amino-acid sequence called POU_S. This latter region is composed of four α helices; the second and third form a classic HTH structure with the third helix lying in the major groove (Fig. 12-1C; 9,10). The first and fourth helices are antiparallel to each other and lie on top of the HTH structure and perpendicular to the second helix. There is a hydrophobic core between these helices. The POU_S domain is homologous to several bacterial repressors, such as the λ and Cro repressors. These inhibitors have an absolute requirement for dimerization for DNA binding; this is accomplished by a fifth helix that acts as a dimerization interface. This helix does not exist in POU_S; rather it is replaced by a variable linker (14–26 amino acids) that couples POU_S to POU_H. This bridge appears to be unstructured because of its susceptibility to proteolysis, and it allows POU_S to bind DNA in either orientation (11). In summary, the POU factors consists of two different covalently linked HTH motifs, instead of the two noncovalently linked homodimers seen in the bacterial homologs.

The recognition sequence for the Oct subfamily is ATGC followed by an AT-rich sequence; POU_S binds ATGC whereas POU_H binds the AT-rich region. Members of the Oct subfamily dimerize weakly in solution, although their binding does exhibit cooperativity when binding to duplicated sequences. Pit-1 forms a much stronger dimer; this phenomenon is probably related to the fact that its DNA-binding site is also usually dimeric. The dimerization is thought to be mediated by the first two helices of POU_H (12).

The final motif was first described in the Myb family (13) and later found in the Ets family (14). Like the homeodomain, the Myb motif has three helices; the third is the recognition helix, while the first two lie on top. However, there are two important differences; first, the second helix is not parallel to the first but lies at an angle so that the three helices form a triangle. Second, highly conserved tryptophan residues in the middle of each helix project out toward the center of the complex in order to form a hydrophobic core.

2. Zinc Finger

Three transcription factor families bind zinc and none have any structural similarity to the others. The first group was discovered in TFIIIA and will be referred to as the true zinc fingers, or simply zinc fingers. This motif consists of 12–14 amino acids bounded by a cysteine pair at the amino terminus and a histidine pair at the carboxy terminus (Fig. 12-2A). These amino acids force the intervening sequence into a loop; the ascending limb is part of a β sheet whereas the descending limb forms an α helix. The helix sits in the major groove at about a 45° angle with its amino-terminal end contacting the DNA. Because only the tip of the finger touches the DNA, each finger can only contact 3–4 bases and many fingers are required to recognize a specific sequence. These fingers are very periodic: each unit rotates 32° along the DNA axis. The ascending limb of β structure makes contacts with the deoxyribose–phosphate backbone.

The nuclear receptors, including the peroxisome proliferator activated receptor (PPAR), constitute a second group containing zinc (15,16). As discussed in Chapter 5, all four coordinating amino acids are cysteines and the overall conformation is that of a loop–helix–extended region (Fig. 12-2B).

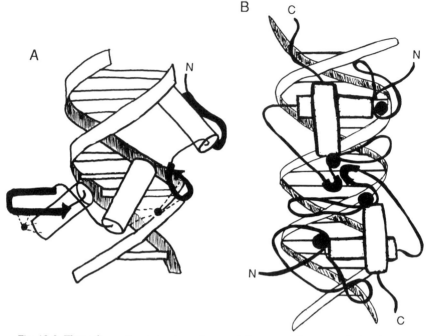

Fig. 12-2. Three-dimensional structure of several zinc-containing transcription factors. (A) zinc finger, (B) zinc twist (nuclear receptors).

There are two "fingers"; the α helix begins in the carboxy-terminal cysteine pair of each and extends into the following sequence. The amino-terminal helix is the recognition helix and lies in the major groove, whereas the preceding loop binds the deoxyribose–phosphate backbone; the second helix lies on top. Both helices are amphipathic and their hydrophobic sides form the core of their association. For this reason, this structure is more accurately referred to as a *zinc twist*; others have called it a *double-loop zinc helix*. Essentially, it is a fancy HTH stabilized by zinc coordination. The nuclear receptors bind DNA as dimers; this association is mediated, in part, by the amino-terminal knuckle of the second zinc twist.

The third group is the zinc cluster. Because it has a coiled coil dimerization motif, it will be discussed in the next section.

3. Coiled Coils

A coiled coil is an oligomerization motif first identified in intermediate filaments. Basically, two α helices line up in parallel and twist into a left-handed supercoil. This interaction is stabilized by hydrophobic binding; indeed, a coiled coil motif can be recognized from its primary sequence, which shows a heptad repeat: every fourth and seventh amino acid is hydrophobic (Fig. 12-3A). In this figure, these positions appear to line up opposite each other; in fact, the amino acids are slightly offset. For example, the leucine at position d is bounded both in front and behind by the a' amino

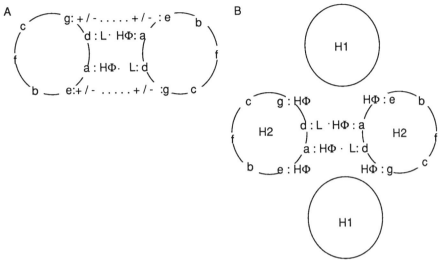

Fig. 12-3. A cross-sectional representation of (A) a coiled coil dimer and (B) a tetramer. a–g, Amino acid positions in a heptad repeat; HΦ, any hydrophobic amino acid; L, leucine.

acids from consecutive repeats on the opposite strand. This leucine is also bounded below by the leucine at d' and above by the amino acid at e'. This four-point enclosure can be constructed around every hydrophobic amino acid in the a/a' and d/d' positions; this arrangement is often referred to as a "knobs-in-holes" structure (17). In dimers, the amino acids at e and g form ionic bonds that determine the specificity of dimerization (18). In tetramers, these residues are hydrophobic and form lipophilic troughs for two additional helices (Fig. 12-3B; 19).

The coiled coils of transcription factors are unique because position d is almost exclusively leucine. This fact led to speculation that the dimer was formed when the forked side-chains of these amino acids interlocked, like a zipper; the motif subsequently became known as a *leucine zipper*. In truth, leucine is the preferred amino acid because its dimensions produce the best and closest packing. Then why do intermediate filaments not have a strict requirement for leucine at d? The reason lies in the pitch, which is very shallow: it takes 16 repeats for one full turn of the supercoil. Transcription factors usually have only 4–6 repeats; this length is only between a quarter turn and a half turn. This very limited entwining facilitates interchange between subunits but also reduces dimer stability; the use of leucine maximizes the dimer interaction over this short distance. The extraordinary length of intermediate filaments results in several supercoil turns; the additional contacts compensate for the use of slightly less optimal hydrophobic amino acids.

The simplest transcription factors in this group have a basic amino-terminal extension of the α helix (*bZIP*). The carboxy terminus dimerizes while the amino terminus bows out to straddle the DNA in the major grooves (Fig. 12-4A). This figure depicts the factor GCN4 (20); the spacing of the HRE for

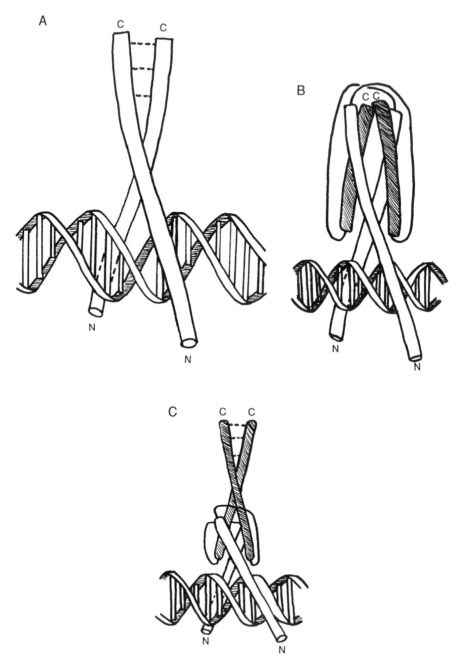

Fig. 12-4. Three-dimensional structure of the coiled coil family of transcription factors. (A) basic zipper (bZIP), (B) basic helix–loop–helix (bHLH); (C) bZIP–HLH.

Jun–Fos is slightly different because the contacts between the basic end of the helix and the DNA cannot be made without bending the DNA. Jun bends the DNA toward the dimer interface while Fos bends it away (21).

The *basic helix–loop–helix* (bHLH) factors have a second coiled coil carboxy-terminal to the first; the two are separated by an Ω loop. The second pair of helices fits into the hydrophobic troughs formed by dimerization of the first pair (Fig. 12-4B; 22). The loop is required to flip the second pair so they are parallel to the first set. Essentially, bHLH is a bZIP in which the carboxy terminus forms a tetramer instead of a dimer. The *helix–span–helix* factors are identical except that the loop is longer. Finally, the second pair of α helices can have a carboxy-terminal extension beyond the tetramer (Fig. 12-4C; 19). These factors have two long helices; the amino-terminal pair forms a classic bZIP. The carboxy-terminal pair also forms a coiled coil at the carboxy-terminal end; however, the amino terminus flares out to fit in the grooves of the first zipper to form a tetramer. Essentially, these factors are bHLH proteins followed by a zipper; as such, they are often abbreviated *bHLH–ZIP*.

The last group possesses characteristics from several classes. The *zinc cluster* has two zinc atoms in a binuclear cluster that stabilizes two short α helices at right angles (Fig. 12-5). The end of the amino-terminal helix is basic and points into the major groove (23–25). An extended linker originating from the carboxy-terminal helix traces the DNA backbone for three-quarters of a turn, where the peptide forms a coiled coil with its dimerization partner. There is evidence for another dimerization region carboxy-terminal to the first; this second oligomerization domain may fold back to form a HLH motif. Basically, these factors are bZIP or bHLH proteins without the DNA-binding amino-terminal extension of the first pair of helices. Instead, the DNA-binding region is a separate module attached to the coiled coil by a tether. This structure allows the components of the HRE to be widely separated; for example, GAL4 recognizes the CCG sequence at the ends of a 17-bp HRE. This distance represents one and a half turns of the DNA helix. Interestingly, the intervening sequence is also recognized by another transcription factor that presumably forms a supercomplex with GAL4.

B. Transcription Activation Motifs

Transcription activation domains have been mapped in several factors; they are often characterized by an abundance of a particular amino acid rather than by a specific sequence (26,27). The most studied motif, one enriched in acidic amino acids, is known as an *acid blob, negative noodle,* or *acid noodle;* the names refer to both the charge and the original belief that these structures formed random coils (28). Later, they were postulated to form amphipathic α helices that interacted with other transcription factors having basic helices. Most recently, they have been predicted to form a hydrophobic β sheet; the negative charges may be necessary to make the lipophilic sheet more accessible (29). Whatever the secondary structure, acidic domains are

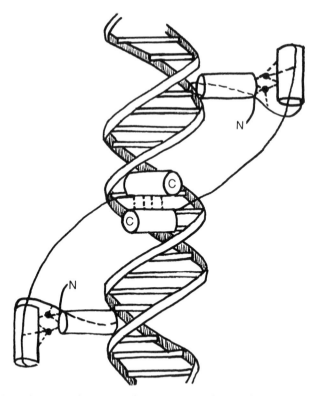

Fig. 12-5. Three-dimensional structure of the zinc cluster family of transcription factors.

known to stimulate RNA polymerase II, and they bind to TATA-box factors TFIIB (30,31) and TFIID (32,33) and to the replication protein A (34,35). The last protein is involved with DNA unwinding. In addition to direct contacts, adaptor molecules that form a bridge between the acidic motifs and other transcription factors have been identified (36).

Other domains rich in glutamine, proline, serine–threonine, or isoleucine (37) have also been documented. Except for the proline-rich regions, these motifs are characterized by their amino acid composition and not their sequence. Some proline-rich regions do contain the sequence Pro–Ser–(+) and form polyproline, or collagen-like, helices (38). These sequences have been shown to bind in the narrow groove of AT-rich domains (39), but it is not known if this interaction occurs in intact cells or whether it has any relationship to transcription activation.

The one characteristic common to all these motifs is their hydrophobicity. Proline and isoleucine are clearly lipophilic; the acidic residues in the acidic domains only serve to increase the accessibility of an otherwise hydrophobic β structure; and glutamine may have a similar function, since mutational studies have shown that the transcriptional activity resides in the hydrophobic amino acids and not in the glutamines (40). Hydrophobic segments in proteins are "sticky" and often participate in protein-protein interactions. As such, TADs may act by attracting critical transcription factors to promoters via their hydrophobic domains.

III. Transcription Factors: Specific

A. Leucine Zipper (bZIP)

1. Activating Transcription Factor (ATF) Family

The ATF family consists of at least two subfamilies (41,42): cAMP response element binding protein (CREB) and cAMP response element modulator (CREM). CREB (Fig. 12-6A) is regulated by protein kinase A (PKA) phosphorylation in a regulatory domain known as the P-box. This modification triggers the subsequent phosphorylation of five adjacent sites by casein kinase II (CKII) and one nearby site by glycogen synthase kinase-3 (GSK-3). This cluster of negative charges interacts with a preceding basic domain to produce a conformational change that enhances transcription activation 10- to 15-fold. It may also increase the affinity of CREB for certain CREs (43). PKC has been reported to modify the same sites *in vitro* (44), but the physiological significance of this event has been questioned (45). In response to elevated calcium levels, calmodulin-dependent protein kinase II (CaMKII) also phosphorylates the same serine as PKA and activates transcription by CREB (46,47). However, this modification by CaMKII is believed to occur only in neurons. Therefore, cAMP is the major activator of CREB and this effect is achieved through PKA-induced phosphorylation.

An alternatively spliced variant of CREB lacks the basic region just prior to the P-box. This variant, also called ATF-1, is actually 5 times more abundant than CREB although it is also 10 times less active (48). ATF-1 may be a natural inhibitor that keeps basal CREB activity low. CREB-2 (or ATF-4) is a homologous protein that lacks both a transcription activation domain (TAD) and a PKA site. It binds CRE but cannot activate transcription; as such, it acts as a repressor (49). Not all members of this family are regulated by PKA. ATF-2 is phosphorylated by mitogen-activated protein kinase (MAPK), which increases the dimerization and DNA binding of ATF-2 (50).

There are five members of the CREM subfamily, all of which are generated by alternative splicing (51). The gene itself is fascinating because several exons are duplicated; therefore, alternative splicing involves not only omitted exons but also choices among two DNA-binding exons and two coiled coil exons. The short forms are all inhibitors. CREMα and CREMβ differ in the DNA-binding exon used and CREMγ lacks a small exon encoding 12 amino acids. All three are missing the pair of glutamine-rich TADs that bracket the P-box; therefore, they cannot activate transcription. Inhibition of intact CREB and CREM requires both dimerization and CRE binding. Interestingly, the short forms still possess the PKA site; this is important, because the P-box

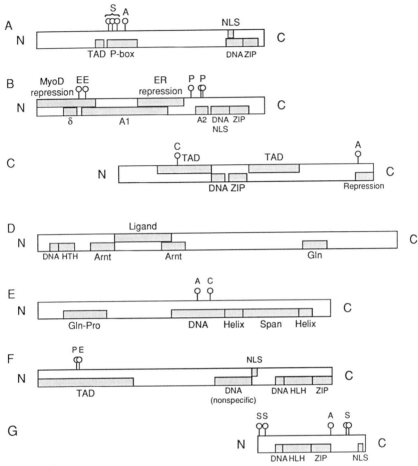

Fig. 12-6. Schematic structure of the coiled coil family of transcription factors. (A) cAMP response element binding protein (CREB); (B) Jun and (C) Fos, which dimerize to form the anterior pituitary factor 1 (AP-1); (D) the aromatic hydrocarbon (Ah) receptor; (E) the anterior pituitary factor 2 (AP-2); (F) Myc and (G) Max, which dimerize. Phosphorylation sites are: A, PKA; C, PKC; E, MAPK; P, GSK-3; S, CKII. Other abbreviations are defined in the text and in the List of Abbreviations at the end of the book.

can activate TADs not only in itself, when present, but also in other transcription factors (52). As such, phosphorylation of this P-box can actually reduce the repression of the short CREMs, presumably by stimulating TADs on adjacent factors. CREMτ is the intact form. It is partially active even without PKA-induced phosphorylation; basal activity is about three times that of CREB. Modification by PKA further increases transcriptional activity but this effect is dampened by simultaneous phosphorylation by Cdc2 (53). S-CREM possesses an alternative start site so the first TAD and the P-box are omitted. This omission results in S-CREM being a repressor, although it is weaker than the short forms that lack both TADs.

2. Jun–Fos (AP-1) Family

Several transcription factors are regulated primarily by PKC; the one in the leucine zipper family is AP-1 (54). Although the most active form of this factor is a heterodimer of Jun and Fos, each protein will first be described separately. Jun has a classic bZIP motif in the carboxy terminus and two TADs, A1 and A2, in the amino terminus (Fig. 12-6). A1 is acidic and A2 is glutamine and proline rich; both have important phosphorylation sites. Transcriptional activity is associated with an increase in phosphorylation in A1 but a decrease in A2. These changes are induced by mitogens, Ras, and activators of PKC; however, PKC does not directly modify Jun. These factors are believed to act at A1 through MAPK (see Fig. 11-2), which directly phosphorylates two critical residues in this region (55). Alternatively, a Jun amino-terminal protein kinase, which has been isolated recently, may be the physiological kinase (56). PKC can activate the dephosphorylated form of this enzyme; as such, the activation of this Jun kinase would represent a more direct pathway than the one involving MAPK. In contrast to A1, A2 is an inhibitory domain when phosphorylated. GSK-3 is the major kinase responsible for constitutively modifying these sites (57,58). PKC can phosphorylate and inhibit GSK-3; since phosphate groups are constantly turning over, the suppression of GSK-3 activity would eventually lead to a reduction in the level of A2 phosphorylation (59). It has also been proposed that PKC may activate a protein phosphatase to accelerate the process, but there are no data on this matter. Whereas A1 primarily affects transcription, the dephosphorylation of A2 increases the binding of Jun to DNA (60).

Note that the phosphorylation of Jun and Fos is very complicated and often depends on the dimerization partner and whether or not AP-1 is bound to DNA. For example, the modification of Jun by PKC, CKII, and cell division cycle kinase 2 (Cdc2) is impaired by DNA binding; however, phosphorylation by the DNA-activated protein kinase (DNA-PK) is enhanced and that by PKA and MAPK is unaffected (61). Phosphorylation by the latter two kinases is also independent of the dimerization partner, but that by CKII is reduced when Jun is coupled with Fos.

There are several other regulatory sites on Jun. A1 is bracketed by two domains that bind a cell-specific inhibitor of this TAD (62); the amino-terminal site, called the δ domain, is also needed for the PKC-induced phosphorylation of A1 (63). Another region that partially overlaps the carboxy terminus of A1 is involved in the repression of estrogen receptor (ER)-induced transcription (64); the zipper region is also believed to be involved in this inhibition. Interactions between the bZIP family and the nuclear receptor family will be discussed in greater detail subsequently. In addition to PKC, AP-1 can be regulated by reactive oxygen intermediates; their target is a conserved cysteine in the DNA-binding domain (DBD) of both Jun and Fos (65,66). Oxidative stress can oxidize these residues and inhibit Jun–Fos.

There are several isoforms of Jun. JunB and JunD bind the same HRE as Jun and can dimerize with Fos, but JunB requires multiple HREs for activity. At singlets, JunB acts as a repressor (67).

Fos is related to Jun, but has its bZIP motif more centrally located in the protein. It also has two TADs that bracket the bZIP structure (Fig. 12-6). Fos is a substrate for many protein kinases, but only one has been shown to be physiologically relevant: a PKA site in the extreme carboxy terminus is required for the transcriptional repression mediated by this domain (68). PKC, CKII, Cdc2, S6 kinase II (S6KII), DNA-PK, and a growth factor-activated Fos kinase have all been shown to phosphorylate Fos, but no effects of these modifications have been documented (69,70).

Like Jun, Fos has several isoforms: FosB, Fra-1, and Fra-2. ΔFosB is a splice variant of FosB that lacks the carboxy-terminal 101 amino acids (60). Since ΔFosB does not have the carboxy-terminal repression domain, it cannot inhibit transcription; however, its transcriptional activity is also reduced.

Jun can homodimerize, bind its HRE, and activate transcription. The Fos zipper sequence is incompatible with homodimerization and this deficiency prevents DNA binding. If Fos is given a Jun zipper, it can homodimerize and bind DNA (71). Fos also has a shorter half-life than Jun; this difference in stability means that Jun–Jun homodimers predominate in the unstimulated state. After Fos induction, Jun–Fos appears. This change in dimer composition is reflected by a switch in HRE preference and gene induction: Jun–Jun prefers the HRE TGACATCA whereas Jun–Fos prefers TGACTCA (54). It also results in a greater stimulation of transcription, since Jun–Fos is a more potent transcription factor than Jun–Jun.

Finally, AP-1 can be regulated by an inhibitor, IP-1 (72,73). This protein loosely binds to AP-1 via the zipper region and blocks DNA binding. It can be phosphorylated and inactivated by either PKA or PKC. This example demonstrates the complexity of transcription factor regulation: although one transduction pathway may appear to dominate the control of a given transcription factor, there are almost always other kinases that can also influence the system.

3. C/EBP Family

Members of the C/EBP family all act at the DNA sequence CCAAT, from which their name is derived: CCAAT/enhancer-binding protein. The one most closely associated with hormonal regulation is called NF-IL6 in humans and C/EBPβ in mice. This transcription factor has an unusual variation of the bZIP motif: a cysteine immediately follows the zipper and is involved in disulfide bond formation (74). Therefore, the coiled coil dimer is reinforced by a covalent link. It is regulated by several kinases: IL-6 activates C/EBPβ by stimulating MAPK to phosphorylate it just before the DBD (75); IL-6 also stimulates a PKC-initiated kinase cascade that phosphorylates and activates the TAD (76); finally, CaMKII can phosphorylate and activate C/EBPβ (77). Because the CaMKII site is located in the zipper, this modification has been postulated to affect dimer selection. However, the site faces away from the protein-protein interface and should not affect dimerization. Also, PKA phosphorylates the proline-rich TAD; however, rather than affecting transcription, this modification stimulates nuclear translocation

(78,79). The several isoforms can all heterodimerize with each other and with C/EBP (80); the heterodimers with C/EBP have greater transcriptional activity than homodimers.

B. Helix–Loop–Helix and Variations

1. Helix–Loop–Helix (bHLH): Ah Receptor and MyoD

The *a*romatic *h*ydrocarbon (Ah) receptor binds several pollutants, the most famous of which is dioxin (81,82). The response element for the Ah receptor is found in genes encoding enzymes that metabolize such compounds. Because it is a ligand-regulated transcription factor and is retained in the cytoplasm by hsp 90 until activation, the Ah receptor was thought to be a member of the nuclear receptor family, perhaps a variation of the peroxisome proliferator activated receptor (PPAR) that bound aromatic instead of aliphatic hydrocarbons. However, cloning of the receptor components revealed them to be bHLH transcription factors. The Ah receptor may still be related to the endocrine system, since the receptor can also be activated by indole derivatives and there are several hormones with indole and other aromatic groups (83).

The Ah receptor is a dimer. Arnt (*A*h *r*eceptor *n*uclear *t*ranslocator) is the hsp 90-binding subunit and is responsible for transporting the LSB (*l*igand-*b*inding *s*ubunit) into the nucleus; both are bHLH proteins, although they share only two small regions of homology (Fig. 12-6D). Arnt binds LSB only after ligand binding has occurred; then hsp 90 dissociates and the dimer migrates into the nucleus and binds DNA. Neither subunit alone can bind DNA.

Another bHLH transcription factor is MyoD, which is involved in muscle differentiation. Growth factors such as fibroblast growth factor (FGF), inhibit differentiation so proliferation can continue; these mitogens inhibit MyoD through two PKC-mediated pathways. First, PKC directly phosphorylates MyoD in the DBD and abolishes DNA binding (84). Second, PKC activates Jun, whose zipper can heterodimerize with the HLH region of MyoD (85); this heterodimer is inactive.

2. Helix–Span–Helix: AP-2

Only one member of the helix–span–helix family is known to be hormonally regulated. AP-2 is found in the *a*nterior *p*ituitary, where it stimulates the transcription of several pituitary hormones (86,87). There is nothing unusual about its structure (Fig. 12-6E). It is stimulated by either PKA or PKC; both sites are located in the DBD, but PKA phosphorylation does not affect DNA binding (88).

3. bHLH-ZIP: Myc–Max

The Myc–Max heterodimer mediates the effects of several mitogens. Myc is an unusual bHLH-ZIP factor because it has a second DBD just amino-terminal to the one associated with the HLH (Fig. 12-6F). This second domain binds DNA nonspecifically and is thought to enable Myc to slide along the DNA to locate its HRE (89). There is some controversy over whether or not Myc can form a homodimer. Even if it does, it is probably not functional, since its DNA affinity is very low (90).

Max, called Myn in mice, is also a bHLH-ZIP factor but is much smaller than Myc because it lacks any known TAD (Fig. 12-6G). Although both the HLH and the zipper regions are required for dimerization, the HLH is a major determinant in Max homodimer formation whereas the zipper is primarily involved with heterodimerization (91). Because Max does not have a TAD, homodimers do not active transcription. In fact, they act as repressors because they can still bind DNA and block its access to other factors. There are several isoforms of Max. Max(s) lacks the first nine amino acids, which are located next to the DBD; this isoform tolerates greater variability at the 5′ end of the HRE (92). ΔMax is a product of alternative splicing that results in a frameshift at amino acid 98 with termination at amino acid 103. Since the zipper is disrupted, dimerization with Myc is less stable and that with Max or ΔMax does not occur at all.

Because Myc homodimerizes poorly and Max lacks a TAD, only Myc–Max heterodimers are transcriptionally active. Based on gel migration studies, Myc–Max bends DNA in a manner similar to Jun–Fos: Max binds DNA away from the HLH-ZIP domain while Myc bends DNA toward this region (93). Surprisingly, this bending is not seen in the three-dimensional structure of Max (94). It is possible that the process of crystallization straightens the DNA to force all the molecules into a repeating structure. The X-ray structure also shows that the loop between the α helices contacts the deoxyribose–phosphate backbone of the minor groove. These added contacts may be necessary to compensate for the reduced flexibility of the bHLH-ZIP; the tetramer is a more rigid structure than the simple dimer of the bZIP factors.

Myc–Max can be regulated by either phosphorylation or inhibitors. PKA impairs Max homodimer formation (95) whereas CKII decreases the DNA-binding affinity of Max homodimers but not of Myc–Max (96). Essentially, Max is activated by modifications that favor heterodimer formation. Both MAPK and GSK-3 phosphorylate the TAD of Myc; the former activates transcription (97) but the function of the latter is unknown (98). In addition to phosphorylation, several homologous inhibitor proteins have been characterized: Mad (*Max dimerization*) (99) and Mxi1 (*Max interactor 1*) (100). These proteins heterodimerize with Max, bind DNA, and repress transcription. It is believed that this alternative heterodimerization acts like a switch. In the uninduced state, Max, which is constitutively synthesized, exists predominantly as homodimers. During growth, Myc is induced, and Myc–Max forms and stimulates the expression of growth-related genes. During differentiation, Mad is induced, and Mad–Max forms and represses the transcription of these same genes.

C. POU Factor: Pit-1

Pit-1 is a pituitary transcription factor that belongs to the POU family. POU_S is responsible for high-affinity DNA binding whereas POU_H only binds DNA with low affinity (Fig. 12-7A). Pit-1 is unusual because it forms dimers more readily than other members of this family; this tendency corresponds to its HRE, which consists of imperfect repeats. Pit-1 can be phosphorylated by either PKA or PKC; however, there are no known consistent effects of PKA. Direct phosphorylation by PKA inhibits Pit-1 by blocking DNA binding, but

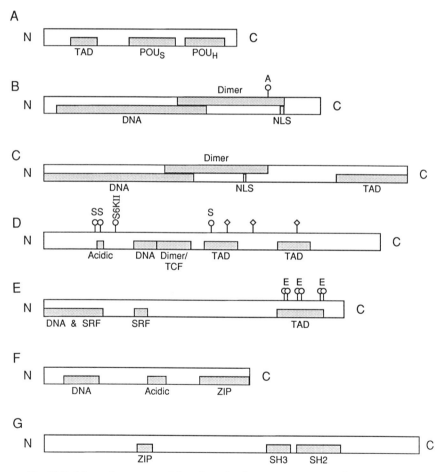

Fig. 12-7. Schematic structure of the other miscellaneous transcription factors. (A) Pit-1; (B) p50 and (C) p65, which dimerize to form the NF-κB factor; (D) serum response factor (SRF) and (E) ternary complex factor (TCF), which oligomerize; (F) interferon-stimulated gene factor γ and (G) 3α (p91), which also oligomerize. Note that the scale of G is two-thirds that of the other factors. Diamonds represent glycosylation sites. Other abbreviations are defined in the text and in Fig. 12-6.

hormones that elevate cAMP *in vivo* enhance Pit-1 activity; the latter effect is indirect and occurs as a result of inducing Pit-1 expression (101).

Thyrotropin-releasing hormone (TRH) stimulates the transcription of the prolactin (PRL) gene through the activation of Pit-1. This activation is mediated by calcium and PKC (102). The resulting phosphorylation alters the HRE preference for Pit-1 (103): the unmodified factor will bind the TATT-CAT core with or without the AT-rich sequence at the 5' end, but phosphorylated Pit-1 shows a requirement for this 5' sequence.

Pit-1 can also be regulated by alternative dimerization. At high Pit-1 concentrations Pit-1 homodimerizes, but at low concentrations Pit-1 will heterodimerize with Oct-1, another member of the POU family (104). Dimerization occurs via the POU_H of Pit-1; Oct-1 replaces POU_H by binding the AT-rich half of the HRE. Certain HREs have a dimer preference, which allows the gene to respond to the concentration of activated Pit-1. For example, the growth hormone (GH) gene prefers the Pit-1 homodimer; this preference means that GH transcription requires high levels of Pit-1. Finally, Pit-1 mRNA is subject to alternative splicing which deletes part of POU_S and converts Pit-1 into a repressor (105).

D. Unknown Class

1. NF-κB

NF-κB is a *n*uclear *f*actor that binds to a response element in the *k* chain gene of the *B* lymphocyte (106; see also Chapter 3). However, this response element has since been shown to be more widespread; it is particularly associated with genes involved in defense mechanisms. NF-κB is a dimer of identical or partially homologous subunits; the most studied form has subunits of 50 and 65 kDa. The entire family composing NF-κB subunits is homologous in the DNA-binding and dimerization domains, which usually form the amino terminus (Figs. 12-7B and 12-7C). p50 has no recognizable TAD and homodimers were thought to be transcriptionally inactive; however, it does activate a variant HRE (Table 12-2; 107). In the closely related subunit p49 (also called p50B), TADs are located in the amino-terminal 100 and carboxy-terminal 150 amino acids (108). Although the sequence in the DBD does not match any known motif, DNA binding does require zinc (109). The p50 precursor has a 550-amino-acid carboxy-terminal extension that acts as an autoinhibitory domain. This extension has seven ankyrin-like repeats; the inhibitory site has been mapped to the last two repeats and the intervening acidic region, which appears to bind the basic nuclear localization signal (NLS) and part of the DBD and mask them (110,111). This carboxy terminus can be generated as a separate molecule by alternative splicing and can still act as an inhibitor; in this form it is referred to as IκBγ (112). Ankyrin domains are also known to bind the cytoskeleton and it has been speculated that this binding may be a second mechanism by which the carboxy terminus of the precursor prevents nuclear migration.

Unlike p50, p65 has a clearly defined TAD located in the carboxy termi-

Table 12-2
DNA Sequence Specificity for Subunits of NF-κB

NF-κB composition	NF-κB response elements[a]			
	GGGGACTTTCC	GGGGAATCTCC	GGGGAATCCC	GGGAAAGTAC
Homodimers				
p49	+	0	0	
p50	B	B	+	
Rel	+	B/0	+	
p65	Weak	0	0	
Heterodimers				
p49–p65	++	B/0	0	
p49–Rel	++	0	0	
p65–Rel	0			B

[a] +, stimulates transcription; 0, does not stimulate transcription; B, binds but transcriptional activation not demonstrated; B/0, binds but does not activate transcription.

nus (Fig. 12-7C). However, it binds DNA poorly as a homodimer, apparently because of steric hindrance by the carboxy terminus, since DNA binding is markedly increased after carboxy-terminal truncation. Binding can also be increased by the presence of multiple HREs or by another subunit, such as p50, that appears to displace the carboxy terminus. p50 and p65 are truly a matched set: p50 binds DNA well but is a weak transcription activator whereas p65 binds DNA poorly but has a strong TAD. p65 binds the 3′ less-conserved end of the HRE and p50 bind the 5′ more-conserved half.

There are several other members of this family. p49 has already been mentioned; it is 60% identical to p50 (113). Rel is more closely related to p65 and appears to bind to a wide range of HRE elements. RelB was originally called I-Rel because no transcriptional activity could be detected and the dimer was thought to be inhibitory. However, other investigators have demonstrated activity; the difference may be a result of the promoter used or of cell specificity. Herein probably lies the explanation for so many subunit variants: each possible combination has a different HRE preference and may also exhibit differences in promoter or cell specificity (Table 12-2; 114,115). Alternative splicing generates even more possibilities; Δp65 lacks a segment in the DBD (116). Although it can still homodimerize with p65, it cannot bind DNA; therefore, it acts as an inhibitor.

Altering subunit composition is only one way that NF-κB can be regulated. Direct phosphorylation of the subunits is possible, but has been demonstrated only for Rel. PKA modification occurs near the NLS and is required for dimerization (117). However, the most common form of regulation is via an inhibitory subunit, IκB, and its variants (118,119). All these inhibitors have ankyrin repeats in the middle of the peptide and function in the same manner as IκBγ: they mask the NLS and trap NF-κB in the cytoplasm until activation. This activation occurs when IκB is phosphorylated by PKC, causing it to dissociate from NF-κB. Evidence for activation by PKA is conflicting: most investigators claim that activation is indirect, since it is slow and phosphorylation is difficult to detect in IκB. However, others report that PKA can directly modify IκB (120,121). There is also evidence for activation by Raf (122) and by the dsRNA kinase (123). Nonetheless, PKC still appears to be the major activator for NF-κB. The activation of some isoforms of IκB may also involve its degradation (124).

The reason for several inhibitors lies in their specificity for the different NF-κB subunits and in their regulation (Table 12-3). For example, IκB is specific for p65; IκBα for p50, and IκBγ for both; the effects of IκBβ are dose dependent. The structural determinants for subunit specificity appear to reside within the first ankyrin repeat (125). However, this scenario is not as simple as it first appears. As noted earlier, p50 homodimers are not very active transcriptionally, although they can still bind DNA well; as a result, they can act as inhibitors. If IκBα inhibits an inhibitor, there will be stimulation. In fact, TADs have been located at both ends of IκBα and some authorities claim that the IκBα–p50 complex directly stimulates transcription (126,127).

Finally, like AP-1, NF-κB is regulated by reactive oxygen intermediates; however, NF-κB is stimulated rather than inhibited by these radicals. The actual targets of these radicals are the soluble tyrosine kinases that stimulate PPI hydrolysis and activate PKC (128). This cascade of events results in the phosphorylation of IκB followed by its proteolytic destruction (129).

2. Serum Response Factor (SRF)

The SRF is another transcription factor whose familial relationship is unknown (130). The DBD is predicted to have either one or two α helices, and the TAD overlaps a serine–threonine-rich region (Fig. 12-7D). This TAD also contains several O-linked glycosylation sites (131). Although strategically located, carbohydrate residues of other factors have never been shown

Table 12-3
Specificity and Regulation of NF-κB Inhibitors

Inhibitor	Alternative name	NF-κB subunit inhibited			Regulating kinase[a]	
		p50	p65	Rel	PKA	PKC
IκB		0	+	+	+	+
IκBα	Bcl-3 variant	+	+/0	0	+/0	+
IκBβ	p40, MAD-3	+[b]	+	+	+	+/0
IκBγ	Carboxy terminus of p50	+	+	+	+	

[a] Effects may not necessarily be direct.
[b] Requires high concentrations.

to affect transcriptional activity (132); however, they may affect localization or stability. The SRF complex is a trimer consisting of two SRFs and one *ternary complex factor* (TCF). It is now known that TCF is identical to Elk1, a member of the Ets family; several members of this family are known to recruit transcription factors to DNA (133,134). TCF also stabilizes the SRF–SRE complex, the half-life of which increases from 1.6–2.5 minutes to 20–30 minutes. TCF is believed to have a Myb-like DBD (14); it binds to the CAGGA sequence just 5′ to the SRE (Fig. 12-7E; 135–137). Several members of this family serve similar functions for other transcription factors; for example, Ets2 is a ternary complex factor for AP-1 on certain HREs (138).

Both SRF and TCF are regulated by phosphorylation. It is clear that MAPK modifies TCF in the carboxy terminus; however, the effects of this phosphorylation are more controversial. Based on gel migration studies, this modification enhances ternary complex formation between TCF and SCF dimers (139), but other researchers point to possible artifacts in the gel experiments and argue that phosphorylation increases transcriptional activity (140,141). CKII phosphorylation of SRF at the amino terminus regulates DNA binding (142), whereas modification of the carboxy terminus is involved in transcriptional repression (143). The mechanism for the effect on DNA binding is controversial: some investigators report that phosphorylation increases the affinity of SRF for SRE, whereas others claim that it only alters exchange rates (144). In addition, S6KII modifies SCF and results in a slight increase in DNA binding (145). Although PKA phosphorylates SRF in the DBD, this modification has no known effects.

3. IFN-Stimulated Gene Factors (ISGFs)

There are several ISGFs. ISGF1 and ISGFγ are the DNA-binding subunits. ISGF1 binds to an inhibitor in the cytosol, and activation involves the dissociation of this inhibitor and the translocation of ISGF1 to the nucleus (146,147). As such, its regulation resembles that of the NF-κB. The DBD is reported to be homologous to that of GAL4, a zinc cluster factor (see preceding discussion). However, two facts cast doubt on this hypothesis. First, ISGF1 binds to the core of the ISRE rather than at the ends, as one would expect for a zinc cluster. Second, the coiled coil is an unusually long distance away from the DBD for a zinc cluster (Fig. 12-7F). ISGF3γ binds to the 5′ end of the ISRE; it also binds to ISGF3α via a coiled coil region (148).

ISGFα actually consists of three peptides: two are alternatively spliced products (p91 and p84) from a single gene and the third is a homologous protein (p113) from a separate gene (149–152). Each has an SH2, an SH3, and a coiled coil domain but no DBD; as such, ISGFα does not bind DNA. ISGFα remains in the cytoplasm until the cell is stimulated by interferon-α (IFN-α), which activates a member of the Jak family of soluble tyrosine kinases (151,153). ISGFα is assumed to associate with Jak via its SH2 domain, after which all three ISGFα proteins become phosphorylated by Jak. This modification is required for nuclear translocation and DNA binding of p91 and p84 (154). It is also required for transcriptional activation by p91;

p84 does not appear to have any transcriptional activity. In the nucleus, ISGFα complexes with ISGFγ and stabilizes the ISGFγ–DNA complex.

p91 occupies a central position in the transcriptional pathway used by many hormones (155–158). As noted already, IFN-α phosphorylates p91 and p113 which, along with ISGF3γ, form ISGF3, which then binds to the ISRE. IFN-γ only phosphorylates p91, whose dimer is also called GAF (IFN-γ-*activated factor*) and binds to the related HRE GAS (IFN-γ-*activated site*). Finally, epidermal growth factor (EGF), platelet-derived growth factor (PDGF), and other growth factors can phosphorylate p91 and at least one other, still unidentified component. This complex forms the SIF (*sis-inducible factor*), which binds another related HRE, the SIE (*sis-inducible element*). At least for the EGFR, the phosphorylation of p91 is direct. p91 is the central character in all these pathways; specificity of action is provided by the other components within the final complex.

E. Summary of Regulation

As the various transcription factors were described here, several mechanisms of regulation were encountered (Table 12-4). It may be useful to summarize them now. First, transcription factors can be induced; this mechanism is particularly important for short-lived factors such as Fos. For example, basal AP-1 activity is due to Jun homodimers because Fos has a much shorter

Table 12-4
General Mechanisms for the Regulation of Transcription Factors

Mechanism	Examples
Transcription	Fos, Myc
Post-transcriptional processing	
Deleted exons	ΔFosB, Δp65, ΔMax
Alternative exons	CREM
Post-translational modifications	
Phosphorylation	See Fig. 12-8
Cleavage	PKC-induced cleavage of p50 precursor
Glycosylation	SRF (?)
Protein–protein interactions	
Inhibitors	IP-1, IκB
Dimers	Jun–Jun vs. Jun–Fos, Myc–Max vs. Mad–Max
Cofactors	TCF for SRF, ISGFα for ISGF1–ISGFγ
Compartmentalization	
Transcription factor phosphorylation status	Rel, C/EBPβ, NF-AT
NLS-masking subunit	IκB, hsp 90
Allosterism	
Hormones	Nuclear receptors
Other ligands	PPAR, Ah receptor

half-life than Jun. With induction, Fos increases, forms heterodimers with Jun, increases its activity, and slightly shifts the HRE preference. Although important, this mechanism requires RNA and protein synthesis and, therefore, is not a primary response.

Another site of regulation occurs at the level of post-transcriptional modification. Many examples of alternative splicing were given. The most common form is the omission of an exon; this deletion usually cripples the factor, resulting in the creation of an inhibitor. Alternatively, the effects may be more selective: the insertion of an extra 26 amino acids in Pit-1 eliminates its ability to induce transcription of the PRL gene, although its stimulation of GH expression is unaltered (159,160). In more elaborate examples, there may be multiple copies of one or more exons, from which a single set is chosen; CREM represents such a paradigm.

However, the regulation most closely linked with the endocrine system is post-translational modification, especially phosphorylation (79,161). Figure 12-8 depicts several of the systems discussed already. Although many kinases may act on any given transcription factor, for clarity only the most prominent kinases are shown for each factor. Glycosylation is another post-translational modification that has been proposed to regulate transcription factors, but the data are still lacking. Finally, p50 can be activated by the proteolytic removal of its inhibitory carboxy terminus; this modification is stimulated by PKC (118) and is obviously irreversible.

Protein–protein interactions represent a fourth mechanism. There are three types of interactions: (i) inhibitors, (ii) dimerization partners, and (iii) cofactors. Inhibitors would include IP-1 and IκB which bind and block the DNA binding of AP-1 and NF-κB, respectively; in both cases, phosphorylation causes dissociation of the inhibitor. The heat shock proteins and steroid receptors represent other examples; here, dissociation follows ligand binding. As noted earlier, most transcription factors are dimers whose partners can come from any member within a particular family; indeed, dimerization between families has also been reported (see subsequent discussion). Transcriptional activity, HRE preference, and regulation are often influenced by the kinds of partners present in the dimer; for example, Myc–Max stimulates transcription whereas Mad–Max inhibits it, and Jun–Jun prefers to bind the sequence TGACATCA whereas Jun–Fos binds TGACTCA. Finally, the transcription factor may require auxiliary proteins, which may be regulated themselves. For example, SCF requires TCF, whose propensity for ternary complex formation is controlled by MAPK; ISGF1–ISGFγ requires ISGFα, whose intracellular localization is regulated by tyrosine phosphorylation.

Fifth, transcription factors can be regulated by compartmentalization (162). This subcellular localization can be controlled by several mechanisms. First, nuclear migration can be induced by the phosphorylation of either the DNA-binding component or some other regulatory subunit; Rel and C/EBPβ are examples of the former, and ISGF3α is an example of the latter. Nuclear localization can also be stimulated by dephosphorylation: NF-AT is a T-cell transcription factor that migrates to the nucleus after it is dephosphorylated

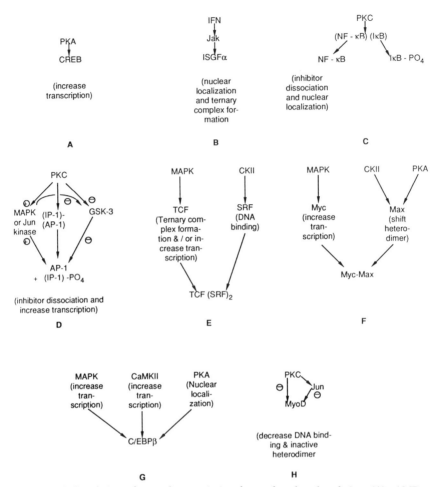

Fig. 12-8. Regulation of several transcription factors by phosphorylation. (A) cAMP response element binding protein (CREB), (B) interferon-stimulated gene factor α (ISGFα), (C) nuclear factor kappa binding protein (NF-κB), (D) anterior pituitary 1 factor (AP-1), (E) serum response factor (SRF), (F) Myc–Max, (G) C/EBPB, (H) MyoD. CaMKII, CaM-dependent kinase II; CKII, casein kinase II; IP-1 and IkB, transcription factor inhibitory subunits; MAPK, MAP kinase; PKA, protein kinase A; PKC, protein kinase C; TCF, ternary complex factor.

by PP-2B. This calcium–CaM regulated phosphatase is activated by the PPI pathway in these cells. Finally, nuclear localization can be achieved by unmasking the NLS: in NF-κB and GR, a masking subunit is removed by phosphorylation or ligand binding, respectively; in p50, the carboxy terminus of the precursor blocks the NLS and unmasking is achieved by proteolysis.

Finally, transcription factors can be regulated allosterically. The regulation of the nuclear receptors for steroids, retinoids, and thyroid hormones has already been extensively discussed (see Chapter 5). PPAR is activated by fatty acids, especially arachidonic acid, which is a second messenger in the PPI pathway. The Ah receptor has no known endogenous ligand, but it is regulated by aromatic hydrocarbons in the environment.

IV. Specificity Problems

A. Promiscuity

By emphasizing only the major kinases regulating each transcription factor, Fig. 12-8 belies the extensive overlap that occurs in the regulation of these proteins. This overlap leads to problems of how specificity is achieved and involves four general areas: (i) many second messengers act through the same transcription factor; (ii) many different transcription factors can hetero-dimerize; (iii) many different factors can bind the same HRE; and (iv) one factor may bind to many different HREs.

For example, PKC is considered to be the major activator of AP-1 be-cause it initiates a cascade that leads to a shift in the phosphorylation of Jun; however, PKA can also stimulate AP-1 by phosphorylating and blocking IP-1, an AP-1 inhibitor. PKC is also considered to be the primary stimulator of NF-κB because its modification of IκB causes the dissociation of the inhibitor; but again, PKA can also remove this inhibitor, although there is still controversy over whether or not this effect is direct. On the other hand, PKA is the major activator of CREB, although PKC and CaMKII can phos-phorylate the same sites on CREB in some tissues, and both PKA and PKC can equally activate AP-2. Therefore, both PKA and PKC can activate AP-1, AP-2, CREB, and NF-κB.

This phenomenon can be further complicated by the promiscuous di-merization of transcription factors that are regulated differently, thereby leading to even greater convergence. For example, there is considerable cross-dimerization within the thyroid hormone receptor family, most of which can bind at least one common HRE. In general, a single ligand can activate the receptor whereas ligands for both components act synergisti-cally. Jun, activated by PKC, can dimerize with CREB or ATF, activated by PKA, and bind the CRE (163). In addition to intrafamily associations, hetero-dimerization can also occur between different families: Jun (leucine zipper) can bind MyoD (bHLH), NF-κB (Rel homology), and nuclear receptors (zinc twist) (164,165); the glucocorticoid receptor (zinc twist) can bind p65 (Rel homology) and Oct-1 (POU) (166,167); and the C/EBP family (leucine zip-per) can bind the NF-κB family (Rel homology) (168).

Although most of these interfamily interactions are inhibitory, C/EBP activity is actually enhanced when it is associated with NF-κB; however, NF-κB activity is reduced (168). Some of the complexes containing nuclear receptors can impart ligand regulation on the entire system; for example, the Jun-TR dimer is regulated by T_3. The Jun activity in this dimer is stimulated in the absence of T_3 but is inhibited in the presence of this ligand (169).

Additional loss of specificity occurs when multiple transcription factors bind the same HRE. The classic example is the glucocorticoid receptor family: the glucocorticoid, progesterone, androgen, and mineralocorticoid receptors all bind the identical HRE, despite having very distinct biological activities. In addition, several transcription factors can bind multiple HREs; for example, Jun-ATF-3 binds both CRE and the AP-1 HRE (149), and the RXR-PPAR heterodimer can bind and activate both the PPAR response element and the ERE (170).

B. Possible Solutions

Several possible solutions to this specificity problem have been proposed; none are mutually exclusive. The first is the *jigsaw puzzle hypothesis* (171): simply stated, this hypothesis claims that the action of a given hormone is determined by the entire constellation of transcription factors that it activates and by the degree of activation. As noted earlier, although many protein kinases may converge on a single transcription factor, only one or two appear to play a dominant role; therefore, the extent of stimulation is as important as the spectrum of factors activated.

The *receptor hypothesis* states that hormone specificity lies in the tissue distribution of that receptor (172,173). For example, although GR and PgR bind the same HRE, progesterone does not induce the glucocorticoid-stimulated genes in liver. However, this lack of response is due to a lack of PgRs in this tissue; progesterone will induce these genes if the liver cells are transfected with PgRs. This hypothesis can be expanded to include the distribution of steroid metabolizing enzymes as well as receptors; the specificity of aldosterone has been shown to be due to the tissue distribution of enzymes that degrade cortisol (see Chapter 4). Unfortunately, this hypothesis does not hold for all systems: in the liver, T_3 induces malic enzyme and the enzymes for fatty acid metabolism (174). In fibroblasts transfected with TR, T_3 only induces the malic enzyme and in transfected QT6 cells T_3 has no effect.

The *ancillary factor hypothesis* claims that other factors interact with the transcription factors to increase specificity. All known accessory factors belong to one of four groups: (i) RXR, (ii) ternary complex factors, (iii) matrix-binding proteins, and (iv) cofactors. The DNA binding of TR and VDR was increased in the presence of nuclear extracts and these activities were named TRAP (T_3 receptor *auxilliary protein*) and NAF (*nuclear accessory factor*), respectively. However, when these factors were further characterized, it was discovered that both TRAP and NAF were identical to RXR. Since then, RXR has been shown to dimerize with every member of the thyroid receptor family and enhance DNA binding and transcriptional selectivity (see Chapter 5).

Several accessory factors recruit transcription factors to HREs by complexing with them and binding flanking sequences. The most noted example is Elk1 and the SRF; however, other accessory factors can perform a similar function for AP-1 (138,175). By binding adjacent nucleotides, these proteins can increase sequence selectivity.

A 10-kDa protein has been isolated from nuclei and increases the binding of PgR 11-fold (176). Its size and partial sequence argue against its being a nuclear receptor. It binds the nuclear matrix and may facilitate the localization of PgR near its HRE. A functionally similar protein associated with the GR has also been purified (177). Some of these factors may also explain tissue specificity; both the CRE and the GRE of the tyrosine aminotransferase gene require liver-specific factors that limit the expression of this gene to the liver despite the presence of PKA and GR in many tissues (178). The GRE in the probasin gene is another example; this GRE is selective for AR versus GR in PC-3 cells (179). In HeLa cells, both receptors are equally active, suggesting that there is some ancillary factor in PC-3 cells that either selectively enhances AR activity or specifically blocks GR function at this site. Some of these accessory proteins may be other transcription factors; for example, glucocorticoid induction of the mouse mammary tumor virus (MMTV) requires the factor NFI, whereas progesterone induction does not. Such an interaction would impart specificity to two hormones that act through the same HRE.

The *position effects hypothesis* states that the binding to an HRE may be influenced by the surrounding sequence and/or spacing with other HREs. The 5' region of the mouse mammary tumor virus (MMTV) genome contains four GREs that can illustrate several aspects of this hypothesis. First, these sites are not equivalent: GR prefers to act through the distal two GREs whereas PgR prefers the proximal two (180). One possible distinguishing feature of these two sets of GREs is the surrounding sequence; for example, it has been shown that both GR and AR recognize an additional 4–7 bp 3' to the GRE and an extra 1–3 bp on the 5' side (181). A similar phenomenon has been described for the ERE (182), the Myc-Max (183), and the T_3 HRE (184). Alternatively, the spacing may be critical: the addition of 5 nucleotides between the two distal GREs increases the response to GR relative to PgR, but the addition of 10, 20, or 30 nucleotides enhances the response to PgR versus GR. The importance of spacing has been more thoroughly studied for the TR family, in which each member has a preference for a particular spacing (Table 12-5; 184–189).

The DNA conformation at the site of the HRE is also important: PgR is more active than GR on transient DNA whereas the reverse is true for minichromosomes. Furthermore, PgR is reported to require negative supercoiling whereas GR does not (190). PgR also prefers to bind GREs on DNA with more ordered structure (191). Finally, different transcription factors may bind to the same HRE but induce different conformations (192). For example, Jun, Fos, and CREB can all bind the AP-1 HRE; however, Jun will bend the DNA toward the major groove; Fos, toward the minor groove; and CREB will not bend the DNA at all. These dramatically different DNA conformations may lead to significant differences in the ultimate effect of each factor.

Table 12-5
Effect of HRE Spacing on Nuclear Receptor Binding Specificity

Number of nucleotides between successive AGGTCA sites	Nuclear receptor binding specificity
1	RXR, COUP, PPAR, PPAR-RXR
2	RXR, TR-RXR
3	VDR-RXR
4	TR, TR-RXR
5	RAR, VDR, RAR-RXR, TR-RXR
6	VDR

V. Mechanisms for Transcription Effects

A. Positive Effects

1. DNA Allostery

Once the transcription factor has bound DNA, what happens next? Two major mechanisms for how these factors work have been proposed: (i) they alter DNA structure and/or (ii) they interact with other transcription factors, particularly those directly involved in transcription initiation. Hormonally regulated transcription factors can change chromatin structure in four ways: (i) DNA unwinding or relaxation, (ii) DNA bending, (iii) DNA looping, or (iv) nucleosomal displacement.

GR induces both relaxation in negatively supercoiled DNA and positive supercoils in relaxed DNA (193); ER can also produce positive supercoiling (194). In both cases, the effects are specific since they require the presence of the appropriate HRE. In addition to its effect on supercoiling, ER stabilizes single-stranded DNA, although there is no evidence that it actually induces melting (195). It is suspected that the changes in supercoiling are direct effects of the binding of the transcription factor to its HRE. However, some of these effects may be mediated through topoisomerases, which can be regulated by several kinases. Topoisomerases catalyze changes in the topology of DNA. Topoisomerase I nicks one strand of the DNA and allows it to relax before ligating the free ends. Topoisomerase II nicks both strands, can introduce negative supercoils, and can knot and unknot DNA (catenate and decatenate). The latter enzyme is stimulated 2- to 3-fold by either CKII or PKC phosphorylation, although the former kinase appears to be the more physiological one (196). Topoisomerase I is also activated by both kinases (197). Finally, the decatenation activity of topoisomerase II has been reported to be stimulated by a direct interaction with several hormonally regulated transcription factors including CREB, ATF-2, and Jun (198).

Many of these factors can also bend DNA; these proteins include TR (199), ER (200), RXR (201), NF-κB (202), and POU factors (203). For TR, there is a correlation between DNA bending and transcriptional activity: variant TR HREs that are not bent by TR do not support transcription. Jun–Fos and Myc–Max bend DNA in a subunit-specific manner. Jun and Myc bend DNA toward the dimer interface; Fos and Max, away from the interface (93,204). As such, Jun homodimers produce a simple bend with the factor bisecting the acute angle, whereas Jun–Fos generates a DNA that roughly maintains a straight structure because the two bends nearly cancel each other out. There is a slight kink at the point that AP-1 binds; it is not clear what role this conformational change plays in transcription; GCN4 is another bZIP factor but it does not bend DNA (Fig. 12-4A).

As will be discussed, HREs often exist as multiple copies at the 5' end of genes; receptor–receptor interactions, either direct or through intermediates, can cause the intervening DNA to loop out. Such loops appear to favor the binding of other transcription factors and have been demonstrated for both PgR bound to the uteroglobin gene (205) and ER bound to the prolactin gene (206).

Finally, the binding of nuclear receptors can result in the displacement of nucleosomes. Nucleosomes are complexes of histones around which DNA is wrapped (see Chapter 13); they act as a physical barrier to transcription initiation. On the MMTV genome, GR displaces a single nucleosome and allows NFI and TFIID to bind (207). A causal relationship is supported by the fact that hyperacetylation of the histones prevents nucleosomal displacement and blocks transcription (208). Furthermore, the MMTV genome can be derepressed by titrating out the nucleosome using competing DNA (209). However, although nucleosomal displacement appears necessary for transcription, it is not sufficient: MMTV on transient DNA does not have nucleosomes but still requires glucocorticoids for induction (210). On the tyrosine aminotransferase gene, GR displaces two nucleosomes (211,212). Nonetheless, this mechanism is not universal: ER binds to its ERE and induces changes in the DNA conformation without displacing any nucleosomes (213).

2. Interaction with Transcription Factors

The second mechanism by which transcription factors can stimulate gene expression is by interacting with components of the transcription initiation machinery. PgR, ER, COUP, Rel, and p50 all bind to TFIIB and stabilize the preinitiation complex (214,215); in the nuclear receptors, this interaction is mediated by the TAD in the LBD. In addition, CREB can bind TFIID and increase the affinity of the latter for the TATA-box (216). Some of these factors can also stimulate transcription by opposing inhibitors; for example, Myc binds to and blocks the action of Yin-Yang-1, a general transcription repressor (217). Therefore, it appears that the hormonally regulated factors, either by direct protein–protein interactions or via changes in the DNA structure, facilitate the assembly of preinitiation factors in the promoter region of target genes.

B. Negative Effects

1. Steric Occlusion

Transcription factors can also inhibit gene expression (218). The simplest mechanism is *steric occlusion*, in which an HRE is located near or may even overlap sites for other positively acting factors, and sterically interferes with either the binding or the activity of these other factors. For example, the expression of the osteocalcin gene is stimulated by 1,25-DHCC and inhibited by both glucocorticoids and PKC. The GRE overlaps the TATA-box (219) and the AP-1 site overlaps the VDRE (220); therefore, the binding of GR would block the binding of preinitiation factors and that of AP-1 would interfere with the binding of VDR. In another example, both Sp1 and TR compete for the same site on the EGFR gene; since Sp1 is required for transcription, occupancy of this site by TR inhibits gene expression (221).

There are two variations on this theme. In the first, inhibition is ligand dependent: in the absence of ligand, the binding of the nuclear receptor results in inhibition, but in the presence of ligand transcription is stimulated. This phenomenon is common in certain members of the TR family, including TR (222), RXR (223), and ecdysone (224). These receptors normally bind tightly to their HREs even without ligand; however, hormone binding is required to stimulate transcription. Originally, this situation was considered to be a form of autosteric occlusion, since the receptor occupies its HRE without doing anything. However, it has recently been shown that the unoccupied TR is not merely a passive obstruction but that it can actively inhibit formation of the preinitiation complex (225).

A second variation is the *negative HRE* (nHRE). This DNA sequence is usually a variant HRE that mediates inhibition. It is thought that if the nuclear receptor does not bind correctly to the DNA, it will not assume a transcriptionally active conformation. For example, many nHREs are half-sites that only allow the monomer to bind, although the dimer is required for activity (see Chapter 5). Spacing is also important; the TRE and ERE only differ in the spacing between the half-sites. Each can bind the HRE of the other but cannot activate gene expression from it (226). Again, the factor occupies an HRE but is inactive.

2. Competition

Competition, or *squelching*, is a second inhibitory mechanism. In this form of repression, the nuclear receptor competes for scarce transcription factors and sequesters them. It can be mimicked by TADs alone and does not require an HRE (227). However, the physiological relevance of this mechanism has recently been called into question: the amounts of receptor required to sequester enough factors to inhibit transcription far exceed levels normally found in tissues. For example, squelching by ER requires concentrations of ER that are 10 times physiological levels (228).

Two examples of ligand-regulated squelching have been postulated.

9-*cis*-RA favors RXR homodimerization which decreases the availability of RXR for heterodimerization with other members of the TR family (229). Since heterodimers are more active, the lack of free RXR would result in reduced transcription. In the second example, unliganded TR can bind DNA and TFIIB (230); without T_3, TR is not transcriptionally active and TFIIB is trapped in an inert complex. However, TFIIB is released when T_3 binds TR.

3. Protein–Protein Antagonism

Two types of protein–protein interactions can result in inhibition: homologous and heterologous. Homologous interactions refer to the binding of transcription factors to defective members from the same family; these inactive subunits include ΔCREB, ΔFosB, and CREMβ. Their effects were discussed earlier.

Heterologous inhibition refers to repression produced when one transcription factor binds another from a second family. The most intensively studied example is the interaction between members of the AP-1 family and the nuclear receptor family (164,231). AP-1 can antagonize the action of GR, PgR, AR, ER, RAR, and TR, but not RXR or MR. Although individual studies may yield slightly differ results, the following basic picture emerges (169,232–238). First, a physical interaction between Jun and the nuclear receptor can be detected, usually by co-immunoprecipitation. This binding requires the coiled coil domain of Jun and possibly part of the amino terminus; both the DBD and the LBD of the nuclear receptor are also required. However, the presence of DNA is not necessary and the DBDs from several nuclear receptors are freely interchangeable; as such, the DBD is not being used to bind DNA. The relationship between Jun and TR is particularly interesting (239): without T_3 this interaction enhances transcription by AP-1, but in the presence of T_3 it becomes inhibitory. A related phenomenon occurs between AP-1 and GR, except that the composition of AP-1 determines the effect: Jun–Fos heterodimers inhibit GR but Jun homodimers or Jun–Fra1 heterodimers are stimulatory (240,241). These and other data implicate Fos as the major inhibitory component of AP-1 (242).

Interactions between other protein families also exist. Jun can bind and inhibit MyoD; the binding occurs between the zipper of Jun and the HLH domain of MyoD (84). In addition, Oct-1 can be suppressed by GR; this interaction requires the second helix in the POU_H domain (166).

4. Silencing

Silencing is a more active type of inhibition. The interactions just discussed merely block the activation by other factors; however, silencers interact with components of the initiation complex to repress transcription directly. Both TR and RAR can exert such an inhibitory effect; the responsible domains have been localized to the amino- and carboxy-terminal ends of the LBD (243).

VI. Hormone Response Elements

Previous sections of this chapter have referred to specific DNA sequences recognized by the individual transcription factors. In this section, the methods for identifying these sequences and some of their characteristics will be covered.

A. Sequences

Several techniques have been employed to identify HREs. The determination of a *consensus sequence* involves the assembly of known sequences for all the genes induced by a particular hormone; one then searches for short sequences that are common to all the 5' regions. The logic is simple: if a certain hormone activates a half dozen or so genes, then its receptor must recognize some common structure in all of them. Unfortunately, this technique is the least intellectually gratifying because the results are not coupled to any binding or functional data. Another problem is that there is no single perfect HRE; rather, many HREs can have several positions that are variable, making their identification even more difficult. For example, following examination of the gene sequences for β casein, MMTV, human GH, and proopiomelanocortin, a 24-nucleotide consensus sequence for the glucocorticoid receptor binding site was postulated (244). However, the sequence was located far upstream (-500 to -300 bp) and the sequence similarity among these sites was only 58–83%. Better methodologies (see subsequent discussion) have shown that the actual binding site consists of six nucleotides (TGTYCT, where Y is any pyrimidine) and is located closer than -200 bp; furthermore, the homology between sequences is 82–100% for any given nucleotide (245). However, this technique can be useful if it is combined with another method that restricts the potential sequences to which the receptor binds.

Histology can be used to localize steroid receptors by immunofluorescence. The first use of this technique was on the insect hormone ecdysone, because it has an $\alpha-\beta$ unsaturated carbonyl within the steroid nucleus. This group can be activated by light having a wavelength of 320 nm, resulting in a covalent bond being formed between the hormone and the receptor; antibodies to ecdysone were then used to localize its receptor to the chromosomal puffs (246). With the purification of steroid receptors, monoclonal antibodies against the receptor itself are now available for these types of studies. Using these antibodies, the estradiol receptor has been found on euchromatin (247). In another example, the unoccupied progesterone receptor is located in the condensed chromatin that becomes euchromatin after occupancy by the steroid (248). Although this technique is the most visually satisfying one, its major drawback is its lack of resolution.

Kinetic analysis measures the association or dissociation constants for the binding of hormone receptors to DNA fragments; binding to DNA reconstituted with histones and to intact chromatin has also been studied. The

fragments with the highest affinity presumably contain the binding sequence. This technique is good for comparing the relative binding affinities
among DNA preparations, but the absolute values are still too low to account
for the specificity observed *in vivo*.

Functional analyses involve altering the 5' region of a gene, reintroducing
the gene into cells, and examining the effects of this modification on the
hormonal control of transcription. For example, one can make successively
larger deletions in the 5' region until hormone inducibility is lost. Unfortunately, a simple deletion is actually two modifications in one: not only are
certain sequences missing, but the spacing between the gene and other
sequences upstream is altered. Such spacing may be critical for the proper
functioning of the regulatory sequences. This problem is overcome by using
linker scanning mutants, which contain unrelated sequences in place of those
deleted so that spacing is preserved. Another modification is *insertion mutation*, in which unrelated sequences are randomly inserted into the 5' region.
The loss of hormone inducibility in a particular mutant would suggest that
the receptor binding site in that mutant has been interrupted. Finally, once
the putative binding site has been restricted to a sufficiently small region of
DNA, *site-directed mutants* can be generated. This technique involves the
introduction of single base-pair mutations in selected positions and results in
the least perturbation of the surrounding DNA.

Footprint analysis involves binding the receptor to DNA and then enzymatically digesting the nucleic acid. The receptor binding site should be
spared because the bound protein interferes with enzymatic digestion. Alternatively, selected guanine residues are methylated and receptor binding is
measured; if a particular base interacts with the receptor, its methylation will
interfere with binding. This latter technique is known as *methylation interference footprinting*.

When a putative HRE has been identified, it can be cut out, spliced onto
a reporter gene, and placed into cells; then gene regulation can be examined.
This is the true test for validating an HRE: if a DNA sequence is the HRE for a
particular hormone, then it should impart hormonal regulation on any gene
to which it is attached.

B. Synergism and Cooperativity

Tables 12-6 and 12-7 list the HREs for several transcription factors regulated
by the endocrine system. Several general characteristics are apparent. First,
most HREs occur as repeats, either direct or inverted. This corresponds to the
dimeric nature of many transcriptional factors. Second, many HREs have
similar or identical sequences; specificity is determined, in part, by spacing
and orientation. The importance of spacing for direct repeats was discussed
already (Table 12-5). The importance of orientation has been studied for the
sequence TGACCTGA (249). As an inverted repeat, called a palindrome, this
sequence binds both TR and RAR, but as a direct repeat it only binds TR. The
introduction of a 3-bp spacer between the direct repeat switches the binding

Table 12-6

HREs for Ligand-regulated Transcription Factors

Hormone	DNA Sequence
Glucocorticoids, progesterone, androgens, aldosterone (GRE)	GGTACAnnnTGTTCT CCATGTnnnACAAGA
Estradiol (ERE)	AGGTCAnnnTGACCT TCCAGTnnnACTGGA
Ecdysone (EcRE)	GGTCAnTGACC CCAGTnACTGG
Triiodothyronine	AGGTAAGnnnAGGGACGTGACCGC^a TCCATTCnnnTCCCTGCACTGGCG
T$_3$/RAR/RXR (TRE$_{pal}$)	TCAGGTCATGACCTGA AGTCCAGTACTGGACT
RAR Laminin	TAACCTnnnTCACCT ATTGGAnnnAGTGGA
RA Receptor	GTTCACnnnnnGTTCAC CAAGTGnnnnnCAAGTG
RXR Apolipoprotein AI	TGAACCCTTGACCCC ACTTGGGAACTGGGG
CRBPII	AGGTCAnAGGTCAnAGGTCAnAGGTCAnAGGTCA TCCAGTnTCCAGTnTCCAGTnTCCAGTnTCCAGT
1,25-DHCC Osteocalcin	TTGGTGACTCACCGGGTGAACGGGGGCAT^b AACCACTGAGTGGCCCACTTGCCCCCGTA
Osteopontin	AGGTTCACGAGGTTCACG TCCAAGTGCTCCAAGTGC
COUP	TGTCAAAGGTCAAA ACAGTTTCCAGTTT
PPRP	TGACCnnTGTCCnGGTCCn$_{16}$GGTTA ACTGGnnACAGGnCCAGGn$_{16}$CCAAT
Ah Receptor (XRE or DRE)	T$_T^A$GCGTG A$_T^A$CGCAC

^{a} Dashed arrow represents half TRE$_{pal}$.
^{b} Dashed arrow represents a RARE; dotted arrow, an AP-1 HRE.

Table 12-7
HREs for Peptide Hormone Mediators

Hormone	DNA Sequence
cAMP (CRE)	TGACGTCA → ← ACTGCAGT
PKC Jun-Fos (AP-1)	TGA $\frac{C}{G}$ TCAG → ← ACT $\frac{G}{C}$ AGTC
NF-κB	GGGACTTTCC CCCTGAAAGG
cAMP/PKC (AP-2)	CCCCAGGC GGGGTCCG
Calcium Pit-1 (positive)	AnTnCATnn $\frac{C}{T}$ TATnCAT TnAnGTAnn $\frac{C}{A}$ ATAnGTA
nCaRE (negative)	TGAGACnnnGTCTCA → ← ACTCTGnnnCAGAGT
CaM (C/EBP-like)	TTATGCAATACACTTGTAGTCTTGCAACA → → ← ← AATACGTTATGTGAACATCAGAACGTTGT
CKII SRF (SRE)	AGATG $\frac{C}{C}$ CCATATTTGG $\frac{C}{C}$ CATCT → ← TCTAC $\frac{C}{G}$ GGTATAAACC $\frac{C}{G}$ GTAGA
Myc-Max	CACGTG → ← GTGCAC
Interferon IFNα (ISRE)	TGAGGAAACGAAACC → → ACTCCTTTGCTTTGG
IFNγ	AGTTTCATATTACTCTAAATC TCAAAGTATAATGAGATTTAG
TNFα	GAGATTCCAC CTCTAAGGTG
TGFβ CTF (inhibition)	TTGGAAnnnATCCAA → ← AACCTTnnnTAGGTT
CTF (stimulation)	TGGCAnnnTGCCAA → ← ACCGTnnnACGGTT
Insulin	G $\frac{T}{A}$ GTTT $\frac{TGC}{CGT}$ A $\frac{C}{A}$ AA C $\frac{A}{T}$ CAAA ^A_A T $\frac{G}{T}$ TT

specificity from TR to RAR. Finally, a 3-bp spacer in the palindrome converts the HRE from a thyroid HRE to an ERE.

Two additional characteristics of HREs are the occurrence of multiple copies of the sequence in genes and the absence of perfect copies; in particular, the 5' half of the HRE usually exhibits considerable variability. Both of these properties are related to how transcription factors bind HREs and how these HREs interact with each other.

Nuclear receptors bind DNA as dimers. Initially, one member binds the 3' more-perfect half (250). Because the second member is tethered to the first, its local concentration is very high and its binding to the 5' half is favored, even though this half of the sequence is more variable. Essentially, the high concentration of the second partner compensates for the imperfect sequence of the HRE. The use of RXR as the second subunit also improves binding to imperfect HREs. RXR appears to be a general filler: it binds to the 5' imperfect half and its presence in a dimer allows its partner to bind to half-sites with a greater variability in spacing (Table 12-5).

In fact, there are several advantages to having imperfect HREs. First, they may alter the responsiveness of genes to transcription factors. For example, the CREB binds imperfect CREs with a lower affinity than perfect sequences; however, they give a greater induction because of their lower baseline (251). Imperfect HREs may also prevent strong inhibition by those nuclear receptors that repress transcription in the absence of their ligand. The perfect HRE may simply have too high an affinity. Third, imperfect HREs may broaden the spectrum of factors that can bind it. For example, the GRE and ERE are highly specific for GR and ER, respectively, but a hybrid ERE–GRE in the uteroglobin gene can bind and be activated by ER, GR, and PgR (252). In another example, a perfect CRE only binds CREB homodimers, whereas imperfect CREs can bind CREB heterodimers (253). Finally, imperfect HREs may differentially affect the conformation of a transcription factor. Oct-1 binds DNA but has no TAD; it must bind other factors with TADs to stimulate transcription. One such factor is V16, which has a TAD but does not bind DNA. V16 will bind Oct-1 only when it is bound to a variant HRE (254). Apparently, Oct-1 assumes different conformations on different HREs and this affects with which proteins it interacts.

In addition to binding cooperativity within an HRE, synergism also occurs among multiple copies of an HRE. For example, the DNA affinity for both GR and PgR increases as much as 100-fold when a second HRE is introduced (255–257). This synergism is more marked for imperfect HREs: the affinity of ER for an imperfect ERE increases 4- to 8-fold by the presence of another ERE, but there is no effect if both EREs are perfect (258,259). This synergism extends to transcription as well; multiple HREs enhance the transcriptional effects of the factors that bind them. This transcriptional synergism is often greater in magnitude than the increase observed in DNA binding. Researchers believe that a single nuclear receptor or transcription factor is not as effective as multiple copies in recruiting and/or stablizing the preinitiation complex.

VII. Summary

The structure of many transcription factors are known and most fall into relatively few families. Nearly all of them use an α helix to make specific contacts with bases in the major groove. The HTH, homeodomains, POU, Myb, and zinc twist factors use a short recognition helix overlaid with one to three additional helices to secure the first helix in place. The coiled coil factors use a long α helix whose carboxy terminus forms a coiled coil and whose amino terminus straddles the major groove. The bZIP, bHLH, helix–span–helix, and bHLH-ZIP factors are all variations on this motif. Most factors form dimers, as is reflected in the DNA sequences that they recognize: most HREs are either direct or inverted repeats.

There is considerable overlap in the activities of these factors. Enhanced specificity is achieved by the selective distribution of hormone receptors, the presence of ancillary factors, and the position and spacing of the HREs. Despite all these mechanisms, some overlap still exists and the final activity of any given hormone may simply reside in the spectrum of activities that it evokes.

Hormonal regulation of these factors involves (i) induction of the factors; (ii) alternative splicing; (iii) phosphorylation by second messenger-regulated kinases; (iv) protein–protein interactions, including variable dimerization partners, inhibitors, cofactors, and hsps; (v) compartmentalization; and (vi) allosterism by ligands. Once activated, these factors stimulate transcription by facilitating the assembly of the preinitiation complex in the promoter region. This may occur either directly by protein–protein binding or via changes in the DNA conformation, including (i) DNA unwinding or relaxation, (ii) DNA bending, (iii) DNA looping, or (iv) nucleosomal displacement. Inhibition of transcription can be accomplished by (i) steric occlusion of stimulatory HREs, TATA-boxes, or other critical sites; (ii) competition for limiting transcription factors; (iii) protein–protein antagonism, in which transcription factors bind and inhibit one another; and (iv) silencing, in which these factor directly inhibit the preinitiation complex.

The DNA sequences recognized by these factors usually occur as direct or inverted repeats, reflecting the dimeric nature of the factors themselves. However, these HREs are rarely perfect; these variations may affect the responsiveness of the gene, keep protein binding low enough to be readily reversible, increase the number of factors that can bind, and differentially affect the conformation of the factors. HREs exist in multiple copies that interact with one another, resulting in synergism of both binding and transcription.

References

General References

Cardenas, M. E., and Gasser, S. M. (1993). Regulation of topoisomerase II by phosphorylation: A role for casein kinase II. *J. Cell Sci.* **104,** 219–225.

de Groot, R. P., and Sassone-Corsi, P. (1993). Hormonal control of gene expression: Multiplicity and versatility of cyclic adenosine 3′,5′-monophosphate-responsive nuclear regulators. *Mol. Endocrinol.* **7,** 145–153.

Edmondson, D. G., and Olson, E. N. (1993). Helix–loop–helix proteins as regulators of muscle-specific transcription. *J. Biol. Chem.* **268,** 755–758.

Gorski, J., Furlow, J. D., Murdoch, F. E., Fritsch, M., Kaneko, K., Ying, C., and Malayer, J. R. (1993). Perturbations in the model of estrogen receptor regulation of gene expression. *Biol. Reprod.* **48,** 8–14.

Grimm, S., and Baeuerle, P. A. (1993). The inducible transcription factor NF-κB: Structure–function relationship of its protein subunits. *Biochem. J.* **290,** 297–308.

Kornberg, T. B. (1993). Understanding the homeodomain. *J. Biol. Chem.* **268,** 26813–26816.

Prendergast, P., Oñate, S. A., Christensen, K., and Edwards, D. P. (1994). Nuclear accessory factors enhance the binding of progesterone receptor to specific target DNA. *J. Steroid Biochem. Mol. Biol.* **48,** 1–13.

Renkawitz, R. (1993). Repression mechanisms of v-ERBA and other members of the steroid receptor superfamily. *Ann. N.Y. Acad. Sci.* **684,** 1–10.

Verrijzer, C. P., and Van der Vliet, P. C. (1993). POU domain transcription factors. *Biochim. Biophys. Acta* **1173,** 1–21.

See also Refs. 1–4, 8, 26, 27, 41, 42, 44, 45, 54, 79, 81, 82, 89, 106, 109, 117, 118, 123, 125, 132, 161, 164, 171, 173, 218, 231, and 241.

Cited References

1. Pabo, C. O., and Sauer, R. T. (1992). Transcription factors: Structural families and principles of DNA recognition. *Annu. Rev. Biochem.* **61,** 1053–1095.
2. Latchman, D. S. (1990). Eukaryotic transcription factors. *Biochem. J.* **270,** 281–289.
3. Harrison, S. C. (1991). A structural taxonomy of DNA-binding domains. *Nature (London)* **353,** 715–719.
4. Cohen, P., and Foulkes, J. G. (eds.) (1991). "The Hormonal Control of Gene Transcription." Elsevier, Amsterdam.
5. Suzuki, M. (1993). Common features in DNA recognition helices of eukaryotic transcription factors. *EMBO J.* **12,** 3221–3226.
6. Leonard, J., Peers, B., Johnson, T., Ferreri, K., Lee, S., and Montminy, M. R. (1993). Characterization of somatostatin transactivating factor-1, a novel homeobox factor that stimulates somatostatin expression in pancreatic islet cells. *Mol. Endocrinol.* **7,** 1275–1283.
7. Miller, C. P., McGehee, R. E., and Lin, J. C. (1993). IDX-1: A new homeodomain transcription factor expressed in rat pancreatic islets and duodenum. *Progr. Abstr. 75th Annu. Meet. Endocr. Soc.,* 374.
8. Rosenfeld, M. G. (1991). POU-domain transcription factors: pou-er-ful developmental regulators. *Genes Dev.* **5,** 897-907.
9. Assa-Munt, N., Mortishire-Smith, R. J., Aurora, R., Herr, W., and Wright, P. E. (1993). The solution structure of the Oct-1 POU-specific domain reveals a striking similarity to the bacteriophage λ repressor DNA-binding domain. *Cell* **73,** 193–205.
10. Dekker, N., Cox, M., Boelens, R., Verrijzer, C. P., van der Vliet, P. C., and Kaptein, R. (1993). Solution structure of the POU-specific DNA-binding domain of Oct-1. *Nature (London)* **362,** 852-855.

11. Li, P., He, X., Gerrero, M. R., Mok, M., Aggarwal, A., and Rosenfeld, M. G. (1993). Spacing and orientation of bipartite DNA-binding motifs as potential functional determinants for POU doman factors. *Genes Dev.* **7**, 2483–2496.
12. Treacy, M. N., Neilson, L. I., Turner, E. E., He, X., and Rosenfeld, M. G. (1992). Twin of I-POU: A two amino acid difference in the I-POU homeodomain distinguishes an activator from an inhibitor of transcription. *Cell* **68**, 491–505.
13. Ogata, K., Hojo, H., Aimoto, S., Nakai, T., Nakamura, H., Sarai, A., Ishii, S., and Nishimura, Y. (1992). Solution structure of a DNA-binding unit of Myb: A helix-turn-helix-related motif with conserved tryptophans forming a hydrophobic core. *Proc. Natl. Acad. Sci. U.S.A.* **89**, 6428–6432.
14. Laget, M. P., Callebaut, I., de Launoit, Y., Stehelin, D., and Mornon, J. P. (1993). Predicted common structural features of DNA-binding domains from Ets, Myb and HMG transcription factors. *Nucleic Acids Res.* **21**, 5987–5996.
15. Luisi, B. F., Xu, W. X., Otwinowski, Z., Freedman, L. P., Yamamoto, K. R., and Sigler, P. B. (1991). Crystallographic analysis of the interaction of the glucocorticoid receptor with DNA. *Nature (London)* **352**, 497–505.
16. Schwabe, J. W. R., Neuhaus, D., and Rhodes, D. (1990). Solution structure of the DNA-binding domain of the oestrogen receptor. *Nature (London)* **348**, 458–461.
17. O'Shea, E. K., Klemm, J. D., Kim, P. S., and Alber, T. (1991). X-Ray structure of the GCN4 leucine zipper, a two-stranded, parallel coiled coil. *Science* **254**, 539–544.
18. O'Shea, E. K., Rutkowski, R., and Kim, P. S. (1992). Mechanism of specificity in the Fos–Jun oncoprotein heterodimer. *Cell* **68**, 699–708.
19. Vinson, C. R., and Garcia, K. C. (1992). Molecular model for DNA recognition by the family of basic-helix–loop–helix-zipper proteins. *New Biol.* **4**, 396–403.
20. Ellenberger, T. E., Brandl, C. J., Struhl, K., and Harrison, S. C. (1992). The GCN4 basic region leucine zipper binds DNA as a dimer of uninterrupted α helices: Crystal structure of the protein-DNA complex. *Cell* **71**, 1223–1237.
21. Kerppola, T. K., and Curran, T. (1991). DNA bending by Fos and Jun: The flexible hinge model. *Science* **254**, 1210–1214.
22. Anthony-Cahill, S. J., Benfield, P. A., Fairman, R., Wasserman, Z. R., Brenner, S. L., Stafford, W. F., Altenbach, C., Hubbell, W. L., and DeGrado, W. F. (1992). Molecular characterization of helix–loop–helix peptides. *Science* **255**, 979–983.
23. Baleja, J. D., Marmorstein, R., Harrison, S. C., and Wagner, G. (1992). Solution structure of the DNA-binding domain of Cd₂-GAL4 from *S. cerevisiae*. *Nature (London)* **356**, 450–453.
24. Kraulis, P. J., Raine, A. R. C., Gadhavi, P. L., and Laue, E. D. (1992). Structure of the DNA-binding domain of zinc GAL4. *Nature (London)* **356**, 448–450.
25. Marmorstein, R., Carey, M., Ptashne, M., and Harrison, S. C. (1992). DNA recognition by GAL4: Structure of a protein–DNA complex. *Nature (London)* **356**, 408–414.
26. Mitchell, P. J., and Tjian, R. (1989). Transcriptional regulation in mammalian cells by sequence-specific DNA binding proteins. *Science* **245**, 371–378.
27. Johnson, P. F., Sterneck, E., and Williams, S. C. (1993). Activation domains of transcriptional regulatory proteins. *J. Nutr. Biochem.* **4**, 368–398.
28. Sigler, P. B. (1988). Acid blobs and negative noodles. *Nature (London)* **333**, 210–212.
29. Leuther, K. K., Salmeron, J. M., and Johnston, S. A. (1993). Genetic evidence that an activation domain of GAL4 does not require acidity and may form a β sheet. *Cell* **72**, 575–585.

30. Lin, Y. S., and Green, M. R. (1991). Mechanism of action of an acidic transcriptional activator *in vitro*. *Cell* **64**, 971–981.
31. Lin, Y. S., Ha, I., Maldonado, E., Reinberg, D., and Green, M. R. (1991). Binding of general transcription factor TFIIB to an acidic activating region. *Nature (London)* **353**, 569–571.
32. Ptashne, M., and Gann, A. A. F. (1990). Activators and targets. *Nature (London)* **346**, 329–331.
33. Stringer, K. F., Ingles, C. J., and Greenblatt, J. (1990). Direct and selective binding of an acidic transcriptional activation domain to the TATA-box factor TFIID. *Nature (London)* **345**, 783–786.
34. Li, R., and Botchan, M. R. (1993). The acidic transcriptional activation domains of VP16 and p53 bind the cellular replication protein A and stimulate *in vitro* BPV-1 DNA replication. *Cell* **73**, 1207–1221.
35. He, Z., Brinton, B. T., Greenblatt, J., Hassell, J. A., and Ingles, C. J. (1993). The transactivator proteins VP16 and GAL4 bind replication factor A. *Cell* **73**, 1223–1232.
36. Berger, S. L., Piña, B., Silverman, N., Marcus, G. A., Agapite, J., Regier, J. L., Triezenberg, S. J., and Guarente, L. (1992). Genetic isolation of ADA2: A potential transcriptional adaptor required for function of certain acidic activation domains. *Cell* **70**, 251–265.
37. Attardi, L. D., and Tjian, R. (1993). Drosophila tissue-specific transcription factor NTF-1 contains a novel isoleucine-rich activation motif. *Genes Dev.* **7**, 1341–1353.
38. Gerber, H. P., Seipel, K., Georgiev, O., Höfferer, M., Hug, M., Rusconi, S., and Schaffner, W. (1994). Transcriptional activation modulated by homopolymeric glutamine and proline stretches. *Science* **263**, 808–811.
39. Churchill, M. E. A., and Travers, A. A. (1991). Protein motifs that recognize structural features of DNA. *Trends Biochem. Sci.* **16**, 92–97.
40. Gill, G., Pascal, E., Tseng, Z. H., and Tjian, R. (1994). A glutamine-rich hydrophobic patch in transcription factor Sp1 contacts the dTAF$_{II}$110 component of the *Drosophila* TFIID complex and mediates transcriptional activation. *Proc. Natl. Acad. Sci. U.S.A.* **91**, 192–196.
41. Lee, K. A. W., and Masson, N. (1993). Transcriptional regulation by CREB and its relatives. *Biochim. Biophys. Acta* **1174**, 221–233.
42. Meyer, T. E., and Habener, J. F. (1993). Cyclic adenosine 3',5'-monophosphate response element binding protein (CREB) and related tarnscription-activating deoxyribonucleic acid-binding proteins. *Endocr. Rev.* **14**, 269–290.
43. Boshart, M., Weih, F., Nichols, M., and Schütz, G. (1991). The tissue-specific extinguisher locus TSE1 encodes a regulatory subunit of cAMP-dependent protein kinase. *Cell* **66**, 849–859.
44. Berk, A. J. (1989). Regulation of eukaryotic transcription factors by post-translational modification. *Biochim. Biophys. Acta* **1009**, 103–109.
45. Karin, M., and Smeal, T. (1992). Control of transcription factors by signal transduction pathways: the beginning of the end. *Trends Biochem. Sci.* **17**, 418–422.
46. Dash, P. K., Karl, K. A., Colicos, M. A., Prywes, R., and Kandel, E. R. (1991). cAMP response element-binding protein is activated by Ca^{2+}/calmodulin- as well as cAMP-dependent protein kinase. *Proc. Natl. Acad. Sci. U.S.A.* **88**, 5061–5065.
47. Sheng, M., Thompson, M. A., and Greenberg, M. E. (1991). CREB: A Ca^{2+}-reg-

ulated transcription factor phosphorylated by calmodulin-dependent kinases. *Science* **252,** 1427–1430.

48. Yamamoto, K. K., Gonzalez, G. A., Menzel, P., Rivier, J., and Montminy, M. R. (1990). Characterization of a bipartite activator domain in transcription factor CREB. *Cell* **60,** 611–617.

49. Karpinski, B. A., Morle, G. D., Huggenvik, J., Uhler, M. D., and Leiden, J. M. (1992). Molecular cloning of human CREB-2: An ATF/CREB transcription factor that can negatively regulate transcription from the cAMP response element. *Proc. Natl. Acad. Sci. U.S.A.* **89,** 4820–4824.

50. Abdel-Hafiz, H. A. M., Heasley, L. E., Kyriakis, J. M., Avruch, J., Kroll, D. J., Johnson, G. L., and Hoeffler, J. P. (1992). Activating transcription factor-2 DNA-binding activity is stimulated by phosphorylation catalyzed by p42 and p54 microtubule-associated protein kinases. *Mol. Endocrinol.* **6,** 2079–2089.

51. Laoide, B. M., Foulkes, N. S., Schlotter, F., and Sassone-Corsi, P. (1993). The functional versatility of CREM is determined by its modular structure. *EMBO J.* **12,** 1179–1191.

52. Brindle, P., Linke, S., and Montminy, M. (1993). Protein-kinase-A-dependent activator in transcription factor CREB reveals new role for CREM repressors. *Nature (London)* **364,** 821–824.

53. de Groot, R. P., Derua, R., Goris, J., and Sassone-Corsi, P. (1993). Phosphorylation and negative regulation of the transcriptional activator CREM by p34^{cdc2}. *Mol. Endocrinol.* **7,** 1495–1501.

54. Karin, M. (1991). The AP-1 complex and its role in transcriptional control by protein kinase C. *In* "The Hormonal Control of Gene Transcription" (P. Cohen and J. G. Foulkes, eds.), pp. 235–253. Elsevier, Amsterdam.

55. Pulverer, B. J., Kyriakis, J. M., Avruch, J., Nikolakaki, E., and Woodgett, J. R. (1991). Phosphorylation of c-*jun* mediated by MAP kinases. *Nature (London)* **353,** 670–674.

56. Adler, V., Polotskaya, A., Wagner, F., and Kraft, A. S. (1992). Affinity-purified c-Jun amino-terminal protein kinase requires serine/threonine phosphorylation for activity. *J. Biol. Chem.* **267,** 17001–17005.

57. DeGroot, R. P., Auwerx, J., Bourouis, M., and Sassone-Corsi, P. (1993). Negative regulation of Jun/AP-1: Conserved function of glycogen synthase kinase-3 and the *Drosophila* kinase *shaggy. Oncogene* **8,** 841–847.

58. Nikolakaki, E., Coffer, P. J., Hemelsoet, R., Woodgett, J. R., and Defize, L. H. K. (1993). Glycogen synthase kinase-3 phosphorylates Jun family members in vitro and negatively regulates their transactivating potential in intact cells. *Oncogene* **8,** 833–840.

59. Plyte, S. E., Hughes, K., Nikolakaki, E., Pulverer, B. J., and Woodgett, J. R. (1992). Glycogen synthase kinase-3: Functions in oncogenesis and development. *Biochim. Biophys. Acta* **1114,** 147–162.

60. Boyle, W. J., Smeal, T., Defize, L. H. K., Angel, P., Woodgett, J. R., Karin, M., and Hunter, T. (1991). Activation of protein kinase C decreases phosphorylation of c-Jun at sites that negatively regulate its DNA-binding activity. *Cell* **64,** 573–584.

61. Abate, C., Baker, S. J., Lees-Miller, S. P., Anderson, C. W., Marshak, D. R., and Curran, T. (1993). Dimerization and DNA binding alter phosphorylation of Fos and Jun. *Proc. Natl. Acad. Sci. U.S.A.* **90,** 6766–6770.

62. Johnson, P. F., Sterneck, E., and Williams, S. C. (1993). Activation domains of transcriptional regulatory proteins. *J. Nutr. Biochem.* **4,** 386–398.

63. Adler, V., Franklin, C. C., and Kraft, A. S. (1992). Phorbol esters stimulate the phosphorylation of c-Jun but not v-Jun: Regulation by the N-terminal δ domain. *Proc. Natl. Acad. Sci. U.S.A.* **89**, 5341–5345.

64. Doucas, V., Spyrou, G., and Yaniv, M. (1991). Unregulated expression of c-Jun and c-Fos proteins but not Jun D inhibits oestrogen receptor activity in human breast cancer derived cells. *EMBO J.* **10**, 2237–2245.

65. Xanthoudakis, S., and Curran, T. (1992). Identification and characterization of Ref-1, a nuclear protein that facilitates AP-1 DNA-binding activity. *Cell* **68**, 653–665.

66. Xanthoudakis, S., Miao, G., Wang, F., Pan, Y. C. E., and Curran, T. (1992). Redox activation of Fos-Jun DNA binding activity is mediated by a DNA repair enzyme. *EMBO J.* **11**, 3323–3335.

67. Chiu, R., Angel, P., and Karin, M. (1989). Jun-B differs in its biological properties from, and is a negative regulator of, c-Jun. *Cell* **59**, 979–986.

68. Dobrzanski, P., Noguchi, T., Kovary, K., Rizzo, C. A., Lazo, P. S., and Bravo, R. (1991). Both products of the *fosB* gene, FosB and its short form, FosB/SF, are transcriptional activators in fibroblasts. *Mol. Cell. Biol.* **11**, 5470–5478.

69. Abate, C., Marshak, D. R., and Curran, T. (1991). Fos is phosphorylated by p34^{cdc2}, cAMP-dependent protein kinase and protein kinase C at multiple sites clustered within regulatory regions. *Oncogene* **6**, 2179–2185.

70. Lees-Miller, S. P., and Anderson, C. W. (1992). The DNA-activated protein kinase, DNA-PK: A potential coordinator of nuclear events. *Cancer Cells* **3**, 341–346.

71. Neuberg, M., Adamkiewicz, J., Hunter, J. B., and Müller, R. (1989). A Fos protein containing the Jun leucine zipper forms a homodimer which binds to the AP1 binding site. *Nature (London)* **341**, 243–245.

72. Auwerx, J., and Sassone-Corsi, P. (1991). IP-1: A dominant inhibitor of Fos/Jun whose activity is modulated by phosphorylation. *Cell* **64**, 983–993.

73. Auwerx, J., and Sassone-Corsi, P. (1992). AP-1 (Fos-Jun) regulation by IP-1: Effect of signal transduction pathways and cell growth. *Oncogene* **7**, 2271–2280.

74. Williams, S. C., Cantwell, C. A., and Johnson, P. F. (1991). A family of C/EBP-related proteins capable of forming covalently linked leucine zipper dimers *in vitro*. *Genes Dev.* **5**, 1553–1567.

75. Nakajima, T., Kinoshita, S., Sasagawa, T., Sasaki, K., Naruto, M., Kishimoto, T., and Akira, S. (1993). Phosphorylation at threonine-235 by a *ras*-dependent mitogen-activated protein kinase cascade is essential for transcription factor NF-IL6. *Proc. Natl. Acad. Sci. U.S.A.* **90**, 2207–2211.

76. Trautwein, C., Caelles, C., van der Geer, P., Hunter, T., Karin, M., and Chojkier, M. (1993). Transactivation by NF-IL6/LAP is enhanced by phosphorylation of its activation domain. *Nature (London)* **364**, 544–547.

77. Wegner, M., Cao, Z., and Rosenfeld, M. G. (1992). Calcium-regulated phosphorylation within the leucine zipper of C/EBPβ. *Science* **256**, 370–373.

78. Metz, R., and Ziff, E. (1991). cAMP stimulates the C/EBP-related transcription factor rNFIL-6 to *trans*-locate to the nucleus and to induce c-*fos* transcription. *Genes Dev.* **5**, 1754–1766.

79. Hunter, T., and Karin, M. (1992). The regulation of transcription by phosphorylation. *Cell* **70**, 375–387.

80. Kinoshita, S., Akira, S., and Kishimoto, T. (1992). A member of the C/EBP family, NF-IL6β, forms a heterodimer and transcriptionally synergizes with NF-IL6. *Proc. Natl. Acad. Sci. U.S.A.* **89**, 1473–1476.

81. Landers, J. P., and Bunce, N. J. (1991). The *Ah* receptor and the mechanism of dioxin toxicity. *Biochem. J.* **276**, 273–287.

82. Swanson, H. I., and Bradfield, C. A. (1993). The AH-receptor: Genetics, structure and function. *Pharmacogenetics* **3**, 213–230.

83. Jellinck, P. H., Forkert, P. G., Riddick, D. S., Okey, A. B., Michnovicz, J. J., and Bradlow, H. L. (1993). Ah receptor binding properties of indole carbinols and induction of hepatic estradiol hydroxylation. *Biochem. Pharmacol.* **45**, 1129–1136.

84. Edmondson, D. G., and Olson, E. N. (1993). Helix–loop–helix proteins as regulators of muscle-specific transcription. *J. Biol. Chem.* **268**, 755–758.

85. Li, L., Chambard, J. C., Karin, M., and Olson, E. B. (1992). Fos and Jun repress transcriptional activation by myogenin and MyoD: The amino terminus of Jun can mediate repression. *Genes Dev.* **6**, 676–689.

86. Williams, T., Admon, A., Lüscher, B., and Tjian, R. (1988). Cloning and expression of AP-2, a cell-type-specific transcription factor that activates inducible enhancer elements. *Genes Dev.* **2**, 1557–1569.

87. Williams, T., and Tjian, R. (1991). Characterization of a dimerization motif in AP-2 and its function in heterologous DNA-binding proteins. *Science* **251**, 1067–1071.

88. Park, K., and Kim, K. H. (1993). The site of cAMP action in the insulin induction of gene expression of acetyl-CoA carboxylase is AP-2. *J. Biol. Chem.* **268**, 17811–17819.

89. Kato, G. J., and Dang, C. V. (1992). Function of the c-Myc oncoprotein. *FASEB J.* **6**, 3065–3072.

90. Papoulas, O., Williams, N. G., and Kingston, R. E. (1992). DNA binding activities of c-Myc purified from eukaryotic cells. *J. Biol. Chem.* **267**, 10470–10480.

91. Reddy, C. D., Dasgupta, P., Saikumar, P., Dudek, H., Rauscher, F. J., and Reddy, E. P. (1992). Mutational analysis of Max: Role of basic, helix–loop–helix/leucine zipper domains in DNA binding, dimerization and regulation of Myc-mediated transcriptional activation. *Oncogene* **7**, 2085–2092.

92. Prochownik, E. V., and VanAntwerp, M. E. (1993). Differential patterns of DNA binding by myc and max proteins. *Proc. Natl. Acad. Sci. U.S.A.* **90**, 960–964.

93. Wechsler, D. S., and Dang, C. V. (1992). Opposite orientations of DNA bending by c-Myc and Max. *Proc. Natl. Acad. Sci. U.S.A.* **89**, 7635–7639.

94. Ferré-D'Amaré, A. R., Prendergast, G. C., Ziff, E. B., and Burley, S. K. (1993). Recognition by Max of its cognate DNA through a dimeric b/HLH/Z domain. *Nature (London)* **363**, 38–45.

95. Kato, G. J., Lee, W. M. F., Chen, L., and Dang, C. V. (1992). Max: Functional domains and interaction with c-Myc. *Genes Dev.* **6**, 81–92.

96. Berberich, S. J., and Cole, M. D. (1992). Casein kinase-II inhibits the DNA-binding activity of Max homodimers but not Myc/Max heterodimers. *Genes Dev.* **6**, 166–176.

97. Seth, A., Gonzalez, F. A., Gupta, S., Raden, D. L., and Davis, R. J. (1992). Signal transduction within the nucleus by mitogen-activated protein kinase. *J. Biol. Chem.* **267**, 24796–24804.

98. Saksela, K., Makela, T. P., Hughes, K., Woodgett, J. R., and Alitalo, K. (1992). Activation of protein kinase C increases phosphorylation of the L-*myc* trans-activator domain at a GSK-3 target site. *Oncogene* **7**, 347–353.

99. Ayer, D. E., Kretzner, L., and Eisenman, R. N. (1993). Mad: A heterodimeric partner for Max that antagonizes Myc transcriptional activity. *Cell* **72**, 211–222.

100. Zervos, A. S., Gyuris, J., and Brent, R. (1993). Mxi1, a protein that specifically interacts with Max to bind Myc–Max recognition sites. *Cell* **72**, 223–232.
101. Sherman, M. R., Tuazon, F. B., Jong, M. T. C., and Samuels, H. H. (1993). Adenosine A1 receptors and protein kinase a mediate changes in Pit-1 gene expression in rat pituitary tumor cells. *Progr. Abstr. 75th Annu. Meet. Endocr. Soc.*, 297.
102. Steinfelder, H. J., Hauser, P., Nakayama, Y., Radovick, S., McClaskey, J. H., Taylor, T., Weintraub, B. D., and Wondisford, F. E. (1991). Thyrotropin-releasing hormone regulation of human *TSHB* expression: Role of a pituitary-specific transcription factor (Pit-1/GHF-1) and potential interaction with a thyroid hormone-inhibitory element. *Proc. Natl. Acad. Sci. U.S.A.* **88**, 3130–3134.
103. Kapiloff, M. S., Farkash, Y., Wegner, M., and Rosenfeld, M. G. (1991). Variable effects of phosphorylation of Pit-1 dictated by the DNA response elements. *Science* **253**, 786–789.
104. Voss, J. W., Wilson, J. W., and Rosenfeld, M. G. (1991). POU-domain proteins Pit-1 and Oct-1 interact to form a heteromeric complex and can cooperate to induce expression of the prolactin promoter. *Genes Dev.* **5**, 1309–1320.
105. Rotin, D., Honegger, A. M., Margolis, B. L., Ullrich, A., and Schlessinger, J. (1992). Presence of SH2 domains of phospholipase $C\gamma_1$ enhances substrate phosphorylation by increasing the affinity toward the epidermal growth factor receptor. *J. Biol. Chem.* **267**, 9678–9683.
106. Grimm, S., and Baeuerle, P. A. (1993). The inducible transcription factor NF-κB: Structure–function relationship of its protein subunits. *Biochem. J.* **290**, 297–308.
107. Kunsch, C., Ruben, S. M., and Rosen, C. A. (1992). Selection of optimal κB/Rel DNA-binding motifs: Interaction of both subunits of NF-κB with DNA is required for transcriptional activation. *Mol. Cell. Biol.* **12**, 4412–4421.
108. Dobrzanski, P., Ryseck, R. P., and Bravo, R. (1993). Both N- and C-terminal domains of RelB are required for full transactivation: Role of the N-terminal leucine zipper-like motif. *Mol. Cell. Biol.* **13**, 1572–1582.
109. Baeuerle, P. A. (1991). The inducible transcription activator NF-κB: Regulation by distinct protein subunits. *Biochim. Biophys. Acta* **1072**, 63–80.
110. Matthews, J. R., Watson, E., Buckley, S., and Hay, R. T. (1993). Interaction of the C-terminal region of p105 with the nuclear localisation signal of p50 is required for inhibition of NF-κB DNA binding activity. *Nucleic Acids Res.* **21**, 4516–4523.
111. Kumar, S., and Gélinas, C. (1993). IκBα-mediated inhibition of v-Rel DNA binding requires direct interaction with the RXXRXRXXC Rel/κB DNA-binding motif. *Proc. Natl. Acad. Sci. U.S.A.* **90**, 8962–8966.
112. Inoue, J., Kerr, L. D., Kakizuka, A., and Verma, I. M. (1992). IκBγ, a 70 kd protein identical to the C-terminal half of p110 NF-κB: A new member of the IκB family. *Cell* **68**, 1109–1120.
113. Schmid, R. M., Perkins, N. D., Duckett, C. S., Andrews, P. C., and Nabel, G. J. (1991). Cloning of an NF-κB subunit which stimulates HIV transcription in synergy with p65. *Nature (London)* **352**, 733–736.
114. Perkins, N. D., Schmid, R. M., Duckett, C. S., Leung, K., Rice, N. R., and Nabel, G. J. (1992). Distinct combinations of NF-κB subunits determine the specificity of transcriptional activation. *Proc. Natl. Acad. Sci. U.S.A.* **89**, 1529–1533.
115. Sica, A., Tan, T. H., Rice, N., Kretzschmar, M., Ghosh, P., and Young, H. A. (1992). The *c-rel* protooncogene product c-Rel but not NF-κB binds to the

intronic region of the human interferon-q gene at a site related to an interferon-stimulable response element. *Proc. Natl. Acad. Sci. U.S.A.* **89,** 1740–1744.

116. Narayanan, R., Klement, J. F., Ruben, S. M., Higgins, K. A., and Rosen, C. A. (1992). Identification of a naturally occurring transforming variant of the p65 subunit of NF-κB. *Science* **256,** 367–370.

117. Mosialos, G., and Gilmore, T. D. (1993). v-Rel and c-Rel are differentially affected by mutations at a consensus protein kinase recognition sequence. *Oncogene* **8,** 721–730.

118. Beg, A. A., and Baldwin, A. S. (1993). The IκB proteins: Multifunctional regulators of Rel/NF-κB transcription factors. *Genes Dev.* **7,** 2064–2070.

119. Gilmore, T. D., and Morin, P. J. (1993). The IκB proteins: Members of a multifunctional family. *Trends Genet.* **9,** 427–433.

120. Link, E., Kerr, L. D., Schreck, R., Zabel, U., Verma, I., and Baeuerle, P. A. (1992). Purified IκB-β is inactivated upon dephosphorylation. *J. Biol. Chem.* **267,** 239–246.

121. Gerondakis, S., Morrice, N., Richardson, I. B., Wettenhall, R., Fecondo, J., and Grumont, R. J. (1993). The activity of a 70 kilodalton IkB molecule identical to the carboxyl terminus of the p105 NF-κB precursor is modulated by protein kinase A. *Cell Growth Diff.* **4,** 617–627.

122. Li, S., and Sedivy, J. M. (1993). Raf-1 protein kinase activates the NF-κB transcription factor by dissociating the cytoplasmic NF-κB-IκB complex. *Proc. Natl. Acad. Sci. U.S.A.* **90,** 9247–9251.

123. Williams, B. R. G. (1991). Transcriptional regulation of interferon-stimulated genes. *Eur. J. Biochem.* **200,** 1–11.

124. Henkel, T., Machleidt, T., Alkalay, I., Krönke, M., Ben-Neriah, Y., and Baeuerle, P. A. (1993). Rapid proteolysis of IκB-α is necessary for activation of transcription factor NF-κB. *Nature (London)* **365,** 182–185.

125. Hatada, E. N., Naumann, M., and Scheidereit, C. (1993). Common structural constituents confer IκB activity to NF-κB p105 and IκB/MAD-3. *EMBO J.* **12,** 2781–2788.

126. Bours, V., Franzoso, G., Azarenko, V., Park, S., Kanno, T., Brown, K., and Siebenlist, U. (1993). The oncoprotein Bcl-3 directly transactivates through κB motifs via association with DNA-binding p50B homodimers. *Cell* **72,** 729–739.

127. Fujita, T., Nolan, G. P., Liou, H. C., Scott, M. L., and Baltimore, D. (1993). The candidate proto-oncogene *bcl-3* encodes a transcriptional coactivator that activates through NF-κB p50 homodimers. *Genes Dev.* **7,** 1354–1363.

128. Schieven, G. L., Kirihara, J. M., Myers, D. E., Ledbetter, J. A., and Uckun, F. M. (1993). Reactive oxygen intermediates activate NF-κB in a tyrosine kinase-dependent mechanism and in combination with vanadate activate the p56^{lck} and p59^{fyn} tyrosine kinases in human lymphocytes. *Blood* **82,** 1212–1220.

129. Beg, A. A., Finco, T. S., Nantermet, P. V., and Baldwin, A. S. (1993). Tumor necrosis factor and interleukin-1 lead to phosphorylation and loss of IκBα: A mechanism for NF-κB activation. *Mol. Cell. Biol.* **13,** 3301–3310.

130. Treisman, R. (1992). The serum response element. *Trends Biochem. Sci.* **17,** 423–426.

131. Reason, A. J., Morris, H. R., Panico, M., Marais, R., Treisman, R. H., Haltiwanger, R. S., Hart, G. W., Kelly, W. G., and Dell, A. (1992). Localization of O-GlcNAc modification on the serum response transcription factor. *J. Biol. Chem.* **267,** 16911–16921.

132. Berk, A. J. (1989). Regulation of eukaryotic transcription factors by post-translational modification. *Biochim. Biophys. Acta* **1009,** 103–109.

133. Klemsz, M. J., McKercher, S. R., Celada, A., Van Beveren, C., and Maki, R. A. (1990). The macrophage and B cell-specific transcription factor PU.1 is related to the *ets* oncogene. *Cell* **61,** 113–124.

134. Pongubala, J. M. R., Van Beveren, C., Nagulapalli, S., Klemsz, M. J., McKercher, S. R., Maki, R. A., and Atchison, M. L. (1993). Effect of PU.1 phosphorylation on interaction with NF-EM5 and transcriptional activation. *Science* **259,** 1622–1625.

135. Hipskind, R. A., Rao, V. N., Mueller, C. G. F., Reddy, E. S. P., and Nordheim, A. (1991). Ets-related protein Elk-1 is homologous to the c-*fos* regulatory factor p62^{TCF}. *Nature (London)* **354,** 531–534.

136. Shaw, P. E. (1992). Ternary complex formation over the c-*fos* serum response element: p62^{TCF} exhibits dual component specificity with contacts to DNA and an extended structure in the DNA-binding domain of p67^{SRF}. *EMBO J.* **11,** 3011–3019.

137. Janknecht, R., and Nordheim, A. (1993). Gene regulation by Ets proteins. *Biochim. Biophys. Acta* **1155,** 346–356.

138. Wu, H., Moulton, K., Horvai, A., Parik, S., and Glass, C. K. (1994). Combinatorial interactions between AP-1 and ets domain proteins contribute to the developmental regulation of the macrophage scavenger receptor gene. *Mol. Cell. Biol.* **14,** 2129–2139.

139. Gille, H., Sharrocks, A. D., and Shaw, P. E. (1992). Phosphorylation of transcription factor p62^{TCF} by MAP kinase stimulates ternary complex formation at c-*fos* promoter. *Nature (London)* **358,** 414–417.

140. Marais, R., Wynne, J., and Treisman, R. (1993). The SRF accessory protein Elk-1 contains a growth factor-regulated transcriptional activation domain. *Cell* **73,** 381–393.

141. Hill, C. S., Marais, R., John, S., Wynne, J., Dalton, S., and Treisman, R. (1993). Functional analysis of a growth factor-responsive transcription factor complex. *Cell* **73,** 395–406.

142. Janknecht, R., Hipskind, R. A., Houthaeve, T., Nordheim, A., and Stunnenberg, H. G. (1992). Identification of multiple SRF N-terminal phosphorylation sites affecting DNA binding properties. *EMBO J.* **11,** 1045–1054.

143. Janknecht, R., Ernst, W. H., Houthaeve, T., and Nordheim, A. (1993). C-Terminal phosphorylation of the serum-response factor. *Eur. J. Biochem.* **216,** 469–475.

144. Marais, R. M., Hsuan, J. J., McGuigan, C., Wynne, J., and Treisman, R. (1992). Casein kinase II phosphorylation increases the rate of serum response factor-binding site exchange. *EMBO J.* **11,** 97–105.

145. Rivera, V. M., Miranti, C. K., Misra, R. P., Ginty, D. D., Chen, R. H., Blenis, J., and Greenberg, M. E. (1993). A growth factor-induced kinase phosphorylates the serum response factor at a site that regulates its DNA-binding activity. *Mol. Cell. Biol.* **13,** 6260–6273.

146. Yan, C., and Tamm, I. (1991). Molecular cloning and characterization of interferon α/β response element binding factors of the murine (2′–5′)oligoadenylate synthetase ME-12 gene. *Proc. Natl. Acad. Sci. U.S.A.* **88,** 144–148.

147. Pellegrini, S., and Schindler, C. (1993). Early events in signalling by interferons. *Trends Biochem. Sci.* **18,** 338–342.

148. Veals, S. A., Maria, T. S., and Levy, D. E. (1993). Two domains of ISGF3γ that

mediate protein–DNA and protein–protein interactions during transcription factor assembly contribute to DNA-binding specificity. *Mol. Cell. Biol.* **13**, 196–206.

149. Fu, X. Y. (1992). A transcription factor with SH2 and SH3 domains is directly activated by an interferon α-induced cytoplasmic protein tyrosine kinase(s). *Cell* **70**, 323–335.

150. Fu, X. Y., Schindler, C., Improta, T., Aebersold, R., and Darnell, J. E. (1992). The proteins of ISGF-3, the interferon α-induced transcriptional activator, define a gene family involved in signal transduction. *Proc. Natl. Acad. Sci. U.S.A.* **89**, 7840–7843.

151. Schindler, C., Shuai, K., Prezioso, V. R., and Darnell, J. E. (1992). Interferon-dependent tyrosine phosphorylation of a latent cytoplasmic transcription factor. *Science* **257**, 809–813.

152. Velazquez, L., Fellous, M., Stark, G. R., and Pellegrini, S. (1992). A protein tyrosine kinase in the interferon α/β signaling pathway. *Cell* **70**, 313–322.

153. Gutch, M. J., Daly, C., and Reich, N. C. (1992). Tyrosine phosphorylation is required for activation of an α interferon-stimulated transcription factor. *Proc. Natl. Acad. Sci. U.S.A.* **89**, 11411–11415.

154. Shuai, K., Stark, G. R., Kerr, I. M., and Darnell, J. E. (1993). A single phosphotyrosine residue of Stat91 required for gene activation by interferon-γ. *Science* **261**, 1744–1746.

155. Larner, A. C., David, M., Feldman, G. M., Igarashi, K., Hackett, R. H., Webb, D. S. A., Sweitzer, S. M., Petricoin, E. F., and Finbloom, D. S. (1993). Tyrosine phosphorylation of DNA binding proteins by multiple cytokines. *Science* **261**, 1730–1733.

156. Sadowski, H. B., Shuai, K., Darnell, J. E., and Gilman, M. Z. (1993). A common nuclear signal transduction pathway activated by growth factor and cytokine receptors. *Science* **261**, 1739–1744.

157. Ruff-Jamison, S., Chen, K., and Cohen, S. (1993). Induction by EGF and interferon-γ of tyrosine phosphorylated DNA binding proteins in mouse liver nuclei. *Science* **261**, 1733–1736.

158. Silvennoinen, O., Schindler, C., Schlessinger, J., and Levy, D. E. (1993). Ras-independent growth factor signaling by transcription factor tyrosine phosphorylation. *Science* **261**, 1736–1739.

159. Konzak, K. E., and Moore, D. D. (1992). Functional isoforms of pit-1 generated by alternative messenger RNA splicing. *Mol. Endocrinol.* **6**, 241–247.

160. Morris, A. E., Kloss, B., McChesney, R. E., Bancroft, C., and Chasin, L. A. (1992). An alternatively spliced Pit-1 isoform altered in its ability to trans-activate. *Nucleic Acids Res.* **20**, 1355–1361.

161. Meek, D. W., and Street, A. J. (1992). Nuclear protein phosphorylation and growth control. *Biochem. J.* **287**, 1–15.

162. Whiteside, S. T., and Goodbourn, S. (1993). Signal transduction and nuclear targeting: Regulation of transcription factor activity by subcellular localisation. *J. Cell Sci.* **104**, 949–955.

163. Hai, T., and Curran, T. (1991). Cross-family dimerization of transcription factors Fos/Jun and ATF/CREB alters DNA binding specificity. *Proc. Natl. Acad. Sci. U.S.A.* **88**, 3720–3724.

164. Schüle, R., and Evans, R. M. (1991). Cross-coupling of signal transduction pathways: Zinc finger meets leucine zipper. *Trends Genet.* **7**, 377–381.

165. Stein, B., Baldwin, A. S., Ballard, D. W., Greene, W. C., Angel, P., and Herrlich,

P. (1993). Cross-coupling of the NF-κB p65 and Fos/Jun transcription factors produces potentiated biological function. *EMBO J.* **12**, 3879–3891.

166. Kutoh, E., Strömstedt, P. E., and Poellinger, L. (1992). Functional interference between the ubiquitous and constitutive octamer transcription factor 1 (OTF-1) and the glucocorticoid receptor by direct protein–protein interaction involving the homeo subdomain of OTF-1. *Mol. Cell. Biol.* **12**, 4960–4969.

167. Ray, A., and Prefontaine, K. E. (1994). Physical association and functional antagonism between the p65 subunit of transcription factor NF-κB and the glucocorticoid receptor. *Proc. Natl. Acad. Sci. U.S.A.* **91**, 752–756.

168. Stein, B., Cogswell, P. C., and Baldwin, A. S. (1993). Functional and physical associations between NF-κB and C/EBP family members: A Rel domain-bZIP interaction. *Mol. Cell. Biol.* **13**, 3964–3974.

169. Lopez, G., Schaufele, F., Webb, P., Holloway, J. M., Baxter, J. D., and Kushner, P. J. (1993). Positive and negative modulation of Jun action by thyroid hormone receptor at a unique AP1 site. *Mol. Cell. Biol.* **13**, 3042–3049.

170. Nunez, S. B., Medin, J. A., Wang, K., Wahli, W., Ozato, K., and Segars, J. H. (1993). Retinoid X receptor beta and peroxisome proliferator-activated receptor alpha activate the A2 estrogen response element. *Prog. Abstr. 75th Annu. Meet. Endocr. Soc.*, 54.

171. Johnson, P. F., and McKnight, S. L. (1989). Eukaryotic transcriptional regulatory proteins. *Annu. Rev. Biochem.* **58**, 799–839.

172. Strähle, U., Boshart, M., Klock, G., Stewart, F., and Schütz, G. (1989). Glucocorticoid- and progesterone-specific effects are determined by differential expression of the respective hormone receptors. *Nature (London)* **339**, 629–632.

173. O'Malley, B. (1990). The steroid receptor superfamily: More excitement predicted for the future. *Mol. Endocrinol.* **4**, 363–369.

174. Hillgartner, F. B., Chen, W., and Goodridge, A. G. (1992). Overexpression of the α-thyroid hormone receptor in avian cell lines: Effects on expression of the malic enzyme gene are selective and cell-specific. *J. Biol. Chem.* **267**, 12299–12306.

175. Jain, J., McCaffrey, P. G., Miner, Z., Kerppola, T. K., Lambert, J. N., Verdine, G. L., Curran, T., and Rao, A. (1993). The T-cell transcription factor NFAT$_p$ is a substrate for calcineurin and interacts with Fos and Jun. *Nature (London)* **365**, 352–355.

176. Schuchard, M., Rejman, J. J., McCormick, D. J., Gosse, B., Ruesink, T., and Spelsberg, T. C. (1991). Characterization of a purified chromatin acceptor protein (receptor binding factor 1) for the avian oviduct progesterone receptor. *Biochemistry* **30**, 4535–4542.

177. Okamoto, K., Hirano, H., and Isohashi, F. (1993). Molecular cloning of rat liver glucocorticoid-receptor translocation promoter. *Biochem. Biophys. Res. Commun.* **193**, 848–854.

178. Nitsch, D., Boshart, M., and Schütz, G. (1993). Activation of the tyrosine aminotransferase gene is dependent on synergy between liver-specific and hormone-responsive elements. *Proc. Natl. Acad. Sci. U.S.A.* **90**, 5479–5483.

179. Rennie, P. S., Bruchovsky, N., Leco, K. J., Sheppard, P. C., McQueen, S. A., Cheng, H., Snoek, R., Hamel, A., Bock, M. E., MacDonald, B. S., Nickel, B. E., Chang, C., Liao, S., Cattini, P. A., and Matusik, R. J. (1993). Characterization of two *cis*-acting DNA elements involved in the androgen regulation of the probasin gene. *Mol. Endocrinol.* **7**, 23–36.

180. Gowland, P. L., and Buetti, E. (1989). Mutations in the hormone regulatory

element of mouse mammary tumor virus differentially affect the response to progestins, androgens, and glucocorticoids. *Mol. Cell. Biol.* **9,** 3999–4008.

181. De Vos, P., Claessens, F., Peeters, B., Rombauts, W., Heyns, W., and Verhoeven, G. (1993). Interaction of androgen and glucocorticoid receptor DNA-binding domains with their response elements. *Mol. Cell. Endocrinol.* **90,** R11–R16.

182. Lannigan, D. A., Tomashek, J. J., Obourn, J. D., and Notides, A. C. (1993). Analysis of estrogen receptor interaction with tertiary-structured estrogen responsive elements. *Biochem. Pharmacol.* **45,** 1921–1928.

183. Solomon, D. L. C., Amati, B., and Land, H. (1993). Distinct DNA binding preferences for the c-Myc/Max and Max/Max dimers. *Nucleic Acids Res.* **21,** 5372–5376.

184. Katz, R. W., and Koenig, R. J. (1993). Nonbiased identification of DNA sequences that bind thyroid hormone receptor $\alpha 1$ with high affinity. *J. Biol. Chem.* **268,** 19392–19397.

185. Mangelsdorf, D. J., Umesono, K., Kliewer, S. A., Borgmeyer, U., Ong, E. S., and Evans, R. M. (1991). A direct repeat in the cellular retinol-binding protein type II gene confers differential regulation by RXR and RAR. *Cell* **66,** 555–561.

186. Umesono, K., Murakami, K. K., Thompson, C. C., and Evans, R. M. (1991). Direct repeats as selective response elements for the thyroid hormone, retinoic acid, and vitamin D_3 receptors. *Cell* **65,** 1255–1266.

187. Forman, B. M., Casanova, J., Raaka, B. M., Ghysdael, J., and Samuels, H. H. (1992). Half-site spacing and orientation determines whether thyroid hormone and retinoic acid receptors and related factors bind to DNA response elements as monomers, homodimers, or heterodimers. *Mol. Endocrinol.* **6,** 429–442.

188. Kadowaki, Y., Toyoshima, K., and Yamamoto, T. (1992). Ear3/COUP-TF binds most tightly to a response element with tandem repeat separated by one nucleotide. *Biochem. Biophys. Res. Commun.* **183,** 492–498.

189. Carlberg, C. (1993). RXR-independent action of the receptors for thyroid hormone, retinoic acid and vitamin D on inverted palindromes. *Biochem. Biophys. Res. Commun.* **195,** 1345–1353.

190. Piña, B., Haché, R. J. G., Arnemann, J., Chalepakis, G., Slater, E. P., and Beato, M. (1990). Hormonal induction of transfected genes depends on DNA topology. *Mol. Cell. Biol.* **10,** 625–633.

191. Smith, C. L., Archer, T. K., Hamlin-Green, G., and Hager, G. L. (1993). Newly expressed progesterone receptor cannot activate stable, replicated mouse mammary tumor virus templates but acquires transactivation potential upon continuous expression. *Proc. Natl. Acad. Sci. U.S.A.* **90,** 11202–11206.

192. Kerppola, T. K., and Curran, T. (1993). Selective DNA bending by a variety of bZIP proteins. *Mol. Cell. Biol.* **13,** 5479–5489.

193. Carballo, M., and Beato, M. (1990). Binding of the glucocorticoid receptor induces a topological change in plasmids containing the hormone-responsive element of mouse mammary tumor virus. *DNA Cell Biol.* **9,** 519–525.

194. Ishibe, Y., Klinge, C. M., Hilf, R., and Bambara, R. A. (1991). Estrogen receptor alters the topology of plasmid DNA containing estrogen responsive elements. *Biochem. Biophys. Res. Commun.* **176,** 486–491.

195. Lannigan, D. A., and Notides, A. C. (1989). Estrogen receptor selectively binds the "coding strand" of an estrogen responsive element. *Proc. Natl. Acad. Sci. U.S.A.* **86,** 863–867.

196. Cardenas, M. E., and Gasser, S. M. (1993). Regulation of topoisomerase II by phosphorylation: A role for casein kinase II. *J. Cell Sci.* **104,** 219–225.

197. Cardellini, E., and Durban, E. (1993). Phosphorylation of human topoisomerase I by protein kinase C *in vitro* and in phorbol 12-myristate 13-acetate-activated HL-60 promyelocytic leukaemia cells. *Biochem. J.* **291**, 303–307.

198. Kroll, D. J., Sullivan, D. M., Gutierrez-Hartmann, A., and Hoeffler, J. P. (1993). Modification of DNA topoisomerase II activity via direct interactions with the cyclic adenosine-3′,5′-monophosphate response element-binding protein and related transcription factors. *Mol. Endocrinol.* **7**, 305–318.

199. Leidig, F., Shepard, A. R., Zhang, W., Stelter, A., Cattini, P. A., Baxter, J. D., and Eberhardt, N. L. (1992). Thyroid hormone responsiveness in human growth hormone-related genes: Possible correlation with receptor-induced DNA conformational changes. *J. Biol. Chem.* **267**, 913–921.

200. Nardulli, A. M., and Shapiro, D. J. (1992). Binding of the estrogen receptor DNA-binding domain to the estrogen response element induces DNA bending. *Mol. Cell. Biol.* **12**, 2037–2042.

201. Lu, X. P., Eberhardt, N. L., and Pfahl, M. (1993). DNA bending by retinoid X receptor-containing retinoid and thyroid hormone receptor complexes. *Mol. Cell. Biol.* **13**, 6509–6519.

202. Schrenk, R., Zorbas, H., Winnacker, E. L., and Baeuerle, P. A. (1990). The NF-κB transcription factor induces DNA bending which is modulated by its 65-kD subunit. *Nucleic Acids Res.* **18**, 6497–6502.

203. Verrijzer, C. P., van Oosterhout, J. A. W. M., van Weperen, W. W., and van der Vliet, P. C. (1991). POU proteins bend DNA via the POU-specific domain. *EMBO J.* **10**, 3007–3014.

204. Kerppola, T. K., and Curran, T. (1991). Fos-Jun heterodimers and Jun homodimers bend DNA in opposite orientations: Implications for transcription factor cooperativity. *Cell* **66**, 317–326.

205. Théveny, B., Bailly, A., Rauch, C., Rauch, M., Delain, E., and Milgrom, E. (1987). Association of DNA-bound progesterone receptors. *Nature (London)* **329**, 79–81.

206. Seyfred, M. A., and Cullen, K. E. (1992). Involvement of DNA looping in estrogen-mediated induction of rat prolactin gene expression. *Progr. Abstr. 74th Annu. Meet. Endocr. Soc.*, 114.

207. Archer, T. K., Cordingley, M. G., Wolford, R. G., and Hager, G. L. (1991). Transcription factor access is mediated by accurately positioned nucleosomes on the mouse mammary tumor virus promoter. *Mol. Cell. Biol.* **11**, 688–698.

208. Bresnick, E. H., John, S., Berard, D. S., LeFebvre, P., and Hager, G. L. (1990). Glucocorticoid receptor-dependent disruption of a specific nucleosome on the mouse mammary tumor virus promoter is prevented by sodium butyrate. *Proc. Natl. Acad. Sci. U.S.A.* **87**, 3977–3981.

209. Perlmann, T., and Wrange, Ö. (1991). Inhibition of chromatin assembly in *Xenopus* oocytes correlates with derepression of the mouse mammary tumor virus promoter. *Mol. Cell. Biol.* **11**, 5259–5265.

210. Archer, T. K., Lefebvre, P., Wolford, R. G., and Hager, G. L. (1992). Transcription factor loading on the MMTV promoter: A bimodal mechanism for promoter activation. *Science* **255**, 1573–1576.

211. Carr, K. D., and Richard-Foy, H. (1990). Glucocorticoids locally disrupt an array of positioned nucleosomes on the rat tyrosine aminotransferase promoter in hepatoma cells. *Proc. Natl. Acad. Sci. U.S.A.* **87**, 9300–9304.

212. Reik, A., Schütz, G., and Stewart, A. F. (1991). Glucocorticoids are required for establishment and maintenance of an alteration in chromatin structure: Induc-

tion leads to a reversible disruption of nucleosomes over an enhancer. *EMBO J.* **10**, 2569–2576.

213. Seyfred, M. A., and Gorski, J. (1990). An interaction between the 5' flanking distal and proximal regulatory domains of the rat prolactin gene is required for transcriptional activations by estrogens. *Mol. Endocrinol.* **4**, 1226–1234.

214. Ing, N. H., Beekman, J. M., Tsai, S. Y., Tsai, M. J., and O'Malley, B. W. (1992). Members of the steroid hormone receptor superfamily interact with TFIIB (S300-II). *J. Biol. Chem.* **267**, 17617–17623.

215. Kerr, L. D., Ransone, L. J., Wamsley, P., Schmitt, M. J., Boyer, T. G., Zhou, Q., Berk, A. J., and Verma, I. M. (1993). Association between proto-oncoprotein Rel and TATA-binding protein mediates transcriptional activation by NF-κB. *Nature (London)* **365**, 412–419.

216. Montminy, M. R., Gonzalez, G. A., and Yamamoto, K. K. (1990). Regulation of cAMP-inducible genes by CREB. *Trends Neurosci.* **13**, 184–188.

217. Shrivastava, A., Saleque, S., Kalpana, G. V., Artandi, S., Goff, S. P., and Calame, K. (1993). Inhibition of transcriptional regulator Yin-Yang-1 by association with c-Myc. *Science* **262**, 1889–1892.

218. Clark, A. R., and Docherty, K. (1993). Negative regulation of transcription in eukaryotes. *Biochem. J.* **296**, 521–541.

219. Strömstedt, P. E., Poellinger, L., Gustafsson, J.Å., and Carlstedt-Duke, J. (1991). The glucocorticoid receptor binds to a sequence overlapping the TATA box of the human osteocalcin promoter: A potential mechanism for negative regulation. *Mol. Cell. Biol.* **11**, 3379–3383.

220. Schüle, R., Umesono, K., Mangelsdorf, D. J., Bolado, J., Pike, J. W., and Evans, R. M. (1990). Jun–fos and receptors for vitamins A and D recognize a common response element in the human osteocalcin gene. *Cell* **61**, 497–504.

221. Xu, J., Thompson, K. L., Shephard, L. B., Hudson, L. G., and Gill, G. N. (1993). T_3 receptor suppression of Sp1-dependent transcription from the epidermal growth factor receptor promoter via overlapping DNA-binding sites. *J. Biol. Chem.* **268**, 16065–16073.

222. Graupner, G., Wills, K. N., Tzukerman, M., Zhang, X., and Pfahl, M. (1989). Dual regulatory role for thyroid-hormone receptors allows control of retinoic-acid receptor activity. *Nature (London)* **340**, 653–656.

223. Widom, R. L., Rhee, M., and Karathanasis, S. K. (1992). Repression by ARP-1 sensitizes apolipoprotein AI gene responsiveness to RXRα and retinoic acid. *Mol. Cell. Biol.* **12**, 3380–3389.

224. Dobens, L., Rudolph, K., and Berger, E. M. (1991). Ecdysterone regulatory elements function as both transcriptional activators and repressors. *Mol. Cell. Biol.* **11**, 1846–1853.

225. Fondell, J. D., Roy, A. L., and Roeder, R. G. (1993). Unliganded thyroid hormone receptor inhibits formation of a functional preinitiation complex: Implications for active repression. *Genes Dev.* **7**, 1400–1410.

226. Hirst, M. A., Hinck, L., Danielsen, M., and Ringold, G. M. (1991). Discrimination of DNA response elements for thyroid and estrogen is dependent upon dimerization or receptor DNA binding domains. *Progr. Abstr. 73rd Annu. Meet. Endocr. Soc.*, 266.

227. Meyer, M. E., Gronemeyer, H., Turcotte, B., Bocquel, M. T., Tasset, D., and Chambon, P. (1989). Steroid hormone receptors compete for factors that mediate their enhancer function. *Cell* **57**, 433–442.

228. Webb, P., Lopez, G. N., Greene, G. L., Baxter, J. D., and Kusher, P. J. (1992). The

limits of the cellular capacity to mediate an estrogen response. *Mol. Endocrinol.* **6**, 157–167.

229. Lehmann, J. M., Zhang, X. K., Graupner, G., Lee, M. O., Hermann, T., Hoffmann, B., and Pfahl, M. (1993). Formation of retinoid X receptor homodimers leads to repression of T₃ response: Hormonal cross talk by ligand-induced squelching. *Mol. Cell. Biol.* **13**, 7698–7707.

230. Baniahmad, A., Ha, I., Reinberg, D., Tsai, S., Tsai, M. J., and O'Malley, B. W. (1993). Interaction of human thyroid hormone receptor β with transcription factor TFIIB may mediate target gene derepression and activation by thyroid hormone. *Proc. Natl. Acad. Sci. U.S.A.* **90**, 8832–8836.

231. Pfahl, M. (1993). Nuclear receptor/AP-1 interaction. *Endocr. Rev.* **14**, 651–658.

232. Jonat, C., Rahmsdorf, J., Park, K. K., Cato, A. C. B., Gebel, S., Ponta, H., and Herrlich, P. (1990). Antitumor promotion and antiinflammation: Down-modulation of AP-1 (Fos/Jun) activity by glucocorticoid hormone. *Cell* **62**, 1189–1204.

233. Schüle, R., Rangarajan, P., Kliewer, S., Ransone, L. J., Bolado, J., Yang, N., Verma, I. M., and Evans, R. M. (1990). Functional antagonism between oncoprotein c-Jun and the glucocorticoid receptor. *Cell* **62**, 1217–1226.

234. Yang-Yen, H. F., Chambard, J. C., Sun, Y. L., Smeal, T., Schmidt, T. J., Drouin, J., and Karin, M. (1990). Transcriptional interference between c-Jun and the glucocorticoid receptor: Mutual inhibition of DNA binding due to direct protein–protein interaction. *Cell* **62**, 1205–1215.

235. Doucas, V., Spyrou, G., and Yaniv, M. (1991). Unregulated expression of c-Jun and c-Fos proteins but not Jun D inhibits oestrogen receptor activity in human breast cancer derived cells. *EMBO J.* **10**, 2237–2245.

236. Schüle, R., Rangarajan, P., Yang, N., Kliewer, S., Ransone, L. J., Bolado, J., Verma, I. M., and Evans, R. M. (1991). Retinoic acid is a negative regulator of AP-1 responsive genes. *Proc. Natl. Acad. Sci. U.S.A.* **88**, 6092–6096.

237. Zhang, X. K., Wills, K. N., Husmann, M., Hermann, T., and Pfahl, M. (1991). Novel pathway for thyroid hormone receptor action through interaction with *jun* and *fos* oncogene activities. *Mol. Cell. Biol.* **11**, 6016–6025.

238. Sharif, M., and Privalsky, M. L. (1992). V-*erb*A and c-*erb*A proteins enhance transcriptional activation by c-*jun*. *Oncogene* **7**, 953–960.

239. Sharif, M., and Privalsky, M. L. (1992). V-*erb*A and c-*erb*A proteins enhance transcriptional activation by c-*jun*. *Oncogene* **7**, 953–960.

240. Maroder, M., Farina, A. R., Vacca, A., Felli, M. P., Meco, D., Screpanti, I., Frati, L., and Gulino, A. (1993). Cell-specific bifunctional role of Jun oncogene family members on glucocorticoid receptor-dependent transcription. *Mol. Endocrinol.* **7**, 570–584.

241. Miner, J. N., and Yamamoto, K. R. (1991). Regulatory crosstalk at composite response elements. *Trends Biochem. Sci.* **16**, 423–426.

242. Kerppola, T. K., Luk, D., and Curran, T. (1993). Fos is a preferential target of glucocorticoid receptor inhibition of AP-1 activity *in vitro*. *Mol. Cell. Biol.* **13**, 3782–3791.

243. Baniahmad, A., Köhne, A. C., and Renkawitz, R. (1992). A transferable silencing domain is present in the thyroid hormone receptor, in the v-*erb*A oncogene product and in the retinoic acid receptor. *EMBO J.* **11**, 1015–1023.

244. Cochet, M., Chang, A. C. Y., and Cohen, S. N. (1982). Characterization of the structural gene and putative 5'-regulatory sequences for human proopiomelanocortin. *Nature (London)* **297**, 335–339.

245. Scheidereit, C., Geisse, S., Westphal, H. M., and Beato, M. (1983). The glucocorticoid receptor binds to defined nucleotide sequences near the promoter of mouse mammary tumour virus. *Nature (London)* **304,** 749–752.
246. Gronemeyer, H., and Pongs, O. (1980). Localization of ecdysone on polytene chromosomes of *Drosophila melanogaster*. *Proc. Natl. Acad. Sci. U.S.A.* **77,** 2108–2112.
247. Press, M. F., Nousek-Goebl, N. A., and Greene, G. L. (1985). Immunoelectron microscopic localization of estrogen receptor with monoclonal estrophilin antibodies. *J. Histochem. Cytochem.* **33,** 915–924.
248. Isola, J. J. (1987). The effect of progesterone on the localization of progesterone receptors in the nuclei of chick oviduct cells. *Cell Tissue Res.* **249,** 317–323.
249. Näär, A. M., Boutin, J. M., Lipkin, S. M., Yu, V. C., Holloway, J. M., Glass, C. K., and Rosenfeld, M. G. (1991). The orientation and spacing of core DNA-binding motifs dictate selective transcriptional responses to three nuclear receptors. *Cell* **65,** 1267–1279.
250. Tsai, S. Y., Carlstedt-Duke, J., Weigel, N. L., Dahlman, K., Gustafsson, J.Å., Tsai, M. J., and O'Malley, B. W. (1988). Molecular interactions of steroid hormone receptor with its enhancer element: Evidence for receptor dimer formation. *Cell* **55,** 361–369.
251. Nichols, M., Weih, F., Schmid, W., DeVack, C., Kowenz-Leutz, E., Luckow, B., Boshart, M., and Schütz, G. (1992). Phosphorylation of CREB affects its binding to high and low affinity sites: Implications for cAMP induced gene transcription. *EMBO J.* **11,** 3337–3346.
252. Alroy, I., and Freedman, L. P. (1992). DNA binding analysis of glucocorticoid receptor specificity mutants. *Nucleic Acids Res.* **20,** 1045–1052.
253. Drust, D. S., Troccoli, N. M., and Jameson, J. L. (1991). Binding specificity of cyclic adenosine 3′,5′-monophosphate-responsive element (CRE)-binding proteins and activating transcription factors to naturally occurring CRE sequence variants. *Mol. Endocrinol.* **5,** 1541–1551.
254. Herr, W. (1991). Regulation of eukaryotic RNA polymerase II transcription by sequence-specific DNA-binding proteins. *In* "The Hormonal Control of Gene Transcription" (P. Cohen and J. G. Foulkes, eds.), pp. 25–56. Elsevier, Amsterdam.
255. Sheridan, P. L., Evans, R. M., and Horwitz, K. B. (1989). Phosphotryptic peptide analysis of human progesterone receptors: New phosphorylated sites formed in nuclei after hormone treatment. *J. Biol. Chem.* **264,** 6520–6528.
256. Tsai, S. Y., Tsai, M. J., and O'Malley, B. W. (1989). Cooperative binding of steroid hormone receptors contributes to transcriptional synergism at target enhancer elements. *Cell* **57,** 443–448.
257. O'Malley, B. (1990). The steroid receptor superfamily: More excitement predicted for the future. *Mol. Endocrinol.* **4,** 363–369.
258. Martinez, E., and Wahli, W. (1989). Cooperative binding of estrogen receptor to imperfect estrogen-responsive DNA elements correlates with their synergistic hormone-dependent enhancer activity. *EMBO J.* **8,** 3781–3791.
259. Ponglikitmongkol, M., White, J. H., and Chambon, P. (1990). Synergistic activation of transcription by the human estrogen receptor bound to tandem responsive elements. *EMBO J.* **9,** 2221–2231.

CHAPTER *13*

Modifications and Conformations of DNA and Nuclear Proteins

I. Introduction

Transcription involves more than simply activating a transcription factor (Chapter 12); the DNA that the factor recognizes may not always be readily accessible. Because of its size and charge, DNA is extensively packaged by chromatin proteins; this complex can impede transcription. Furthermore, both these proteins and the DNA itself can be covalently modified; these alterations can change chromatin structure and affect transcription. The nature of the packaging and these modifications will now be examined.

II. Chromatin Structure

A. Nucleosomes

1. Components

DNA presents the cell with two packaging problems: (i) a very negatively charged molecule and (ii) a very long polymer. The *histones* are designed to solve these problems: they are small, very basic proteins that are involved in DNA packaging (1,2). The histones are classified according to the abundance of their basic amino acids: histones H3 and H4 are the arginine-rich histones because they have slightly more arginine than lysine (Table 13-1). They are also among the most highly conserved proteins in nature: histone H4 sequences from cows and peas reveal only two amino acid differences and both of these substitutions are conservative. A conservative substitution occurs when one amino acid is replaced by a structurally similar one so the overall function of the protein remains unperturbed. Histones H2A and H2B are the moderately lysine-rich histones and are moderately conserved in evolution. All four of these proteins have the same charge distribution: a strongly basic amino terminus comprising one-third to one-half of the molecule, a basic carboxy terminus, and a neutral central region. The positive ends of the histones are thought to bind the negative DNA, whereas the center is involved in histone–histone interactions.

These four proteins are called the *core histones* because they form the nucleus around which the DNA winds. This nucleus, or *nucleosome*, has three parts: a $(H3)_2(H4)_2$ tetramer and two (H2A) (H2B) dimers. The tetramer forms a shallow spiraling circle that resembles a locking washer (3); the DNA will run along the back of this tetramer. Its direct interaction with DNA explains why H3 and H4 are the most conserved of the histones. Each (H2A) (H2B) dimer forms a wedge above and below the spiral to give the entire nucleosome a flatter disk-like shape. The disk is 55 Å by 110 Å and is encircled by 140 bp of DNA or about 1.75 turns (Fig. 13-1A). Although they may interfere with transcription initiation, nucleosomes do not impede elongation. The (H2A) (H2B) dimers may temporarily leave to open up the nucleosome and reduce any potential physical hindrance to the transcriptional machinery. Such a hypothetical structure consisting of only the $(H3)_2(H4)_2$ tetramer is called a *lexosome*.

Table 13-1

Characteristics and Modifications of Histones and HMG Proteins

	Molecular weight (kDa)	Lys/Arg	Nuclear protein modification[a]				
			Acetylation[b]	Phosphorylation	Poly(ADP-ribosyl)ation	Methylation	Glycosylation
Substrates							
Histone H1	21.0	63/3	0	++	++	0	0
Histone H2A	14.0	14/12	+	+	+	0	0
Histone H2B	13.8	20/8	+	0	+	0	0
Histone H3	15.3	13/18	++	+	0	++(Lys)	0
Histone H4	11.3	11/14	++	+	0	++(Lys)	0
HMG 1–2	31.7	50/10	+	0	++	+(Arg)	+
HMG 14–17	11.2	21/5	+	++/+	+	?	+
Control							
Turnover			Rapid	Rapid	Rapid	Slow	
RNA/protein synthesis required			No	No	No	?	
Hormonally regulated			++	++	++	±	

[a] For intact normal cells or tissues.
[b] N^{ϵ}-Lysine only.

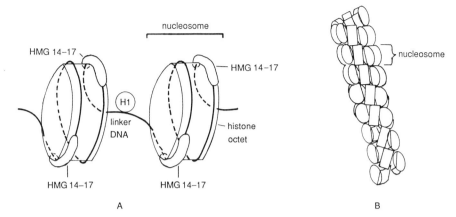

Fig. 13-1. Nucleosomes. (A) The histone octet with the intervening linker DNA and histone H1. (B) Aggregation of nucleosomes into a solenoid structure.

Successive nucleosomes are connected by 20–100 bp of DNA, called *linker DNA;* such an arrangement resembles beads on a string. The last histone, histone H1, is a lysine-rich histone that binds to the linker DNA and is essential to the further condensation of chromatin. H1 is known to inhibit the initiation, but not elongation, of transcription; this repression is due, in part, to the chromatin condensation induced by H1 (4). In addition, H1 may displace some transcription factors from DNA. Originally, it was thought that H1 was itself displaced from linker DNA during transcription; researchers now believe that it merely loosens its grip. H1 contains a central globular domain of four α helices in a barrel. In inactive chromatin, H1 is closely associated with DNA, but in transcriptionally active regions only the amino- and carboxy-terminal tails touch the DNA. This reduced interaction apparently favors chromatin decondensation and does not interfere with transcription factors.

Another way to remove the inhibitory effects of H1 is to replace it with an H1 variant. Histone variants, called *isohistones,* have been identified for all histones except histone H4, the most evolutionarily conserved histone (5). Histone H1° binds to the linker DNA more tightly than histone H1 and, in fact, displaces it in terminally differentiated but not actively dividing tissue. Histone H1° is also less effective in chromatin condensation than histone H1 (6). Finally, histone H1° is hormonally regulated (7); this variant is lost in target organs following hormone deprivation and returns with hormone replacement. This effect is specific, since histone H1 does not change in these same tissues and histone H1° in nontarget tissues is unaffected by the hormone status of the animal. Therefore, some hormones may act, in part, by replacing histone H1 with histone H1° so the chromatin will relax and the DNA can be transcribed.

Other histones also have variants: one is a protein conjugate between histone H2A and HMG 20 (8). Furthermore, since HMG 20 is identical to ubiquitin, the complex is presently called uH2A. As the name implies, *ubiquitin* is a ubiquitous protein that is covalently attached via an isopeptide (amide) bond to other proteins destined for degradation. As such, it is a molecular condemnation notice. In histone uH2A, the carboxy-terminal glycine of ubiquitin forms an isopeptide bond with the ϵ-amino group of K-119 in histone H2A (Fig. 13-2).

As much as 10% of histone H2A and 1.5% of histone H2B is conjugated to ubiquitin; amazingly, the addition of this 76-amino-acid peptide does not appear to alter the nucleosomal structure, although it may impede refolding once the nucleosome is opened (9). However, as a molecular marker for degradation, it does result in a rapid turnover of these histones. Histones normally have very long half-lives: 9–15 days for histones H3 and H4, 4–6 days for histones H2A and H2B, and ~2 days for histone H1 in terminally differentiated kidney cells (10). Therefore, what this modification may do is increase the turnover of ordinary histones to facilitate the insertion of isohistones that are more conducive to transcription. Indeed, in *Drosophila,* uH2A levels are highest in actively transcribed regions (11).

Other nuclear proteins are also important in chromatin structure. One such class was initially extracted into 0.35 *M* NaCl and remained soluble in 2% trichloroacetic acid. The supernatant contained proteins with a high mobility in polyacrylamide gels; therefore, they were named the *high-mobility group* (HMG) proteins. High-mobility group proteins 14 and 17 are so similar to each other that they will be considered a single group (HMG 14–17); HMG 1 and 2 will be treated likewise (HMG 1–2). The HMG 14–17 proteins have an uneven charge distribution: the amino terminus is very basic whereas the carboxy terminus is very negative. There are two HMG 14–17 binding sites on each nucleosome, and the proteins are believed to secure the DNA where it enters and exits the nucleosome; the basic amino terminus binds the DNA and the negative carboxy terminus binds the histones (12). As a result, HMG 14–17 stabilizes the nucleosome, whether in the condensed or the unraveled state (13). These proteins are also partially responsible for inducing regular spacing in nucleosomes (14). Finally, they are also thought to interact with the nuclear matrix through their sugar residues (15); unlike histones, HMG proteins are glycosylated (Table 13-1).

The HMG 1–2 proteins are larger than the HMG 14–17 proteins and have a very different structure. HMG 1–2 proteins have a central hydropho-

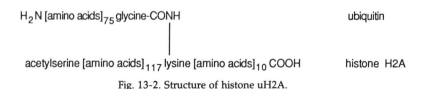

Fig. 13-2. Structure of histone uH2A.

bic domain containing duplicated DNA-binding motifs known as HMG boxes. Each motif is composed of three α helices (16): the first two are antiparallel and perpendicular to the third so they form an "L." This structure is somewhat reminiscent of the POU domains: two covalently linked dimers, each having one helix lying in the major group and two or more helices lying on top nearly perpendicular to the first. However, the method by which HMG boxes bind DNA is still unknown. The carboxy terminus is extremely acidic; in fact, the last 30 residues are either glutamic or aspartic acid (17). The physiological function for this carboxy terminus is unknown, but *in vitro* it is capable of unwinding the DNA helix (18); it is also very efficient in bending DNA (19). Several facts implicate these proteins in gene activation:

1. They partially unwind the DNA helix (20).

2. They bind specific DNA sequences, especially at cruciform structures, where they remove the transcriptional block that these structures create (21).

3. They stimulate transcription *in vitro*, where they facilitate the formation of the active initiation complex (22,23).

2. Organization

One of the more controversial topics involving nucleosomes is whether or not they occupy specific, fixed positions along the DNA (24,25). Certain mechanisms would allow this positioning to occur. First, certain sequences favor bending in one plane and binding to nucleosomes: for example, AT-rich sequences are preferred where the minor groove is compressed. Second, proteins that bind specific DNA sequences can form boundaries, after which nucleosomes would line up in phase. In general, the shorter the linker DNA, the more persistent the phasing. If these bound proteins occurred periodically, they could shepherd the nucleosomes over a considerable distance. Z-DNA can also act as a boundary, since nucleosomes cannot bind Z-DNA. Third, chromatin folding can influence nucleosomal spacing.

The existence of nucleosomal positioning has important regulatory implications. For example, in several genes nucleosomes lie over the promoter and must be removed before transcription can begin (see Chapter 12). Nucleosomes do not impede elongation, but they do repress initiation. Nucleosomes may also favor the binding of certain proteins; for example, the PgR prefers to bind at the edge of nucleosomes (26).

The nucleosomes themselves can condense into a higher ordered structure called a solenoid (Fig. 13-1B). This superstructure is 200–300 Å in diameter and has six to eight nucleosomes per per turn. About 50 kilobases (kb) of the solenoid, or about 35 turns, twist into a loop; these loops can then form an even larger solenoid called a *coil* (27). Six loops form a single turn of the coil, each turn is called a *rosette*, and 30 rosettes make up the entire coil. A chromatid contains about 10 coils.

B. Histone Modifications

Histones are susceptible to innumerable modifications, only four of which will be considered in this chapter: acetylation, phosphorylation, poly(ADP–ribosyl)ation, and methylation (28). Which characteristics might indicate that a particular modification is likely to be involved in gene activation? First, since gene induction is usually rapid, the modification should have a rapid turnover to allow for the rapid modulation of the modification. Second, if the modification is to be a primary event in hormone action, it should be independent of RNA and protein synthesis. Finally, there should be evidence for hormonal regulation. Of the modifications just listed, only methylation is a poor candidate (see Table 13-1).

Before examining in detail the various post-translational modifications that histones can undergo, it is important to identify the substrate positively; this may not be easy, since many modifications alter the size and/or the charge of the substrate. Second, it is important to identify the particular site on the substrate, since different sites may be functionally distinct; this is especially true for phosphorylation and acetylation and there is some evidence that it may also be true for methylation. Third, pharmacological agents are frequently used to perturb these modifications, but all drugs have undesirable side effects that are not always controlled for in these investigations.

The final problem relates to the physiological interpretation of the data. First, an increase in the incorporation of a labeled precursor, such as radioactive phosphate or acetate, may only represent an increased turnover of this modification. In other words, a faster turnover would allow a greater *percentage* of the modified units to become labeled, even though the *total* level of the modification remains unchanged. Second, hormone-altered modifications may, in fact, only represent hormone-altered label uptake, equilibrium, or substrate turnover. Third, there are always problems with artifacts, especially during processing; homogenization may reveal previously unexposed sites that would normally never be modified *in vivo*. Finally, in studies using intact animals the question of direct versus indirect action always arises. Insulin has been reported to induce histone H1 phosphorylation *in vivo*, but in intact animals insulin induces hypoglycemia, which triggers the release of glucagon. Glucagon also stimulates histone H1 phosphorylation. Is insulin acting directly on histone H1 or indirectly through elevated glucagon levels? These caveats will be discussed in greater detail later, as appropriate.

1. Acetylation

Acetylation refers to the covalent addition of an acetate to a free amino group: CH_3CONHR (29–31). The free amino group may be either at the amino terminus (N^α) or on the side chain of lysine (N^ϵ). Acetylation is performed by several acetyltransferases, which exhibit the following histone substrate specificity: $H3 \cong H4 > H2A \cong H2B > H1$. N^α-Acetyltransferase attaches acetyl groups to proteins during synthesis (for example, histone H1); such groups are very stable, do not appear to be associated with gene activation, and will not be considered further. N^ϵ-Acetylation, however, has a rapid turnover and can be performed by two acetyltransferases, A and B. Like the N^α-acetyltransferase, N^ϵ-acetyltransferase B occurs in the cytoplasm and acetylates nascent proteins; it prefers lysines adjacent to neutral amino acids, such as those in histone H4. In contrast, acetyltransferase A is tightly bound to chromatin and prefers lysines adjacent to other basic amino acids. Both enzymes require ATP, magnesium, and acetyl coenzyme A, which is the source of the acetate.

These enzymes are complemented by a deacetylase that removes acetyl groups. The deacetylase is noncompetitively inhibited by butyrate, resulting in the hyperacetylation of all histones except histone H1. Since butyrate easily traverses the cell membrane, it can be used to study the function of acetylation in living cells. However, this chemical is not without important side effects (32):

1. In some systems such as the mammary gland, butyrate can also inhibit the acetyltransferase, resulting in a net hypoacetylation (33).

2. Butyrate may stimulate the phosphorylation of HMG 14–17 and some histones, as well as induce poly(ADP–ribosyl)ation. Since acetylation relaxes chromatin structure (see subsequent discussion), this stimulation is thought to be secondary to the exposure of previously hidden phosphorylation or ribosylation sites.

3. Butyrate may provoke differentiation apart from its effects on acetylation. Indeed, a butyrate hormone response element (HRE) has been identified (34), suggesting that it may directly activate a transcription factor. Such a factor may be related to peroxisome proliferator nuclear receptor (PPAR), which can be activated by fatty acids.

4. Butyrate may inhibit DNA synthesis. This effect may simply be a result of its induction of differentiation.

5. Butyrate may alter DNA methylation patterns by inhibiting the DNA methylase.

6. Finally, butyrate may alter hormone receptor levels; for example, it reduces estradiol (35) and triiodothyronine (T_3) receptors (36).

Further complications can arise because butyrate treatment may not always increase acetylation levels to those observed under physiological conditions (37). Finally, butyrate induces a global acetylation whereas natural acetylation is more selective. This difference is important, since modifications at specific positions are associated with distinct functions. In *Drosophila*, lysines 5 and 8 in histone H4 are acetylated in active euchromatin whereas lysine 12 is acetylated in inactive heterochromatin and lysine 16 is modified in the hyperactive X chromosome of male flies (38). In the amphibian *Triturus*, lysines 8, 12, and 16 in histone H4 are acetylated at the base of the transcriptionally active loops, but lysine 5 is the only modified residue in the loops themselves (39).

The hormonal regulation of histone acetylation has been well documented (Table 13-2; 33, 40–44), but the actual mechanisms for this control have been less well studied. *In vivo,* estradiol is capable of stimulating acetylation 10- to 12-fold within 10 minutes (40), intriguingly suggesting that this steroid is acting directly (see Chapter 5). This hypothesis is further supported by the report that estradiol, in concentrations between 10^{-7} and 10^{-9} M, can stimulate acetyltransferase in homogenates of uteri from immature rats (45) and that the estrogen receptor (ER) is required (44). In rat mammary explants, prolactin (PRL) also stimulates an acetyltransferase (33), but its action must be indirect since peptide hormones cannot cross the plasma membrane. One possible mechanism utilizes spermidine as an intermediate: at physiological concentrations, spermidine can activate acetyltransferase (46) and inhibit deacetylase (47); furthermore, this polyamine is elevated by PRL (see Chapter 10).

The major effect of acetylation is DNA decondensation. Butyrate-induced acetylation in excess of 10 groups per nucleosome results in a more relaxed chromatin structure as evidenced by increased DNase I susceptibility and by data from gel electrophoresis, electric dichroism, and sedimentation studies (48). For example, acetylated histones are more easily displaced from the nucleosome in the protamine competition assay than from unmodified histones (33,49). Conversely, chromosomes that are highly condensed, such as the inactive X chromosome, are devoid of certain acetylated histones (50). There are several possible mechanisms for this effect. First, acetylation decreases the effectiveness of H1 to induce the solenoid structure (51). Second, it reduces the affinity of the tails of HMG proteins and histone H4 for DNA (52,53). Third, it leads to the release of negative supercoils (54). All these effects result in a more open structure that facilitates the binding of transcription factor such as TFIIIA (55).

However, the question still remains: How active a role does acetylation play in this process? In particular, does acetylation actually induce DNA relaxation, or does it simply destabilize the structure so that other factors can

Table 13-2
Hormonal Stimulation of Histone Acetylation[a]

Hormone	Histones	System
Estradiol	H2, H3, H4, HMG 14	Guinea pig uterus
Aldosterone	H4	Kidneys of adrenalectomized rats
Cortisol[b]	HMG 14-17	Rat liver
EGF	H2B, H4	Chang liver cells
hCG	H2A, H4	Immature rat ovary
Prolactin	H2A, H2B, H3, H4	Rat mammary gland

[a] See text for references.
[b] Decreases acetylation of HMG 1–2.

unravel the solenoid, or does it do nothing but fix the open structure once the decondensation has occurred? These questions are still unresolved, but current opinion favors one of the last two possibilities.

2. Phosphorylation

Phosphorylation is another modification that has a rapid turnover and is independent of protein and RNA synthesis (56–58); furthermore, it is hormonally regulated (Table 13-3; 59–62). Thyroid-stimulating hormone (TSH) (63), glucagon (64), human chorionic gonadotropin (hCG) (40), the β-adrenergic agonists (65), angiotensin, and adrenocorticotropic hormone (ACTH) (66) all act through cAMP and protein kinase A (PKA); their phosphorylation sites conform to the typical substrate specificity for PKA (see Table 11-1). These sites include S-37 in histone H1, S-10 in histone H3, and S-6 in HMG 14. Note that one of the histone H1 variants has an alanine in place of S-37. Such an isohistone could obviously not be phosphorylated by PKA, which could have a significant effect on the ability of the DNA associated with nucleosomes containing this variant to be transcribed. In contrast to the cAMP-mediated hormones, PRL stimulates phosphorylation at a different site in the amino-terminal half of histone H1 (67); neither the exact site nor the responsible kinase has been identified. The phosphorylation induce by epidermal growth factor (EGF), fibroblast growth factor (FGF), insulin, and bombesin can be mimicked by 12-O-tetradecanoylphorbol-13-acetate (TPA), suggesting that PKC may mediate the action of these hormones (68).

Like acetylation, the phosphorylation of specific sites has different functions. Although heavy phosphorylation, particularly of histone H1, is asso-

Table 13-3
Hormonal Stimulation of Nuclear Protein Phosphorylation[a]

Hormone	Substrates	System
TSH	H1, H3, HMG 14	Calf thyroid slices
Glucagon	H1, H3, HMG 14	Rat liver
hCG	H1, H2A	Immature rat ovary
Catecholamines (β)	H1	Rat pineal gland
Angiotensin[b]	H3	Glomerulosa cells
ACTH[b]	H3	Glomerulosa cells
EGF	H3	Fibroblasts
FGF	H3	Fibroblasts
Bombesin	H3	Fibroblasts
Insulin	H3	Fibroblasts
Prolactin	H1, H2A, H2B	Murine mammary gland
Thyroxine	H1, H2A	Tadpole liver
Dexamethasone[c]	H1, H2A	GR and L cell lines
Aldosterone	H1	Kidney

[a] See text for references.
[b] Blocked by ANF.
[c] Synthetic glucocorticoid.

ciated with chromatin condensation and mitosis (69), selective phosphorylation by PKA of histone H5 (a histone H1 variant) and histone H3 leads to chromatin relaxation, as judged by electron microscopy (70). This phosphorylation weakens the binding of H1 to the linker DNA and allows DNA decondensation (71). Furthermore, the hormones known to elevate endogenous cAMP levels both stimulate phosphorylation and induce transcription, suggesting an important relationship (58).

3. Poly(ADP–Ribosyl)ation

Poly(ADP–ribosyl)ation involves the attachment of a branched polymer of ADP–ribose units, which are derived from NAD (72–75). The nicotinamide is removed and the now available 1' carbon of the ribose is coupled to a negative residue such as the side chain of glutamic acid or the carboxy terminus (see Fig. 13-3). The 1' carbon of the next subunit is then attached to the first via the 2' carbon of the other ribose.

The major substrates for this modification vary from system to system. Histone H1 is generally preferred over histones H2A and H2B, although in wheat embryos this pattern is reversed. Histones H3 and H4 are never modified. The HMG 1–2 proteins are usually preferred over HMG 14–17. However, the best substrate is the enzyme responsible for this modification: the poly(ADP–ribosyl)synthetase. This enzyme has 15 attachment sites, each of which may have side chains over 80 units long; this modification would add a minimum of 650 kDa to a protein that was originally only 110 kDa in size. The RNA polymerase is another potential substrate. Both the synthetase and the RNA polymerase are inhibited by this modification.

The poly(ADP–ribosyl)synthetase catalyzes chain initiation, elongation, and branching. It is a single-chain globular protein containing just over 1000 amino acids. The enzyme is divided into three approximately equal sections: an amino-terminal DNA-binding domain, a central automodification domain, and a carboxy-terminal NAD-binding site (76,77). The enzyme has a basic isoelectric point and is located on the linker DNA. The enzymatic activity requires double-stranded DNA, magnesium, histones, and a reducing agent such as β-mercaptoethanol. Regulation of the synthetase is still poorly understood; for example, the data on the role of the polyamines are confusing. Spermidine and spermine can fulfill the requirement for histones and divalent cations, but in fibroblasts inhibitors of polyamine synthesis stimulate the enzyme 2- to 3-fold (78). Phorbol esters can stimulate the enzyme 10-fold in these same cells (79), but *in vitro* PKC stoichiometrically phosphorylates and inhibits the enzyme (80). Finally, the enzyme can be inhibited by analogs of NAD such as 3-aminobenzamide and 3-methoxybenzamide. These compounds are very useful in studying the role of poly(ADP–ribosyl)ation in tissues, but they also have potential toxicity, including the inhibition of thymidine incorporation, lactate dehydrogenase, and glucose oxidase (81). Fortunately, such untoward effects require inhibitor concentrations of 1 m*M* or more, and frequently the activity of

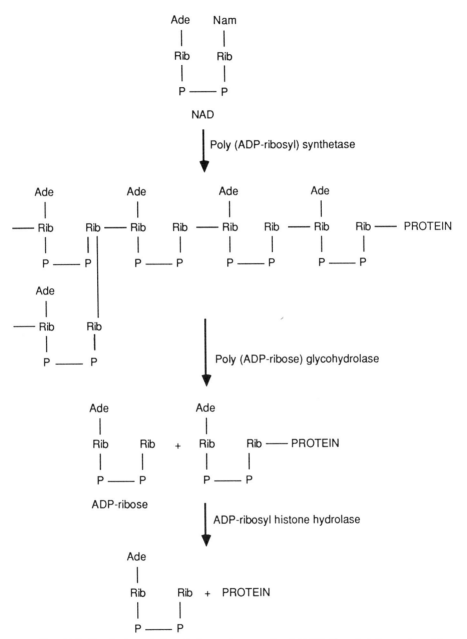

Fig. 13-3. Synthetic and degradative pathways of poly(ADP-ribosyl)ated proteins. Ade, Adenine; Nam, nicotinamide; P, phosphate; Rib, ribose.

poly(ADP–ribosyl)synthetase is adequately suppressed at lower concentrations.

The degradation of this polymer is accomplished by two enzymes (Fig. 13-3). The poly(ADP–ribose)glycohydrolase cleaves ribose–ribose bonds, including those at the branching points; as a consequence, it can remove all but the last subunit. This enzyme has two isoforms: II is cytoplasmic and inhibited by cAMP (82); I is nuclear, more active, and prefers histone H1 and the RNA polymerase (83). The second enzyme, ADP–ribosyl histone hydrolase, cleaves the ribose–protein bond, thereby freeing the last subunit. The degradative enzymes vary reciprocally with the polymerizing activity (84).

Assays for poly(ADP–ribosyl)synthetase are fraught with difficulties. In general, cells or nuclei are exposed to a labeled precursor such as NAD or adenosine, and radioactive incorporation into protein or histones is determined. The first problem involves the inability of NAD to enter intact cells. One can either permeabilize cells with a hypotonic solution or perform the assay in nuclei. In both cases, one must be very careful not to introduce nicks into the DNA during homogenization (85), because DNA breaks will activate the synthetase which, in addition to its role in gene expression, is also important in DNA repair (86). Labeled adenosine will enter intact cells, but it is a less specific precursor. Therefore, only a small fraction of the radioactive nucleoside becomes attached to protein, so more label must be used and the substrates must be carefully purified. Furthermore, it requires at least 18 hours for the adenosine to equilibrate with the intracellular NAD pool. The assay system chosen is of more than academic interest; labeling patterns differ between intact and broken cell preparations (87) and even the concentrations of NAD used can affect chain lengths (88).

Other problems that must also be solved are those of labile bonds, product identification, and competing reactions. Some of the polymer bonds are labile in alkali, so tissue processing should be performed rapidly at 4°C in slightly acidic buffers. The charge and molecular weight of the product can be substantially altered; however, short incubation times will prevent the polymer from becoming so long that the product is no longer recognizable when compared with unmodified standards. Finally, other nonhistone–non-HMG substrates can become heavily labeled, including the synthetase itself. Adequate purification and identification of the reaction products will allow extraneous reactions to be segregated and analyzed separately.

As noted earlier, this enzyme is involved in DNA repair (89,90). It binds nicked DNA and protects the DNA from recombination or spurious transcription. Researchers also believe that the histones may be shuttled to the automodified poly(ADP–ribosyl)synthetase to expose the DNA to the repairing enzymes. The structure of poly(ADP–ribose) is helicoidal, like other nucleic acids, and is capable of binding histones. After the damage is repaired, the polymers are digested and the histones are return to the DNA. The poly(ADP–ribosyl)synthetase also inhibits DNA synthesis and transcription until the repair has occurred.

However, the association between this modification and gene expression is not as clear. In many hormonal systems, poly(ADP–ribosyl)ation is linked to differentiation (Table 13-4). The effect of steroids requires at least several hours (91) and, in the case of progesterone-induced oocyte maturation, requires RNA and protein synthesis (92). However, this action requires several days, whereas hormones in other systems act more acutely. In contrast to the sex steroids, which stimulate the synthetase (91–94), TSH probably increases poly(ADP–ribosyl)ation by inhibiting the glychoydrolase (95). This degradative enzyme is inhibited by cAMP, and the action of TSH on this modification is mimicked by this second messenger.

On the other hand, there are many examples in which this modification is negatively related to differentiation. One might question the study on chick embryo livers (96) because of the teratogenic doses used (100–200 μg cortisol *in ovo*); however, the studies in mammary epithelium are not as easily dismissed (97,98). One possibility is that poly(ADP–ribosyl)ation in mammary cells is not taking place on the nucleosomes containing the transcribed genes, such as the mouse mammary tumor virus or milk proteins, but on chromatin harboring negative regulatory elements. Inhibition of poly(ADP–ribosyl)ation at such genes could decrease the transcription of a repressor and enhance the expression of other genes normally under the control of that repressor.

Another possible explanation may be found in the structural effects elicited by this modification. Like acetylation and cAMP-dependent phosphorylation, poly(ADP–ribosyl)ation is associated with chromatin relaxation. For example, pancreatic polynucleosomes that have been modified by the purified synthetase will not recondense in high salt solutions, whereas

Table 13-4
Hormonal Regulation of Poly(ADP-ribosyl)ation in Histones and HMG Proteins[a]

Hormone	Substrates	Effect	System	Comments
Testosterone	?	Stimulation	Mouse kidney	
Progesterone	?	Stimulation	*Xenopus* oocyte	Requires RNA, protein synthesis
TSH	?	Stimulation	Dog thyroid slices	Mimicked by cAMP
Cortisol	?	Inhibition	Chick embryo liver	Toxic doses used
Estradiol	H1, H2B, H3, HMG 14–17	Stimulation	Rat uterus	Reduced by progesterone
Dexamethasone[b]	HMG 14–17	Inhibition	Mouse mammary tumor cells	Stimulates degradation
Insulin	H1, HMG 1–2	Inhibition	Mouse mammary gland explants	Stimulates degradation; blocked by cAMP analogs
Prolactin	H1, HMG 1–2	Inhibition	Mouse mammary gland explants	Inhibits synthesis

[a] See text for references.
[b] Synthetic glucocorticoid.

control polynucleosomes will (99). Some poly(ADP–ribosyl)ated histones may even dissociate from DNA (75). There are also reports, however, that this polymer can cross-link histone H1 to form dimers that stabilize the condensed structure (100); still other investigations show that poly(ADP–ribosyl)ated histones are associated with both active and inactive chromatin (101). These studies were performed under different conditions, so the data may not be comparable. However, one cannot eliminate the possibility that both effects might be physiologically manifested in different tissues or even different regions of the chromatin in the same cell. If this modification favors condensation in the mammary gland, then hormones inducing differentiation would certainly be expected to inhibit poly(ADP–ribosyl)ation.

In addition to its role in DNA repair and transcription, this modification facilitates nucleosomal assembly during DNA replication (102). The synthetase is also located in ribonucleoprotein (RNP) particles that sequester mRNA (see Chapter 14). Investigators believe that poly(ADP–ribosyl)ation may neutralize the positive charge on proteins and aid in the release of the trapped mRNA (103).

4. Methylation

Methylation refers to the attachment of one to three methyl groups to the nitrogen of either lysine (N^ϵ) or arginine (N^ω). The former occurs in histones H3 and H4, and the latter is found in HMG 1-2 proteins; in both, dimethylation is the most common state. Three enzymes catalyze this reaction: methylases I and II methylate arginines and carboxy groups, respectively, and are found in low levels in the cytoplasm; methylase III is nuclear and methylates lysines. All three enzymes use S-adenosylmethionine as the methyl donor. Because methylation has such a slow turnover, demethylating enzymes were not thought to exist; however, N^ϵ-alkyllysinase activity has been detected in some tissues, although the levels vary considerably. Allosteric regulation of these enzymes has not been extensively studied. Spermidine does inhibit the methylation of histone H4 in rat brain, but the site of action for this polyamine is unknown.

Evidence for the hormonal regulation is meager. Estradiol stimulates and epinephrine inhibits the methylation of histones in rat brain, but the data are marginal (104,105). T_3 stimulates histone methylation in rat liver, but this effect appears to be secondary to hormone-induced DNA replication (106); histone methylation is closely associated with mitosis and is independent of the mitotic agent. Indeed, although the kidney and spleen are also target organs of this hormone, T_3 stimulates neither DNA replication nor histone methylation in these tissues.

Histone methylation has always been associated with chromatin condensation and mitosis. This association, along with a slow turnover and little or no evidence for direct hormonal regulation, suggests that methylation does not play a significant role in gene expression. However, some data have argued for a role in gene repression (107). When *Drosophila* Kc cells are exposed to 37°C, heat shock proteins are induced, normal proteins are suppressed, and histones H2B and H3 are methylated. Exposure to 32°C or ethanol still induces the heat shock proteins, but normal proteins continue to be expressed and methylation patterns do not change. In this system, histone methylation appears to be correlated with the repression of normal house-keeping proteins. Attempts have been made to show a direct association between methylation and active or inactive chromatin, but the results have not been consistent (108,109).

C. High-Mobility-Group Protein Modifications

The modifications of the HMG proteins parallel those of histones. Several hormones can stimulate the acetylation of HMG proteins (Table 13-2; 44,110). Acetylated HMG 1 binds to and activates DNA polymerase (111) and facilitates nucleosomal assembly (112).

The endogenous phosphorylation of HMG 14–17 reduces the affinity of these proteins for DNA (113,114), but determination of the physiological kinase has been difficult. Of the four HMG proteins, only HMG 14 has a cAMP-dependent phosphorylation site, which is modified in intact tissues exposed to hormones that elevate cAMP concentrations; examples include TSH in thyroid slices and glucagon in liver (58). Furthermore, this phosphorylation can be mimicked by cAMP analogs. Other sites can be phosphorylated *in vitro* by other kinases, but the physiological relevance is unclear. For example, both PKG and casein kinase II (CKII) can phosphorylate HMG 14, and PKC can modify HMG 17 and HMG 1 (115–117). However, except for CKII, which increases the DNA affinity of HMG 14, the effects of these phosphorylations are unknown.

The poly(ADP–ribosyl)ation of HMG proteins has been extensively studied in mammary epithelium. In a mammary tumor cell line, dexamethasone, a synthetic glucocorticoid, decreases the level of this modification in HMG 14–17 within minutes and well before the induction of mouse mammary tumor virus RNA. Furthermore, inhibitors of the poly(ADP–ribosyl)synthetase enhance the dexamethasone induction of this virus. However, pre-existing polymers of ADP–ribose are stable for over 3 hours even though the half-time for the dexamethasone response is only 10–15 minutes. These results suggest that dexamethasone is not inhibiting the synthetase but instead is stimulating the enzymes involved in degrading this polymer (97,118).

Similar results were found in mammary gland explants (98). Again, inhibitors of the synthetase augment the hormonal induction of differentiation; in this system, α-lactalbumin and casein were used as markers for differentiation and were induced by insulin, cortisol, and PRL. Furthermore, insulin stimulates the poly(ADP–ribose)glycohydrolase, the major degradative enzyme. The following data suggest that this stimulation is achieved by lowering cAMP levels: (i) this enzyme is inhibited by cAMP, (ii) insulin reduces cAMP levels in mammary gland explants, and (iii) cAMP analogs block the effect of insulin. However, in mammary gland explants, modulation of the synthetase is also important and it is inhibited by PRL. In summary, a decrease in poly(ADP–ribosyl)ation is associated with differentiation in mammary epithelium. In explants, this reduction is a result of two pathways, each of which is under separate hormonal control: PRL inhibits the synthetase and insulin stimulates the glycohydrolase.

Very little work has been done on methylation in HMG proteins. Approximately 2.9% of HMG 1 and 8.9% of HMG 2 are methylated. Nothing is known about the hormonal regulation, if any, of this modification nor of the possible effects on HMG function.

III. Template Activity

A. DNase Sensitivity

As noted earlier, the modification of histones and HMG proteins can affect chromatin structure; these different conformations can affect how efficiently the resident genes are transcribed. This variable ability to be transcribed is referred to as *template activity.* For example, the tightly coiled solenoid is often referred to as *condensed* DNA and forms the transcriptionally inactive *heterochromatin,* whereas the unraveled structure is known as *relaxed* DNA and forms the transcriptionally active *euchromatin.* These two types of DNA conformation can be detected by limited digestion with various DNases (119): the more open the DNA structure, the more susceptible it is to digestion. Therefore, DNase sensitivity can be used as a crude indicator of DNA structure. The following examples demonstrate the association between hormone-induced gene expression and DNA conformation.

Micrococcal nuclease is a DNase that specifically cleaves the linker DNA. In the oviduct of immature chicks, no ovalbumin mRNA is detectable, and the gene is insensitive to the nuclease. After primary stimulation with diethylstilbestrol, a synthetic estrogen, ovalbumin mRNA accumulates and the DNA is digested into single or small clusters of nucleosomes (120). The gene once again becomes resistant to micrococcal nuclease 4–5 days after hormone withdrawal, and no transcription takes place. Secondary induction restores both transcription and DNA susceptibility to digestion.

The vitellogenin genes in *Xenopus* liver show a similar, although not identical, effect (121). These genes are divided into two groups known as the A genes and the B genes. The B genes are always sensitive to digestion with DNase I, a nonspecific nuclease, and are always readily inducible. The A genes are resistant to DNase I in the untreated male frog and primary induction with estradiol is slow. The A genes exhibit DNase I sensitivity and are rapidly inducible following secondary stimulation 1 month after primary stimulation and hormone withdrawal. However, if 8 months are allowed to elapse between primary and secondary induction, the A genes return to a nuclease-resistant state and the induction of transcription is slow.

These experiments suggest that transcription is associated with relaxed DNA and that if the DNA is already relaxed before induction, induction occurs more quickly. This latter effect may explain why secondary induction in many systems is faster and greater in magnitude than primary induction, that is, this memory effect may reside in the DNA structure. The second example also illustrates the point that, although a change in chromatin structure may facilitate transcription, it is not sufficient.

B. DNA Methylation

1. Introduction and Methodology

Another postulated mechanism for hormonally altering template activity is the methylation of cytidines at position 5 (122–125). This methylation usually occurs in C_PG sequences, has been associated with gene repression, and can be inherited. The latter characteristic is due to a methylase that is linked to DNA synthesis and is relatively specific for hemimethylated DNA. After DNA replication, the parental strand is still methylated but the daughter strand is not; this hemimethylated site is then fully methylated by the enzyme. If a site was not originally methylated in the parental strand, both strands will be unmethylated; such a site is a poor substrate for this methylase. Therefore, methylated sites remain methylated and unmethylated sites remain unmethylated. This methylase can also produce *de novo* methylation, but this activity is much slower and is influenced by the base sequence and chromatin structure.

One can locate these methylation sites by restriction mapping. Bacteria are susceptible to infection by certain viruses, called *bacteriophages;* resistant bacterial strains develop enzymes, called *restriction endonucleases,* that cleave viral DNA at highly specific sequences. Similar sequences in the host are protected by methylation, that is, methylation at these sites renders them resistant to endonuclease cleavage (Table 13-5). Using these enzymes, cleavage sites can be mapped within any given piece of DNA. If this is done before and after hormone treatment and if additional sites appear after the treatment, then it is concluded that the hormone must have stimulated demethylation at these new sites, thereby rendering them susceptible to restriction endonucleases. The major caveat of this technique is that only a few sites are being sampled: there could be numerous sites at which methylation status is changing that are not recognized by any of the enzymes that one may be using. For example, HpaII produces more fragments in the α-globin gene in erythrocytes than in brain or sperm, suggesting that the gene is hypomethy-

Table 13-5

Sequence Specificity for Selected Restriction Endonucleases

Methylation effect	Restriction endonuclease		
	*Hpa*II	*Hha*I	*Msp*I
Endonuclease sensitive	$^{(m)}$C↓CGG	GCG↓C	C↓$^{(m)}$CGG
Endonuclease resistant	$^{(m)}$C^{m}CGG	G^{m}CGC	^{m}C$^{(m)}$CGG

lated in erythrocytes (126). This observation is consistent with the fact that the α-globin gene is active only in erythrocytes. However, no difference in cleavage patterns is noted when HhaI is used; if one had only tested this latter restriction endonuclease, one might have concluded that methylation patterns were identical in all tissues. The more enzymes one uses, the more complete a picture one sees. Methylation sites can also be determined by direct sequencing (127); however, this technique is more laborious than the use of restriction nucleases.

In addition to observing the natural changes in methylation patterns, these patterns can be experimentally manipulated. The simplest method is to use *5-azacytidine*, a suicide inhibitor of the methylase. To be effective, it must be incorporated into the DNA where it causes hypomethylation. For example, the metallothionein I gene is normally inducible by glucocorticoids or cadmium in several lines but not in mouse thymoma cells; however, it does become inducible following treatment with 5-azacytidine (128). These are fairly typical results: the drug, either by itself or in combination with other inducers, stimulates gene transcription in cells that normally do not express that gene. Such data have led to the hypothesis that methylation represses genes and demethylation is involved in their induction. Unfortunately, the drug is nonspecific and hypomethylates extensive regions of the genome; furthermore, it may also inhibit other methylation reactions, such as phospholipid methylation.

A more selective way of altering methylation patterns is to use cloned genes. For example, various portions of the γ-globin gene were methylated and the gene was then transfected into cells (129). Methylation of the structural gene or the vector did not interfere with expression, but methylation of the 5' flanking sequences totally blocked transcription. Other experiments have confirmed that repression is most effective when methylation occurs in the preinitiation domain of a gene (130).

2. Examples

Unfortunately, the association of demethylation with transcription is far from perfect; for example, the vitellogenin gene is still expressed in *Xenopus* liver, even though it remains fully methylated (131), and 5-azacytidine specifically *inhibits* milk protein synthesis in the mouse mammary gland (132). However, the chick vitellogenin gene has been among the most extensively studied methylation systems and can provide some of the most useful insights into this process.

Estradiol treatment of immature chicks results in both the transcription of the vitellogenin gene and the appearance of DNase hypersensitive sites in the 5' region (133); a *hypersensitive site* is a site of DNA cleavage induced by a brief incubation with low concentrations of DNase I. Another site in the 5' region is demethylated, but this occurs *after* transcription begins. The coding strand is the first to be demethylated; the complementary nonsense strand follows about 24 hours later. The demethylation does not require DNA synthesis, so it is not a result of repeated DNA replication combined with a failure to remethylate. This passive mechanism has been postulated by others, who suggest that transcription factors bound to active genes prevent methylation so that the original methylation pattern is eventually diluted out. Instead, this system demonstrates that an active mechanism is required. One hypothesis is that 5-methylcytidine is demethylated directly; another is that gene induction is accompanied by DNA nicks that stimulate repair-type synthesis and the removal of the methylated nucleotides.

After hormone withdrawal, the demethylated site is not remethylated, although one hypersensitive site is lost and transcription ceases. This result might indicate that, in this system, some of the hypersensitive sites are related to transcription whereas demethylation is involved in the memory effect. However, this latter hypothesis was not supported by experiments in chick embryos (134). When chick embryos are given a single dose of estradiol, the vitellogenin genes respond as just described. However, after 25 weeks the hypersensitive site is lost and the demethylated site has undergone variable remethylation. Despite this event, the memory effect is still present in many of the birds and is not correlated with the degree of methylation. Furthermore, the other hypothesis linking the hypersensitive sites to transcription is not supported by other experiments in the immature chick: both the hypersensitive sites and demethylation appear in the vitellogenin gene in all estrogen-responsive tissues, such as the oviduct, even though the gene is only expressed in the liver. The gene is not altered in tissues unresponsive to estradiol. This is not an uncommon finding: the gene for SVS IV, an androgen-dependent protein, is hypomethylated in the seminal vesicles and the prostrate gland; both tissues are androgen responsive. However, the SVS IV gene is only expressed in the seminal vesicles. Therefore, both hypersensitive sites and demethylation appear to be generalized responses by tissues sensitive to a particular hormone. They apparently occur in all genes inducible by that hormone and in all the tissues responsive to the hormone, despite the fact that only a particular subset of these genes will actually be activated in any given tissue.

Vitellogenin, like all the other proteins discussed already, is a tissue-specific protein that is made only when induced. For such genes, methylation and demethylation are discrete events at restricted locations in the 5′ region. This pattern does not hold for *housekeeping genes;* these are the genes that are constitutively transcribed in virtually all cells. These latter genes are associated with large islands (500–2000 bp) that are very rich in the sequence C_pG. These islands are located in the 5′ region and are inevitably nonmethylated, except for those genes on the inactive X chromosome (135). Further support for the association of island methylation and gene inactivation come from transfection experiments with an artificially methylated gene for amidophosphoribosyl transferase; only methylation of the 5′ region inhibited gene expression. Researchers have postulated that, when these genes are active, the islands are protected from methylation by certain proteins, perhaps related to transcription. Furthermore, because this class of genes is almost always active, methylation is a rare event.

3. Function

What then is the role of methylation? In all systems examined thus far, methylation in the 5′ region inhibits gene expression, but demethylation occurs in all tissues responsive to a particular hormone, whether or not those genes will be transcribed. Most authorities agree that changes in methylation patterns are not primary events in gene expression or repression. Rather, methylation merely serves to imprint inactivity on a gene that was initially repressed by some other mechanism. Furthermore, because of its persistence and its relatively low level in somatic cells, methylation may be more important in developmental processes than in acute gene regulation.

How might methylation maintain gene repression? There are two major mechanisms. The first and simplest is that methylation of an HRE blocks the binding of some transcription factors. For example, the HREs for cAMP response element binding protein (CREB), Myc–Max, and nuclear factor κB (NF-κB) contain C_pG; if these sequences are methylated, these transcription factors will not bind. However, it is also possible that methylation may block the binding of a repressor and actually stimulate gene transcription. This possibility has been advanced to explain the association between the induction of the human PRL gene and its methylation (136). Note that not all transcription factors are affected by this modification; the methylation of the binding site for Sp1 does not block Sp1 binding.

A second mechanism involves the specific binding of methylated DNA by proteins that repress transcription (137,138). These proteins can be hormonally regulated. For example, in the immature hen, the ovalbumin gene is repressed by the binding of these proteins to methylated sites (139). Estrogen stimulation lowers the levels of these proteins and exposes the sites to demethylation; these changes permit the expression of ovalbumin. During molting or the egg-laying pause, the estrogen levels fall and the methylated DNA-binding proteins increase to repress ovalbumin once again. Although the sites in the ovalbumin gene are still unmethylated, the higher repressor concentration compensates for its lower affinity for the unmethylated sequences.

C. Z-DNA

In the preceding discussion, the relationship between template activity and both DNA packaging and methylation were explored. One other determinant of template activity has also been postulated: DNA helical structure. DNA can assume several conformations. B-DNA is the classic Watson–Crick model, whereas A-DNA resembles the structure of RNA and is found in DNA–RNA hybrids. Z-DNA is a very elongated, left-handed helix that can be found in DNA regions rich in guanine and cytosine. Such regions frequently occur in the 5′ regions of genes, particularly at transcription initiation sites (140). Furthermore, the formation of Z-DNA is favored by polyamines, which are known to be elevated by many hormones (see Chapter 10). Finally, the estrogen response element (ERE) appears to assume a non-B conformation based on chemical reactivity and S1 nuclease digestion (141). This structure is intrinsic to the sequence, since it does not require chromatin proteins and is not observed in related HREs. However, there is not yet any convincing evidence that the presence of alternative DNA conformations is correlated with transcription (142).

IV. Summary

The major effects of histone and HMG protein modifications appear to be on chromatin structure: relaxed chromatin is associated with active transcription whereas condensed chromatin is not. Methylation and the heavy phosphorylation of histone H1 appear to favor condensation and gene repression; acetylation and cAMP-dependent phosphorylation are more conducive to relaxation and transcription. Poly(ADP–ribosyl)ation is usually associated with relaxation but, as discussed earlier, this conclusion is still controversial. Finally, the interrelationships among these modifications tend to support this division (Fig. 13-4). For example, acetylation facilitates poly(ADP–ribosyl)ation and phosphorylation of histones other than H1; acetylation and poly(ADP–ribosyl)ation both inhibit histone H1 phosphorylation; finally, spermidine stimulates acetylation whereas it inhibits methylation.

Many of these modifications represent primary hormone action, since they occur rapidly and do not require RNA or protein synthesis. For example, the cAMP-dependent hormones appear to act through PKA, which can either directly phosphorylate histones or indirectly affect other modifications by phosphorylating the responsible enzymes. The mechanism of steroid and thyroid hormone actions is more problematic, since the notion of nongenomic effects of these hormones is still viewed with great skepticism. These modifications then affect chromatin structure. Those that relax chromatin make the DNA easier to transcribe, whereas those promoting condensation inactivate genes. These structures can often be detected by monitoring DNase sensitivity: relaxed chromatin is more susceptible to these enzymes than condensed chromatin. These nuclear protein modifications may also be important phenomena responsible for the memory effect in secondary induction by maintaining once-activated genes in the relaxed conformation.

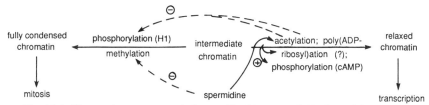

Fig. 13-4. Chromatin structure as influenced by histone and HMG modifications and the interrelationship of their modifications.

Finally, template activity can be altered by DNA methylation, which is usually associated with gene inactivation. However, hypomethylation is not closely related to transcription; instead, it appears to be a general marker for potential hormone sensitivity. Also, DNA methylation appears to fix gene inactivity brought about by some other factor. Methylated sequences can repress transcription either directly by failing to bind certain transcription factors or indirectly by binding repressor proteins.

References

General References

Jost, J. P., and Saluz, H. P. (eds.) (1993). "DNA Methylation: Molecular Biology and Biological Significance." Birkhäuser Verlag, Basel.

Lautier, D., Lagueux, J., Thibodeau, J., Ménard, L., and Poirier, G. G. (1993). Molecular and biochemical features of poly(ADP–ribose) metabolism. *Mol. Cell. Biol.* **122**, 171–193.

López-Rodas, G., Brosch, G., Georgieva, E. I., Sendra, R., Franco, L., and Loidl, P. (1993). Histone deacetylase: A key enzyme for the binding of regulatory proteins to chromatin. *FEBS Lett.* **317**, 175–180.

Tordera, V., Sendra, R., and Pérez-Ortín, J. E. (1993). The role of histones and their modifications in the informative content of chromatin. *Experientia* **49**, 780–788.

Turner, B. M. (1993). Decoding the nucleosome. *Cell* **75**, 5–8.

Volpe, P., Iacovacci, P., Butler, R. H., and Eremenko, T. (1993). 5-Methylcytosine in genes with methylation-dependent regulation. *FEBS Lett.* **329**, 233–237.

See also Refs. 1, 2, 4, 5, 13, 24, 25, 28–32, 56–58, 72–75, 86, 89, 90, 119, 122–125, and 135.

Cited References

1. Alberts, B., Bray, D., Lewis, J., Raff, M., Roberts, K., and Watson, J. D. (1994). "The Molecular Biology of the Cell." 3rd Ed. Garland Publishing, New York.

2. Reeves, R. (1984). Transcriptionally active chromatin. *Biochim. Biophys. Acta* **782**, 343–393.

3. Arents, G., Burlingame, R. W., Wang, B. C., Love, W. E., and Moudrianakis, E. N. (1991). The nucleosomal core histone octamer at 3.1 Å resolution: A tripartite protein assembly and a left-handed superhelix. *Proc. Natl. Acad. Sci. U.S.A.* **88**, 10148–10152.

4. Zlatanova, J. (1990). Histone H1 and the regulation of transcription of eukaryotic genes. *Trends Biochem. Sci.* **15**, 273–276.

5. Cole, R. D. (1987). Microheterogeneity in H1 histones and its consequences. *Int. J. Pept. Protein Res.* **30**, 433–449.

6. Marion, C., Roche, J., Roux, B., and Gorka, C. (1985). Differences in the condensation of chromatin by individual subfractions of histone H1: Implications for the role of H1° in the structural organization of chromatin. *Biochemistry* **24**, 6329–6335.

7. Gierset, R., Gorka, C., Hasthorpe, S., Lawrence, J. J., and Eisen, H. (1982).

Developmental and hormonal regulation of protein H1° in rodents. *Proc. Natl. Acad. Sci. U.S.A.* **79,** 2333–2337.

8. Busch, H. (1984). Ubiquitination of protein. *Meth. Enzymol.* **106,** 238–262.
9. Davie, J. R., and Murphy, L. C. (1990). Level of ubiquitinated histone H2B in chromatin is coupled to ongoing transcription. *Biochemistry* **29,** 4752–4757.
10. Djondjurov, L. P., Yancheva, N. Y., and Ivanova, E. C. (1983). Histones of terminally differentiated cells undergo continuous turnover. *Biochemistry* **22,** 4095–4102.
11. Levinger, L., and Varshavsky, A. (1982). Selective arrangement of ubiquitinated and D1 protein-containing nucleosomes within the *Drosophila* genome. *Cell* **28,** 375–385.
12. Martian, J. K. W., Paton, A. E., Bunich, G. J., and Olins, D. E. (1980). Nucleosome cores have two specific binding sites for nonhistone chromosomal proteins HMG 14 and HMG 17. *Science* **209,** 1534–1536.
13. Ausio, J. (1992). Structure and dynamics of transcriptionally active chromatin. *J. Cell Sci.* **102,** 1–5.
14. Tremethick, D. J., and Drew, H. R. (1993). High mobility group proteins 14 and 17 can space nucleosomes *in vitro*. *J. Biol. Chem.* **268,** 11389–11393.
15. Reeves, R., and Chang, P. (1983). Investigations of the possible functions of glycosylation in the high mobility group proteins: Evidence for a role in nuclear matrix association. *J. Biol. Chem.* **258,** 679–687.
16. Bianchi, M. E., Falciola, L., Ferrari, S., and Lilley, D. M. J. (1992). The DNA binding site of HMG1 protein is composed of two similar segments (HMG boxes), both of which have counterparts in other eukaryotic regulatory proteins. *EMBO J.* **11,** 1055–1063.
17. Lee, K. L. D., Pentecost, B. T., D'Anna, J. A., Tobey, R. A., Gurley, L. R., and Dixon, G. H. (1987). Characterization of DNA sequences corresponding to three distinct HMG-1 mRNA species in line CHO Chinese hamster cells and cell cycle expression of the HMG-1 gene. *Nucleic Acids Res.* **15,** 5051–5068.
18. Yoshida, M. (1987). High glutamic and aspartic region in nonhistone protein HMG(1+2) unwinds DNA double helical structure. *J. Biochem. (Tokyo)* **101,** 175–180.
19. Paull, T. T., Haykinson, M. J., and Johnson, R. C. (1993). The nonspecific DNA-binding and DNA-bending proteins HMG1 and HMG2 promote the assembly of complex nucleoprotein structure. *Genes Dev.* **7,** 1521–1534.
20. Javaherian, L., Liu, L. F., and Wang, J. C. (1980). Nonhistone protein HMG1 and HMG2 change the DNA helical structure. *Science* **199,** 1345–1346.
21. Waga, S., Mizuno, S., and Yoshida, M. (1990). Chromosomal protein HMG1 removes the transcriptional block caused by the cruciform in supercoiled DNA. *J. Biol. Chem.* **265,** 19424–19428.
22. Tremethick, D. J., and Molloy, P. L. (1986). High mobility group proteins 1 and 2 stimulate transcription *in vitro* by RNA polymerases II and III. *J. Biol. Chem.* **261,** 6986–6992.
23. Singh, J., and Dixon, G. H. (1990). High mobility group proteins 1 and 2 function as general class II transcription factors. *Biochemistry* **29,** 6295–6302.
24. Grunstein, M. (1990). Histone function in transcription. *Annu. Rev. Cell Biol.* **6,** 643–678.
25. Thoma, F. (1992). Nucleosome positioning. *Biochim. Biophys. Acta* **1130,** 1–19.
26. Pham, T. A., McDonnell, D. P., Tsai, M. J., and O'Malley, B. W. (1992). Modula-

tion of progesterone receptor binding to progesterone response elements by positioned nucleosomes. *Biochemistry* **31**, 1570–1578.

27. Filipski, J., Leblanc, J., Youdale, T., Sikorska, M., and Walker, P. R. (1990). Periodicity of DNA folding in higher order chromatin structures. *EMBO J.* **9**, 1319–1327.
28. Wu, R. S., Panusz, H. T., Hatch, C. L., and Bonner, W. M. (1986). Histones and their modifications. *CRC Crit. Rev. Biochem.* **20**, 201–264.
29. Csordas, A. (1990). On the biological role of histone acetylation. *Biochem. J.* **265**, 23–38.
30. Pfeffer, U., and Vidali, G. (1991). Histone acetylation: Recent approaches to a basic mechanism of genome organization. *Int. J. Biochem.* **23**, 277–285.
31. Turner, B. M. (1991). Histone acetylation and control of gene expression. *J. Cell Sci.* **99**, 13–20.
32. Doenecke, D., and Gallwitz, D. (1982). Acetylation of histones in nucleosomes. *Mol. Cell. Biochem.* **44**, 113–128.
33. Hirose, M., Sarui, K., and Sunagawa, A. (1985). Correlation between nuclear histone acetylation and casein messenger RNA induction in the mammary gland. *J. Biochem. (Tokyo)* **97**, 781–789.
34. Gill, R. K., and Christakos, S. (1993). Identification of sequence elements in mouse calbindin-D$_{28k}$ gene that confer 1,25-dihydroxyvitamin D$_3$- and butyrate-inducible responses. *Proc. Natl. Acad. Sci. U.S.A.* **90**, 2984–2988.
35. Stevens, M. S., Aliabadi, Z., and Moore, M. R. (1984). Associated effects of sodium butyrate on histone acetylation and estrogen receptor in the human breast cancer cell line MCF-7. *Biochem. Biophys. Res. Commun.* **119**, 132–138.
36. Ortiz-Caro, J., Montiel, F., Pascual, A., and Aranda, A. (1986). Modulation of thyroid hormone receptors by short-chain fatty acids in glial C6 cells: Role of histone acetylation. *J. Biol. Chem.* **261**, 13997–14004.
37. Piñeiro, M., Hernández, F., Puerta, C., and Palacián, E. (1993). Transcription of mononucleosomal particles acetylated in the presence of *n*-butyrate. *Mol. Biol. Rep.* **18**, 37–41.
38. Turner, B. M., Birley, A. J., and Lavender, J. (1992). Histone H4 isoforms acetylated at specific lysine residues define individual chromosomes and chromatin domains in *Drosophila* polytene nuclei. *Cell* **69**, 375–384.
39. Sommerville, J., Baird, J., and Turner, B. M. (1993). Histone H4 acetylation and transcription in amphibian chromatin. *J. Cell Biol.* **120**, 277–290.
40. Jungmann, R. A., and Schweppe, J. S. (1972). Mechanisms of action of gonadotropin. I. Evidence for gonadotropin-induced modifications of ovarian nuclear basic and acidic protein biosynthesis. *J. Biol. Chem.* **247**, 5535–5542.
41. Liew, C. C., Suria, D., and Gornall, A. G. (1973). Effect of aldosterone on acetylation and phosphorylation of chromosomal proteins. *Endocrinol. (Baltimore)* **93**, 1025–1034.
42. Pasqualini, J. R., Cosquer-Clavreul, C., Vidali, G., and Allfrey, V. G. (1981). Effects of estradiol on the acetylation of histones in the fetal uterus of the guinea pig. *Biol. Reprod.* **25**, 1035–1039.
43. Kaneko, Y. (1983). Epidermal growth factor enhances acetylation of nuclear proteins in cultured human liver cells. *Biochim. Biophys. Acta* **762**, 111–118.
44. Bertrand-Mercat, P., and Pasqualini, J. R. (1991). Antagonistic effect of the antiestrogen 4-hydroxytamoxifen on estradiol-stimulated acetylation of nuclear high mobility group (HMG) proteins in the uterus of newborn guinea-pigs. *Life Sci.* **48**, 2081–2087.

45. Libby, P. R. (1968). Histone acetylation by cell-free preparations from rat uterus: *In vitro* stimulation by estradiol-17β *Biochem. Biophys. Res. Commun.* **31**, 59–65.
46. Estepa, I., and Pestana, A. (1983). Isolation and partial characterization of three histone-specific acetyltransferases from *Artemia. Eur. J. Biochem.* **132**, 249–254.
47. Vu, Q. A., Zhang, D., Chroneos, Z. C., and Nelson, D. A. (1987). Polyamines inhibit the yeast histone deacetylase. *FEBS Lett.* **220**, 79–83.
48. Bode, J., Gómez-Lira, M. M., and Schröter, H. (1982). Nucleosomal particles open as the histone core becomes hyperacetylated. *Eur. J. Biochem.* **130**, 437–445.
49. Loidl, P., and Gröbner, P. (1987). Postsynthetic acetylation of histones during the cell cycle: A general function for the displacement of histones during chromatin rearrangements. *Nucleic Acids Res.* **15**, 8351–8366.
50. Jeppesen, P., and Turner, B. M. (1993). The inactive X chromosome in female mammals is distinguished by a lack of histone H4 acetylation, a cytogenic marker for gene expression. *Cell* **74**, 281–289.
51. Ridsdale, J. A., Hendzel, M. J., Delcuve, G. P., and Davie, J. R. (1990). Histone acetylation alters the capacity of the H1 histones to condense transcriptionally active/competent chromatin. *J. Biol. Chem.* **265**, 5150–5156.
52. Bode, J. (1984). Nucleosomal conformations induced by the small HMG proteins or by histone hyperacetylation are distinct. *Arch. Biochem. Biophys.* **228**, 364–372.
53. Hong, L., Schroth, G. P., Matthews, H. R., Yau, P., and Bradbury, E. M. (1993). Studies of the DNA binding properties of histone H4 amino terminus: Thermal denaturation studies reveal that acetylation markedly reduces the binding constant of the H4 "tail" to DNA. *J. Biol. Chem.* **268**, 305–314.
54. Norton, V. G., Imai, B. S., Yau, P., and Bradbury, E. M. (1989). Histone acetylation reduces nucleosome core particle linking number change. *Cell* **57**, 449–457.
55. Lee, D. Y., Hayes, J. J., Pruss, D., and Wolffe, A. P. (1993). A positive role for histone acetylation in transcription factor access to nucleosomal DNA. *Cell* **72**, 73–84.
56. Hohmann, P. (1983). Phosphorylation of H1 histones. *Mol. Cell. Biochem.* **57**, 81–92.
57. Matthews, H. R., and Huebner, V. D. (1984). Nuclear protein kinases. *Mol. Cell. Biochem.* **59**, 81–99.
58. Cooper, E., and Spaulding, S. W. (1985). Hormonal control of the phosphorylation of histones, HMG proteins and other nuclear proteins. *Mol. Cell. Endocrinol.* **39**, 1–20.
59. Turkington, R. W., and Riddle, M. (1969). Hormone-dependent phosphorylation of nuclear proteins during mammary gland differentiation *in vitro. J. Biol. Chem.* **244**, 6040–6046.
60. Prentice, D. A., Taylor, S. E., Newmark, M. Z., and Kitos, P. A. (1978). The effects of dexamethasome on histone phosphorylation in L cells. *Biochem. Biophys. Res. Commun.* **85**, 541–550.
61. Morris, S. M., and Cole, R. D. (1980). Thyroxine stimulation of tadpole liver phosphorylation *in vivo. Dev. Biol.* **74**, 379–386.
62. Wurtz, T. (1985). Events in glucocorticoid hormone action: A correlation of histone H1 variant pattern changes, hormone binding to cell nuclei, and induction of mouse mammary tumor virus RNA. *Eur. J. Biochem.* **152**, 173–178.
63. Walton, G. M., Gill, G. N., Cooper, E., and Spaulding, S. W. (1984). Thyroid-stimulated phosphorylation of high mobility group protein 14 *in vivo* at the site

catalyzed by cyclic nucleotide-dependent protein kinases *in vitro. J. Biol. Chem.* **259**, 601–607.

64. Iynedjian, P. B., and Arslan, Y. (1984). Phosphorylation of histones and non-histone nuclear proteins in liver cells stimulated by glucagon and cyclic AMP. *FEBS Lett.* **178**, 143–148.

65. Hashimoto, S., and Guroff, G. (1982). Norepinephrine and nerve growth factor: Similar proteins phosphorylated in the nuclei of target cells. *Biochem. Biophys. Res. Commun.* **104**, 1477–1483.

66. Elliott, M. E. (1990). Phosphorylation of adrenal histone H3 is affected by angiotensin, ACTH, dibutyryl cAMP, and atrial natriuretic peptide. *Life Sci.* **46**, 1479–1488.

67. Hohmann, P., and Hughes, C. (1987). H1 histone synthesis and phosphorylation in mouse mammary gland in vitro. *Mol. Cell. Endocrinol.* **54**, 35–41.

68. Mahadevan, L. C., Willis, A. C., and Barratt, M. J. (1991). Rapid histone H3 phosphorylation in response to growth factors, phorbol esters, okadaic acid, and protein synthesis inhibitors. *Cell* **65**, 775–783.

69. Banerjee, S., Bennion, G. R., Goldberg, M. W., and Allen, T. D. (1991). ATP dependent histone phorphorylation and nucleosome assembly in a human cell free extract. *Nucleic Acids Res.* **19**, 5999–6006.

70. Marion, C., Martinage, A., Tirard, A., Roux, B., Daune, M., and Mazen, A. (1985). Histone phorphorylation in native chromatin induces local structural changes as probed by electric birefringence. *J. Mol. Biol.* **186**, 367–379.

71. Hill, C. S., Rimmer, J. M., Green, B. N., Finch, J. T., and Thomas, J. O. (1991). Histone-DNA interactions and their modulation by phosphorylation of –Ser–Pro–X–Lys/Arg– motifs. *EMBO J.* **10**, 1939–1948.

72. Hayaishi, O., and Ueda, K. (eds) (1982). "ADP-Ribosylation Reactions: Biology and Medicine." Academic Press, New York.

73. Gaal, J. C., and Pearson, C. K. (1985). Eukaryotic nuclear ADP-ribosylation reactions. *Biochem. J.* **230**, 1–18.

74. Ueda, K., and Hayaishi, O. (1985). ADP-ribosylation. *Annu. Rev. Biochem.* **54**, 73–100.

75. Lautier, D., Lagueux, J., Thibodeau, J., Ménard, L., and Poirier, G. G. (1993). Molecular and biochemical features of poly(ADP-ribose) metabolism. *Mol. Cell. Biol.* **122**, 171–193.

76. Uchida, K., Morita, T., Sato, T., Ogura, T., Yamashita, R., Noguchi, S., Suzuki, H., Nyunoya, H., Miwa, M., and Sugimura, T. (1987). Nucleotide sequence of a full-length cDNA for human fibroblast poly(ADP-ribose) polymerase. *Biochem. Biophys. Res. Commun.* **148**, 617–622.

77. Mazen, A., Menissier-de Murcia, J., Molinete, M., Simonin, F., Gradwohl, G., Poirier, G., and de Murcia, G. (1989). Poly(ADP-ribose) polymerase: A novel finger protein. *Nucleic Acids Res.* **17**, 4689–4698.

78. Wallace, H. M., Gordon, A. M., Keir, H. M., and Pearson, C. K. (1984). Activation of ADP-ribosyltransferase in polyamine-depleted mammalian cells. *Biochem. J.* **219**, 211–221.

79. Singh, N., Poirier, G., and Cerutti, P. (1985). Tumor promoter phorbol-12-myristate-13-acetate induces poly(ADP)-ribosylation in fibroblasts. *EMBO J.* **4**, 1491–1494.

80. Bauer, P. I., Farkas, G., Buday, L., Mikala, G., Meszaros, G., Kun, E., and Farago, A. (1992). Inhibition of DNA binding by the phosphorylation of poly

ADP-ribose polymerase protein catalysed by protein kinase C. *Biochem. Biophys. Res. Commun.* **187,** 730–736.

81. Milam, K. M., and Cleaver, J. E. (1984). Inhibitors of poly(adenosine diphosphate-ribose) synthesis: Effect on other metabolic processes. *Science* **223,** 589–591.

82. Maruta, H., Inageda, K., Aoki, T., Nishina, H., and Tanuma, S. (1991). Characterization of two forms of poly(ADP-ribose) glycohydrolase in guinea pig liver. *Biochemistry* **30,** 5907–5912.

83. Uchida, K., Suzuki, H., Maruta, H., Abe, H., Aoki, K., Miwa, M., and Tanuma, S. (1993). Preferential degradation of protein-bound (ADP-ribose)$_n$ by nuclear poly(ADP-ribose) glycohydrolase from human placenta. *J. Biol. Chem.* **268,** 3194–3200.

84. Tanuma, S., and Otsuka, F. (1991). Change in activity of nuclear poly(ADP-ribose) glycohydrolase during the HeLa 93 cell cycle. *Arch. Biochem. Biophys.* **284,** 227–231.

85. Li, J. C., and Kaminskas, E. (1987). DNA fragmentation in permeabilized cells. *Biochem. J.* **247,** 805–806.

86. Sugimura, T., and Miwa, M. (1983). Poly(ADP-ribose) and cancer research. *Carcinogenesis (London)* **4,** 1503–1506.

87. Tanuma, S., Kawashima, K., and Endo, H. (1985). Comparison of ADP-ribosylation of chromosomal proteins between intact and broken cells. *Biochem. Biophys. Res. Commun.* **127,** 896–902.

88. Kirsten, E., Jackowski, G., McLick, J., Hakam, A., Decker, K., and Kun, E. (1985). Cellular regulation of poly(ADP) ribosylation of proteins. I. Comparison of hepatocytes, cultured cells and liver nuclei and the influence of varying concentrations of NAD. *Exp. Cell Res.* **161,** 41–52.

89. Satoh, M. S., and Lindahl, T. (1992). Role of poly(ADP-ribose) formation in DNA repair. *Nature (London)* **356,** 356–358.

90. Althaus, F. R. (1992). Poly ADP-ribosylation: A histone shuttle mechanism in DNA excision repair. *J. Cell Sci.* **102,** 663–670.

91. Suzuki, H., Buonamassa, T., and Weisz, A. (1990). Inverse relationship between poly (ADP-ribose) polymerase activity and 2',5'-oligoadenylates core level in estrogen-treated immature rat. *Mol. Cell. Biochem.* **99,** 33–39.

92. Burzio, L. O., and Koide, S. S. (1977). Stimulation of poly(adenosine diphosphate ribose) synthetase activity of *Xenopus* germinal vesicle by progesterone. *Ann. N.Y. Acad. Sci.* **286,** 398–407.

93. Guo, J. Z., and Gorski, J. (1989). Estrogen effects on modifications of chromatin proteins in the rat uterus, *J. Steroid Biochem.* **32,** 13–20.

94. Gartemann, A., Brederhorst, R., Wielckens, K., Stratking, W. H. H., and Hilz, H. (1981). Mono- and poly-ADP-ribosylation of proteins in mouse kidney after castration and testosterone treatment. *Biochem. J.* **198,** 37–44.

95. Pisarev, M. A., Hepburn, A., and Dumont, J. E. (1985). Action of TSH on nuclear ADP-ribosylation in dog thyroid slicers. *Experientia* **41,** 1453–1455.

96. Shimoyama, M., Kitamura, A., and Tanigawa, Y. (1982). Glucocorticoid effects on poly(ADP-ribose) metabolism. *In* "ADP-Ribosylation Reactions: Biology and Medicine" (O. Hayaishi and K. Uedo, eds.), pp. 465–475. Academic Press, New York.

97. Tanuma, S., Johnson, L. D., and Johnson, G. S. (1983). ADP-ribosylation of chromosomal proteins and mouse mammary tumor virus gene expression: Glu-

cocorticoids rapidly decrease endogenous ADP-ribosylation of nonhistone high mobility group 14 and 17 proteins. *J. Biol. Chem.* **258**, 15371–15375.

98. Bolander, F. F. (1985). The relationship between adenosine diphosphate-ribosylation and mammary gland differentiation. *J. Cell. Biochem.* **29**, 361–372.

99. Poirier, G. G., de Murcia, G., Jongstra-Bilen, J., Niedergang, C., and Mandel, P. (1982). Poly(ADP-ribosyl)ation of polynucleosomes causes relaxation of chromatin structure. *Proc. Natl. Acad. Sci. U.S.A.* **79**, 3423–3427.

100. Stone, P. R., Lorimer, W. S., and Kidwell, W. R. (1977). Properties of the complex between histone H1 and poly(ADP-ribose) synthesized in HeLa cell nuclei. *Eur. J. Biochem.* **81**, 9–18.

101. Hough, C. J., and Smulson, M. E. (1984). Association of poly(adenosine diphosphate ribosylated) nucleosomes with transcriptionally active and inactive regions of chromatin. *Biochemistry* **23**, 5016–5023.

102. Boulikas, T. (1990). Poly(ADP-ribosylated) histones in chromatin replication. *J. Biol. Chem.* **265**, 14638–14647.

103. Chypre, C., Le Calvez, C., Hog, F., Revel, M. O., Jesser, M., and Mandel, P. (1989). Phosphorylation de la poly(ADP-ribose) polymérase cytoplasmique liée à des particules ribonucléoprotéiques libres par une protéine kinase C associée. *C. R. Acad. Sci. Sér. III* **309**, 471–476.

104. Das, R., and Kanungo, M. S. (1980). *In vitro* methylation of chromosomal proteins of the brain of rats of various ages and its modulation by epinephrine. *Indian J. Biochem. Biophys.* **17**, 429–431.

105. Thakur, M. K., and Kanungo, M. S. (1981). Methylation of chromosomal proteins and DNA of rat brain and its modulation by estradiol and calcium during aging. *Exp. Gerontol.* **16**, 331–336.

106. Short, J., and Kibert, L. (1980). Enhanced hepatic chromatin protein methylation induced by triiodothyronine treatment of the rat. *Endocrine Res. Commun.* **7**, 113–119.

107. Desrosiers, R., and Tanguay, R. M. (1985). The modifications in the methylation patterns of H2B and H3 after heat shock can be correlated with the inactivation of normal gene expression. *Biochem. Biophys. Res. Commun.* **133**, 823–829.

108. Hendzel, M. J., and Davie, J. R. (1989). Distribution of methylated histones and histone methyltransferases in chicken erythrocyte chromatin. *J. Biol. Chem.* **264**, 19208–19214.

109. Reneker, J., and Brotherton, T. W. (1991). Postsynthetic methylation of core histones in K562 cells is associated with bulk acetylation but not with transcriptional activity. *Biochemistry* **30**, 8402–8407.

110. Prasad, S., and Thakur, M. K. (1988). Age-dependent effects of sodium butyrate and hydrocortisone on acetylation of high mobility group proteins of rat liver. *Biochem. Int.* **16**, 375–382.

111. Alexandrova, E. A., and Beltchev, B. G. (1988). Acetylated HMG1 protein interacts specifically with homologous DNA polymerase alpha *in vitro*. *Biochem. Biophys. Res. Commun.* **154**, 918–927.

112. Dimov, S. I., Alexandrova, E. A., and Beltchev, B. G. (1990). Differences between some properties of acetylated and nonacetylated forms of HMG1 protein. *Biochem. Biophys. Res. Commun.* **166**, 819–826.

113. Spaulding, S. W., Fucile, N. W., Bofinger, D. P., and Sheflin, L. G. (1991). Cyclic adenosine 3′,5′-monophosphate-dependent phosphorylation of HMG 14 inhibits its interactions with nucleosomes. *Mol. Endocrinol.* **5**, 42–50.

114. Lund, T., and Berg, K. (1991). Metaphase-specific phosphorylations weaken the association between chromosomal proteins HMG 14 and 17, and DNA. *FEBS Lett.* **289**, 113–116.

115. Palvimo, J., and Mäenpää, P. H. (1988). Binding of high-mobility-group proteins HMG 14 and HMG 17 to DNA and histone H1 as influenced by phosphorylation. *Biochim. Biophys. Acta* **952**, 172–180.

116. Fedorova, N. A. (1991). High-mobility group proteins: Structure, localization, functions. *Biokhimiya* **56**, 9–18.

117. Kimura, K., Katoh, N., Sakurada, K., and Kubo, S. (1985). Phosphorylation of high mobility group 1 protein by phospholipid-sensitive Ca^{2+}-dependent protein kinase from pig testis. *Biochem. J.* **227**, 271–276.

118. Tsai, Y. J., Aoki, T., Maruta, H., Abe, H., Sakagami, H., Hatano, T., Okuda, T., and Tanuma, S. (1992). Mouse mammary tumor virus gene expression is suppressed by oligomeric ellagitannins, novel inhibitors of poly(ADP-ribose) glycohydrolase. *J. Biol. Chem.* **267**, 14436–14442.

119. Telford, D. J., and Steward, B. W. (1989). Micrococcal nuclease: Its specificity and use for chromatin analysis. *Int. J. Biochem.* **21**, 127–137.

120. Bloom, K. S., and Anderson, J. N. (1982). Hormonal regulation of the conformation of the ovalbumin gene in chick oviduct chromatin. *J. Biol. Chem.* **257**, 13018–13027.

121. Williams, J. L., and Tata, J. R. (1983). Simultaneous analysis of conformation and transcription of A and B groups of vitellogenin genes in male and female *Xenopus* during primary and secondary activation by estrogen. *Nucleic Acids Res.* **11**, 1151–1166.

122. Cedar, H., and Razin, A. (1990). DNA methylation and development. *Biochim. Biophys. Acta* **1049**, 1–8.

123. Weissbach, A., Ward, C., and Bolden, A. (1990). Eukaryotic DNA methylation and gene expression. *Curr. Top. Cell Regul.* **30**, 1–21.

124. Hergersberg, M. (1991). Biological aspects of cytosine methylation in eukaryotic cells. *Experientia* **47**, 1171–1185.

125. Lewis, J., and Bird, A. (1991). DNA methylation and chromatin structure. *FEBS Lett.* **285**, 155–159.

126. Haigh, L. S., Owens, B. B., Hellewell, S., and Ingram, V. M. (1982). DNA methylation in chicken α-globin gene expression. *Proc. Natl. Acad. Sci. U.S.A.* **79**, 5332–5336.

127. Doerfler, W., Toth, M., Kochanek, S., Achten, S., Freisem-Rabien, U., Behn-Krappa, A., and Orend, G. (1990). Eukaryotic DNA methylation: Facts and problems. *FEBS Lett.* **268**, 329–333.

128. Compere, S. J., and Palmiter, R. D. (1981). DNA methylation controls the inducibility of the mouse metallothionein-I gene in lymphoid cells. *Cell* **25**, 233–240.

129. Stein, R., Gruenbaum, Y., Razin, A., and Cedar, H. (1982). Methylation and the regulation of globin gene expression. *Cell* **34**, 197–206.

130. Levine, A., Cantoni, G. L., and Razin, A. (1992). Methylation in the preinitiation domain suppresses gene transcription by an indirect mechanism. *Proc. Natl. Acad. Sci. U.S.A.* **89**, 10119–10123.

131. Gerber-Huber, S., May, F. E. B., Westley, B. R., Felber, B. K., Hosbach, H. A., Andres, A. C., and Ryffel, G. U. (1983). In contrast to other *Xenopus* genes the estrogen-inducible vitellogenin genes are expressed when totally methylated. *Cell* **33**, 43–51.

132. Bolander, F. F. (1983). The effect of 5-azacytidine on mammary gland differentiation *in vitro. Biochem. Biophys. Res. Commun.* **111**, 150–155.
133. Burch, J. B. E., and Weintraub, H. (1983). Temporal order of chromatin structural changes associated with activation of the major chicken vitellogenin gene. *Cell* **33**, 65–76.
134. Burch, J. B. E., and Evans, M. I. (1986). Chromatin structural transitions and the phenomenon of vitellogenin gene memory in chickens. *Mol. Cell. Biol.* **6**, 1886–1893.
135. Bird, A. P. (1986). CpG-rich islands and the function of DNA methylation. *Nature (London)* **321**, 209–213.
136. Gellersen, B., and Kempf, R. (1990). Human prolactin gene expression: Positive correlation between site-specific methylation and gene activity in a set of human lymphoid cell lines. *Mol. Endocrinol.* **4**, 1874–1886.
137. Boyes, J., and Bird, A. (1991). DNA methylation inhibits transcription indirectly via a methyl-CpG binding protein. *Cell* **64**, 1123–1134.
138. Levine, A., Cantoni, G. L., and Razin, A. (1991). Inhibition of promoter activity by methylation: Possible involvement of protein mediators. *Proc. Natl. Acad. Sci. U.S.A.* **88**, 6515–6518.
139. Jost, J. P., Saluz, H. P., and Pawlak, A. (1991). Estradiol down regulates the binding activity of an avian vitellogenin gene repressor (MDBP-2) and triggers a gradual demethylation of the mCpG pair of its DNA binding site. *Nucleic Acids Res.* **19**, 5771–5775.
140. Schroth, G. P., Chou, P. J., and Ho, P. S. (1992). Mapping Z-DNA in the human genome: Computer-aided mapping reveals a nonrandom distribution of potential Z-DNA-forming sequences in human genes. *J. Biol. Chem.* **267**, 11846–11855.
141. Lannigan, D. A., Koszewski, N. J., and Notides, A. C. (1993). Estrogen-responsive elements contain non-B DNA. *Mol. Cell. Endocrinol.* **94**, 47–54.
142. Lancillotti, F., Lopez, M. C., Arias, P., and Alonso, C. (1987). Z-DNA in transcriptionally active chromosomes. *Proc. Natl. Acad. Sci. U.S.A.* **84**, 1560–1564.

CHAPTER **14**

Post-transcriptional Control

CHAPTER OUTLINE

I. Introduction

The previous chapters in this part have primarily analyzed gene control from a transcriptional perspective; in this chapter, other post-transcriptional control points will be covered. The three major focal points will be RNA processing, translational control, and post-translational modifications.

II. RNA Processing

A. Stability

In the rat mammary gland, prolactin (PRL) stimulates the accumulation of casein mRNA 34-fold but the absolute rate of transcription increases only 2-fold. The difference is made up by the change in half-life, which increases from 5.4 hours in cultures without PRL to 96 hours in cultures with this hormone (1). In this system, gene expression as evidenced by mRNA accumulation is primarily evoked by altering mRNA half-life. This mechanism operates in many systems: in chick oviduct, estrogens increase the mRNA half-life of ovalbumin from 4–5 to 24 hours (2) and that of conalbumin from 3 to 8 hours (3); in *Xenopus* liver, these same steroids increase the half-life of vitellogenin mRNA from 16 hours to 3 weeks (4). Decreasing the half-life of mRNAs is also possible. In cultures of chick embryo hepatocytes, triiodothyronine (T_3) induces the malic enzyme whereas glucagon inhibits it (5). T_3 elevates the malic enzyme mRNA 11- to 14-fold, although the transcriptional rate only doubles, suggesting an increased half-life. However, glucagon definitely affects the half-life by reducing it from 8–11 hours to only 1.5 hours; glucagon has no effect on the transcription of this enzyme. Finally, a single hormone can affect the half-lives of two different mRNAs in opposite ways: in a pituitary cell line, thyrotropin-releasing hormone (TRH) stimulates PRL mRNA accumulation but inhibits growth hormone (GH) mRNA accumulation (6). TRH increases the half-life of the PRL mRNA from 17 to 27 hours and reduces that of the GH mRNA from 24 to 15 hours. TRH does not affect mRNA processing in this system.

Several factors can affect mRNA stability; the first is the length of the poly(A) tail. A group of poly(A)-binding proteins combines with this tail to form nucleosome-like structures; these particles are relatively resistant to nuclease attack (7). Protein kinase C (PKC) lengthens the poly(A) tract on corticotropin-releasing factor (CRF) mRNA by 100 nucleotides and cAMP does the same for vasopressin mRNA (8); on the other hand, T_3 decreases the length of the poly(A) tail on thyroid-stimulating hormone β (TSHβ) mRNA (9). The most obvious target for these hormones and second messengers is the poly(A) polymerase; numerous reports have been made of hormones affecting the activity of this enzyme. Unfortunately, most studies are done under nonsaturating conditions. To understand this problem, assume that under basal conditions only 25% of the enzyme is being utilized; after hormone exposure, RNA synthesis triples. Now 75% of the enzyme is being utilized and its total endogenous activity will increase even though enzyme number and intrinsic activity are unchanged. In other words, the hormone is not directly stimulating enzyme activity but is only increasing substrate levels. To determine whether a hormone is actually altering enzyme number or specific activity, the enzyme should be assayed under conditions in which it is maximally utilized, that is, substrate should be saturating.

As alluded to already, there are two mechanisms for increasing the activity of poly(A) polymerase. Steroids increase enzyme number as evidenced by the requirement for protein synthesis; the effect of glucocorticoids on the poly(A) tail of GH mRNA would be an example (10). On the other hand, PKC increases the specific activity of the polymerase in T lymphocytes (11). This action certainly suggests phosphorylation as a mechanism for regulating enzyme activity; however, *in vitro* the enzyme is a very poor substrate for PKC. Only a cyclic nucleotide-independent protein kinase similar to the NI kinase has been shown to phosphorylate quantitatively and to activate poly(A) polymerase significantly (12). It is possible that PKC triggers *in vivo* a kinase cascade that ends with the NI-like kinase.

mRNA can be destabilized by the presence of A/U-rich repeats in the 3' untranslated region. Once again, these sequences are recognized by specific RNA-binding proteins; the difference is that these A/U-binding proteins result in the degradation of the mRNA (13). Hormones can affect this system in four ways. First, they can alter the level of these proteins. β-Agonists down-regulate the β-adrenergic receptor (βAR), in part by inducing these proteins, whereas insulin and dexamethasone elevate βAR mRNA by repressing the A/U-binding proteins (14). Second, hormones can alter the activity of these proteins. cAMP can increase the half-life of phosphoenolpyruvate carboxykinase mRNA 10-fold by causing these proteins to dissociate from the mRNA (15). This effect is rapid and phosphorylation-dependent, suggesting that PKA is involved with inactivating some of these proteins. Another mechanism involves the elimination of these sequences: cAMP response element modulator τ (CREMτ) is induced in the testis by follicle-stimulating hormone (FSH) by using an alternative poly(A) site, which eliminates 9 of the 10 A/U-rich regions in the 3' tail (16). Finally, estradiol preferentially lowers albumin mRNA levels in *Xenopus* liver by inducing an endonuclease that favors the albumin mRNA as substrate (17).

Hormones may also affect mRNA stability indirectly. By stimulating translation initiation (see subsequent discussion), the ribosome density increases and protects the mRNA. In addition, there may be a shift in poly(A) binding proteins. As noted already, estradiol increases vitellogenin mRNA and decreases albumin mRNA; the massive elevation of vitellogenin mRNA will outcompete the albumin mRNA for the limiting amount of poly(A)-binding protein, leaving the latter exposed to RNases (18).

B. Modifications

The addition of a poly(A) track is not the only modification that RNA undergoes after transcription: many RNA species are also subjected to cleavage, splicing, and base modifications. In liver nucleoli from Leghorn roosters, the conversion of rRNA from a 32 S precursor to the 28 S mature form can be followed in pulse–chase experiments (19). In the absence of estrogen, this processing requires 20 minutes, but following estrogen treatment the conversion only requires a few minutes. Another type of processing requires nucleotide modifications such as methylation. Both estradiol (20) and PRL (21) stimulate tRNA methylase 2- to 3-fold in immature rat uteri and mouse mammary explants, respectively. Unfortunately, most of these data were obtained under nonsaturating conditions; therefore, it is not clear whether the processing machinery was really being changed or was just being utilized more effectively.

C. Nuclear Egression

Eukaryotes have their genetic material enclosed within a nuclear membrane, which acts as a barrier between transcription and translation. Its effectiveness is attested to by the fact that most mRNAs never leave the nucleus and are eventually degraded. Therefore, nuclear egression of mRNA is certainly a potential control point. Dexamethasone induces α_{2u}-globulin in rat liver (22); after adrenalectomy, the mRNA for this protein accumulates in the nucleus whereas the mRNA content in polysomes falls. Within 2 hours of dexamethasone administration, nuclear mRNA levels decline whereas those in the polysomes rise; researchers assumed that this transfer was too fast to be mediated by transcription, although no transcription inhibitors were tested. Furthermore, the size of these mRNA species is unchanged, suggesting that processing is not involved. The conclusion is that glucocorticoids could directly stimulate the nucleocytoplasmic transport of mRNA.

Other investigators have studied the effects of hormones on the nuclear efflux of endogenous mRNA or the nuclear influx of dextran. In isolated liver nuclei, insulin and cAMP stimulate mRNA efflux 60–80% but the insulin concentrations were supraphysiological (23). In a similar system, both insulin and epidermal growth factor (EGF) increased dextran influx 200–300%; the effect appeared to be specific, since neither the denatured hormones nor intact glucagon had any effect (24). Nonetheless, the hormone concentrations required to elicit this response were still extremely high.

How might this nuclear egression be regulated? Research has implicated a nuclear nucleotide triphosphatase in the transfer of mRNA from the nucleus to the cytoplasm. Human chorionic gonadotropin (hCG) stimulated this enzyme 2- to 3-fold in the isolated nuclear membranes of luteal cells (25). This stimulation does not occur in the nuclear membranes of nontarget organs nor in the nonnuclear membranes of luteal cells. Similar results have been reported in other systems: estradiol stimulates the ATPase almost 40-fold in isolated uterine nuclei (26) whereas insulin and cAMP have more modest effects in liver nuclei (27). Where examined, these hormones affect only the V_{max} of the enzyme; the K_m is not significantly altered. Another mechanism involves a nuclear envelope protein called p110 (28). Phosphorylation by PKC is associated with the transport of mRNA.

In contrast to mRNA, the egression of pre-rRNA involves the protein nucleolin. Insulin in picomolar concentrations rapidly stimulates the phosphorylation of nucleolin via casein kinase II (CKII). This modification correlates with pre-rRNA efflux (29).

III. Translation

A. Introduction

The transport of mRNA into the cytoplasm does not automatically result in its translation. PRL injection into pseudopregnant rabbits induces both casein mRNAs and casein proteins, but in virgin rabbits almost no casein is synthesized, although its mRNA is induced 58-fold and is found attached to ribosomes (30). In another example, the C57BL mouse strain is infected with the mouse mammary tumor virus but only exhibits a low mammary tumor incidence. During lactation, the viral RNA is produced in abundance and is transported to the cytoplasm, where it co-sediments with polysomes. However, no viral peptides are produced. The RNA is normal, since it can be purified from these glands and be translated in the reticulocyte lysate system (31).

B. Regulation of General Translation

Many hormones are known to facilitate protein synthesis by inducing the cellular machinery for translation. This is particularly notable in systems in which hormones stimulate large amounts of protein secretion, as in milk production. In the mammary gland, both cortisol and PRL have been shown to induce tRNAs (21), 28 S rRNA (32), and the formation of rough endoplasmic reticulum (33).

In other systems this effect can be semiselective. For example, if the protein to be made has a biased amino acid composition, the hormone may stimulate only the tRNAs for those amino acids, thereby favoring the synthesis of that protein. Alanine, serine, and glycine represent 80% of all the amino acids in silk fibroin. In the silk glands of the fifth instar silkworm, the tRNAs for these three amino acids are induced along with their respective acyl tRNA synthetases (34). This alteration in tRNA abundance is required for the efficient translation of this protein. The antifreeze protein in winter flounder represents a hormonally regulated system; 60% of the amino acids in the antifreeze protein are alanines. The onset of winter causes GH to decline; this decrease leads to an increase in both the mRNA for the antifreeze protein and in a single alanine isoacceptor (35,36). This isoacceptor is presumed to be the one that recognizes the codon GCC, which encodes 70–75% of all the alanines in the mRNA for the antifreeze protein.

C. Regulation of Selective Translation

In addition to tRNA abundance, there are other examples of even more selective control. 1,25-Dihydroxycholecalciferol (1,25-DHCC) doubles the rate of chain elongation of chromogranin A in the parathyroid gland without affecting the translation of parathormone (37). In another example, polyamines inhibit the enzymes responsible for their synthesis by decreasing enzyme number. However, since the mRNAs for these enzymes do not change, the effect must be post-transcriptional (38). Indeed, in a reticulocyte lysate system, polyamines selectively inhibit the translation of the mRNAs for ornithine decarboxylase (ODC) and S-adenosylmethionine (SAM) decarboxylase; the translation of total protein or serum albumin is unaffected (39). In other words, in some systems it is possible for a hormone to direct the protein synthetic machinery to translate one mRNA or a small group of mRNAs while ignoring others. A similar phenomenon occurs in plants, where jasmonic acid induces defense genes while it inhibits the translation of pre-existing mRNAs. These mRNAs appear normal, but chain initiation is reduced (40).

Where is this control exerted? The induction of heat shock proteins provides a clue (41). When *Drosophila* cells are incubated at 36°C, special heat shock genes are transcribed and their mRNAs are translated; no other mRNA is translated. This latter mRNA is not degraded and is normally translated when the temperature returns to 25°C. This system can be dissected further by incubating cells at either 25 or 36°C and separating the lysates, which contain the protein synthetic machinery, from the mRNAs; the fractions can then be recombined in different ways. The high-temperature mRNA contains both normal and heat shock mRNAs but, when it is recombined with the high-temperature lysate, only the heat shock mRNAs are translated. This result is expected based on the experiments in whole cells. The low-temperature mRNA contains only normal mRNA and, when recombined with the high-temperature lysate, is still not translated. This result eliminates the possibility that the normal mRNAs were reversibly inactivated at the elevated temperature. When high-temperature mRNA is mixed with a low-temperature lysate, both normal and heat shock proteins are synthesized. This result suggests that the selectivity resides in the translational machinery.

D. Molecular Mechanisms

What are the molecular bases for affecting the activity of the translational machinery? Covalent modifications of the initiation factors, the elongation factors, or the ribosome may explain this phenomenon (Table 14-1; 42). Of the initiation factors, eIF-2[1] has been the most extensively studied; this factor is responsible for putting the first tRNA in place. It is a heterotrimer: the α subunit binds GTP, the β subunit is involved in the GTP exchange, and the γ subunit binds Met–tRNA$^{Met}_f$. The phosphorylation of eIF-2α constitutes one aspect of the physiological control of hemoglobin (44). Hemoglobin consists of an iron-containing porphyrin ring, *heme*, and a protein, *globin*. In iron-de-

---

[1] The terminology used in this chapter conforms to the recommendations of the Nomenclature Committee of the International Union of Biochemistry (43).

Table 14-1

Occurrence and Effects of Phosphorylation on the Translation Machinery

Translation factor	Function	Phosphorylation					Effect
		PKC	S6KI	CKII	PKA	Other	
eIF-2α	Complexes with GTP and initiator Met-tRNA; binds to 40S preinitiation complex	+	+	+		Heme-controlled inhibitor; dsRNA kinase; dephosphorylated by insulin	Decreases translation by decreasing GTP exchange and recycling; forms nonfunctional complex with eIF-2β
eIF-2Bε	GTP exchange			+		GSK-3	Increases GTP exchange 5-fold (partially overcome phosphorylation of eIF-2α)
eIF-4B	eIF-4 recycling and mRNA binding to 40S preinitiation complex	+	+	+		Insulin; EGF	Selective translation
eIF-4Fα	Binds m^{7}G cap of mRNA	+	+		+	Insulin; EGF; PDGF; TNFα (via protamine kinase)	Increases binding to mRNA and increases translation 3- to 5-fold
eEF-1β and δ	Amino acyl tRNA binding	+					Increases translation 3-fold
eEF-1γ	Amino acyl tRNA binding					Cdc2	Inhibits GTP exchange
eEF-2	Translocation					CaMKIII; dephosphorylated, by cAMP	Blocks translocation (CaMKIII); activation (cAMP)
S6	mRNA binding site on ribosome	+	+		+	PKG and CaMKII	Increases AUG binding and translation 4-fold

479

ficient anemia, there is little iron and heme; in the absence of iron and heme, it is senseless to synthesize the globin. Therefore, low heme concentrations activate a protein kinase that phosphorylates the α subunit and inhibits all translation; in reticulocytes, globin is virtually the only protein being made. Interferon acts in a similar manner to shut down all translation; in this case, the purpose is to abort a viral infection. Several other hormonally regulated kinases can also modify eIF-2α with similar, but less dramatic, effects (Table 14-1). However, since most of these kinases are activated by growth factors whose actions would need enhanced translation, their effects are paradoxical and their physiological role is uncertain.

Another intensively studied initiation factor is eIF-4Fα (formerly called eIF-4E), which binds the mRNA cap structure. Its phosphorylation is stimulated by several growth factors and results in increased translation. Recently, one of the responsible kinases has been identified as protamine kinase, a downstream component of the mitogen-activated protein kinase (MAPK) cascade (45). One of the reasons for the interest in eIF-4Fα is its potential for selectivity; its function is to melt secondary structures in mRNA to facilitate translation. This effect would be greatest in those mRNAs with such structures. For example, the mRNA for ODC, the rate-limiting enzyme in polyamine synthesis, has such secondary structures and is preferentially translated following insulin stimulation (46). If the 5' end of this mRNA is spliced onto other mRNAs, they too will become insulin responsive.

Elongation factors and ribosomal proteins can also be phosphorylated. Calmodulin-dependent protein kinase III (CaMKIII) modifies eEF-2 and reduces the rate of translation; this effect may have selective consequences since it could allow less efficiently translated mRNA better access to the translational machinery (47). In addition to its regulation by calcium and calmodulin, CaMKIII can be phosphorylated and activated by protein kinase A (PKA) (48). cAMP can also reverse the effect of CaMKIII by inducing the dephosphorylation of eEF-2 (49). Ribosomal protein S6 has been the focus of many studies, both because it is the mRNA binding site on the ribosome and because its phosphorylation is stimulated by so many growth factors. Such modifications enhance translation.

Not all modifications are phosphorylations: eIF-5A (formerly called eIF-4D) is modified by butylamine, which is derived from spermidine. The butylamine is attached to a lysine and then hydroxylated to form hypusine (see Chapter 10). Although this modification is not required for general translation, it is required for cell division (50). Therefore, regulation of the synthesis of hypusine may control the translation of mRNAs for genes involved with mitosis. Since this reaction is dependent on the polyamine concentration, those hormones that elevate polyamine levels could trigger this modification and facilitate the synthesis of proteins needed for cell division.

In addition to covalent modifications, translation can be affected by mRNA binding factors. As noted earlier, polyamines suppress the translation of the mRNA for the polyamine synthetic enzymes; in the SAM decarboxylase gene, this effect is a result of polyamine binding to the GC-rich region in the 5' end (51). In another example, cortisol stimulates the translation of myelin basic protein in reticulocyte lysates by enhancing the formation of an initiation complex (52). It requires a specific sequence in the mRNA; researchers assume that a cortisol-binding protein recognizes this sequence and that its subsequent binding to the mRNA enhances translation. However, this protein does not appear to be the classic glucocorticoid receptor (GR), since its ligand and nucleotide-binding specificities are different.

A similar phenomenon occurs in genes involved in iron metabolism (53,54). These genes have a specific sequence, the iron response element (IRE), that is bound by the iron response factor (IRF). When the IRE is at the 5' end of the mRNA, IRF binding blocks translation, but at the 3' end IRF binding stabilizes the mRNA. IRF is actually aconitase, an enzyme in the tricarboxylic acid cycle; it has an iron–sulfur cluster that is required for enzymatic activity but that must be removed for IRF activity. The generation of apoaconitase is accomplished by nitric oxide (NO). The mechanism is unknown but NO does activate the soluble guanylate cyclase by binding to the heme iron and stimulating its dissociation. NO may have the same effect on iron–sulfur clusters. Alternatively, it may react with sulfhydryl groups, another common target of NO, and trigger a conformation change that favors the removal of iron. In either case, the resulting apoaconitase can bind the IRE and this binding can be further increased by PKC phosphorylation (55). Therefore, this system represents an example in which hormonally generated second messengers can specifically affect the translation of a restricted set of genes.

Finally, translation can be regulated by compartmentalization of the mRNA into ribonucleoprotein (RNP) particles. For example, mRNAs for ribosomal proteins are distributed between polysomes and RNP particles; the latter are translationally inactive. The degree of translation is, therefore, determined by a balance between the two pools. In lymphosarcoma cells, dexamethasone inhibits the translation of these mRNAs by shifting them into RNP particles (56).

IV. Post-translational Regulation

A. Protein Modifications

Once a protein is synthesized, it may undergo many modifications . These alterations are performed in a very orderly sequence as the protein traverses several cellular organelles on its way to being secreted (Table 14-2). This section will only discuss *N*-linked glycosylation. This modification involves the attachment of sugar residues onto an asparagine, as opposed to *O*-linked glycosylation, in which monosaccharides are coupled to a serine or a threonine. In the former, an entire oligosaccharide side chain is synthesized on a carrier lipid, which then transfers this core structure *en bloc* to the nascent

Table 14-2
Location of Some Post-translational Modifications

Location	Modification
Rough endoplasmic reticulum	Cleavage of the signal sequence; hydroxylation; some end-group blockers; cross-linking by disulfide bonds; core glycosylation; addition of core PI-glycan; myristoylation
Golgi apparatus	Terminal glycosylation; O-linked glycosylation; phosphorylation; palmitoylation; sulfation
Secretory vesicles	Cleavage (e.g., of the C peptide in insulin)
Extracellular	Cleavage (e.g., in zymogens), cross-linking (e.g., in collagen and fibrin)

polypeptide. This event is called *core glycosylation*. While the protein is still in the rough endoplasmic reticulum, some of the sugars at the ends are removed; this process continues in the Golgi apparatus. Finally, new sugars are added to the ends; each type of protein receives a unique sequence. This process is called *terminal glycosylation*. As will be illustrated in this discussion, core glycosylation appears to be automatic, but terminal glycosylation is frequently under hormonal regulation and is associated with secretion.

The hormonal control of post-translational modification has been investigated in a number of systems, only two of which will be discussed: the mouse mammary tumor virus and TSH. The virus is a standard retrovirus having five genes (57):

1. The *gag* gene encodes two structural polyproteins.

2. The *pol* gene encodes the reverse transcriptase.

3. The *env* gene encodes a single glycosylated polyprotein that will be split into two envelope proteins.

4. The *pro* gene overlaps the *gag* and *pol* genes and encodes a protease used in processing some of the other gene products.

5. The ORF (*open reading frame*) in the 3' end of the genome encodes a superantigen that interacts with the immune system of the mouse.

The processing of the polyproteins is somewhat variable, but the following schemata appear to represent the predominant pathways (58). One of the *gag* products, pr74^{gag}, first must be phosphorylated to pr76^{gag} before cleavage can take place; the numbers refer to the protein molecular masses in kilodaltons. This phosphorylation is stimulated by dexamethasone; indirectly, so is the subsequent processing by cleavage since the precursor, pr74^{gag}, accumulates in the absence of dexamethasone. In a similar manner, the *env* product, pr60^{env}, must be glycosylated before further processing can occur. The core glycosylation to pr74^{env} is automatic, but the terminal glycosylation to gp78 requires dexamethasone.

In another example, TRH stimulates the secretion of TSH from rat pitui-tary cell cultures (59). TSH is, however, inhibited by T_3 or somatotropin release-inhibiting factor (SRIF). The former represents specific negative feedback inhibition, whereas the latter is a general inhibitor of hormone release. None of these factors affects TSH synthesis or core glycosylation; however, TRH stimulates and T_3 and SRIF inhibit terminal glycosylation. These effects are selective, since terminal glycosylation of other proteins is not affected. Finally, if terminal glycosylation is pharmacologically inhibited by monensin, TRH-induced TSH release is also suppressed; inhibition of core glycosylation by tunicamycin has no effect on TRH-stimulated TSH secre-tion. The conclusions are:

1. TSH is constitutively synthesized and core glycosylated.

2. Factors affecting secretion act at the terminal glycosylation step.

3. Terminal glycosylation immediately leads to secretion.

The coupling between terminal glycosylation and secretion appears to be a general phenomenon; for example, in mouse mammary explants, T_3 stimu-lates the terminal glycosylation and release of α-lactalbumin (60).

The molecular mechanisms underlying these effects are unknown but two obvious ones come to mind. First, hormones could induce the enzymes involved in these modifications. This is probably how glucocorticoids affect the processing of mouse mammary tumor virus peptides, since this effect requires protein synthesis (61). In particular, glucocorticoids have been shown to induce mannosidase II, an enzyme that trims the core (62). Estrogens can also elevate the levels of glycosylating enzymes (63–65): N-acetylgalactosyltransferase, the first step in O-linked glycosylation; oligo-saccharyltransferase, which transfers the core to the protein; mannosylphos-phoryldolichol synthase, which is involved in the synthesis of the core; and sulfotransferases, which cap and protect terminal sugar residues. Second, these enzymes could be more acutely regulated by phosphorylation. For example, the mannosylphosphodolichol synthase is stimulated by phospho-rylation by PKA (66). Finally, these enzymes may be affected by allosteric modulators. For example, calcium is a second messenger and can activate α1,2-mannosidase, another trimming enzyme (67). Furthermore, the subunit that recognizes the N-glycosylation site in proteins is identical to protein disulfide isomerase, a protein that binds T_3 (see Chapter 5). However, the effect of T_3 binding on glycosylation is unknown.

B. Protein Stability

Hormones can also affect protein stability. In the first example given here, phytohormones influence the proper folding of α-amylase. In the second example, hormones affect the proteolytic degradation of milk proteins.

Seeds contain a starchy center surrounded by a cellular layer, the *aleur-*

one layer. During germination, the cells of the aleurone synthesize α-amylase, which breaks the starch down so it can provide energy for early growth. These events are hormonally regulated: abscisic acid maintains dormancy whereas gibberellic acid triggers germination. Gibberellic acid stimulates the influx of calcium, which is required for the proper folding and stabilization of α-amylase (68). Abscisic acid blocks this elevation in calcium; α-amylase is misfolded and rapidly degraded.

In mouse mammary explants, cortisol will progressively stimulate casein accumulation over a concentration range of 10 ng/ml to 1 μg/ml; however, the actual rate of synthesis is no higher at 1 μg/ml than at 10 ng/ml (69). On the other hand, the half-life of the casein is markedly longer at the higher steroid concentration. At the lower hormone concentration, about half of all milk proteins are degraded in 40 hours; however, in the presence of 1 μg of cortisol/ml, only 10% of the casein is degraded, although the destruction of the other proteins remains at around 50%. Glucocorticoids are known to stabilize lysosomes; this action was advanced as a possible mechanism to explain the increased half-life of casein. However, it is not clear why lysosomal stabilization would selectively favor casein.

V. Summary

This and the preceding unit have demonstrated that (i) cellular phenotypes are usually controlled by multiple hormones and (ii) these hormones interact at several levels. Therefore, transcription is only one facet of a continuum. To illustrate these points further, the effects of four hormones on PRL induction of milk proteins will be reviewed; most of the data have been presented separately in previous chapters (Table 14-3).

Table 14-3
Interactions of Insulin, Cortisol, Progesterone, and T_3 on PRL Action in the Murine Mammary Gland

Parameter	Insulin	Cortisol	Progesterone	T_3
PRL receptor	+	+	−	+
Second messengers				
Polyamines		+		
Prostaglandins			−	
mRNA accumulation				
Casein	+	+	−	
α-Lactalbumin	+	+	−	+
Translation	+	+	−	+[a]
Post-translational modification				+
Casein half-life		+		

[a] Data from rabbits only.

At the receptor level, insulin and cortisol are required to maintain normal levels of the PRL receptor; T_3 further elevates these levels and progesterone lowers them. Receptor concentrations are important, since they will determine the sensitivity of the cell to any particular hormone. Progesterone also lowers the insulin receptor number and is capable of binding, but not activating, the cortisol receptor; essentially, progesterone at the elevated levels observed during pregnancy acts as a competitive antagonist. Additional sites of progesterone interference include (i) blocking PRL stimulation of prostaglandin synthesis, (ii) suppressing PRL induction of casein gene transcription, and (iii) inhibiting the translation of milk proteins. Both insulin and cortisol stimulate casein and α-lactalbumin gene transcription; the latter hormone also stabilizes the resulting mRNAs. Insulin, cortisol, and T_3 also induce components of the translational machinery. Cortisol has the additional effects of increasing the half-life of casein and of augmenting the PRL stimulation of polyamine synthesis by increasing both SAM decarboxylase and spermidine synthetase activities. Finally, T_3 selectively stimulates α-lactalbumin terminal glycosylation.

The rationale behind such a complex regulation is not known. In part, it may be related to the necessity of coordinating lactation with parturition, suckling, and maternal metabolism. In any event, the fact remains that one cannot entirely understand or appreciate the actions of a hormone by only examining one of its effects on gene expression in the absence of all other synergistic and antagonistic factors.

References

General References

Beinert, H., and Kennedy, M. C. (1993). Aconitase, a two-faced protein: Enzyme and iron regulatory factor. *FASEB J.* **7**, 1442–1449.
Pantopoulos, K., Weiss, G., and Hentze, M. W. (1994). Nitric oxide and the post-transcriptional control of cellular iron traffic. *Trends Cell Biol.* **4**, 82–86.
Rhoads, R. E. (1993). Regulation of eukaryotic protein synthesis by initiation factors. *J. Biol. Chem.* **268**, 3017–3020.
See also Refs. 7 and 47.

Cited References

1. Guyette, W. A., Matusik, R. J., and Rosen, J. M. (1979). Prolactin-mediated transcriptional and posttranscriptional control of casein gene expression. *Cell* **17**, 1013–1023.
2. Palmiter, R. D., and Carey, N. H. (1974). Rapid inactivation of ovalbumin messenger ribonucleic acid after acute withdrawal of estrogen. *Proc. Natl. Acad. Sci. U.S.A.* **71**, 2357–2361.
3. McKnight, G. S., and Palmiter, R. D. (1979). Transcriptional regulation of the ovalbumin and conalbumin genes by steroid hormones in chick oviduct. *J. Biol. Chem.* **254**, 9050–9058.

4. Brock, M. L., and Shapiro, D. J. (1983). Estrogen stabilizes vitellogenin mRNA against cytoplasmic degradation. *Cell* **34**, 207–214.

5. Back, D. W., Wilson, S. B., Morris, S. M., and Goodridge, A. G. (1986). Hormonal regulation of lipogenic enzymes in chick embryo hepatocytes in culture: Thyroid hormone and glucagon regulate malic enzyme mRNA level at post-transcriptional steps. *J. Biol. Chem.* **261**, 12555–12561.

6. Laverriere, J. N., Morin, A., Tixier-Vidal, A., Truong, A. T., Gourdji, D., and Martial, J. A. (1983). Inverse control of prolactin and growth hormone gene expression: Effect of thyroliberin on transcription and RNA stabilization. *EMBO J.* **2**, 1493–1499.

7. Bernstein, P., and Ross, J. (1989). Poly(A), poly(A) binding protein and the regulation of mRNA stability. *Trends Biochem. Sci.* **14**, 373–377.

8. Adler, G. K., Rosen, L. B., Fiandaca, M. J., and Majzoub, J. A. (1992). Protein kinase-C activation increases the quantity and poly(A) tail length of corticotropin-releasing hormone messenger RNA in HPLC cells. *Mol. Endocrinol.* **6**, 476–484.

9. Krane, I. M., Spindel, E. R., and Chin, W. W. (1991). Thyroid hormone decreases the stability and the poly(A) tract length of rat thyrotropin β-subunit messenger RNA. *Mol. Endocrinol.* **5**, 469–475.

10. Paek, I., and Axel, R. (1987). Glucocorticoids enhance stability of human growth hormone mRNA. *Mol. Cell. Biol.* **7**, 1496–1507.

11. Schröder, H. C., Rottmann, M., Wenger, R., and Müller, W. E. G. (1990). Dramatic increase in poly(A) synthesis after infection of Molt-3 cells with HIV. *Virus Res.* **15**, 251–266.

12. Stetler, D. A., Seidel, B. L., and Jacob, S. T. (1984). Purification and characterization of a nuclear protein kinase from rat liver and a hepatoma that is capable of activating poly(A) polymerase. *J. Biol. Chem.* **259**, 14481–14485.

13. Hentze, M. W. (1991). Determinants and regulation of cytoplasmic mRNA stability in eukaryotic cells. *Biochim. Biophys. Acta* **1090**, 281–292.

14. Port, J. D., Huang, L. Y., and Malbon, C. C. (1992). β-Adrenergic agonists that down-regulate receptor mRNA up-regulate a M_r 35,000 protein(s) that selectively binds to β-adrenergic receptor mRNAs. *J. Biol. Chem.* **267**, 24103–24108.

15. Nachaliel, N., Jain, D., and Hod, Y. (1993). A cAMP-regulated RNA-binding protein that interacts with phosphoenolpyruvate carboxykinase (GTP) mRNA. *J. Biol. Chem.* **268**, 24203–24209.

16. Foulkes, N. S., Schlotter, F., Pévet, P., and Sassone-Corsi, P. (1993). Pituitary hormone FSH directs the CREM functional switch during spermatogenesis. *Nature (London)* **362**, 264–267.

17. Orava, M. M., Isomaa, V. V., and Jänne, O. A. (1980). Early changes in nucleoplasmic poly(A) polymerase activity in immature rabbit uterus after estradiol administration. *Steroids* **36**, 689–696.

18. Pastori, R. L., Moskaitis, J. E., Buzek, S. W., and Schoenberg, D. R. (1991). Coordinate estrogen-regulated instability of serum protein-coding messenger RNAs in *Xenopus laevis*. *Mol. Endocrinol.* **5**, 461–468.

19. van den Berg, J. A., Gruber, M., and Ab, G. (1976). Estradiol-induced enhancement of the processing of the 32S ribosomal precursor in rooster liver. *FEBS Lett.* **63**, 65–60.

20. Munns, T. W., Sims, H. F., and Katzman, P. A. (1975). Effects of estradiol on uterine ribonucleic acid metabolism. Assessment of transfer ribonucleic acid methylation. *Biochemistry* **14**, 4758–4764.

21. Green, M. R., Hatfield, D. L., Miller, M. J., and Peacock, A. C. (1985). Prolactin homogeneously induces the tRNA population of mouse mammary explants. *Biochem. Biophys. Res. Commun.* **129**, 233–239.

22. Fulton, R., Birnie, G. D., and Knowler, J. T. (1985). Post-transcriptional regulation of rat liver gene expression by glucocorticoids. *Nucleic Acids Res.* **13**, 6467–6482.

23. Schumm, D., and Webb, T. E. (1981). Insulin-modulated transport of RNA from isolated liver nuclei. *Arch. Biochem. Biophys.* **210**, 275–279.

24. Schindler, N., and Jiang, L. W. (1987). Epidermal growth factor and insulin stimulate nuclear pore-mediated macromolecular transport in isolated rat liver nuclei. *J. Cell Biol.* **104**, 849–853.

25. Ramani, N., and Rao, C. V. (1987). Direct stimulation of nucleoside triphosphatase activity in bovine luteal nuclear membranes by human chorionic gonadotropin. *Endocrinol. (Baltimore)* **120**, 2468–2473.

26. Thampan, R. V. (1988). Estradiol-stimulated nuclear ribonucleoprotein transport in the rat uterus: A molecular basis. *Biochemistry* **27**, 5019–5026.

27. Goldfine, I. D., Clawson, G. A., Smuckler, E. A., Purrello, F., and Vigneri, R. (1982). Action of insulin at the nuclear envelope. *Mol. Cell. Biochem.* **48**, 3–14.

28. Schafer, P., Aitken, S. J. M., Bachmann, M., Agutter, P. S., Müller, W. E. G., and Prochnow, D. (1993). Immunological evidence for the localization of a 110-kDa poly(A) binding protein from rat liver in nuclear envelopes and its phosphorylation by protein kinase C. *Cell. Mol. Biol.* **39**, 703–714.

29. Csermely, P., Schnaider, T., Cheatham, B., Olson, M. O. J., and Kahn, C. R. (1993). Insulin induces the phosphorylation of nucleolin: A possible mechanism of insulin-induced RNA efflux from nuclei. *J. Biol. Chem.* **268**, 9747–9752.

30. Houdebine, L. M. (1979). Role of prolactin in the expression of casein genes in the virgin rabbit. *Cell Diff.* **8**, 49–59.

31. Vaidya, A. B., Taraschi, N. E., Tancin, S. L., and Long, C. A. (1983). Regulation of endogenous murine mammary tumor virus expression in C57BL mouse lactating mammary glands: Transcription of functional mRNA with a block at the translational level. *J. Virol.* **46**, 818–828.

32. Teyssot, B., and Houdebine, L. M. (1980). Role of prolactin in the transcription of β-casein and 28-S ribosomal genes in the rabbit mammary gland. *Eur. J. Biochem.* **110**, 263–272.

33. Oka, T., and Topper, Y. J. (1971). Hormone-dependent accumulation of rough endoplasmic reticulum in mouse mammary epithelium cells *in vitro*. *J. Biol. Chem.* **246**, 7701–7707.

34. Garel, J. P. (1976). Quantitative adaptation of isoacceptor tRNAs to mRNA codons of alanine, glycine and serine. *Nature (London)* **260**, 805–806.

35. Pickett, M. H., White, B. N., and Davies, P. L. (1983). Evidence that translational control mechanisms operate to optimize antifreeze protein production in the winter flounder. *J. Biol. Chem.* **258**, 14762–14765.

36. Idler, D. R., Fletcher, G. L., Belkhode, S., King, M. J., and Hwang, S. J. (1989). Regulation of antifreeze protein production in winter flounder: A unique function for growth hormone. *Gen. Comp. Endocrinol.* **74**, 327–334.

37. Mouland, A. J., and Hendy, G. N. (1992). 1,25-dihydroxycholecalciferol regulates chromogranin-A translatability in bovine parathyroid cells. *Mol. Endocrinol.* **6**, 1781–1788.

38. Porter, C. W., Berger, F. G., Pegg, A. E., Ganis, B., and Bergerone, R. J. (1987). Regulation of ornithine decarboxylase activity by spermidine and the spermidine analogue N^1N^8-bis(ethyl)spermidine. *Biochem. J.* **242**, 433–440.

39. Kameji, T., and Pegg, A. E. (1987). Inhibition of translation of mRNAs for ornithine decarboxylase and S-adenosylmethionine decarboxylase by polyamines. *J. Biol. Chem.* **262**, 2427–2430.

40. Reinbothe, S., Reinbothe, C., and Parthier, B. (1993). Methyl jasmonate-regulated translation of nuclear-encoded chloroplast proteins in barley (*Hordeum vulgare* L. cv. Salome). *J. Biol. Chem.* **268**, 10606–10611.

41. Kruger, C., and Benecke, B. J. (1981). *In vitro* translation of *Drosophila* heat-shock and non-heat-shock mRNA in heterologous and homologous cell-free systems. *Cell* **23**, 595–603.

42. Hershey, J. W. B. (1991). Translational control in mammalian cells. *Annu. Rev. Biochem.* **60**, 717–755.

43. Safer, B. (1989). Nomenclature of initiation, elongation and termination factors for translation in eukaryotes: Recommendations 1988. *Eur. J. Biochem.* **186**, 1–3.

44. Samuel, C. E. (1993). The eIF-2α protein kinases, regulators of translation in eukaryotes from yeasts to humans. *J. Biol. Chem.* **268**, 7603–7606.

45. Amick, G. D., and Damuni, Z. (1992). Protamine kinase phosphorylates eukaryotic protein synthesis initiation factor 4E. *Biochem. Biophys. Res. Commun.* **183**, 431–437.

46. Manzella, J. M., Rychlik, W., Rhoads, R. E., Hershey, J. W. B., and Blackshear, P. J. (1991). Insulin induction of ornithine decarboxylase: Importance of mRNA secondary structure and phosphorylation of eucaryotic initiation factors eIF-4B and eIF-4E. *J. Biol. Chem.* **266**, 2383–2389.

47. Redpath, N. T., and Proud, C. G. (1994). Molecular mechanisms in the control of translation by hormones and growth factors. *Biochim. Biophys. Acta* **1220**, 147–162.

48. Redpath, N. T., and Proud, C. G. (1993). Cyclic AMP-dependent protein kinase phosphorylates rabbit reticulocyte elongation factor-2 kinase and induces calcium-independent activity. *Biochem. J.* **293**, 31–34.

49. Sitikov, A. S., Simonenko, P. N., Shestakova, E. A., Ryazanov, A. G., and Ovchinnikov, L. P. (1988). cAMP-dependent activation of protein synthesis correlates with dephosphorylation of elongation factor 2. *FEBS Lett.* **228**, 327–331.

50. Park, M. H., Wolff, E. C., and Folk, J. E. (1993). Is hypusine essential for eukaryotic cell proliferation? *Trends Biochem. Sci.* **18**, 475–479.

51. Suzuki, T., Kashiwagi, K., and Igarashi, K. (1993). Polyamine regulation of S-adenosylmethionine decarboxylase synthesis through the 5′-untranslated region of its mRNA. *Biochem. Biophys. Res. Commun.* **192**, 627–634.

52. Verdi, J. M., and Campagnoni, A. T. (1990). Translational regulation by steroids: Identification of a steroid modulatory element in the 5′-untranslated region of the myelin basic protein messenger RNA. *J. Biol. Chem.* **265**, 20314–20320.

53. Drapier, J. C., Hirling, H., Wietzerbin, J., Kaldy, P., and Kühn, L. C. (1993). Biosynthesis of nitric oxide activates iron regulatory factor in macrophages. *EMBO J.* **12**, 3643–3649.

54. Weiss, G., Goossen, B., Doppler, W., Fuchs, D., Pantopoulos, K., Werner-Felmayer, G., Wachter, H., and Hentze, M. W. (1993). Translational regulation via iron-responsive elements by the nitric oxide/NO-synthase pathway. *EMBO J.* **12**, 3651–3657.

55. Eisenstein, R. S., Tuazon, P. T., Schalinske, K. L., Anderson, S. A., and Traugh, J. A. (1993). Iron-responsive element-binding protein: Phosphorylation by protein kinase C. *J. Biol. Chem.* **268**, 27363–27370.

56. Meyuhas, O., Thompson, E. A., and Perry, R. P. (1987). Glucocorticoids selectiv-

ity inhibit translation of ribosomal protein mRNAs in P1798 lymphosarcoma cells. *Mol. Cell. Biol.* **7,** 2691–2699.

57. Bolander, F. F. (1993). The mouse mammary tumor virus as a model for human breast cancer. *Curr. Trends Exp. Endocrinol.* **1,** 1–9.

58. Firestone, G. L., Payvar, F., and Yamamoto, K. R. (1982). Glucocorticoid regulation of protein processing and compartmentalization. *Nature (London)* **300,** 221–225.

59. Ponsin, G., and Mornex, R. (1983). Control of thyrotropin glycosylation in normal rat pituitary cells in culture: Effect of thryotropin-releasing hormone. *Endocrinol. (Baltimore)* **113,** 549–556.

60. Ziska, S. E., Bhattacharjee, M., Herber, R. L., Qasba, P. K., and Vonderhaar, B. K. (1988). Thyroid hormone regulation of α-lactalbumin: Differential glycosylation and messenger ribonucleic acid synthesis in mouse mammary glands. *Endocrinol. (Baltimore)* **123,** 2242–2248.

61. Karlsen, K., Vallerga, A. K., Hone, J., and Firestone, G. L. (1986). A distinct glucocorticoid hormone response regulates phosphoprotein maturation in rat hepatoma cells. *Mol. Cell. Biol.* **6,** 574–585.

62. Snider, L. D., Corey, J. L., Rabindran, S. K., and Stallcup, M. R. (1990). Characterization of oligosaccharide chains on mouse mammary tumor virus envelope proteins and the implications for the mechanism of their glucocorticoid regulated processing. *Mol. Endocrinol.* **4,** 749–757.

63. Carson, D. D., Farrar, J. D., Laidlaw, J., and Wright, D. A. (1990). Selective activation of the N-glycosylation apparatus in uteri by estrogen. *J. Biol. Chem.* **265,** 2947–2955.

64. Chilton, B. S., Kaplan, H. A., and Lennarz, W. J. (1988). Estrogen regulation of the central enzymes involved in O- and N-linked glycoprotein assembly in the developing and the adult rabbit endocervix. *Endocrinol. (Baltimore)* **123,** 1237–1244.

65. Dharmesh, S. M., and Baenziger, J. U. (1993). Estrogen modulates expression of the glycosyltransferases that synthesize sulfated oligosaccharides on lutropin. *Proc. Natl. Acad. Sci. U.S.A.* **90,** 11127–11131.

66. Banerjee, D. K., Kousvelari, E. E., and Baum, B. J. (1987). cAMP-mediated protein phosphorylation of microsomal membranes increases mannosylphosphodolichol synthase activity. *Proc. Natl. Acad. Sci. U.S.A.* **84,** 6389–6393.

67. Schutzbach, J. S., and Forsee, W. T. (1990). Calcium ion activation of rabbit liver α1,2-mannosidase. *J. Biol. Chem.* **265,** 2546–2549.

68. Jones, R. L., Gilroy, S., and Hillmer, S. (1993). The role of calcium in the hormonal regulation of enzyme synthesis and secretion in barley aleurone. *J. Exp. Bot.* **44** *(Suppl.),* 207–212.

69. Nagamatsu, Y., and Oka, T. (1983). The differential actions of cortisol on the synthesis and turnover of α-lactalbumin and casein and on accumulation of their mRNA in mouse mammary gland in organ culture. *Biochem. J.* **212,** 507–515.

PART **5**

Special Topics

CHAPTER **15**

Molecular Evolution of the Endocrine System

CHAPTER OUTLINE

I. Introduction

As the structures of more hormones and receptors are determined, interesting evolutionary relationships begin to emerge. These relationships provide valuable insights into how the endocrine system developed. In this context, it is important to realize that hormones rarely have any inherent biological activity: only two are known to have enzymatic activity and none are transport proteins or structural molecules. Their action is manifested only through their receptors; and if their receptors are membrane bound, the effector responsibility is further transferred to a second messenger. Therefore, a change in a hormone can only be understood in terms of how it alters receptor binding; if there is pressure for a hormone to change, its receptor may also have to change in a complementary manner. In essence, this is an evolution of an entire system and requires the coevolution of many of its components.

Because no humans have been around for the last billion years to record evolution, evolutionary relationships must be inferred. Sequence analysis provides many clues. In addition, species surveys are helpful; by knowing the distribution of a particular component of the endocrine system, one can make reasonable estimates of when it first appeared and from what it may have been derived. However, this method assumes that the evolutionary relationships of the species are known. Such phylogenic trees were originally derived from morphological data; more recently, biochemical and genetic information have augmented the original analyses. It is reassuring that all these data basically support the initial tree (Fig. 15-1). Certainly there are still disputes: Are sponges really animals? Are green alga really plants? However, this text will use the original scheme and comment on alternative interpretations as the material warrants.

II. Hormones

A. Origin

Peptides form the largest and most variable class of hormones (see Chapter 1). Furthermore, since peptide hormones evolve more rapidly than other components of the endocrine system (see subsequent discussion), divergence quickly obliterates evolutionary relationships. A few hormones are related to enzymes. Thrombin and the hepatocyte growth factor are associated with blood clotting: thrombin cleaves fibrinogen to form the clot whereas hepatocyte growth factor (HGF) is an inactive homolog of plasminogen, which digests the clot. Platelet-derived endothelial cell growth factor is homologous to and mimics the activity of thymidine phosphorylase. Other hormones are related to elements of the extracellular matrix; for example, the structural homology between epidermal growth factor (EGF) and some of these matrix components is so notable that they have come to be known as *EGF repeats*.

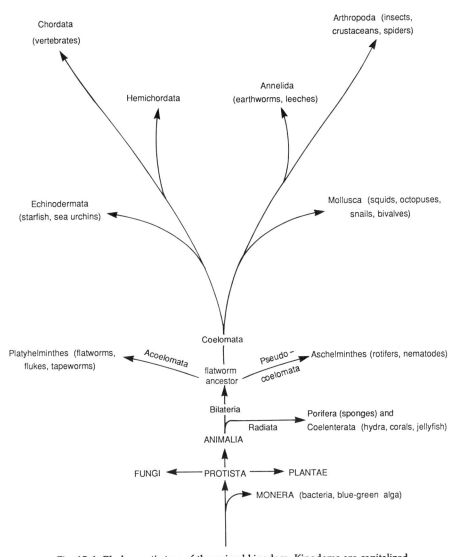

Fig. 15-1. Phylogenetic tree of the animal kingdom. Kingdoms are capitalized.

The origin of nonpeptide hormones is even more difficult to determine since there is no amino acid sequence to trace. The amines probably arose from nutrients; amines are common breakdown products of proteins and are used by animals to locate food. In addition, amine receptors belong to the serpentine family, which is also used for sensory perception including light, smell, and probably taste. Other nonpeptide hormones are components of secondary metabolism that were apparently appropriated as signaling molecules because of some advantageous property.

B. Evolution

1. Caveats

The construction of evolutionary relationships is fraught with dangers, especially when based on species surveys. The sophisticated and highly sensitive assays available today can seemingly detect minute quantities of proteins almost everywhere. For example, such results have been used to support the *unification* theory, which states that all the hormones present throughout the biota have always existed; they were present in the first unicellular organisms and have persisted to the modern era with relatively little change. Furthermore, although the major synthesis of these hormones may be concentrated in certain specialized glands, they are also made in many other tissues. In other words, all hormones are synthesized in all tissues of all organisms.

Such a theory is tenable for steroids, prostaglandins, and amines because they are simple compounds that can be synthesized in only a few steps from common precursors. Unfortunately, for this very reason it is difficult to evaluate the significance of their presence or absence in nonvertebrates. Data from peptide hormones should be more reliable in the determination of evolutionary relationships. However, before accepting these data, the following criteria should be met.

1. The hormone should actually be present in the invertebrate or extraglandular tissue. To satisfy this criterion, the possibility of contamination should be eliminated. There is a report of a steroid radioimmunoassay (RIA) suddenly giving erratic results; the problem was traced to the technician, who had begun to use birth control pills. Presumably, the steroids in the oral contraceptive were being excreted in her perspiration or other bodily fluid and were contaminating the samples. Radioimmunoassays are so sensitive that it does not require much contamination to be detected. In a related example, polycarbonate flasks were found to be the source of an estrogenic compound that was leached from them during autoclaving (1).

A second component of this criterion is that the hormone be present in reasonable amounts. Insulin is reported to be present in *Tetrahymena* at a concentration of 75 pg/g cell (2); the concentration in human pancreas is 45 μg/g tissue and in serum is 1–5 ng/ml. The lower the concentration, the greater the chance that its presence is due to contamination.

Third, incomplete ablation of the gland must be ruled out; if the secretion is being chemically suppressed, residual secretion must be ruled out; if cell lines are being tested, the serum, which contains many hormones, must be removed for a sufficiently long period of time to insure no carryover.

Fourth, the results of the RIA should be validated. Antibodies can recognize as few as two or three amino acids, resulting in the possibility of cross-reactions with unrelated material. The use of multiple antisera directed against different parts of the protein would yield more reassuring results.

Samples should also produce displacements parallel to the standards. Finally, with respect to RIAs, the decreased binding of tracer should be shown to be due to displacement and not to tracer degradation. There was a report of opiate peptides in *Escherichia coli* because extracts "displaced" the tracer. The work was later retracted when it was discovered that the unknown substance was, in fact, a peptidase that was destroying the tracer.

Fifth, short peptides identical to or very similar to vertebrate hormones may actually be found in nonvertebrates or plants, but sequence similarities among very small peptides are difficult to evaluate. When examining such sequences, the arguments for homology (that is, identity due to evolutionary descent) can be strengthened when (i) the sequence is longer, (ii) critical residues are conserved, or (iii) unusual amino acid modifications are preserved. For example, a prothoracicotropic hormone of the silkworm (PTTH-S) has two nonidentical subunits containing 20 and 28 amino acids (3). More important, it has a 35% identity to insulin including an identical distribution of all six cysteines. Finally, computer modeling predicts a three-dimensional structure similar to that for other members of the insulin family (4). The quaternary structure and cysteine placements substantially enhance the hypothesis of overall sequence homology. In another example, leucosulfakinin, a cockroach neuropeptide, is 75% identical to cholecystokinin (CCK), including the presence of a sulfated tyrosine, an unusual amino acid modification that is required for both leucosulfakinin and CCK activity (5). Not all examples are so clear: α-mating factor from yeast has a 60% similarity to gonadotropin-releasing hormone (GnRH), a decapeptide (6). However, one glaring omission is the absence of glycine in position six. This glycine is conserved in all vertebrate GnRHs and structure–function studies suggest that it is involved in a β-II type turn; as such, no other naturally occurring amino acid can substitute for it (7). This amino acid deletion results in the α-mating factor having very little activity in stimulating the release of luteinizing hormone (LH) from pituitary cells; in fact, GnRH is 10,000 times more active. However, the phylogenic distance between yeasts and vertebrates is so great that one cannot eliminate the possibility that the two hormones are related but have different structure–function relationships. A purported human chorionic gonadotropin (hCG) from bacteria demonstrates another problem (8): first, the overall identity is only 25%; more importantly, numerous gaps had to be introduced into the sequence to achieve even this low level of identity. The fewer gaps there are, the more convincing the homology.

2. The hormone should actually be synthesized by the invertebrate or nonglandular tissue. Classically, this condition could be established by exposing the tissue to labeled amino acids and precipitating the putative hormone with specific antibodies. However, hormone synthesis is frequently too low to be detected by this technique. Methods to detect the mRNA are more sensitive, and perhaps too sensitive. The genome appears to be slightly leaky, that is, there is a very low rate of transcription of most genes in virtually all tissues. This phenomenon is called *illegitimate transcription* and yields less than one copy per 500–1000 cells (9,10). Such concentrations are probably not physiologically relevant, but are easily measured by the polymerase chain reaction technique.

Should the presence of the peptide or its mRNA be unequivocally demonstrated, three other considerations must be addressed: (i) the developmental state of the tissue, (ii) whether the tissue is normal, and (iii) the transfer of genetic material across species. First, embryonic and fetal tissues have various degrees of totipotency, that is, they have the ability to differentiate into a large number of structures. When still undifferentiated, these tissues may exhibit characteristics associated with all these adult structures. However, when the tissue becomes committed to a particular lineage, it only retains those characteristics associated with that adult tissue. For example, mRNA for insulin can be detected in the yolk sac and fetal liver which, like the pancreas, are of endodermal origin (11). However, insulin mRNA cannot be detected in the adult liver. In another example, proenkephalin mRNA is widely expressed in the neonatal rat, although its expression in the adult is much more restricted (12). Therefore, evidence for the expression of a hormone in early developmental stages cannot be used as proof that the tissue synthesizes the hormone in the adult. Similarly, tumors and derived cell lines are notorious for the production of ectopic hormones; this is usually a result of random gene activation and, again, cannot be reliably related to normal tissues in adults.

Finally, vertebrate hormones and their mRNA may become secondarily incorporated into invertebrates. Many pathogenic organisms can acquire host proteins; for example, *Mycoplasma* can pick up angiotensin receptors from host cells (13) whereas trypanosomes acquire epidermal growth factor receptors (EGFRs) from their host (14). This phenomenon is acute and transient; however, the transfer of genetic material can permanently alter the genome of either the pathogen or the host. Such *lateral* (or *horizontal*) *gene transfer* has been documented in several species (15,16): the glyceraldehyde 3-phosphate dehydrogenase and glucose 6-phosphate isomerase in *E. coli* originated from eukaryotes. Bacteria are known to acquire nucleic acids from their environment, but how might such an exchange of genetic material occur among eukaryotes? Parasites may provide a mechanism. A mite feeds on *Drosophila* eggs in a manner that allows the mite to retain cellular inclusions, including DNA (17). These inclusions can then be transferred to the next egg, including those of another species.

3. Finally, the hormone should have demonstrable and relevant effects in the nonvertebrates. This requirement would include the presence of an appropriate receptor as well as an appropriate biological effect. For example, many pathogens have evolved a sensitivity to the hormones of higher animals to adapt more effectively to their hosts: the fungi responsible for vaginal infections often possess "receptors" for steroids and react to their presence, but such receptors have no homology at all to their mammalian counterparts (18). In another example, analogs of ecdysone and juvenile hormone are

made by plants as a defense against insect predation and not for any internal use as hormones. The same can be said for prostaglandins in corals. In contrast, *Drosophila* has both an insulin-like hormone, PTTH-S, and an insulin-like receptor that possesses tyrosine kinase activity (19). The structure, activity, immunogenicity, and insulin sensitivity of this receptor resemble those of the vertebrate insulin receptor (20,21). Furthermore, PTTH has important defined functions in insects (3).

There is one final consideration when evaluating the physiological relevance of the presence of a hormone in nonglandular tissues: Is the hormone a remnant from the processing of polyproteins? Adrenocorticotropic hormone (ACTH) is frequently reported to be synthesized in nonpituitary tissues (22), but it is part of the polyprotein proopiomelanocortin (POMC), which also contains the endorphins (see Chapter 3). The latter are parahormones, which have a wide distribution. Is the occurrence of ACTH secondary to the processing of POMC for the endorphins? Is this ACTH ever secreted or is it simply degraded? For example, the ACTH from lymphocytes is synthesized in very small quantities and cannot be detected in the culture medium (23).

2. Peptide Hormones

Having discussed the caveats in identifying extraglandular or nonvertebrate hormones, the distribution of insulin and glucagon will be examined. Insulin is clearly present throughout the coelomates; in addition to the insect homolog (PTTH-S), a molluscan homolog has been isolated and sequenced. The conserved cysteines, predicted three-dimensional structure, and cleavage to remove the C-peptide all attest to this molecule being an insulin homolog (24–26). A homolog has also been reported for sponges (27). This peptide has an unexpectedly high identity to human insulin: 85% in the A and B peptides, compared with 35–40% between humans and insects or mollusks, who are evolutionarily much closer to humans. This homolog lacks an intrachain disulfide bridge in the A peptide and a basic residue at the A–C junction; as a result, it can only be cleaved at the B–C site. It is present in certain cells of the sponge at concentrations approximately 50% of those in the pancreas. Initially, insulin-like activity was reported in *Neurospora crassa*; in addition to biological, physiochemical, and immunological similarities, low capacity insulin receptors were also detected; vertebrate insulin affects both glucose oxidation and glycogen metabolism in this fungus (28,29). However, no real gene for insulin could be cloned, and a purported pseudogene has such a low identity that its relationship to insulin is questionable (30). Finally, although the insulin receptor has not yet been sequenced, it has been sufficiently purified to determine that it is significantly smaller than the vertebrate receptor and lacks any kinase activity (31). In summary, insulin occurs throughout the coelomates but there is still no evidence for its presence outside the animal kingdom. A lack of studies prevents a determination of where in this kingdom insulin first appeared.

The study of the evolution of glucagon represents a different approach. Glucagon is one of several members of a peptide hormone family; by analyzing the sequence differences and estimating rates of evolution, one can calculate how long ago various members diverged. For example, this technique estimates that an ancestral glucagon gene arose 0.8–1 bya (billion years ago), when the earliest invertebrates were evolving, and that a discrete glucagon gene appeared about 430 mya, along with the earliest vertebrates (32).

3. Nonpeptide Hormones

The evolution of steroids is less an evolution of hormones than it is an evolution of steroidogenic enzymes. Although steroids are nearly ubiquitous, their use as hormones is more sporadic. The simplest organism to use these compounds is a water mold whose pheromones, antheridiol and oogoniol, are steroids (33). In addition, plants synthesize brassinosteroids, which they use as hormones (see Chapter 3). However, the systematic use of steroids as messenger molecules only occurs in the animal kingdom; even here, hormonal steroids have only been documented in the phyla Arthropoda and Chordata (Fig. 15-2). The enzymatic machinery to synthesize the sex steroids (progesterone, estradiol, and testosterone) is present in the phyla Mollusca and Echinodermata, and estrogens stimulate egg-laying in gastropods and both vitellogenesis and ovarian development in shrimp (34,35). The additional enzymes required to make glucocorticoids appear in the elasmobranchs (sharks and rays); the glucocorticoids are also used as hormones in this class. Aldosterone first appears in the bony fishes. Since the enzyme synthesizing glucocorticoids and mineralocorticoids is the same, this development suggests that the P450c11 enzyme either modified its catalytic site or added a second active site to acquire the 18-ol-dehydrogenase activity (see Chapter 2).

The eicosanoids constitute another group of nonpeptide molecules that are relatively easy to synthesize, and therefore enjoy a wide distribution in nature. However, like steroids, their use as hormones is more restricted. Prostaglandins (PGs) are present in vertebrates, in which they act both as parahormones and as amplification systems. Their distribution in invertebrates is spotty and their concentrations are low. Although they can elicit various effects in insects (36), there is no evidence that they act as parahormones or transducers in any invertebrate. They are synthesized in corals in concentrations so high that corals were once a commercial source for these compounds. However, the PGs in corals were probably developed as a defense mechanism akin to the ecdysone analogs in plants.

The hydroxyeicosatetraenoic acids, another group of eicosanoids (see Chapter 3), are present throughout the coelomates. In the echinoderms, they function in the transduction pathway for 1-methyladenine, a hormone in starfish (37); they are also synthesized in sea urchins (38). In *Aplysia*, a mollusk, PMRFamide is a neuroactive peptide that inhibits electrical activity (39). Its activity is blocked by an inhibitor of the lipoxygenase pathway but not by an inhibitor of the cyclooxygenase pathway. Finally, FMRFamide stimulates the production of one of the hydroxyeicosatetraenoic acids, and

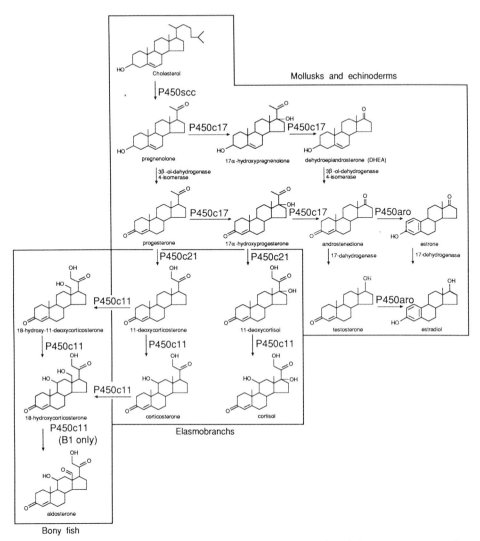

Fig. 15-2. Steroid hormone biosynthetic pathway showing the phylogenic emergence of the different groups of enzymes.

the effect of this peptide on electrical activity can be mimicked by that acid. In crustaceans, the barnacle-hatching substance has been structurally determined to be an eicosatetraenoic acid derivative (41). There is also a report of 11-HETE in an acoelomate, *Hydra*, where it enhances tentacle regeneration (40). Therefore, it appears that the use of eicosanoids in the endocrine system came rather late in evolution: the lipoxygenase pathway developed first and occurs throughout the coelomates, whereas the PG pathway is restricted to vertebrates.

Although the plants do not have eicosanoids, they do have a parallel pathway. Higher plants lack arachidonic acid, but do possess analogous enzymes that act on linolenic acid to produce traumatic and jasmonic acid (Fig. 3-15). Essentially, jasmonic acid is a short-chain version of (PGB) and traumatic acid of leukotriene B_2. Interestingly, these compounds are used for much the same purpose in these widely different kingdoms: both the animal and the plant derivatives are elevated in response to injury or infection and, in turn, induce defense responses (42). This is probably an example of convergent evolution and implies that there is some advantage to using this structure to mediate inflammatory responses.

III. Receptors

A. Origin

1. Nuclear Receptors

There are two major hypotheses concerning the origin of nuclear receptors. The first suggests that the receptors originated as steroid-metabolizing enzymes that acquired DNA-binding domains (DBDs) and transcriptional activation domains (TADs). There is precedent for an allosteric site developing from a catalytic one: the cyclic nucleotide allosteric site in the phosphodiesterase is believed to have evolved from a duplication of the active site of the enzyme (43). In addition, there is a common sequence between the steroid receptors and the steroid-metabolizing enzymes (44); however, subsequent functional studies have shown that these sequences are not involved in ligand binding (45).

Alternatively, nuclear receptors may have originated from pre-existing transcription factors that developed allosteric steroid-binding sites. Such factors were initially regulated by some other mechanism, and there is evidence that some of them may still be operative. For example, the progesterone receptor (PgR), the retinoic acid receptor (RAR), and the vitamin D receptor (VDR) can be activated by protein kinase A (PKA) in the absence of ligand and both the glucocorticoid receptor (GR) and the PgR can be translocated to the nucleus in response to heat or chemical stress (see Chapter 5). The first allosteric site may have been designed for hydrophobic metabolites, such as those that bind the peroxisome proliferator-activated receptor (PPAR); in coelomates, these metabolites were replaced by lipophilic hormones. The heat shock proteins came later; hsp 90 is associated only with the estrogen receptor (ER) and GR family (vertebrates) and hsp 59 only exists in mammals.

2. Membrane Receptors

One of the first hypotheses on the origin of membrane receptors was based on the fact that anticodons generally designate amino acids that are structurally complementary to the one specified by the codons. Therefore, peptides synthesized off opposite strands should bind one another; more specifically, the antisense strand to a peptide hormone gene could encode the receptor for that hormone. This became known as the *sense–antisense complementarity theory* or the *molecular recognition theory* (46). However, peptides synthesized from the predicted sequence of the antisense strand only show limited specificity and low binding toward the complementary hormones. Finally, as more and more receptors are actually cloned, it has become clear that there is no homology between receptor sequences and those from the antisense strand (47–50).

Another possible origin for membrane receptors is from the group of adhesion molecules that mediates cell–cell and cell–substratum interactions. Even most unicellular organisms attach to their substratum; these binding proteins could be recruited to bind soluble ligands. For example, the cytokine receptors are composed of modified fibronectin III domains (see Chapter 6), which are also involved in cell–substratum interactions; some receptors still need matrix cofactors, such as betaglycan (TGFβ-R) and heparin (FGFR). In addition, several hormones are synthesized as membrane precursors and are active without cleavage: they include EGF, transforming growth factor α (TGFα), colony-stimulating factor-1 (CSF-1), tumor necrosis factor α (TNFα), stem cell growth factor (SCF), and the heregulin receptor-2 (HER-2) ligand. Such proteins may have initially mediated cell–cell interactions via binding proteins on adjacent cells; later, the membrane-bound hormone may have been cleaved to extend the range of its activity.

Finally, some of the receptors for amines may have arisen from primitive food or sensory receptors (51,52). Many organisms today have amine exoceptors to locate food, since amines are a common breakdown product of protein. In addition, both the amine receptors and most of the known sensory receptors belong to the same family of serpentine receptors. Other receptors may have evolved from transport proteins for these amines: both the metabotropic and ion channel receptors for glutamate have extracellular domains homologous to the periplasmic binding protein of bacteria (53). This latter protein binds amino acids in the periplasmic space and presents them to the amino acid transporter.

B. Diversification

The simplest way for a receptor gene to diversify is by duplication. Evidence for this mechanism comes from the many examples of homologous hormone receptors occurring either in tandem or clustered on a restricted region of a chromosome: platelet-derived growth factor receptor (PDGFR), CSF-1R, and Kit on chromosome 5q (54); prolactin receptor (PRLR) and growth hormone receptor (GHR) on 5p (55); and several of the serpentine receptors on 5q (56). A more controversial mechanism is *reverse transcription*, by which a processed or partially processed mRNA from one gene is somehow transcribed into DNA and reintegrated into the genome to form a second gene called a *retroposon.* Such genes can often be recognized by a deficiency of introns, a poly(A) tail, and a chromosomal location widely separated form the original gene; highly homologous genes arising from gene duplication should be located very close to each other. Most retroposons are nonfunctional because they lack a promoter. However, expression from a retroposon could occur if the original mRNA had an aberrant start site that was upstream from the promoter or if it had been inserted near another promoter.

There are two proposed examples of reverse transcription in endocrinology: the murine insulins and the serpentine receptors. Unlike all other mammals, rats and mice have two insulin genes; they are both expressed and are highly homologous (57). However, insulin gene I lacks one of the two introns in gene II, has a poly(A) tail, and is located either on a separate chromosome from that containing gene II (mice) or on the same chromosome but more than 9 kb from gene II (rats). The conclusion is that gene I is a functional retroposon of gene II. Similarly, the genes for both the α_2AR (58) and the muscarinic receptors (MRs) (59) lack introns and have other characteristics compatible with their being retroposons.

A third mechanism is *exon shuffling*. Eukaryotic genes are split into short coding regions, called exons, widely separated by long introns. It is thought that each exon encodes a functional unit (60,61). For example, in the insulin receptor gene, the ligand-binding domain, the tyrosine kinase, and the transmembrane region are all encoded on separate groups of exons (62). Since these exons are usually separated by very long introns, it is easy to imagine how they may undergo aberrant recombination resulting in a particular exon, with its intrinsic activity, being transferred to the gene of another protein. This process is called exon shuffling and allows a protein to accrue many functions by accumulating selected exons.

As noted earlier, most of the serpentine receptors lack introns; however, the glycoprotein hormone and the metabotropic glutamate receptors (mGluRs) are exceptions. The transmembrane helices and the carboxy terminus are still encoded on a single exon; only the new, unusually long amino terminus is encoded by several exons. It appears as if a serpentine receptor core acquired a new ligand-binding domain from an unknown source (63). In the case of the mGluR, the source may have been the amino terminus of the kainate-type glutamate receptor since the two amino termini are homologous (64-66). As noted already, this homology is also seen in the bacterial permeases, proteins involved in transport. As such, these exons may represent a primitive amino-acid-binding domain. The cytokine receptors and receptor tyrosine kinases (RTKs) represent another potential example of exon shuffling. In this case, the shuffling resulted in the incorporation of immunoglobulin-like loops into the extracellular domain (Fig. 15-3; 67).

A final mechanism of diversification is *branch jumping*, which is best illustrated by the GH–PRL family. This family has two major branches, GH and PRL, which arose by gene duplication in the earliest vertebrates. The receptors appear to have duplicated at about the same time. With one exception, there is no cross-binding of either GH or PRL to the receptor of the

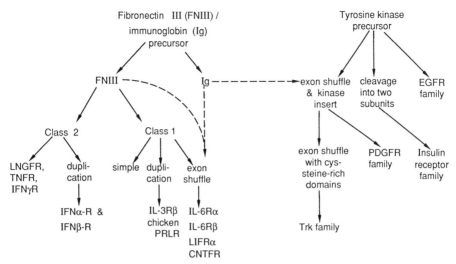

Fig. 15-3. Hypothetical evolutionary scheme for the fibronectin-like receptors. Solid lines indicate direct lineage, whereas dashed lines represent exon shuffling.

other; this is surprising since the receptor binding sites on both hormones overlap (68–70). The exception is the primate GH, which binds and activates the PRLR as well as the GHR. Because the binding sites overlap, a common core of residues must have been conserved in both GHs and PRLs, necessitating the change of only a few amino acids for GH to reacquire PRL-binding activity (71). At this point, primate GH is straddling the branches. Recently, primate GH has duplicated to form a new hormone expressed in the placenta; this placental lactogen is 85% identical to GH but has absolutely no GH activity. Additional mutations made the placental lactogen incapable of binding the GH receptor, although binding to the PRL receptor is unaffected. The placental lactogen has now completely switched over to another receptor.

The serpentine receptors may represent another example of branch jumping (Fig. 15-4; 72). There are many ways to construct a phylogenic tree for these receptors (73,74) and most of them will show the βARs and MRs clustered together. However, other isoforms are inexplicably split; for example, the α-agonists, dopamine, and serotonin can bind to receptor isoforms scattered among several distinctly separate subfamilies. Since all these hormones are amines and make similar contacts with the receptor (see Fig. 6-4), a slight change in the ligand-binding pocket of one receptor may favor the binding of an amine that normally binds to a totally different receptor subfamily.

It is interesting to speculate on the possibility of branch jumping also occurring between receptors and second messengers. For example, a mutation in the sequence around a phosphotyrosine in RTKs may alter the SH2-containing proteins that are attracted to and activated by the receptor,

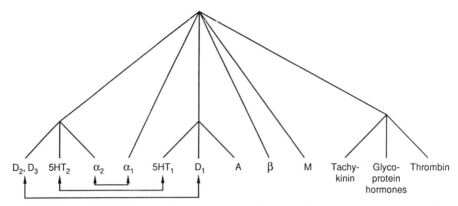

Fig. 15-4. Hypothetical evolutionary scheme for the serpentine receptors. Arrows indicate receptors from different subfamilies that bind the same ligand, suggesting branch jumping. A, Adenosine receptors; α, α-adrenergic receptors; β, β-adrenergic receptors; D, dopamine receptors; 5HT, 5-hydroxytryptamine (serotonin) receptors; M, muscarinic receptors.

thereby changing the system output. A mutation in the intracellular regions of serpentine receptors may change the G protein to which it is coupled. Branch jumping, at whatever level, allows a hormone to acquire new functions and/or tissue distributions.

C. Evolution

The construction of an evolutionary scheme for receptors is influenced by the methodology used. For example, biochemical and genetic techniques have been unable to identify any serpentine receptors before the coelomates (75). However, pharmacologists can detect responses to the ligands for these receptors as far back as the flatworms and coelenterates (76). Finally, based on sequence divergence, it has been calculated that the βARs and MRs separated 0.6–1 bya at the time of the earliest invertebrates and that the βARs and rhodopsin split 1–1.5 bya when only the protists and bacteria existed (77). The mathematical analysis predicts that serpentine receptors were present in unicellular organisms, whereas the structural data fail to find any such receptors outside the coelomates. It is possible that the earliest serpentine receptors have changed so much over the eons that they are no longer recognizable. For example, the yeast pheromone receptors have seven transmembrane helices and couple to G proteins but have absolutely no sequence homology to the serpentine receptors (78–80). Even bacteria have membrane proteins with similar topology but no homology, including bacteriorhodopsin.

1. Nuclear Receptors

The phylogeny of the nuclear receptors is not as confused because of their relatively recent emergence; they are present throughout the coelomates, since nuclear receptors have been cloned from *Drosophila* and echino-derms (79,80). A nuclear receptor has also been purported to be cloned from a nematode, although no data were given (81). Because every family of nuclear receptor is present in both vertebrates and *Drosophila*, it is reasonable to conclude that these molecules must have existed and split before the coelomates arose. Although steroid-like hormones are found in water molds and plants (see preceding discussion), receptors for these agents have not yet been characterized. Yeast do not have nuclear receptors for many of the mammalian hormones including estradiol, glucocorticoids, triiodothyronine, 1,25-DHCC, and retinoids.

Based on the analysis of the DNA-binding domain (DBD) and the lig-and-binding domain (LBD), the nuclear receptors appear to have a common ancestor that gave rise to three major branches (Fig. 15-5; (82). As expected from their biological characteristics (see Chapter 5), the GR and the thyroid receptor (TR) families constitute two of these branches. The third branch is represented by the retinoic acid X receptor (RXR) and the chicken ovalbumin upstream promoter (COUP), whereas the ER is shown as separating early from the GR family. Biologically, ER and COUP have similar properties and were grouped together (Table 5-1).

It is interesting that the evolution of the hormone response elements (HREs) generally parallels that of the nuclear receptors. The original HRE is believed to have been TGACC(T), which occurred singly or in tandem repeats (83); this sequence corresponds to the TR response element. The introduction of variable spacing created the VDRE and RARE. In an alterna-

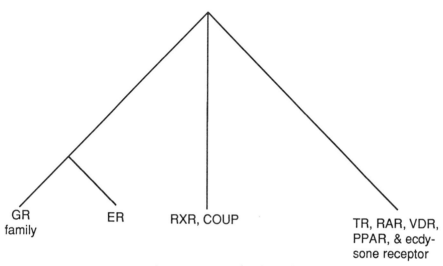

Fig. 15-5. Hypothetical evolutionary scheme for the nuclear receptors. COUP, Chicken upstream promoter (binding protein); ER, estradiol receptor; GR, glucocorticoid receptor; PPAR, peroxisome proliferator receptor; RAR, retinoic acid receptor; RXR, retinoic acid X receptor; VDR, vitamin D receptor.

tive pathway, the original HRE was inverted and a single base pair spacer was inserted; this sequence became the ecdysone response element. Increasing the spacer to 3 bp generated the ERE. Finally, mutation of the HRE to TGTTCT created the GRE. As the nuclear receptors became more complex, they may also have become more unstable so the most recent ones, ER and the GR family, required protein chaperones. At this point, the heat shock proteins were incorporated into the nonactivated complexes.

2. Membrane Receptors

The evolution of the cytokine receptors represents an excellent example of the evolution of proteins, since it includes complete gene duplication, duplication with fusion, and exon shuffling (Fig. 15-3; 66). The fibronectin type III domain and the immunoglobulin loop both contain a β structure adapted for binding and are thought to have arisen from a common ancestor. In immunoglobulins, the seven β strands form two sheets between which antigens bind. In the class 1 cytokine receptors, this unit was duplicated and altered to create two small disulfide loops at the amino terminus and a WS box at the carboxy terminus: this became known as the cytokine motif (see Chapter 6). The hormone is bound to loops at the end of the β strands. Further duplication occurred in the interleukin-3 receptor β (IL-3Rβ) and the chicken PRLR (84).

In class 2 receptors, the FNIII unit was also duplicated and some degeneracy appears to have occurred, since only five strands are discernible in each of the four domains. Another difference is the arrangement of these domains: in the class 1 receptors, the β structures abut each other at right angles to form a niche for hormone binding (see Fig. 6-5). In class 2 receptors, the domains line up end-to-end to form long fingers that wrap around the hormone. Interestingly, the major contact points remain at the terminal loops. This structure is found in the TNFR, the interferon-γ receptor (IFNγ-R), and the low-affinity NGF receptor (LNGFR). The receptors for IFNα and IFNβ underwent a further duplication of the extracellular domain only.

In other cytokine receptors, immunoglobulin loops and/or additional unmodified FNIII domains were picked up, presumably by exon shuffling (see Fig. 6-6). Exon shuffling probably also accounts for the introduction of immunoglobulin loops in the PDGF and Trk families. In addition, the Trk receptors appear to have acquired other cysteine-rich domains, some of which resemble the kringle domain of blood clotting factors (Fig. 15-3).

IV. Transducers

A. Cyclic Nucleotides and G Proteins

The small G proteins involved in translation and organelle trafficking are ubiquitous; this is no surprise considering the vital nature of these processes. However, this may not be true of the signal-transducing Ras. Ras is present throughout the animals, fungi, and protists (85). Indeed, the Grb2 adaptor system used by the RTKs to activate Ras not only is present in mammals, *Drosophila*, and the nematode *Caenorhabditis elegans*, but the components are interchangeable (86,87). Ras has not yet been reported in plants; antibodies against this protein are unable to detect anything in the alga *Dunaliella* (88). Although a sequence for a purported Ras protein in bacteria has been published, its low identity to other Ras proteins (19%) makes its designation as Ras difficult (89).

The trimeric G proteins are also widely distributed; sequences from mollusks (90), *C. elegans* (91), fungi (92), plants (93), and a protist (94) have been reported. Although identities vary between 35 and 45%, functional interactions are highly conserved; for example, the mammalian α subunit can bind the yeast $\beta\gamma$ dimer (95), and the *Drosophila* α subunit can replace the mammalian α subunit in stimulating adenylate cyclase (96). In addition, the mammalian βAR can activate insect adenylate cyclase via the insect G protein (97). However, the role of plant G proteins in signal transduction is still uncertain (98); the α subunits cloned to date more closely resemble the Rab family (see Chapter 8) than the mammalian α subunits, and a functional link between plant hormones and any of these putative α subunits has not yet been proven.

One of the targets of the trimeric G proteins is the adenylate cyclase. This enzyme resembles the voltage-gated ion channels in its topology; in fact, in *Paramecium* it functions as a potassium channel, from which it may have been derived (99–101). The active site in the enzymes from animals, fungi, and protists are all homologous; bacteria also have an adenylate cyclase, but this protein appears to have had a separate origin (102). The catalytic site of the guanylate cyclase is also homologous to that of the adenylate cyclase, although it has only one transmembrane helix; this may have arisen by exon shuffling, wherein the catalytic domain was transferred to another membrane protein. The soluble guanylate cyclase has only been found in vertebrates and insects (103), and may be the result of another exon shuffling event.

The presence of a cAMP pathway in plants is still controversial. The system is clearly present and operational in green alga (104–106), but some authorities place these organisms within the kingdom Protista. The concentrations of cAMP in higher plants are very low, in the picomolar range (107,108), although in the lily they do fluctuate during meiosis and can inhibit this process with an IC_{50} of 3.5 pM (109). Several PKA-like clones have also been isolated from plants, but their regulation and activity have not yet been investigated (110). Finally, a transcription factor with a 48% identity to cAMP response element binding protein (CREB) in the DBD and zipper region has been found; but again its regulation has not been examined (111).

In contrast to plants, PKA has been unequivocally demonstrated in protists, fungi, and animals. In protists, the regulatory (R) and catalytic (C) components are part of the same protein (112); in these organisms the kinase is still a monomer (113). After PKG split off, R and C became separated into individual genes. By the time the fungi appeared, an amino-terminal extension had been added to allow for R dimerization.

B. Calcium and Phospholipids

1. Calcium and the Polyphosphoinositide Pathway

The classic polyphosphoinositide (PPI) pathway exists in animals, fungi, and protists. In animals, it can be traced as far down as the sponges, where an aggregation factor stimulates phosphoinositide (PI) turnover, inositol 1,4,5-trisphosphate (IP$_3$) release, and cytosolic calcium elevation (114). In addition, the effects of this factor are mimicked by a calcium ionophore. In *Dictyostelium*, IP$_3$ is used as the second messenger of extracellular cAMP, an ectohormone in this species (115). Its production is coupled to a PI-specific phospholipase C (PLC) whose sequence resembles that of mammalian PLCδ (116).

However, the existence of this pathway in plants is controversial. There is no question that calcium is an important cellular regulator in plants (117–119), but it is not clear whether IP$_3$ is responsible for elevating levels of this cation. The difficulty in obtaining an answer lies in the problems associated with plants. First, inositol is more widely used in plants, making precursor–product relationships more difficult to determine. Second, the phosphoinositides are labeled more rapidly than other lipids, leading to possible artifacts (120). Third, plant responses are slow so cause-and-effect relationships are not as apparent. Finally, PPI levels are far below those seen in mammalian systems, usually accounting for only 0.5% of PI (121).

Major evidence for a PPI pathway in plants is provided by the numerous reports of the ability of IP$_3$ to release calcium from tonoplasts (122,123). However, there are also data that question the physiological importance of this release: (i) the levels of phosphoinositol bisphosphate (PIP$_2$) are low in plants, (ii) the concentrations of IP$_3$ required to release the calcium are 10 times those effective in animals, (iii) calcium release is less efficient than in animals, (iv) the release is not observed in all plant systems, and (v) the release can be mimicked by phytic acid, suggesting that the IP$_3$ effect is a nonspecific one secondary to its negative charge (124). In addition, no PI-specific PLC has been purified and sequenced from plants. Although PLC activities have been reported, few are specific for PIP$_2$ or regulated by G proteins (125–128). The only exception is the green alga, in which the concentrations of PIP$_2$ are comparable to those in animals and in which a PLC activity with mammalian characteristics has been detected (129–131). However, as noted earlier, the placement of these organisms is uncertain; they have been classified as either plants or protists.

If calcium is important in plants, how is it regulated? Most plant hormones elevate calcium by increasing influxes. Abscisic acid (ABA) closes stomata by stimulating calcium influx (132) and the gibberellic acid (GA) elevation of calcium in barley aleurone protoplasts requires extracellular calcium (133). However, the most direct evidence comes from studies using calcium-binding fluorescent dyes in carrot protoplasts, in which the increased calcium levels induced by elicitors comes from the medium (134).

2. Protein Kinases

PKC has been cloned from species throughout the animal kingdom (135–138) as well as from yeast (139). PKC activity has been reported in plants, but these phospholipid-stimulated kinases were eventually shown to be a form of the calmodulin (CaM)-dependent kinases (see subsequent discussion). Identification of PKC by immunological techniques is also risky considering the close homology among kinase catalytic sites. Finally, this homology complicates the interpretation of kinase clones, whose products have not yet been evaluated with respect to regulation.

On the other hand, CaM and the CaM-dependent kinases are ubiquitous. CaM has been highly conserved: mammalian and *Drosophila* CaM are 99% identical and mammalian and plant CaM are 92% identical (140). The presence of CaM in prokaryotes is more controversial (141). A peptide with the physiochemical, immunological, and biological activity of CaM has been identified in prokaryotes, but only one sequence has been reported. The peptide from *Saccharopolyspora* is homologous to CaM only in the four calcium-binding sites (142).

CaMKII-like clones have been isolated from fungi (143,144) and plants (145–148). There are two forms in plants: one is the equivalent of the animal CaMKII; the other form incorporates a CaM domain in its carboxy terminus. Although this kinase is calcium dependent, it is not technically CaM dependent since it possesses its own CaM. This latter form is also stimulated by phospholipids and was initially mistaken for the plant PKC.

C. Miscellaneous Protein Kinases

Casein kinase II (CKII) is also ubiquitous and highly conserved. Most kinases from mammals and yeasts or plants have between 40 and 50% identity in the catalytic domains; however, for CKII the residues are 75–80% identical (149–153). In fungi and peas, the kinase is a tetramer and is stimulated by polyamines (154–157); however, the β subunit is not required for kinase activity in plants (158,159) as it is in animals and fungi (160). Polyamines themselves are present in all life forms. In plants, polyamines are important in growth, the stabilization of cell membranes, and the retardation of senescence (161). They appear to operate as hormone mediators for some of the actions of indoleacetic acid, the cytokinins, and the gibberellins. Unfortunately, there are not sufficient data from any single system to satisfy all the requirements for designating a second messenger; however, data from several different studies indicate that these hormones do elevate polyamine levels and ornithine decarboylase (ODC) activity. Furthermore, their effects are inhibited by methylglyoxal *bis* (guanylhydrazone) (MGBG); this inhibition is relieved by spermidine. Finally, polyamines alone can at least cause growth. In plants, polyamines are also negatively controlled. Both ABA and ethylene promote senescence, and tend to have effects on polyamine metabolism that are opposite to those just described.

The proline-directed kinases are also widely distributed. MAPK and its activation cascade have been documented in yeast and plants (162,163). Indeed, the plant MAPKK can phosphorylate and activate *Xenopus* MAPK. In addition, mammalian Raf can phosphorylate yeast MAPKK and bind yeast Ras (164,165). Glycogen synthase kinase (GSK) and cell division cycle dependent kinase 2 (Cdc2) are other proline-directed kinases present in plants and fungi (166,167).

The tyrosine kinases are more controversial. Both membrane-bound and soluble tyrosine kinases exist throughout the animal kingdom. Src has also been detected in the slime mold, a protist (168) but not in plants (169). However, plants do possess kinases that have a dual specificity (169). Nonetheless, serine–threonine–tyrosine kinases do not form a discrete evolutionary group but are scattered throughout the kinase family; this distribution suggests that the acquisition of tyrosine kinase activity by a serine–threonine kinase is a chance occurrence and cannot be used to predict the presence of more typical tyrosine kinases.

D. Protein Phosphatases

The serine–threonine protein phosphatases are nearly ubiquitous. PP-1, PP-2A, and PP-2C have been identified in plants (170,171). PP-1, PP-2A, and PP-2B are also present in fungi and protists, and the *Neurospora* PP-2B can form functional heterodimers with the mammalian enzyme (172). The fungal phosphatases are between 50 and 86% identical to their mammalian counterparts (172–175). Tyrosine protein phosphatases (PTP) are similarly widespread in animals, fungi (176,177), and protists (178). However, no PTP sequences have been reported from plants, although PTP activity has been detected in the potato tuber (179).

E. Summary

The distribution of transducers across the biota tends to conform to one of two patterns (Fig. 15-6). CaM, CaMKII, CKII, MAPK, the serine–threonine phosphatases, and the trimeric G proteins are present in all eukaryotes. On the other hand, the cyclic nucleotide and PPI pathways, at least in their classical forms, are absent from plants, and neither Ras, specific tyrosine kinases, nor PTPs have been unequivocally demonstrated in this kingdom. Several other conclusions can be drawn regarding the phylogenic relationship of various groups. First, the transduction apparatus in sponges is very similar to that in animals, that is, the endocrinological data support the original placement of sponges in this kingdom. Second, the green algae much more closely resemble the protists than the plants. If one assumes that the Chlorophyta belong in the plant kingdom, then the more advanced plants had to have lost or severely modified a number of their second messenger

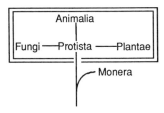

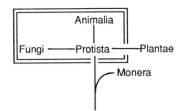

Trimeric G proteins
Calmodulin
CaM-dependent kinase II
Casein kinase II
MAP kinase
Serine-threonine phosphatases

Ras
cAMP and cGMP pathways
Classical PPI pathway
PKC
Tyrosine kinases and phosphatases

Fig. 15-6. Distribution of components of transduction pathways in the biological kingdoms. The transducers present in the boxed kingdoms are listed below each figure.

systems. If the green algae are protists, then the plants could simply have diverged before the development of these transducers. Finally, the remarkable similarity between the animal and fungal kingdoms would tend to support the view that these groups had a monophyletic origin (180,181).

By examining the degree of conservation among these various systems, one can also speculate on how the system was originally established and then coevolved (182). Table 15-1 gives the percentage identity among various components of the endocrine systems in *Drosophila* and mammals. The peptide hormones are the least conserved at 30–35%; membrane receptors are more conserved at 50–60%; and transducers are highly conserved at 70–99%. The following scheme is speculative but compatible with these data: second messengers began as intracellular regulators and are, therefore, as old as cells. As organisms became multicellular, hormones were developed

Table 15-1

Percentage Identity between the Components of the Endocrine Systems of *Drosophila* and Mammals

Hormones	Receptors[a]	Transducers[a]	Transcription factors[b]
35 (Insulin)	53 (IR)	99 (CaM)	48 (CREB)
33 (EGF/Notch)[c]	55 (EGFR)	71 (G_α)	47 (NF-κB)
	60 (MR)	82 (PKA)	
	50 (GABA$_A$R)	88 (PKG)	
		85 (CaMKII)	
		86 (CKII)	
		90 (PP-1)	
		94 (PP-2B)	

[a] For kinases, only the catalytic domains were compared.
[b] Only the DNA-binding and dimerization domains were compared.
[c] Only the EGF-like repeats were compared.

to coordinate cells and tissues; the easiest mechanism by which hormones could act was for the hormone to hook up to the pre-existing machinery. Receptors were developed at the same time as an interface between the two components. Once established, receptors evolved more slowly than peptide hormones because of greater constraints on the former. Hormones only must bind to their receptors; receptors, however, must bind their ligands, must interact with one or more transducers, may have to interact with each other (for example, through clustering or allosterism), and may have to be regulated in other ways, for example, by phosphorylation or recycling.

The system could then be expanded by gene duplication or, more rarely, by reverse transcription. For example, multiple receptors could develop to increase the spectrum of effects of a hormone; hormone duplication and specialization of function would then follow. Alternatively, the hormone could duplicate first. Although the new hormone would have to act on pre-existing receptors, it may have sufficiently different metabolism or binding kinetics to maintain itself until its own receptor evolved. In addition, new functions could be acquired by receptor jumping or by exon shuffling among the receptors.

Other investigators have postulated that the various components evolved separately and coupled by chance. For example, receptors may have been developed for cell anchorage or sensory perception; G proteins functioned in translation and organelle trafficking; and the adenylate cyclase may have evolved as an ion or voltage regulator, as it appears to have done in *Paramecium* (see preceding discussion). Only later did chance coupling occur. Both hypotheses may have some validity depending on the particular system.

V. Transcription Factors

A. Conservation of Transcriptional Machinery

Although yeasts do not have any detectable nuclear receptors for mammalian steroids, T_3, 1,25-DHCC, or retinoids, these receptors can be introduced into yeasts and will activate transcription (183–186). This activity suggests that the factors necessary for nuclear receptor function are present in yeasts and can interact with the mammalian receptors. In fact, the glucocorticoid receptor will even function in plant cells (187). This phenomenon is not restricted to nuclear receptors: mammalian Jun–Fos can stimulate the transcription of wheat glutenin, which has two AP-1 sites (188).

B. Transcription Factors

The reason mammalian transcription factors can function so effectively in different kingdoms is that many of these factors are themselves present and highly conserved in these organisms. The bZIP factors are ubiquitous: proteins homologous to CREB in the DBD and dimerization domain have been isolated from tobacco and wheat and recognize CRE sequences (111). However, because of the low concentration of cAMP and complete absence of PKA in plants, these factors must be regulated in some alternative fashion. The ABA response element binding protein is also a bZIP factor, although it is not known how ABA regulates its function (189). The control of another plant bZIP factor is known: the G-box binding factor 1 is activated by phosphorylation by CKII (190,191).

bHLH–ZIP factors are somewhat more restricted. For example, Myc is present in many coelomates, where the CKII sites are conserved (192); however, they are not found in yeasts (193). The aromatic hydrocarbon (Ah) receptor, a bHLH factor, has only been identified in vertebrates (194). These data suggest an interesting evolutionary progression in which the initial ubiquitous bZIP domain duplicated and the amino terminus of the second helix became modified to bind the zipper of the first helix instead of DNA. This bHLH–ZIP factor was created sometime prior to the coelomates and provided a more rigid structure. Early in vertebrate evolution, carboxy-terminal extension was lost, producing a bHLH structure that was a little more flexible. The basic helix–span–helix may have arisen from the bHLH by expansion of the intervening loop. Recent three-dimensional studies of Max show that this loop contacts the deoxyribose–phosphate backbone of the minor groove (195) and expansion of this loop could provide additional binding specificity that was lost when the bHLH–ZIP was shortened.

Like bZIP transcription factors, serum response factor (SRF)-like factors are widely distributed (196). In yeast, this family includes MCM1 and ARG80, which are involved in the pheromone response and arginine metabolism, respectively. Furthermore, MCM1 will both heterodimerize with mammalian SRF and bind ternary complex factor (TCF) on a modified HRE. In plants, the homologs include DEF A and AG, which are both involved in flowering; however, these factors will not dimerize with SRF or recruit TCF to an HRE. The latter finding may be due to the fact that TCF, or Elk, cannot be detected in plants or fungi (197); therefore, TCF may have been a late addition to the SRF complex.

Other transcription factors have been less well studied. The POU factors have been found at least as far back as nematodes and planaria and probably arose by exon shuffling between a homeodomain and another DBD resembling POU_S (198,199). The Brn subfamily appears to have been generated by reverse transcription, since its members have no introns and have remnants of a poly(A) tail. NF-κB has been identified in insects and can be activated by PKC; it is conserved enough to bind the HRE from mammalian immunoresponsive genes (200,201).

VI. Evolution of Function

The examples just given demonstrate how hormones, receptors, transducers, and transcription factors can evolve and alter their functions, but because hormones are removed from their effects, it is also possible for a hormone to remain structurally stable and still have its function change dramatically during evolution. In essence, as old functions become less important, the hormone can be recruited to regulate new functions. Prolactin is an excellent example of such a hormone (202).

PRL is best known for its function in lactation; indeed, this activity has given the hormone its name. However, only mammals synthesize milk, and PRL is an ancient hormone that is present in most vertebrates, including bony fish. There are usually five functions attributed to PRL, several of which show a definite phylogenic trend.

1. PRL is important in osmoregulation, especially in those species whose life cycles bring them into dramatically different environments. For example, certain fish migrate between fresh and salt water, and amphibians undergo early development in water before moving onto land. PRL is involved in both these transitions.

2. PRL has several reproductive functions in higher vertebrates: it is gonadotropic in rodents, mammotropic in all mammals, and induces brooding behavior in birds.

3. PRL has been reported to have epidermal functions, but most of these can be reclassified into one of the first two categories. For example, the effects of PRL on ion and water permeability in skin can be related to osmoregulation.

4. A fourth function is growth, which may be either specific, such as mammary hyperplasia, or general, such as larval growth. Juvenile and adult growth are governed by GH.

5. PRL has several metabolic functions, but most of them simply support the other activities listed and show no phylogenic specificity.

Figure 15-7 shows a gradual shift from one function to another as different vertebrate classes appeared. The first function PRL had was osmoregulation. This activity continued in amphibians because their life cycle required them to return to the water for reproduction and their larvae developed in water, that is, osmoregulation became linked to reproduction via the water drive and larval growth. Little is known about the actions of PRL in reptiles, but in mammals and birds the osmoregulatory functions have nearly disappeared because both classes are primarily terrestrial. Lactation can be considered an extension of the function of larval growth; the gonadotropic function, which is required for the maintenance of pregnancy in rodents, can be interpreted in the same manner. Finally, it has been suggested that the newest member of this family, placental lactogen, may play some direct role in fetal growth. PRL, therefore, is a hormone that has gradually assumed new functions and shed old ones during its history.

VII. Summary

Evolution implies a pre-existing structure or system. Kinases and transcription factors are essential for any type of internal regulation and, therefore,

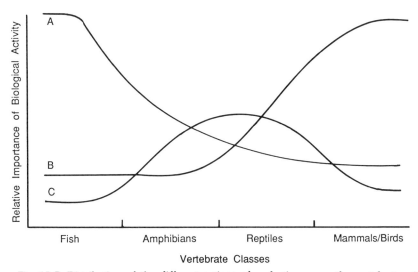

Fig. 15-7. Distribution of the different actions of prolactin among the vertebrates: (A) osmoregulation, (B) reproduction, and (C) larval growth.

were present in the earliest organisms. In the unicellular organisms, there was also a need to interact with the environment and to local food sources. As such, membrane proteins developed to bind the substratum and to detect nutrients, especially amines. When unicellular organisms became multicellular, there was a further need to coordinate activities, and messenger molecules were developed. Because of their endless variability and ease of synthesis (all organisms have translational machinery), peptides became one of the earliest and most versatile groups of hormones; amines and secondary metabolites were other sources. These external messengers recruited membrane proteins to plug into a pre-existing regulatory system, consisting of second messengers and transcription factors.

Because peptide hormones only needed to interact with their receptors, they had the least structural constraints and evolved rapidly. Receptors had to interact with more components and evolved more slowly. The transducers were critically involved with so many regulatory processes that their evolution was the slowest of any component in the signaling pathway. The mechanisms of diversification include gene duplication, exon shuffling, and branch jumping. In addition to the structural evolution of the endocrine system, hormones can also undergo functional evolution.

References

General References

Coté, G. G., and Crain, R. C. (1993). Biochemistry of phosphoinositides. *Annu. Rev. Plant Physiol. Plant Mol. Biol.* **44,** 333–356.

De Loof, A., and Schoofs, L. (1990). Homologies between the amino acid sequences of some vertebrate peptide hormones and peptides isolated from invertebrate sources. *Comp. Biochem. Physiol.* **95B,** 459–468.

Drøbak, B. K. (1993). Plant phosphoinositides and intracellular signaling. *Plant Physiol.* **102,** 705–709.

Fingerman, M., Nagabhushanam, R., and Sarojini, R. (1993). Vertebrate-type hormones in crustaceans: Localization, identification and functional significance. *Zool. Sci.* **10,** 13–29.

Kuma, K., Iwabe, N., and Miyata, T. (1993). Motifs of cadherin- and fibronectin type III-related sequences and evolution of the receptor-type–protein tyrosine kinases: Sequence similarity between proto-oncogene *ret* and cadherin family. *Mol. Biol. Evol.* **10,** 539–551.

Lummis, S. C. R., Galione, A., and Taylor, C. W. (1990). Transmembrane signalling in insects. *Annu. Rev. Entomol.* **35,** 345–377.

Nietfeld, J. J. (1993). Cytokines and proteoglycans. *Experientia* **49,** 456–469.

Pertseva, M. (1991). The evolution of hormonal signalling systems. *Comp. Biochem. Physiol.* **100A,** 775–787.

Renaud, F. L., Chiesa, R., De Jesús, J. M., López, A., Miranda, J., and Tomassini, N. (1991). Hormones and signal transduction in protozoa. *Comp. Biochem. Physiol.* **100A,** 41–45.

Trewavas, A., and Gilroy, S. (1991). Signal transduction in plant cells. *Trends Genet.* **7,** 356–361.

Van Haastert, P. J. M., Janssens, P. M. W., and Erneux, C. (1991). Sensory transduction in eukaryotes: A comparison between *Dictyostelium* and vertebrate cells. *Eur. J. Biochem.* **195,** 289–303.

Walker, R. J., and Holden-Dye, L. (1991). Evolutionary aspects of transmitter molecules, their receptors and channels. *Parasitology* **102,** S7–S29.

See also Refs. 15, 16, 32, 36, 41, 44, 51, 52, 67, 75, 77, 81, 83, 99, 101, 102, 113, 117–119, 121, 124, 141, 161, 173, 175, and 202.

Cited References

1. Krishnan, A. V., Stathis, P., Permuth, S. F., Tokes, L., and Feldman, D. (1993). Bisphenol-A: An estrogenic substance is released from polycarbonate flasks during autoclaving. *Endocrinol. (Baltimore)* **132,** 2279–2286.

2. LeRoith, D., Shiloach, J., Roth, J., and Lesniak, M. A. (1980). Evolutionary origins of vertebrate hormones: Substances similar to mammalian insulins are native to unicellular eukaryotes. *Proc. Natl. Acad. Sci. U.S.A.* **77,** 6184-6188.

3. Nagasawa, H., Kataoka, H., Isogai, A., Tamura, S., Suzuki, A., Mizoguchi, A., Fujiwara, Y., Suzuki, A., Takahashi, Y., and Ishizaki, H. (1986). Amino acid sequence of a prothoracicotropic hormone of the silkworm *Bombyx mori*. *Proc. Natl. Acad. Sci. U.S.A.* **83,** 5840–5843.

4. Jhoti, H., McLeod, A. N., Blundell, T. L., Ishizaki, H., Nagasawa, H., and Suzuki, A. (1987). Prothoracicotropic hormone has an insulin-like tertiary structure. *FEBS Lett.* **219,** 419–425.

5. Nachman, R. J., Holman, G. M., Cook, B. J., Haddon, W. F., and Ling, N. (1986). Leucosulfakinin-II, a blocked sulfated insect neuropeptide with homol-

ogy to cholecystokinin and gastrin. *Biochem. Biophys. Res. Commun.* **140**, 357–364.

6. Loumaye, E., Thorner, J., and Catt, K. J. (1982). Yeast mating pheromone activates mammalian gonadotrophs: Evolutionary conservation of a reproductive hormone. *Science* **218**, 1323–1325.

7. Karten, M. J., and Rivier, J. E. (1986). Gonadotropin-releasing hormone analog design. Structure–function studies toward the development of agonists and antagonists: Rationale and perspective. *Endocr. Rev.* **7**, 44–66.

8. Grover, S., Woodward, S. R., and Odell, W. D. (1993). A bacterial protein has homology with human chorionic gonadotropin (hCG). *Biochem. Biophys. Res. Commun.* **193**, 841–847.

9. Sarkar, G., and Sommer, S. S. (1989). Access to a messenger RNA sequence or its protein product is not limited by tissue or species specificity. *Science* **244**, 331–334.

10. Chelly, J., Concordet, J. P., Kaplan, J. C., and Kahn, A. (1989). Illegitimate transcription: Transcription of any gene in any cell type. *Proc. Natl. Acad. Sci. U.S.A.* **86**, 2617–2621.

11. Muglia, L., and Locker, J. (1984). Extrapancreatic insulin gene expression in the fetal rat. *Proc. Natl. Acad. Sci. U.S.A.* **81**, 3635–3639.

12. Kew, D., and Kilpatrick, D. L. (1990). Widespread organ expression of the rat proenkephalin gene during early postnatal development. *Mol. Endocrinol.* **4**, 337–340.

13. Bergwitz, C., Madoff, S., Abou-Samra, A. B., and Jüppner, H. (1991). Specific, high-affinity binding sites for angiotensin II on *Mycoplasma hyorhinis*. *Biochem. Biophys. Res. Commun.* **179**, 1391–1399.

14. Lima, M. F., Junior, P. F., and Villalta, F. (1992). Receptors for epidermal growth factor in intracellular forms of *Trypanosoma cruzi*. *FASEB J.* **6**, A1352.

15. Smith, M. W., Feng, D. F., and Doolittle, R. F. (1992). Evolution by acquisition: The case for horizontal gene transfers. *Trends Biochem. Sci.* **17**, 489–493.

16. Amábile-Cuevas, C. F., and Chicurel, M. E. (1993). Horizontal gene transfer. *Am. Sci.* **81**, 332–341.

17. Houck, M. A., Clark, J. B., Peterson, K. R., and Kidwell, M. G. (1991). Possible horizontal transfer of *Drosophila* genes by the mite *Proctolaelaps regalis*. *Science* **253**, 1125–1129.

18. Madani, N. D., Malloy, P. J., Rodriguez-Pombo, P., Krishnan, A. V., and Feldman, D. (1994). *Candida albicans* estrogen-binding protein gene encodes an oxidoreductase that is inhibited by estradiol. *Proc. Natl. Acad. Sci. U.S.A.* **91**, 922–926.

19. Petruzzelli, L., Herrera, R., Garcis-Arenas, R., and Rosen, O. M. (1985). Acquisition of insulin-dependent protein tyrosine kinase activity during *Drosophila* embryogenesis. *J. Biol. Chem.* **260**, 16072–16075.

20. Petruzzelli, L., Herrera, R., Arenas-Garcia, R., Fernandez, R., Birnbaum, M. J., and Rosen, O. M. (1986). Isolation of a *Drosophila* genomic sequence homologous to the kinase domain of the human insulin receptor and detection of the phosphorylated *Drosophila* receptor with an anti-peptide antibody. *Proc. Natl. Acad. Sci. U.S.A.* **83**, 4710–4714.

21. Arpagaus, M. (1987). Vertebrate insulin induces diapause termination in *Pieris brassicae* pupae. *Roux's Arch. Dev. Biol.* **196**, 527–530.

22. Saito, E., and Odell, W. D. (1983). Corticotropin/lipotropin common precursor-like material in normal rat extrapituitary tissues. *Proc. Natl. Acad. Sci. U.S.A.* **80**, 3792–3796.

23. Olsen, N. J., Nicholson, W. E., DeBold, C. R., and Orth, D. N. (1992). Lympho-cyte-derived adrenocorticotropin is insufficient to stimulate adrenal steroido-genesis in hypophysectomized rats. *Endocrinol. (Baltimore)* **130**, 2113–2119.
24. Smit, A. B., Geraerts, W. P. M., Meester, I., van Heerikhuizen, H., and Joosse, J. (1991). Characterization of a cDNA clone encoding molluscan insulin-related peptide II of *Lymnaea stagnalis*. *Eur. J. Biochem.* **199**, 699–703.
25. Li, K. W., Geraerts, W. P. M., Ebberink, R. H. M., and Joose, J. (1992). Purifica-tion and sequencing of molluscan insulin-related peptide I (MIP I) from the neuroendocrine light green cells of *Lymnaea stagnalis*. *Mol. Cell. Endocrinol.* **85**, 141–150.
26. Li, K. W., Geraerts, W. P. M., and Joosse, J. (1992). Purification and sequencing of molluscan insulin-related peptide II from the neuroendocrine light green cells in *Lymnaea stagnalis*. *Endocrinol. (Baltimore)* **130**, 3427–3432.
27. Robitzki, A., Schröder, H. C., Ugarkovic, D., Pfeifer, K., Uhlenbruck, G., and Müller, W. E. G. (1989). Demonstration of an endocrine signaling circuit for insulin in the sponge *Geodia cydonium*. *EMBO J.* **8**, 2905–2909.
28. McKenzie, M. A., Fawell, S. E., Cha, M., and Lenard, J. (1988). Effects of mammalian insulin on metabolism, growth, and morphology of a wall-less strain of *Neurospora crassa*. *Endocrinol. (Baltimore)* **122**, 511–517.
29. Fawell, S. E., McKenzie, M. A., Greenfield, N. J., Adebodun, F., Jordan, F., and Lenard, J. (1988). Stimulation by mammalian insulin of glycogen metabolism in a wall-less strain of *Neurospora crassa*. *Endocrinol. (Baltimore)* **122**, 518–523.
30. Muthukumar, G., and Lenard, J. (1991). A preproinsulin-like pseudogene from *Neurospora crassa*. *Mol. Cell. Endocrinol.* **82**, 275–283.
31. Kole, H. K., Muthukumar, G., and Lenard, J. (1991). Purification and properties of a membrane-bound insulin binding protein, a putative receptor, from *Neu-rospora crassa*. *Biochemistry* **30**, 682–688.
32. Campbell, R. M., and Scances, C. G. (1992). Evolution of the growth hormone-releasing factor (GRF) family of peptides. *Growth Regul.* **2**, 175–191.
33. Kochert, G. (1978). Sexual pheromones in algae and fungi. *Annu. Rev. Plant Physiol.* **29**, 461–486.
34. Sandor, T., and Mehdi, A. Z. (1979). Steroids and evolution. *In* "Hormones and Evolution" (E. J. W. Barrington, ed.), pp. 1–72. Academic Press, New York.
35. Quinitio, E. T., Yamauchi, K., Hara, A., and Fuji, A. (1991). Profiles of proges-terone- and estradiol-like substances in the hemolymph of female *Pandalus kessleri* during an annual reproductive cycle. *Gen. Comp. Endocrinol.* **81**, 343–348.
36. Stanley-Samuelson, D. W., and Loher, W. (1990). Evolution aspects of prosta-glandins and other eicosanoids in invertebrates. *In* "Progress in Comparative Endocrinology" (A. Epple, C. G. Scanes, and M. H. Stetson, eds.), pp. 614–619. John Wiley & Sons, New York.
37. Meijer, L., Maclouf, J., and Bryant, R. W. (1986). Arachidonic acid metabolism in starfish oocytes. *Dev. Biol.* **114**, 22–33.
38. Perry, G., and Epel, D. (1985). Fertilization stimulates lipid peroxidation in the sea urchin egg. *Dev. Biol.* **107**, 58–65.
39. Piomelli, D., Volterra, A., Dale, N., Siegelbaum, S. A., Kandel, E. R., Schwartz, J. H., and Belardetti, F. (1987). Lipoxygenase metabolites of arachidonic acid as second messengers for presynaptic inhibition of *Aplysia* sensory cells. *Nature (London)* **328**, 38–43.
40. Di Marzo, V., De Petrocellis, L., Gianfrani, C., and Cimino, G. (1993). Biosyn-

thesis, structure and biological activity of hydroxyeicosatetraenoic acids in *Hydra vulgaris. Biochem. J.* **295**, 23–29.

41. Gerhart, D. J., Clare, A. S., Eisenman, K., Rittschof, D., and Forward, R. B. (1990). Eicosanoids in corals and crustaceans: Primary metabolites that function as allelochemicals and pheromones. *In* "Progress in Comparative Endocrinology" (A. Epple, C. G. Scanes, and M. H. Stetson, eds.), pp. 598–602. John Wiley & Sons, New York.

42. Farmer, E. E., and Ryan, C. A. (1992). Octadecanoid precursors of jasmonic acid activate the synthesis of wound-inducible proteinase inhibitors. *Plant Cell* **4**, 129–134.

43. Shabb, J. B., and Corbin, J. D. (1992). Cyclic nucleotide-binding domains in proteins having diverse functions. *J. Biol. Chem.* **267**, 5723–5726.

44. Picado-Leonard, J., and Miller, W. L. (1988). Homologous sequences in steroidogenic enzymes, steroid receptors and a steroid binding protein suggest a consensus steroid-binding sequence. *Mol. Endocrinol.* **2**, 1145–1150.

45. Fawell, S. E., Lees, J. A., and Parker, M. G. (1989). A proposed consensus steroid-binding sequence—A reply. *Mol. Endocrinol.* **3**, 1002–1005.

46. Slootstra, J. W., and Roubos, E. W. (1991). Two receptor binding regions of human FSH show sense–antisense similarity to the human FSH receptor. *Biochem. Biophys. Res. Commun.* **179**, 266–271.

47. Goldstein, A., and Brutlag, D. L. (1989). Is there a relationship between DNA sequences encoding peptide ligands and their receptors? *Proc. Natl. Acad. Sci. U.S.A.* **86**, 42–45.

48. Guillemette, G., Boulay, G., Gagnon, S., Bosse, R., and Escher, E. (1989). The peptide encoded by angiotensin II complementary RNA does not interfere with angiotensin II action. *Biochem. J.* **261**, 309.

49. de Gasparo, M., Whitebread, S., Einsle, K., and Heusser, C. (1989). Are the antibodies to a peptide complementary to angiotensin II useful to isolate the angiotensin II receptor? *Biochem. J.* **261**, 310–311.

50. Jurzak, M., Pavo, I., and Fahrenholz, F. (1993). Lack of interaction of vasopressin with its antisense peptides: A functional and immunological study. *J. Recept. Res.* **13**, 881–902.

51. Csaba, G. (1990). Presence and development of hormone receptors in unicellular organisms. *In* "Progress in Comparative Endocrinology" (A. Epple, C. G. Scanes, and M. H. Stetson, eds.), pp. 116–126. John Wiley & Sons, New York.

52. Spudich, J. L. (1993). Color sensing in the *Archaea*: A eukaryotic-like receptor coupled to a prokaryotic transducer. *J. Bacteriol.* **175**, 7755–7761.

53. O'Hara, P. J., Sheppard, P. O., Thgersen, H., Venezia, D., Haldeman, B. A., McGrane, V., Houamed, K. M., Thomsen, C., Gilbert, T. L., and Mulvihill, E. R. (1993). The ligand-binding domain in metabotropic glutamate receptors is related to bacterial periplasmic binding proteins. *Neuron* **11**, 41–52.

54. Roberts, W. M., Look, A. T., Roussel, M. F., and Sherr, C. J. (1988). Tandem linkage of human CSF-1 receptor (c-*fms*) and PDGF receptor genes. *Cell* **55**, 655–661.

55. Arden, K. C., Boutin, J. M., Djiane, J., Kelly, P. A., and Cavenee, W. K. (1990). The receptors for prolactin and growth hormone are localized in the same region of human chromosome 5. *Cytogenet. Cell Genet.* **53**, 161–165.

56. Sunahara, R. K., Niznik, H. B., Weiner, D. M., Stormann, T. M., Brann, M. R., Kennedy, J. L., Gelernter, J. E., Rozmahel, R., Yang, Y., Israel, Y., Seeman, P.,

and O'Dowd, B. F. (1990). Human dopamine D_1 receptor encoded by an intron-less gene on chromosome 5. *Nature (London)* **347**, 80–83.

57. Lomedico, P., Rosenthal, N., Efstratiadis, A., Gilbert, W., Kolodner, R., and Tizard, R. (1979). The structure and evolution of the two nonallelic rat pre-proinsulin genes. *Cell* **18**, 545–558.

58. Dohlman, H. G., Caron, M. G., and Lefkowitz, R. J. (1987). A family of receptors coupled to guanine nucleotide regulatory proteins. *Biochemistry* **26**, 2657–2664.

59. Bonner, T. I., Buckley, N. J., Young, A. C., and Brann, M. R. (1987). Identification of a family of muscarinic acetylcholine receptor genes. *Science* **237**, 527–532.

60. Traut, T. W. (1988). Do exons code for structural or functional units in proteins? *Proc. Natl. Acad. Sci. U.S.A.* **85**, 2944–2948.

61. Seidel, H. M., Pompliano, D. L., and Knowles, J. R. (1992). Exons as microgenes? *Science* **257**, 1489–1490.

62. Seino, S., Seino, M., Nishi, S., and Bell, G. I. (1989). Structure of the human receptor gene and characterization of its promoter. *Proc. Natl. Acad. Sci. U.S.A.* **86**, 114–118.

63. Heckert, L. L., Daley, I. J., and Griswold, M. D. (1992). Structural organization of the follicle-stimulating hormone receptor gene. *Mol. Endocrinol.* **6**, 70–80.

64. Houamed, K. M., Kuijper, J. L., Gilbert, T. L., Haldeman, B. A., O'Hara, P. J., Mulvihill, E. R., Almers, W., and Hagen, F. S. (1991). Cloning, expression, and gene structure of a G protein-coupled glutamate receptor from rat brain. *Science* **252**, 1318–1321.

65. Masu, M., Tanabe, Y., Tsuchida, K., Shigemoto, R., and Nakanishi, S. (1991). Sequence and expression of a metabotropic glutamate receptor. *Nature (London)* **349**, 760–765.

66. Nakanishi, N., Shneider, N. A., and Axel, R. (1991). A family of glutamate receptor genes: Evidence for the formation of heteromultimeric receptors with distinct channel properties. *Neuron* **5**, 569–581.

67. Yamamori, T., and Sarai, A. (1992). Coevolution of cytokine receptor families in the immune and nervous systems. *Neurosci. Res.* **15**, 151–161.

68. Cunningham, B. C., and Wells, J. A. (1989). High-resolution epitope mapping of hGH-receptor interactions by alanine-scanning mutagenesis. *Science* **244**, 1081–1085.

69. Cunningham, B. C., Mulkerrin, M. G., and Wells, J. A. (1991). Dimerization of human growth hormone by zinc. *Science* **253**, 545–548.

70. Cunningham, B. C., and Wells, J. A. (1991). Rational design of receptor-specific variants of human growth hormone. *Proc. Natl. Acad. Sci. U.S.A.* **88**, 3407–3411.

71. Lowman, H. B., Cunningham, B. C., and Wells, J. A. (1991). Mutational analysis and protein engineering of receptor-binding determinants in human placental lactogen. *J. Biol. Chem.* **266**, 10982–10988.

72. Simon, G., Pasztelyi, Z., and Zelles, T. (1992). Cross reactivity among the ligands of the 7-helix family. *Acta Physiol. Hung.* **79**, 147–152.

73. Linden, J., Tucker, A. L., and Lynch, K. R. (1991). Molecular cloning of adenosine A_1 and A_2 receptors. *Trends Pharmacol. Sci.* **12**, 326–328.

74. Vu, T. K. H., Hung, D. T., Wheaton, V. I., and Coughlin, S. R. (1991). Molecular cloning of a functional thrombin receptor reveals a novel proteolytic mechanism of receptor activation. *Cell* **64**, 1057–1068.

75. Venter, J. C., di Porzio, U., Robinson, D. A., Shreeve, S. M., Lai, J., Kerlavage, A.

R., Fracek, S. P., Lentes, K. U., and Fraser, C. M. (1988). Evolution of neurotransmitter receptor systems. *Prog. Neurobiol.* **30**, 105–169.

76. Awad, E. W., and Anctil, M. (1993). Identification of β-like adrenoceptors associated with bioluminescence in the sea pansy *Renilla koellikeri. J. Exp. Biol.* **177**, 181–200.

77. Yokoyama, S., Isenberg, K. E., and Wright, A. F. (1989). Adaptive evolution of G-protein coupled receptor genes. *Mol. Biol. Evol.* **6**, 342–353.

78. Nakayama, N., Miyajima, A., and Arai, K. (1985). Nucleotide sequences of *STE2* and *STE3*, cell type-specific sterile genes from *Saccharomyces cerevisiae. EMBO J.* **4**, 2643–2648.

79. Konopka, J. B., Jenness, D. D., and Hartwell, L. H. (1988). The C-terminus of the *S. cerevisiae* α-pheromone receptor mediates an adaptive response to pheromone. *Cell* **54**, 609–620.

80. Reneke, J. E., Blumer, K. J., Courchesne, W. E., and Thorner, J. (1988). The carboxy-terminal segment of the yeast α-factor receptor is a regulatory domain. *Cell* **55**, 221–234.

81. Laudet, V., Hänni, C., Coll, J., Catzeflis, F., and Stéhelin, D. (1992). Evolution of the nuclear receptor gene family. *EMBO J.* **11**, 1003–1013.

82. Chan, S. M., Xu, N., Niemeyer, C. C., Bone, J. R., and Flytzanis, C. N. (1992). SpCOUP-TF: A sea urchin member of the steroid/thyroid hormone receptor family. *Proc. Natl. Acad. Sci. U.S.A.* **89**, 10568–10572.

83. Wahli, W., and Martinez, E. (1991). Superfamily of steroid nuclear receptors: Positive and negative regulators of gene expression. *FASEB J.* **5**, 2243–2249.

84. Tanaka, M., Maeda, K., Okubo, T., and Nakashima, K. (1992). Double antenna structure of chicken prolactin receptor deduced from the cDNA sequence. *Biochem. Biophys. Res. Commun.* **188**, 490–496.

85. Gandarillas, A., Renart, J., and Quintanilla, M. (1992). Biochemical characterization of *Artemia* ras p21. *Mol. Cell. Biochem.* **112**, 29–33.

86. Egan, S. E., Giddings, B. W., Brooks, M. W., Buday, L., Sizeland, A. M., and Weinberg, R. A. (1993). Association of Sos Ras exchange protein with Grb2 is implicated in tyrosine kinase signal transduction and transformation. *Nature (London)* **363**, 45–51.

87. Olivier, J. P., Raabe, T., Henkemeyer, M., Dickson, B., Mbamalu, G., Margolis, B., Schlessinger, J., Hafen, E., and Pawson, T. (1993). A Drosophila SH2-SH3 adaptor protein implicated in coupling the sevenless tyrosine kinase to an activator of Ras guanine nucleotide exchange, Sos. *Cell* **73**, 179–191.

88. Palme, K., Diefenthal, T., and Moore, I. (1993). The *ypt* gene family from maize and *Arabidopsis*: Structural and functional analysis. *J. Exp. Bot.* **44** *(Suppl)*, 183–195.

89. Ahnn, J., March, P. E., Takiff, H. E., and Inouye, M. (1986). A GTP-binding protein of *Escherichia coli* has homology to yeast RAS proteins. *Proc. Natl. Acad. Sci. U.S.A.* **83**, 8849–8853.

90. Knol, J. C., Weidemann, W., Planta, R. J., Vreugdenhil, E., and van Heerikhuizen, H. (1992). Molecular cloning of G protein α subunits from the central nervous system of the mollusc *Lymnaea stagnalis. FEBS Lett.* **314**, 215–219.

91. van der Voorn, L., Gebbink, M., Plasterk, H. A., and Ploegh, H. L. (1990). Characterization of a G-protein β-subunit gene from the nematode *Caenorhabditis elegans. J. Mol. Biol.* **213**, 17–26.

92. Whiteway, M., Hougan, L., Dignard, D., Thomas, D. Y., Bell, L., Saari, G. C., Grant, F. J., O'Hara, P., and MacKay, V. L. (1989). The *STE4* and *STE18* genes of

yeast encode potential β and γ subunits of the mating factor receptor-coupled G protein. *Cell* **56**, 467–477.

93. Ma, H., Yanofsky, M. F., and Meyerowitz, E. M. (1990). Molecular cloning and characterization of *GPA1*, a G protein α subunit gene from *Arabidopsis thaliana*. *Proc. Natl. Acad. Sci. U.S.A.* **87**, 3821–3825.

94. Okaichi, K., Cubitt, A. B., Pitt, G. S., and Firtel, R. A. (1992). Amino acid substitutions in the *Dictyostelium* Gα subunit Gα2 produce dominant negative phenotypes and inhibit the activation of adenylyl cyclase, guanylyl cyclase, and phospholipase C. *Mol. Biol. Cell* **3**, 735–747.

95. Kang, Y. S., Kane, J., Kurjan, J., Stadel, J. M., and Tipper, D. J. (1990). Effects of expression of mammalian Gα and hybrid mammalian-yeast Gα proteins on the yeast pheromone response signal transduction pathway. *Mol. Cell. Biol.* **10**, 2582–2590.

96. Quan, F., Thomas, L., and Forte, M. (1991). *Drosophila* stimulatory G protein α subunit activates mammalian adenylyl cyclase but interacts poorly with mammalian receptors: Implications for receptor-G protein interaction. *Proc. Natl. Acad. Sci. U.S.A.* **88**, 1898–1902.

97. Kleymann, G., Boege, F., Hahn, M., Hampe, W., Vasudevan, S., and Reiländer, H. (1993). Human β₂-adrenergic receptor produced in stably transformed insect cells is functionally coupled via endogenous GTP-binding protein to adenylyl cyclase. *Eur. J. Biochem.* **213**, 797–804.

98. Terryn, N., Van Montagu, M., and Inzé, D. (1993). GTP-binding proteins in plants. *Plant Mol. Biol.* **22**, 143–152.

99. Jan, L. Y., and Jan, Y. N. (1992). Tracing the roots of ion channels. *Cell* **69**, 715–718.

100. Schultz, J. E., Klumpp, S., Benz, R., Schürhoff-Goeters, W. J. C., and Schmid, A. (1992). Regulation of adenylyl cyclase from *Paramecium* by an intrinsic potassium conductance. *Science* **255**, 600–603.

101. Tang, W. J., and Gilman, A. G. (1992). Adenylyl cyclases. *Cell* **70**, 869–872.

102. Chinkers, M., and Garbers, D. L. (1991). Signal transduction by guanylyl cyclases. *Annu. Rev. Biochem.* **60**, 553–575.

103. Elphick, M. R., Green, I. C., and O'Shea, M. (1993). Nitric oxide synthesis and action in an invertebrate brain. *Brain Res.* **619**, 344–346.

104. Pijst, H. L. A., van Driel, R., Janssens, P. M. W., Musgrave, A., and van den Ende, H. (1984). Cyclic AMP is involved in sexual reproduction of *Chlamydomonas eugametos*. *FEBS Lett.* **174**, 132–136.

105. Francko, D. A. (1989). Modulation of photosynthetic carbon assimilation in *Selenastrum capricornutum* (Chlorophyceae) by cAMP: an electrogenic mechanism? *J. Phycol.* **25**, 305–313.

106. Carré, I. A., and Edmunds, L. N. (1992). cAMP-dependent kinases in the algal flagellate *Euglena gracilis*. *J. Biol. Chem.* **267**, 2135–2137.

107. Gangwani, L., Tamot, B. K., Khurana, J., and Maheshwari, S. C. (1991). Identification of 3′,5′-cyclic AMP in axenic cultures of *Lemna paucicostata* by high-performance liquid chromatography. *Biochem. Biophys. Res. Commun.* **178**, 1113–1119.

108. Yavorskaya, V. K., Dragovoz, I. V., Savinsky, S. V., Markova, V. E., and Kofman, I. S. (1991). Determination of cyclic 3′,5′-adenosine monophosphate in plant tissues by high performance liquid chromatography. *Phytochem. Anal.* **2**, 204–207.

109. Sato, S., Tabata, S., and Hotta, Y. (1992). Changes in intracellular cAMP level and activities of adenylcylase and phosphodiesterase during meiosis of lily microsporocytes. *Cell Struct. Funct.* **17,** 335–339.

110. Lin, X., Feng, X. H., and Watson, J. C. (1991). Differential accumulation of transcripts encoding protein kinase homologs in greening pea seedlings. *Proc. Natl. Acad. Sci. U.S.A.* **88,** 6951–6955.

111. Katagiri, F., Lam, E., and Chua, N. H. (1989). Two tobacco DNA-binding proteins with homology to the nuclear factor CREB. *Nature (London)* **340,** 727–730.

112. Lin, P. P. C., and Volcani, B. E. (1989). Novel adenosine 3′,5′-cyclic monophosphate dependent protein kinases in a marine diatom. *Biochemistry* **28,** 6624–6631.

113. Hokmann, F., Dostmann, W., Keilbach, A., Landgraf, W., and Ruth, P. (1992). Structure and physiological role of cGMP-dependent protein kinase. *Biochim. Biophys. Acta* **1135,** 51–60.

114. Müller, W. E. G., Rottmann, M., Diehl-Seifert, B., Kurelec, B., Uhlenbruck, G., and Schröder, H. C. (1987). Role of the aggregation factor in the regulation of phosphoinositide metabolism in sponges: Possible consequences on calcium efflux and on mitogenesis. *J. Biol. Chem.* **262,** 9850–9858.

115. Europe-Finner, G. N., and Newell, P. C. (1987). Cyclic AMP stimulates accumulation of inositol trisphosphate in *Dictyostelium*. *J. Cell Sci.* **87,** 221–229.

116. Drayer, A. L., and van Haastert, P. J. M. (1992). Molecular cloning and expression of a phosphoinositide-specific phospholipase C of *Dictyostelium discoideum*. *J. Biol. Chem.* **267,** 18387–18392.

117. Poovaiah, B. W., and Reddy, A. S. N. (1993). Calcium and signal transduction in plants. *Crit. Rev. Plant Sci.* **12,** 185–211.

118. Bush, D. S. (1993). Regulation of cytosolic calcium in plants. *Plant Physiol.* **103,** 7–13.

119. Gilroy, S., Bethke, P.C., and Jones, R.L. (1993). Calcium homeostasis in plants. *J. Cell Sci.* **106,** 453–462.

120. Coté, G. G., and Crain, R. C. (1992). Artifactual elevation of the apparent levels of phosphatidic acid and phosphatidylinositol 4,5-biphosphate during short-term labeling of plant tissue with radioactive precursor. *Plant Physiol.* **100,** 1042–1043.

121. Hetherington, A. M., and Drøbak, B. K. (1992). Inositol-containing lipids in higher plants. *Prog. Lipid Res.* **31,** 53–63.

122. Reddy, A. S. N., and Poovaiah, B. W. (1987). Inositol 1,4,5-trisphosphate induced calcium release from corn coleoptile microsomes. *J. Biochem. (Tokyo)* **101,** 569–573.

123. Schumaker, K. S., and Sze, H. (1987). Inositol 1,4,5-trisphosphate releases Ca^{2+} from vacuolar membrane vesicles of oat roots. *J. Biol. Chem.* **262,** 3944–3946.

124. Buckhout, T. J. (1990). Mechanism and regulation of Ca^{2+} uptake and release in higher plants: Role of calmodulin and inositol-1,4,5-trisphosphate. *In* "Inositol Metabolism in Plants" (D. J. Morré, W. F. Boss, and F. A. Loewus, eds.), pp. 277–287. John Wiley & Sons, New York.

125. Tate, B. F., Schaller, G. E., Sussman, M. R., and Crain, R. C. (1989). Characterization of a polyphosphoinositide phospholipase C from the plasma membrane of *Avena sativa*. *Plant Physiol.* **91,** 1275–1279.

126. Melin, P. M., Pical, C., Jergil, B., and Sommarin, M. (1992). Polyphosphoinosi-

tide phospholipase C in wheat root plasma membranes. Partial purification and characterization. *Biochim. Biophys. Acta* **1123,** 163–169.

127. Pical, C., Sandelius, A. S., Melin, P. M., and Sommarin, M. (1992). Polyphosphoinositide phospholipase C in plasma membranes of wheat (*Triticum aestivum* L.): Orientation of active site and activation by Ca^{2+} and Mg^{2+}. *Plant Physiol.* **100,** 1296–1303.

128. Yotsushima, K., Nakamura, K., Mitsui, T., and Igaue, I. (1992). Purification and characterization of phosphatidylinositol-specific phospholipase C in suspension-cultured cells of rice (*Oryza sativa* L.). *Biosci. Biotech. Biochem.* **56,** 1247–1251.

129. Einspahr, K. J., Peeler, T. C., and Thompson, G. A. (1989). Phosphatidylinositol 4,5-bisphosphate phospholipase C and phosphomonoesterase in *Dunaliella salina* membranes. *Plant Physiol.* **90,** 1115–1120.

130. Förster, B. (1990). Injected inositol 1,4,5-trisphosphate activates Ca^{2+}-sensitive K^{+} channels in the plasmalemma of *Eremosphaera viridis*. *FEBS Lett.* **269,** 197–201.

131. Irvine, R. F., Letcher, A. J., Stephens, L. R., and Musgrave, A. (1992). Inositol polyphosphate metabolism and inositol lipids in a green alga, *Chlamydomonas eugametos*. *Biochem. J.* **281,** 261–266.

132. Fairley-Grenot, K., and Assmann, S. M. (1991). Evidence for G-protein regulation of inward K^{+} channel current in guard cells of fava bean. *Plant Cell* **3,** 1037–1044.

133. Gilroy, S., and Jones, R. L. (1992). Gibberellic acid and abscisic acid coordinately regulate cytoplasmic calcium and secretory activity in barley aleurone protoplasts. *Proc. Natl. Acad. Sci. U.S.A.* **89,** 3591–3595.

134. Messiaen, J., Read, N. D., Van Cutsem, P., and Trewavas, A. J. (1993). Cell wall oligogalacturonides increase cytosolic free calcium in carrot protoplasts. *J. Cell Sci.* **104,** 365–371.

135. Parker, P. J., Coussens, L., Totty, N., Rhee, L., Young, S., Chen, E., Stabel, S., Waterfield, M. D., and Ullrich, A. (1986). The complete primary structure of protein kinase C-the major phorbol ester receptor. *Science* **233,** 853–859.

136. Rosenthal, A., Rhee, L., Yadegari, R., Paro, R., Ullrich, A., and Goeddel, D. V. (1987). Structure and nucleotide sequence of a *Drosophila melanogaster* protein kinase C gene. *EMBO J.* **6,** 433–441.

137. Tabuse, Y., Nishiwaki, K., and Miwa, J. (1989). Mutations in a protein kinase C homolog confer phorbol ester resistance on *Caenorhabditis elegans*. *Science* **243,** 1713–1716.

138. Sossin, W. S., Diaz-Arrastia, R., and Schwartz, J. H. (1993). Characterization of two isoforms of protein kinase C in the nervous system of *Aplysia californica*. *J. Biol. Chem.* **268,** 5763–5768.

139. Levin, D. E., Fields, O., Kunisawa, R., Bishop, J. M., and Thorner, J. (1990). A candidate protein kinase C gene, *PKC1*, is required for the *S. cerevisiae* cell cycle. *Cell* **62,** 213–224.

140. Jena, P. K., Reddy, A. S. N., and Poovaiah, B. W. (1989). Molecular cloning and sequencing of a cDNA for plant calmodulin: Signal-induced changes in the expression of calmodulin. *Proc. Natl. Acad. Sci. U.S.A.* **86,** 3644–3648.

141. Onek, L. A., and Smith, R. J. (1992). Calmodulin and calcium mediated regulation in prokaryotes. *J. Gen. Microbiol.* **138,** 1039–1049.

142. Swan, D. G., Cortes, J., Hale, R. S., and Leadlay, P. F. (1989). Cloning, characterization, and heterologous expression of the *Saccharopolyspora erythraea*

(*Streptomyces erythraeus*) gene encoding an EF-hand calcium-binding protein. *J. Bacteriol.* **171,** 5614–5619.

143. Pausch, M. H., Kaim, D., Kunisawa, R., Admon, A., and Thorner, J. (1991). Multiple Ca^{2+}/calmodulin-dependent protein kinase genes in a unicellular eukaryote. *EMBO J.* **10,** 1511–1522.

144. Ulloa, R. M., Torres, H. N., Ochatt, C. M., and Téllez-Iñón, M. T. (1991). Ca^{2+} calmodulin-dependent protein kinase activity in the ascomycetes *Neurospora crassa. Mol. Cell. Biochem.* **102,** 155–163.

145. Harper, J. F., Sussman, M. R., Schaller, G. E., Putnam-Evans, C., Charbonneau, H., and Harmon, A. C. (1991). A calcium-dependent protein kinase with a regulatory domain similar to calmodulin. *Science* **252,** 951–954.

146. Suen, K. L., and Choi, J. H. (1991). Isolation and sequence analysis of a cDNA clone for a carrot calcium-dependent protein kinase: Homology to calcium/calmodulin-dependent protein kinases and to calmodulin. *Plant Mol. Biol.* **17,** 581–590.

147. Harper, J. F., Binder, B. M., and Sussman, M. R. (1993). Calcium and lipid regulation of an *Arabidopsis* protein kinase expressed in *Escherichia coli. Biochemistry* **32,** 3282–3290.

148. Watillon, B., Kettmann, R., Boxus, P., and Burny, A. (1993). A calcium/calmodulin-binding serine/threonine protein kinase homologous to the mammalian type II calcium/calmodulin-dependent protein kinase is expressed in plant cells. *Plant Physiol.* **101,** 1381–1384.

149. Chen-Wu, J. L. P., Padmanabha, R., and Glover, C. V. C. (1988). Isolation, sequencing, and disruption of the *CKA1* gene encoding the alpha subunit of yeast casein kinase II. *Mol. Cell. Biol.* **8,** 4981–4990.

150. Hu, E., and Rubin, C. S. (1990). Casein kinase II from *Caenorhabditis elegans*: Properties and developmental regulation of the enzyme: Cloning and sequence analyses of cDNA and the gene for the catalytic subunit. *J. Biol. Chem.* **265,** 5072–5080.

151. Dobrowolska, G., Boldyreff, B., and Issinger, O. G. (1991). Cloning and sequencing of the casein kinase 2 α subunit from *Zea mays. Biochim. Biophys. Acta* **1129,** 139–140.

152. Ole-Moi Yoi, O. K., Sugimoto, C., Conrad, P. A., and Macklin, M. D. (1992). Cloning and characterization of the casein kinase II α subunit gene from the lymphocyte-transforming intracellular protozoan parasite *Theileria parva. Biochemistry* **31,** 6193–6202.

153. Mizoguchi, T., Yamaguchi-Shinozaki, K., Hayashida, N., Kamada, H., and Shinozaki, K. (1993). Cloning and characterization of two cDNAs encoding casein kinase II catalytic subunits in *Arabidopsis thaliana. Plant Mol. Biol.* **21,** 279–289.

154. Pardo, P., and Moreno, S. (1988). Characterization of two casein kinase activities in the fungus *Mucor rouxii. Sec. Mess. Phosphoprot.* **12,** 183–196.

155. Kandror, K. V., Vasiliev, A. O., Kapkov, D. V., and Stepanov, A. S. (1990). Casein kinase II from *Verticillium dahliae*: Isolation and characterization. *Biochem. Int.* **20,** 59–69.

156. Favre, B., and Ojha, M. (1991). Purification and properties of a casein kinase II-like enzyme from *Neurospora crassa. FEMS Microbiol. Lett.* **78,** 21–24.

157. Li, H., and Roux, S. J. (1992). Purification and characterization of a casein kinase 2-type protein kinase from pea nuclei. *Plant Physiol.* **99,** 686–692.

158. Dobrowolska, G., Meggio, F., Szczegielniak, J., Muszynska, G., and Pinna, L. A.

(1992). Purification and characterization of maize seedling casein kinase IIB, a monomeric enzyme immunologically related to the α subunit of animal casein kinase-2. *Eur. J. Biochem.* **204**, 299–303.

159. Li, H., and Roux, S. J. (1992). Purification and characterization of a casein kinase 2-type protein kinase from pea nuclei. *Plant Physiol.* **99**, 686–692.

160. Roussou, I., and Draetta, G. (1994). The *Schizosaccharomyces pombe* casein kinase II α and β subunits: Evolutionary conservation and positive role of the β subunit. *Mol. Cell. Biol.* **14**, 576–586.

161. Galston, A. W., and Sawhney, R. K. (1990). Polyamines in plant physiology. *Plant Physiol.* **94**, 406–410.

162. Duerr, B., Gawienowski, M., Ropp, T., and Jacobs, T. (1993). MsERK1: A mitogen-activated protein kinase from a flowering plant. *Plant Cell* **5**, 87–96.

163. Nishida, E., and Gotoh, Y. (1993). The MAP kinase cascade is essential for diverse signal transduction pathways. *Trends Biochem. Sci.* **18**, 128–131.

164. Hughes, D. A., Ashworth, A., and Marshall, C. J. (1993). Complementation of *byr1* in fission yeast by mammalian MAP kinase kinase requires coexpression of Raf kinase. *Nature (London)* **364**, 349–352.

165. Van Aelst, L., Barr, M., Marcus, S., Polverino, A., and Wigler, M. (1993). Complex formation between RAS and RAF and other protein kinases. *Proc. Natl. Acad. Sci. U.S.A.* **90**, 6213–6217.

166. Hughes, K., Nikolakaki, E., Plyte, S. E., Totty, N. F., and Woodgett, J. R. (1993). Modulation of the glycogen kinase-3 family by tyrosine phosphorylation. *EMBO J.* **12**, 803–808.

167. Miao, G. H., Hong, Z., and Verma, D. P. S. (1993). Two functional soybean genes encoding $p34^{cdc2}$ protein kinases are regulated by different plant developmental pathways. *Proc. Natl. Acad. Sci. U.S.A.* **268**, 943–947.

168. Tan, J. L., and Spudich, J. A. (1990). Developmentally regulated protein-tyrosine kinase genes in *Dictyostelium discoideum*. *Mol. Cell. Biol.* **10**, 3578–3583.

169. Hirayama, T., and Oka, A. (1992). Novel protein kinase of *Arabidopsis thaliana* (APK1) that phosphorylates tyrosine, serine and threonine. *Plant Mol. Biol.* **20**, 653–662.

170. MacKintosh, C., and Cohen, P. (1989). Identification of high levels of type 1 and type 2A protein phosphatases in higher plants. *Biochem. J.* **262**, 335–339.

171. MacKintosh, C., Coggins, J., and Cohen, P. (1991). Plant protein phosphatases: Subcellular distribution, detection of protein phosphatase 2C and identification of protein phosphatase 2A as the major quinate dehydrogenase phosphatase. *Biochem. J.* **273**, 733–738.

172. Ueki, K., and Kincaid, R. L. (1993). Interchangeable associations of calcineurin regulatory subunit isoforms with mammalian and fungal catalytic subunits. *J. Biol. Chem.* **268**, 6554–6559.

173. Cohen, P. T. W., Brewis, N. D., Hughes, V., and Mann, D. J. (1990). Protein serine/threonine phosphatases: An expanding family. *FEBS Lett.* **268**, 355–359.

174. Cyert, M. S., Kunisawa, R., Kaim, D., and Thorner, J. (1991). Yeast has homologs (*CNA1* and *CNA2* gene products) of mammalian calcineurin, a calmodulin-regulated phosphoprotein phosphatase. *Proc. Natl. Acad. Sci. U.S.A.* **88**, 7376–7380.

175. Bollen, M., and Stalmans, W. (1992). The structure, role, and regulation of type 1 protein phosphatases. *Crit. Rev. Biochem. Mol. Biol.* **27**, 227–281.

176. Guan, K., Deschenes, R. J., Qiu, H., and Dixon, J. E. (1991). Cloning and expression of a yeast protein tyrosine phosphatase. *J. Biol. Chem.* **266**, 12964–12970.

177. Saito, H., and Streuli, M. (1991). Molecular characterization of protein tyrosine phosphatases. *Cell Growth Differ.* **2**, 59–65.

178. Ramalingam, R., Shaw, D. R., and Ennis, H. L. (1993). Cloning and functional expression of a *Dictyostelium discoideum* protein tyrosine phosphatase. *J. Biol. Chem.* **268**, 22680–22685.

179. Polya, G. M., and Wettenhall, R. E. H. (1992). Rapid purification and N-terminal sequencing of a potato tuber cyclic nucleotide binding phosphatase. *Biochim. Biophys. Acta* **1159**, 179–184.

180. Wainright, P. O., Hinkle, G., Sogin, M. L., and Stickel, S. K. (1993). Monophyletic origins of the metazoa: An evolutionary link with fungi. *Science* **260**, 340–342.

181. Baldauf, S. L., and Palmer, J. D. (1993). Animals and fungi are each other's closest relatives: Congruent evidence from multiple proteins. *Proc. Natl. Acad. Sci. U.S.A.* **90**, 11558–11562.

182. Murphy, P. M. (1993). Molecular mimicry and the generation of host defense protein diversity. *Cell* **72**, 823–826.

183. Metzger, D., White, J. H., and Chambon, P. (1988). The human oestrogen receptor functions in yeast. *Nature (London)* **334**, 31–36.

184. Wright, A. P. H., Carlstedt-Duke, J., and Gustafsson, J.Å. (1990). Ligand-specific transactivation of gene expression by a derivative of the human glucocorticoid receptor expressed in yeast. *J. Biol. Chem.* **265**, 14763–14769.

185. Purvis, I. J., Chotai, D., Dykes, C. W., Lubahn, D. B., French, F. S., Wilson, E. M., and Hobden, A. N. (1991). An androgen-inducible expression system for *Saccharomyces cerevisiae*. *Gene* **106**, 35–42.

186. Heery, D. M., Zacharewski, T., Pierrat, B., Gronemeyer, H., Chambon, P., and Losson, R. (1993). Efficient transactivation by retinoic acid receptors in yeast requires retinoid X receptors. *Proc. Natl. Acad. Sci. U.S.A.* **90**, 4281–4285.

187. Schena, M., Lloyd, A. M., and Davis, R. W. (1991). A steroid-inducible gene expression system for plant cells. *Proc. Natl. Acad. Sci. U.S.A.* **88**, 10421–10425.

188. Hilson, P., de Froidmont, D., Lejour, C., Hirai, S. I., Jacquemin, J. M., and Yaniv, M. (1990). Fos and Jun oncogenes transactivate chimeric or native promoters containing AP1/GCN4 binding sites in plant cells. *Plant Cell* **2**, 651–658.

189. Guiltinan, M. J., Marcotte, W. R., and Quatrano, R. S. (1990). A plant leucine zipper protein that recognizes an abscisic acid response element. *Science* **250**, 267–271.

190. Klimczak, L. J., Schindler, U., and Cashmore, A. R. (1992). DNA binding activity of the Arabidopsis G-box binding factor GBF1 is stimulated by phosphorylation by casein kinase II from broccoli. *Plant Cell* **4**, 87–98.

191. Schindler, U., Menkens, A. E., Beckmann, H., Ecker, J. R., and Cashmore, A. R. (1992). Heterodimerization between light-regulated and ubiquitously expressed *Arabidopsis* GBF bZIP proteins. *EMBO J.* **11**, 1261–1273.

192. Walker, C. W., Boom, J. D. G., and Marsh, A. G. (1992). First non-vertebrate member of the *myc* gene family is seasonally expressed in an invertebrate testis. *Oncogene* **7**, 2007–2012.

193. Meichle, A., Philipp, A., and Eilers, M. (1992). The functions of Myc proteins. *Biochim. Biophys. Acta* **1114**, 129–146.

194. Hahn, M. E., Poland, A., Glover, E., and Stegeman, J. J. (1992). The Ah receptor in marine animals: Phylogenetic distribution and relationship to cytochrome P4501A inducibility. *Mar. Environ. Res.* **34**, 87–92.

195. Ferré-D'Amaré, A. R., Prendergast, G. C., Ziff, E. B., and Burley, S. K. (1993).

Recognition by Max of its cognate DNA through a dimeric b/HLH/Z domain. *Nature (London)* **363**, 38–45.

196. Mueller, C. G. F., and Nordheim, A. (1991). A protein domain conserved between yeast MCM1 and human SRF directs ternary complex formation. *EMBO J.* **10**, 4219–4229.

197. Degnan, B. M., Degnan, S. M., Naganuma, T., and Morse, D. E. (1993). The *ets* multigene family is conserved throughout the metazoa. *Nucleic Acids Res.* **21**, 3479–3484.

198. Verrijzer, C. P., and Van der Vliet, P. C. (1993). POU domain transcription factors. *Biochim. Biophys. Acta* **1173**, 1–21.

199. Orii, H., Agata, K., and Watanabe, K. (1993). POU-domain genes in planarian *Dugesia japonica*: The structure and expression. *Biochem. Biophys. Res. Commun.* **192**, 1395–1402.

200. Bose, H. R. (1992). The Rel family: Models for transcriptional regulation and oncogenic transformation. *Biochim. Biophys. Acta* **1114**, 1–17.

201. Sun, S. C., and Faye, I. (1992). Cecropia immunoresponsive factor, an insect immunoresponsive factor with DNA-binding properties similar to nuclear-factor κB. *Eur. J. Biochem.* **204**, 885–892.

202. Nicoll, C. S. (1980). Ontogeny and evolution of prolactin's functions. *Fed. Proc. Fed. Am. Soc. Exp. Biol.* **39**, 2563–2566.

CHAPTER **16**

Pathogen – Endocrine System Interactions

I. Introduction

Hormones have long been associated with certain cancers (1,2): in humans, estrogens have been linked to breast and uterine tumors whereas prolactin (PRL) is associated with mammary tumors in rodents. Furthermore, certain endocrine deficiencies are known to have protective effects: untreated eunuchs do not develop prostate cancer and patients with untreated Turner's syndrome, which includes nonfunctional ovaries, do not develop breast cancer. Still, there has always been the question of whether these effects are direct or indirect. Are these hormones actually carcinogenic or do they merely induce a proliferative state that renders the tissue more susceptible to other agents?

Although the role of hormones in tumor induction is not clear, they are involved in the growth of certain tumors, most notably estrogens in breast and uterine cancers and androgens in prostate cancer. Furthermore, the appropriate endocrinectomy leads to remission. Unfortunately, even this association is variable; not all tumors are responsive and even those that initially respond frequently relapse. These discrepancies might be explained by proposing that hormones could have induced hormone-dependent tumors, which then developed the ability to synthesize their own hormones; at this point, the tumors became independent of exogenous hormones (3,4). Certainly, many tumors do produce peptide hormones not made in the original tissue, and although no nonadrenal nongonadal tumor can make steroids *de novo*, some mammary tumors do possess steroid-metabolizing enzymes that allow them to synthesize active steroids from circulating precursors. However, the presence of these ectopic hormones or enzymes does not always correlate with the hormone-independent state. Because of counterregulatory mechanisms in animals, the simple ectopic production of hormones may induce hyperplasia but does not appear to be sufficient for malignant transformation.

Rather, it appears necessary to modify these hormones, or some other component of their transduction pathway, so they remain active even in the face of counterregulatory measures. The genes encoding the normal proteins are called *proto-oncogenes* whereas those generating constitutively active signaling molecules are called *oncogenes*. However, one oncogene is still not sufficient; usually there must be at least two (5,6). The first oncogene is plasma membrane associated and induces *transformation*; transformation is the process by which cells become independent of environmental checks on cell growth. Such cells, for example, will grow in soft agar or will ignore cell–cell contacts and form multilayered cultures. The second oncogene is nucleus associated and induces *immortalization*; this is the process by which cells overcome senescence and is correlated with premalignancy. Most malignancies are associated with such pairs of oncogenes.

Certain viruses can also cause tumors and do so via the same mechanisms. Viruses are thought to be derived from pieces of the host genome that have acquired an independent existence. If these pieces contain a proto-oncogene, the potential exists for its mutation into an oncogene that can induce cancers. Indeed, all known viral oncogenes (v-*onc*) have cellular counterparts (c-*onc*). This is an excellent strategy: viruses only have limited space in their genome, but cell growth is a complex phenomenon requiring the coordination of many cellular processes. Rather than trying to control all these processes individually, the virus merely plugs into a pre-existing regulatory system: the mitogenic pathway (7).

II. Viral and Bacterial Genes

A. Virulence Genes and the Immune System

Many bacteria and viruses possess genes that do not directly cause toxicity or malignancy; instead, they facilitate the infection process. Such genes are called *virulence* genes and their products usually interfere with the immune system (Table 16-1; 8). Several viral proteins affect cytokine and steroid production. For example, interleukin-1β (IL-1β) is synthesized as a precursor that must be cleaved to its active form, like proinsulin and angiotensinogen (see Chapter 2). crmA is a *serine protease inhibitor (serpin)* that inhibits the IL-1β-converting enzyme. In a second example, IL-10 is a counterregulatory cytokine that keeps the immune system in check by inhibiting the synthesis of other cytokines; BCRF1 is an IL-10 homolog from the Epstein–Barr virus. Third, the vaccinia virus produces a homolog of the 3β-hydroxysteroid dehydrogenase (9); although its exact function is unknown, it would be reasonable to assume that it elevates glucocorticoids, which are known to be immunosuppressive. Finally, cytokines can also be neutralized by sequestration. Many viruses encode soluble cytokine receptors that are believed to act as sinks for the cytokines. These receptors include those for ILs, tumor necrosis factor (TNF) (8), and interferon γ (IFNγ) (10). Bacteria can use a similar strategy: the *Yersinia* genome contains a gene that encodes a homolog of the platelet membrane protein GPIbα (11). This protein is a general receptor for several components of the blood clotting system, including thrombin and von Willebrand factor, and mediates platelet activation. It is thought that the GPIbα homolog sequesters thrombin and blocks its role in inflammatory reactions.

Other pathogen products interfere with the signaling pathways: some bind C4b or C3b to block the complement pathway whereas others prevent the plasma membrane translocation of β_2-microglobulin or the major histocompatibility complex class I. Several viral products inhibit the interferon-induced protein kinase, which normally limits viral infection by phosphorylating eIF-2 and freezing translation (8,12). Others bind soluble tyrosine kinases, such as Lyn and Fyn, and prevent their activation of the polyphosphoinositide (PPI) pathway in B lymphocytes (13). Soluble tyrosine kinases are critical components of cytokine receptor transduction (see Chapter 6) and can be neutralized by protein tyrosine phosphatases, which several pathogenic bacteria produce (14).

Table 16-1

Some Pathogen–Immune Interactions

Target	Protein	Pathogen	Action
Cytokine synthesis	crmA	Cowpox[a]	Serpin that inhibits IL-1β converting enzyme
	BCRF1	Epstein–Barr[b]	IL-10 homolog; inhibits cytokine synthesis
	Sa1F7L	Vaccinia[a]	3β-Hydroxysteroid dehydrogenase
Cytokine sequestration	B15R, B18R	Vaccinia[a]	IL-1/IL-6-like receptors
	T2	Myxoma[a]	TNF receptor type I (soluble)
	T7	Myxoma[a]	IFNγ receptor (soluble)
	YOPM	*Yersinia*	GPIbα homolog; binds thrombin
Complement	VCP	Vaccinia[a]	Binds C4b; inhibits classical pathway
	CCPH	Herpes saimiri	Binds C4b; inhibits classical pathway
	gC-1	Herpes simplex	Binds C3b; inhibits both pathways
	gE-gI	Herpes simplex	Binds Fc of IgE
Antigen recognition	E3-gp19K	Adenovirus	Binds MHC-I and prevent translocation to surface
	UL18	Cytomegalovirus[b]	MHC-I homolog; binds β_2-microglobulin and prevent translocation surface
Phosphorylation[c]	VA	Adenovirus	Inhibits phosphorylation of eIF-2
	EBER	Epstein–Barr[b]	Inhibits phosphorylation of eIF-2
	LMP2A	Epstein–Barr[b]	Binds soluble tyrosine kinases; blocks calcium mobilization
	σ3	Reovirus	Inhibits phosphorylation of eIF-2
	TAR	Human immunodeficiency virus (HIV)[d]	Inhibits phosphorylation of eIF-2
	YOP2b, YOP51	*Yersinia*	Protein tyrosine phosphatases
Transcription	v-Re1	Reticuloendotheliosis virus[d]	NF-κB-like transcription factor (dominant inhibitor); may stimulate at some sites

[a] DNA poxviruses.

[b] DNA herpes viruses.

[c] VA (and possibly TAR) RNA binds to and inactivates the IFN-induced kinase. σ3 is a capsid protein that binds dsRNA.

[d] Retroviruses.

The major transduction pathways for immune cells often terminates with the transcription factor NF-κB. The hormone response element (HRE) for this factor appears in the 5' end of many defense genes and its inactivation would severely cripple the immune system. One viral protein, Rel, is a dominant inhibitor of this transcription factor.

B. Oncogenes and the Mitotic Pathway

Viral and bacterial products that actually induce tumor formation are related to the mitogenic pathway (Table 16-2; 15–18). First, these oncogene products are either mitogens, including fibroblast growth factor (FGF) and platelet-derived growth factor (PDGF), or enzymes that synthesize nonpeptide mitogens. The latter situation occurs in plants infected with *Agrobacterium tumefaciens*, which contains the Ti plasmid (19). This bacterium causes crown gall tumor, which can grow in culture without the plant growth hormones cytokinin and indoleacetic acid. The reason is simple: three of the seven genes on the plasmid encode enzymes that can synthesize these hormones from common precursors. Gene 4 encodes an isopentenyl transferase, which transfers an isopentenyl group to AMP to form a cytokinin (Fig. 16-1A; 20). The products of genes 1 and 2 are involved in the synthesis of indoleacetic acid (21). Gene 2 encodes an amidohydrolase and, although the product of gene 1 has not been positively identified, it is probably a tryptophan monooxygenase (Fig. 16-1B). This two-step pathway does occur in certain bacteria; however, in plants the synthesis of indoleacetic acid normally proceeds through indole-3-pyruvic acid and indole-3-acetaldehyde. *Agrobacterium rhizogenes* uses a different strategy: its oncogenes encode for glucosidases that liberate these plant mitogens form their inactive conjugates. The *rolB* and *rolC* genes produce indole β-glucosidase and cytokinin β-glucosidase, respectively (22,23).

Oncogenes can also encode receptors. Most of these receptors are receptor tyrosine kinases (RTKs) because of the central role they play in mitogenesis. All these receptors harbor some mutation that renders them constitutively active. The only exception is Erb-A, which is a truncated triiodothyronine (T_3) receptor and a dominant inhibitor. Since T_3 often induces developmental programs, it may be considered a differentiative hormone (see Chapter 2); as such, its inhibition would favor growth.

Many components of the transduction system are also found among the oncogene products: small and trimer G proteins, soluble tyrosine kinases, SH2 adaptors, and some protein kinases. For example, a mutant protein kinase Cα (PKCα) has been found in invasive pituitary adenomas (24). In addition, a chemical co-carcinogen targets PKC; the receptor for 12-O-tetradecanoylphorbol-13-acetate (TPA), a potent tumor promoter, is identical to this kinase (25).

Finally, oncogenes can encode transcription factors, only a few of which are shown in Table 16-2. Again, many of them are regulated by kinases

Table 16-2
Some Oncogene Products Associated with the Endocrine System

Group	Oncogene proteins[a]	Cellular homolog
Hormones	Int-2, Hst	FGF-like
	Sis	PDGF-like
	Ti plasmid[b]	Synthetic enzymes for cytokinin and indoleacetic acid, and glucosidases that release them from inactive conjugates
	NZ2, NZ7[c]	VEGF-like
Receptors		
Cytokine	Mp1	Hematopoietic factor receptor
Nuclear	Erb-A	T_3 receptor (dominant inhibitor)
Serpentine	ECRF3[d]	IL-8 receptor B
	US27, US28, UL33[d]	Macrophage inflammatory protein 1-α receptor
Tyrosine kinase	Erb-B, Neu	EGF-like receptors
	Flg, Bek	FGF-like receptor
	Fms	CSF-1 receptor
	Kit	PDGF-like receptor
	Met	Hepatic growth factor receptor
	Sea	Insulin-like receptor
	Trk, TrkB	Neurotropin receptors (high affinity)
Transducers	Crk	SH2 adaptor
	Ras	G-like protein (small)
	Gsp, Gip[e]	G-like protein (trimer)
	Raf(= Mil), Mos	Ser–Thr kinases that phosphorylate MAPKK
	Src, Lck, Fyn, etc.	Soluble tyrosine kinases associated with membrane receptors
Transcription factors	Elk-1	TCF (part of serum response factor complex)
	Fos, Jun	PKC-regulated transcription factor (AP-1)
	Myc, Max	CKII- and MAPK-regulated transcription factor

[a] From retroviruses unless otherwise noted.
[b] From *Agrobacterium tumefaciens* and *A. rhizogenes*.
[c] From orf virus (poxvirus).
[d] From human cytomegalovirus and herpesvirus saimiri (DNA herpesvirus).
[e] Mutated proto-oncogene; no viral counterpart known.

associated with the mitogenic pathway, including PKC, mitogen-activated protein kinase (MAPK), and casein kinase II (CKII).

All the proteins in Table 16-2 are mutated proto-oncogenes or microbial homologs of these proto-oncogenes. Viruses and other pathogens can also bind to, and in some cases activate, several hormone receptors without directly producing tumors, that is, they are not oncogenes but still represent a way of manipulating the endocrine system of the host (Table 16-3; 26–32). Two functions have been proposed for this interaction. First, it may represent a point of entry into the cell. Infection begins when the virus binds to a cell surface protein and hormone receptors are a good choice, since their distri-

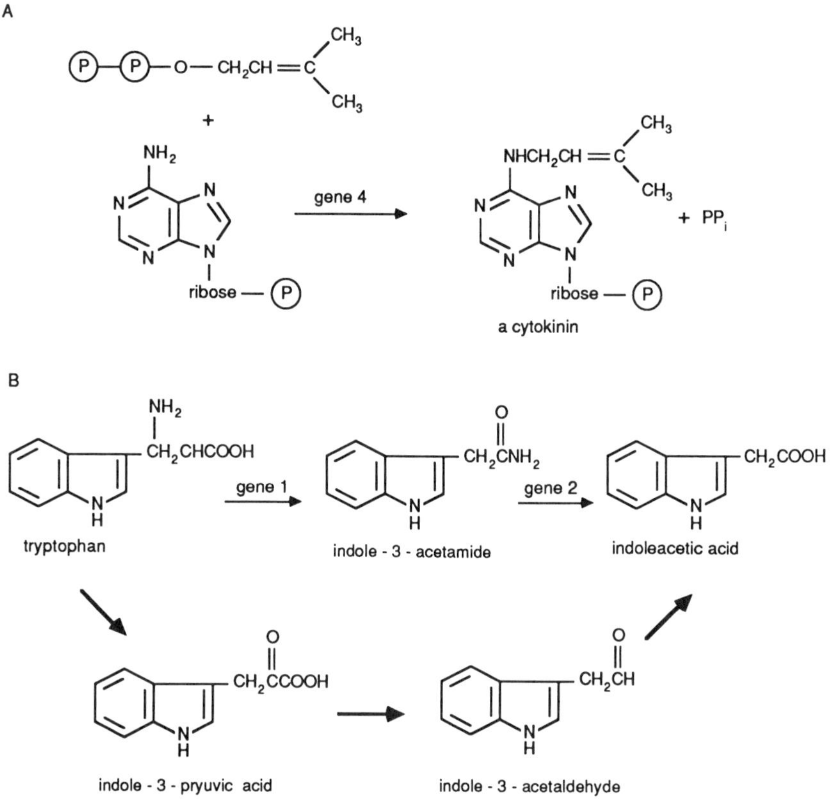

A

a cytokinin

B

tryptophan

indole - 3 - acetamide

indoleacetic acid

indole - 3 - pryuvic acid

indole - 3 - acetaldehyde

Fig. 16-1. Biosynthetic pathways for (A) cytokinins and (B) indoleacetic acid. Thin lines represent steps catalyzed by products of the Ti plasmid; heavy lines represent those steps that normally occur in plants.

Table 16-3
Some Hormone Receptors Bound by Pathogen Proteins for Activation or Cell Entry

Virus	Hormone receptor
Epstein–Barr virus	IFNα-C3d
Fibropapillomavirus	Platelet-derived growth factor
Friend spleen focus-forming virus	Erythropoietin
Herpes simplex type 1	Fibroblast growth factor[a]
Human immunodeficiency virus	CD4, nicotinic acetylcholine, glutamate
Plasmodium vivax (malaria)	IL-8-MGSA
Poxviruses	Epidermal growth factor
Rabies	Nicotine acetylcholine
Reovirus	β-Adrenergic; EGF

[a] Low affinity receptor (heparin) only.

bution is often restricted to certain target tissues. Second, it may stimulate the metabolic machinery of the cell in a way that favors viral replication. The cholera and pertussis toxins from bacteria may have a related function, although they act at the level of G proteins; cAMP is mitogenic in many tissues. These effects are similar to those evoked by the oncogenes; indeed, the difference may simply be one of degree.

In summary, the effects of pathogens on the endocrine system can be grouped into three major functions: (i) to gain entry into the cell (infection), (ii) to disable the immune system of the host (virulence), and (iii) to create an environment conducive to microbial reproduction (from mitogenesis to oncogenesis).

C. Hormone Regulation of Viral Expression

The relationship between hormones and oncogenes is bidirectional: not only do some oncogenes mimic the actions of hormones, but hormones can regulate the expression of oncogenes. Many viruses have HREs in the regulatory regions of their genomes (Table 16-4; 33–54). However, appearances can be deceiving: this is less an example of the host controlling the virus than of the virus sensing the endocrine status of the host to determine the best time to replicate.

The mouse mammary tumor virus (MMTV) is an excellent example. MMTV is a retrovirus that is propagated from mother to pups (55). The virus is induced primarily in the mammary gland during late pregnancy and lactation, when it is secreted into the milk; the pups are infected via suckling. The virus is then carried by T lymphocytes from the intestine to the mammary gland, where its RNA is transcribed into DNA that randomly integrates into the host genome (56). When the female pups mature and become pregnant, the cycle repeats itself. Actually, MMTV infects many tissues in the mouse and can be naturally expressed in the immune and reproductive systems, as well as in the salivary gland. However, expression in the mammary gland far exceeds that in any other tissue (57).

Based on this method of propagation, it is to the advantage of the virus to coordinate its reproductive cycle with that of its host; for example, viral production in the virgin would be futile. To this effect, the MMTV genome has a progesterone HRE in its 5' long terminal repeat (LTR) (33,38); progesterone levels are elevated in pregnancy and may initiate viral transcription at a time when milk production and suckling are imminent. The human papilloma virus also has HREs for sex steroid receptors and infects reproductive tissues (37). In this example, the virus would be activated at the same time that the tissue is stimulated by these steroids; this stimulated state may favor viral replication.

Reproduction in other tissues may require a different endocrine milieu. For example, in addition to mammary tumors, MMTV can cause T cell lymphomas. However, tumorigenesis in this tissue requires a deletion in the 5' LTR; this deletion removes a tissue-specific inhibitory region and creates a

Table 16-4
Some Tumor-Associated Viruses Containing HREs

Virus	HRE	Associated tumors
Mouse mammary tumor virus (MMTV)	Glucocorticoid–progesterone	Mammary
MMTV (deletion variant)	AP-1	T cell lymphomas
Human papilloma virus type 16	Glucocorticoid–progesterone	Anogenital
	Estrogen	
Human immunodeficiency virus	Glucocorticoid[a]	Kaposi's sarcoma
	RXR	
	NF-κB	
	Thyroid hormone	
	AP-1	
	C/EBPβ	
Epstein–Barr virus	Glucocorticoid[a]	Burkitt's lymphoma, nasopharyngeal carcinoma
Moloney murine leukemia virus	Glucocorticoid[b]	Leukemia
	Thyroid hormone	
Human T-cell leukemia virus type 1	cAMP	Leukemia
Herpes simplex virus	cAMP	Cervical carcinoma
	Thyroid hormone	
Polyoma virus	AP-1	Many
	Glucocorticoid-progesterone	
	Estrogen	
Hepatitis B virus	Retinoic acid (RXR)	Hepatocellular carcinoma

[a] Progesterone not tested.
[b] MLV provirus is also androgen inducible; progesterone not tested.

new AP-1 site (35,47). The immune system is primarily dependent on the PKC transduction system and many viruses that infect these tissues have HREs for AP-1 or NF-kB; an example of the latter would be the human immunodeficiency virus.

III. Anti-oncogenes

Mitosis is a complex process that is under both positive and negative control. In this section, the negative regulators will be considered. Because they inhibit mitosis, whereas oncogenes stimulate it, these mitotic inhibitors are often referred to as products of *anti-oncogenes* (58–61).

A. Transcription Regulators

Several anti-oncogene products affect transcription. The *retinoblastoma* (Rb) gene encodes a 105-kDa phosphoprotein whose loss can lead to the development of retinoblastomas (62,63). In its active hypophosphorylated state, Rb can bind and inhibit Abl, a soluble tyrosine kinase (64); Rb can also complex with several transcription factors and affect their activity. It binds to and inhibits Myc (65), DRTF1 (66), and Elf-1 (67), and converts E2F from a transcription activator to an inhibitor (68,69). However, Rb is not an exclusive inhibitor: it is a positive cofactor for MyoD (70). These effects are entirely consistent, since Rb inhibits those factors that stimulate mitosis (Myc) and facilitates those factors that suppress proliferation and induce differentiation (MyoD). There is some controversy over whether Rb itself can bind DNA and activate transcription. Most data suggest that its DNA binding is nonspecific; however, mutations in its DNA-binding domain (DBD) reduce growth, demonstrating a critical role for DNA binding in the action of Rb (71).

Rb can also inhibit mitosis by binding and inhibiting cyclin D, a regulatory subunit of the mitosis-associated kinase cell division cycle dependent kinase 2 (Cdc2) (72). However, this relationship is bidirectional: cyclin E binds both Rb and Cdc2, allowing the latter to phosphorylate and inactivate Rb (73,74). Phosphorylation may prevent the nuclear translocation of Rb (75). Rb levels can also be regulated: transforming growth factor-β (TGF-β) inhibits growth and elevates Rb levels. Furthermore, TGFβ, along with IFNα and IL-6, inhibits the phosphorylation of Rb (76,77).

Finally, Rb can be targeted by viral oncogene products. The active hypophosphorylated Rb is bound by E1A from the adenovirus, the large T antigen from SV40, E7 from the papilloma virus, and EBNA-5 from the Epstein–Barr virus (78–81). These oncogene products pull Rb off of the transcription factors and stabilize the free form. E1A also binds cyclin A–Cdc2 and may recruit the kinase to phosphorylate and inactivate Rb.

Another anti-oncogene product, *p53*, is a transcription factor whose loss is associated with colorectal cancers (62,82–84). It has an acidic amino-terminal transcriptional activation domain (TAD), a central region that can inhibit transcription, and a carboxy-terminal DBD that recognizes direct repeats of the TGCCT sequence (85). In addition to activating its own set of genes, it blocks the DNA binding and helicase activities of the T antigen DNA polymerase α, perhaps by binding to the replication protein A (86). It also binds to the TATA-binding protein (TBP) and interferes with the stable binding of both TBP and TFIIA to the TATA-box (87); however, p53 does not affect preformed initiation complexes or elongation (88). Finally, p53 is induced after DNA damage; these data have suggested that one of the physiological functions of p53 may be to block the cell cycle after DNA damage has occurred to allow for the repair of DNA (89).

Like Rb, p53 can be regulated by both phosphorylation and compartmentalization. DNA binding requires the phosphorylation of p53 by CKII (90,91). In addition, p53 may be sequestered in the cytoplasm during periods of rapid growth or metabolism; for example, p53 is excluded from the nucleus of lactating epithelial cells (92). This compartmentalization may be achieved by membrane receptors, since it has been reported that p53 binds to the cytoplasmic tail of the IFNα–C3d receptor (93); this association could provide a mechanism by which hormones may directly affect p53 localization.

p53 complexes with several oncogene products, including the large T antigen, E1B, E6, EBNA-5 (80), Mdm-2 (94), and the X antigen from the hepatitis B virus (95). The large T antigen and E1B trap p53 in inactive complexes, E6 tags p53 for destruction by ubiquitin (96), and Mdm-2 inhibits p53-mediated transcription by binding to the amino-terminal TAD of p53 (97). Actually, the nononcogenic form of Mdm-2 appears to be a physiological regulator of p53; the two proteins are mutually inhibitory and the net effect is determined by a balance between the two factors.

The *WT1* (Wilms' Tumor 1) gene is a zinc finger transcription factor; its loss is associated with Wilms' tumor (58,98,99). The amino terminus represses transcription and its central region activates transcription (100). These effects are often affected by its physical interaction with p53. For example, WT1 alone activates the transcription factor EGR-1, but the WT1–p53 complex converts EGR-1 to a repressor (101). However, the interaction between WT1 and p53 can be positive: WT1 enhances the transcriptional activity of p53 at the creatine kinase promoter. Part of its tumor-suppressing activity appears to be a result of its ability to repress the expression of several growth factors (102,103).

B. Protein Phosphatases

If many oncogene products are tyrosine kinases, then protein tyrosine phosphatases (PTPs) could be considered anti-oncogene products. Indeed, PTP genes are lost in a high percentage of some tumors (104), and overexpression of PTPs can suppress or even reverse transformation (105). Occasionally, the situation in malignancies is confused by the compensatory PTP increase, which occurs when the tumor is induced by a tyrosine kinase oncogene. In these cases, both the kinase and the PTP activities are elevated; however, the greater the ratio of kinase to PTP activity, the greater the aggressiveness of the tumor because there is a relative PTP deficiency (106). Other factors that can influence the effects of PTPs are substrate specificity and localization; unlike the serine–threonine phosphatases, some PTPs tend to be much more specialized with respect to substrate preferences, tissue distribution, and cellular localization (107).

Serine–threonine phosphatases are also anti-oncogene products (108,109). The A subunit of PP-2A can be bound by the small t antigen of SV40 and the polyoma middle T antigen. The latter is an integral membrane protein that sequesters the normally cytosolic PP-2A. The small t antigen decreases the phosphatase activity 50–70% on certain substrates, although total activity is unchanged. For example, PP-2A activities toward MAP kinase and its activator are reduced (110); persistent phosphorylation of these mitogen-associated kinases may favor oncogenesis. Activity toward Rb is also diminished, maintaining Rb in an inactive hyperphosphorylated state. In addition, these antigens may change the substrate specificity of PP-2A; for example, the PTP activity of PP-2A increases 10-fold relative to the serine – threonine phosphatase activity (111).

In addition to oncogene products, a chemical co-carcinogen targets serine – threonine phosphatases. *Okadaic acid*, a tumor promoter, is a potent inhibitor of both PP-1 and PP-2A.

C. Other Anti-oncogenes

Several other prominent anti-oncogene products do not fall into any of the already-mentioned classes. As noted earlier, mutated Ras, which is constitutively active, is oncogenic. However, another way to elevate Ras activity would be to inactivate GTPase-activating protein (GAP), which facilitates the hydrolysis of GTP bound to normal Ras and inactivates this G protein. No such mutations have been reported for RasGAP, but they have been identified in a GAP-like protein in patients with *neurofibromatosis type 1* (112). The physiological role for this protein is unknown, but it has a GAP-like domain and can enhance the GTPase activity of Ras; therefore, it may keep Ras in check. Most genomic mutations are located in the GAP-like region, and the clinical picture reflects growth and hyperactivity: neurofibromas and an increased risk of malignancies. Somatic mutations in this gene have also been reported in colon adenocarcinomas and anaplastic astrocytomas.

Since cell – cell and cell – substratum contacts are important in controlling cell growth, any factor promoting these contacts could also be considered a product of an anti-oncogene. The product of the *DCC* (*deleted in colon carcinoma*) gene is probably such a protein. DCC is a transmembrane protein with numerous fibronectin type III and immunoglobulin-like domains characteristic of cell adhesion molecules. NF2 may be another anti-oncogene in this class. A defective NF2 gene product is associated with vestibular schwannomas and multiple meningiomas, and is homologous to several proteins involved in coupling the integrin receptor to the cytoskeleton (113). A third candidate is *APC* (*adenomatous polyposis of the colon*); it binds β-catenin which is part of the cell junction complex (114,115). Finally, *VHL* (*von Hippel-Lindau disease*) inactivation is associated with vascular malformation in the retina and cerebellum. Its sequence contains several tandem repeats known to be involved in protein association and cell adhesion (116). All these anti-oncogenes may play roles in contact inhibition.

IV. Summary

Pathogens exploit the endocrine system to facilitate their infection and replication. They can use hormone receptors to gain entry into the cell, disable the immune system by blocking cytokine actions, and hijack the mitotic apparatus to create an environment conducive to replication. The last effect is usually accomplished by a viral homolog to a normal component of the growth factor signaling cascade; however, this homolog is mutated so it is constitutively active. Such proteins are called oncogenes; their normal cellular counterparts are called proto-oncogenes, because spontaneous mutations can render them oncogenic as well. These oncogene products can act at any level from hormones to transcription factors, but usually two are required: a membrane-associated protein that overcomes environmental checks and a nuclear one that overcomes senescence.

In addition to stimulating the mitogenic pathway, oncogenes can inhibit regulatory checks on this process. Such checks are the products of anti-oncogenes and involve blocking the effects of proliferation-associated transcription factors, reversing the phosphorylation of kinases, inactivating G proteins, and mediating contact inhibition. The loss of these anti-oncogenes or the inactivation of their products is often associated with malignancies.

References

General References

Beckage, N. E. (1993). Endocrine and neuroendocrine host–parasite relationship. *Receptor* **3**, 233–245.

Bryant, P. J. (1993). Towards the cellular functions of tumour suppressors: An introduction. *Trends Cell Biol.* **3**, 31–35.

Goodrich, D. W., and Lee, W. H. (1993). Molecular characterization of the retinoblastoma susceptibility gene. *Biochim. Biophys. Acta* **1155**, 43–61.

Kouzarides, T. (1993). Transcriptional regulation by the retinoblastoma protein. *Trends Cell Biol.* **3**, 211–213.

Marsh, M., and Pelchen-Matthews, A. (1993). Entry of animal viruses into cells. *Rev. Med. Virol.* **3**, 173–185.

Smith, M. R., Matthews, N. T., Jones, K. A., and Kung, H. (1993). Biological actions of oncogenes. *Pharmacol. Ther.* **58**, 211–236.

Walter, G., and Mumby, M. (1993). Protein serine/threonine phosphatases and cell transformation. *Biochim. Biophys. Acta* **1155**, 207–226.

See also Refs. 1–8, 15–18, 25, 44, 58–61, 83, 84, 98, 99, 108, 109, 111, and 113.

Cited References

1. Lippman, M. E., and Swain, S. M. (1992). Endocrine-responsive cancers of humans. *In* "Textbook of Endocrinology" (J. D. Wilson and D. W. Foster, eds.), 8th Ed., pp. 1577-1597. Saunders, Philadelphia.
2. Odell, W. D., and Appleton, W. S. (1992). Humoral manifestations of cancer. *In* "Textbook of Endocrinology" (J. D. Wilson and D. W. Foster, eds.), 8th ed., pp. 1599–1617. Saunders, Philadelphia.
3. Kasid, A., and Lippman, M. E. (1987). Estrogen and oncogene mediated growth regulation of human breast cancer cells. *J. Steroid Biochem.* **27**, 465–470.
4. Dickson, R. B., Johnson, M. D., Bano, M., Shi, E., Kurebayashi, J., Ziff, B., Martinez-Lacaci, I., Amundadottir, L. T., and Lippman, M. E. (1992). Growth factors in breast cancer: Mitogenesis to transformation. *J. Steroid Biochem. Mol. Biol.* **43**, 69–78.

5. Herrlich, P., and Ponta, H. (1989). "Nuclear" oncogenes convert extracellular stimuli into changes in the genetic program. *Trends Genet.* **5**, 112–116.
6. Weinberg, R. A. (1989). Oncogenes, antioncogenes, and the molecular bases of multistep carcinogenesis. *Cancer Res.* **49**, 3713–3721.
7. Todaro, G. J. (1982). Autocrine secretion of peptide growth factors by tumor cells. *Natl. Cancer Inst. Monogr.* **60**, 139–147.
8. Gooding, L. R. (1992). Virus proteins that counteract host immune defenses. *Cell* **71**, 5–7.
9. Moore, J. B., and Smith, G. L. (1992). Steroid hormone synthesis by a vaccinia enzyme: A new type of virus virulence factor. *EMBO J.* **11**, 1973–1980.
10. Upton, C., Mossman, K., and McFadden, G. (1992). Encoding of a homolog of the IFN-γ receptor by myxoma virus. *Science* **258**, 1369–1372.
11. Bliska, J. B., Galán, J. E., and Falkow, S. (1993). Signal transduction in the mammalian cell during bacterial attachment and entry. *Cell* **73**, 903–920.
12. Lloyd, R. M., and Shatkin, A. J. (1992). Translational stimulation by reovirus polypeptide σ3: Substitution for VAI RNA and inhibition of phosphorylation of the α subunit of eukaryotic initiation factor 2. *J. Virol.* **66**, 6878–6884.
13. Miller, C. L., Longnecker, R., and Kieff, E. (1993). Epstein–Barr virus latent membrane protein 2A blocks calcium mobilization in B lymphocytes. *J. Virol.* **67**, 3087–3094.
14. Guan, K., and Dixon, J. E. (1990). Protein tyrosine phosphatase activity of an essential virulence determinant in *Yersinia. Science* **249**, 553–556.
15. Macara, I. G. (1989). Oncogenes and cellular signal transduction. *Physiol. Rev.* **69**, 797–820.
16. Storms, R. W., and Bose, H. R. (1989). Viral oncogenes and signal transduction. *Virus Res.* **12**, 251–282.
17. Aaronson, S. A. (1991). Growth factors and cancer. *Science* **254**, 1146–1153.
18. Cantley, L. C., Auger, K. R., Carpenter, C., Duckworth, B., Graziani, A., Kapeller, R., and Soltoff, S. (1991). Oncogenes and signal transduction. *Cell* **64**, 281–302.
19. Weiler, E. W., and Schroder, J. (1987). Hormone genes and crown gall disease. *Trends Biochem. Sci.* **12**, 271–275.
20. Buchmann, I., Marner, F. J., Schröder, G., Waffenschmidt, S., and Schröder, J. (1985). Tumour genes in plants: T-DNA encoded cytokinin biosynthesis. *EMBO J.* **4**, 853–859.
21. Thomashow, M. F., Hugly, S., Buchholz, W. G., and Thomashow, L. S. (1986). Molecular basis for the auxin-independent phenotype of crown gall tumor tissues. *Science* **231**, 616–618.
22. Estruch, J. J., Chriqui, D., Grossman, K., Schell, J., and Spena, A. (1991). The plant oncogene *rolC* is responsible for the release of cytokinins from glucoside conjugates. *EMBO J.* **10**, 2889–2895.
23. Estruch, J. J., Schell, J., and Spena, A. (1991). The protein encoded by the *rolB* plant oncogene hydrolyses indole glucosides. *EMBO J.* **10**, 3125–3128.
24. Alvaro, V., Lévy, L., Dubray, C., Roche, A., Peillon, F., Quérat, B., and Joubert, D. (1993). Invasive human pituitary tumors express a point-mutated α-protein kinase-C. *J. Clin. Endocrinol. Metab.* **77**, 1125–1129.
25. Ashendel, C. L. (1985). The phorbol ester receptor: A phospholipid-regulated protein kinase. *Biochim. Biophys. Acta* **822**, 219–242.
26. Bracci, L., Lozzi, L., Rustici, M., and Neri, P. (1992). Binding of HIV-1 gp120 to the nicotinic receptor. *FEBS Lett.* **311**, 115–118.

27. Goldstein, D. J., Andersson, T., Sparkowski, J. J., and Schlegel, R. (1992). The BPV-1 E5 protein, the 16 kDa membrane pore-forming protein and the PDGF receptor exist in a complex that is dependent on hydrophobic transmembrane interactions. *EMBO J.* **11**, 4851–4859.

28. Shieh, M. T., WuDunn, D., Montgomery, R. I., Esko, J. D., and Spear, P. G. (1992). Cell surface receptors for herpes simplex virus are heparan sulfate proteoglycans. *J. Cell Biol.* **116**, 1273–1281.

29. Zon, L. I., Moreau, J. F., Koo, J. W., Mathey-Prevot, B., and D'Andrea, A. D. (1992). The erythropoietin receptor transmembrane region is necessary for activation by the Friend spleen focus-forming virus gp55 glycoprotein. *Mol. Cell. Biol.* **12**, 2949–2957.

30. Hanham, C. A., Zhao, F., and Tignor, G. H. (1993). Evidence from the anti-idiotypic network that the acetylcholine receptor is a rabies virus receptor. *J. Virol.* **67**, 530–542.

31. Ushijima, H., Ando, S., Kunisada, T., Schroder, H. C., Klocking, H. P., Kijjoa, A., and Muller, W. E. G. (1993). HIV-1 gp120 and NMDA induce protein kinase C translocation differentially in rat primary neuronal culture. *J. Acq. Immune Def. Syndr.* **6**, 339–343.

32. Horuk, R., Chitnis, C. E., Darbonne, W. C., Colby, T. J., Rybicki, A., Hadley, T. J., and Miller, L. H. (1993). A receptor for the malarial parasite *Plasmodium vivax*: The erythrocyte chemokine receptor. *Science* **261**, 1182–1184.

33. Cato, A. C. B., Henderson, D., and Ponta, H. (1987). The hormone response element of the mouse mammary tumour virus DNA mediates the progestin and androgen induction of transcription in the proviral long terminal repeat region. *EMBO J.* **6**, 363–368.

34. Speck, N. A., and Baltimore, D. (1987). Six distinct nuclear factors interact with the 75-base-pair repeat of the Moloney murine leukemia virus enhancer. *Mol. Cell. Biol.* **7**, 1101–1110.

35. Ball, J. K., Diggelmann, H., Dekaban, G. A., Grossi, G. F., Semmler, R., Waight, P. A., and Fletcher, R. F. (1988). Alterations in the U_3 region of the long terminal repeat of an infectious thymotropic type B retrovirus. *J. Virol.* **62**, 2985–2993.

36. Martin, M. E., Piette, J., Yaniv, M., Tang, W. J., and Folk, W. R. (1988). Activation of the polyomavirus enhancer by a murine activator protein 1 (AP1) homolog and two contiguous proteins. *Proc. Natl. Acad. Sci. U.S.A.* **85**, 5839–5843.

37. Pater, M. M., Hughes, G. A., Hyslop, D. E., Nakshatri, H., and Pater, A. (1988). Glucocorticoid-dependent oncogenic transformation by type 16 but not type 11 human papilloma virus DNA. *Science* **335**, 832–835.

38. Bradham, B. M., and Bolander, F. F. (1989). The role of sex steroids in the expression of MMTV in the normal mouse mammary gland. *Biochem. Biophys. Res. Commun.* **159**, 1020–1025.

39. Poteat, H. T., Kadison, P., McGuire, K., Park, L., Park, R. E., Sodroski, J. G., and Haseltine, W. A. (1989). Response of the human T-cell leukemia virus type 1 long terminal repeat to cyclic AMP. *J. Virol.* **63**, 1604–1611.

40. Furth, P. A., Westphal, H., and Hennighausen, L. (1990). Expression from the HIV-LTR is stimulated by glucocorticoids and pregnancy. *AIDS Res. Hum. Retroviruses* **6**, 553–560.

41. Kupfer, S. R., and Summers, W. C. (1990). Identification of a glucocorticoid-responsive element in Epstein–Barr virus. *J. Virol.* **64**, 1984–1990.

42. Leib, D. A., Nadeau, K. C., Rundle, S. A., and Schaffer, P. A. (1991). The promoter of the latency-associated transcripts of herpes simplex virus type 1

contains a functional cAMP-response element: Role of the latency-associated transcripts and cAMP in reactivation of viral latency. *Proc. Natl. Acad. Sci. U.S.A.* **88**, 48–52.

43. Schuster, C., Chasserot-Golaz, S., Urier, G., Beck, G., and Sergeant, A. (1991). Evidence for a functional glucocorticoid responsive element in the Epstein – Barr virus genome. *Mol. Endocrinol.* **5**, 267–272.
44. zur Hausen, H. (1991). Viruses in human cancers. *Science* **254**, 1167–1173.
45. Ghosh, D. (1992). Glucocorticoid receptor-binding site in the human immunodeficiency virus long terminal repeat. *J. Virol.* **66**, 586–590.
46. Huan, B., and Sidiqui, A. (1992). Retinoid X receptor RXRα binds to and transactivates the hepatitis B virus enhancer. *Proc. Natl. Acad. Sci. U.S.A.* **89**, 9059–9063.
47. Miller, C. L., Garner, R., and Paetkau, V. (1992). An activation-dependent, T-lymphocyte-specific transcriptional activator in the mouse mammary tumor virus *env* gene. *Mol. Cell. Biol.* **12**, 3262–3272.
48. Park, H. Y., Davidson, D., Raaka, B. M., and Samuels, H. H. (1993). The herpes simplex virus thymidine kinase gene promoter contains a novel thyroid hormone response element. *Mol. Endocrinol.* **7**, 319–330.
49. Desai-Yajnik, V., and Samuels, H. H. (1993). The NF-κB and Sp1 motifs of the human immunodeficiency virus type 1 long terminal repeat function as novel thyroid hormone response elements. *Mol. Cell. Biol.* **13**, 5057–5069.
50. Soudeyns, H., Geleziunas, R., Shyamala, G., Hiscott, J., and Wainberg, M. A. (1993). Identification of a novel glucocorticoid response element within the genome of the human immunodeficiency virus type 1. *Virology* **194**, 758–768.
51. Tesmer, V. M., Rajadhyaksha, A., Babin, J., and Bina, M. (1993). NF-IL6-mediated transcriptional activation of the long terminal repeat of the human immunodeficiency virus type 1. *Proc. Natl. Acad. Sci. U.S.A.* **90**, 7298–7302.
52. Tesmer, V. M., Rajadhyaksha, A., Babin, J., and Bina, M. (1993). NF-IL6-mediated transcriptional activation of the long terminal repeat of the human immunodeficiency virus type 1. *Proc. Natl. Acad. Sci. U.S.A.* **90**, 7298–7302.
53. Ladias, J. A. A. (1994). Convergence of multiple nuclear receptor signaling pathways onto the long terminal repeat of human immunodeficiency virus-1. *J. Biol. Chem.* **269**, 5944–5951.
54. Moens, U., Subramaniam, N., Johansen, B., Johansen, T., and Traavik, T. (1994). A steroid hormone response unit in the late leader of the noncoding control region of the human polyomavirus BK confers enhanced host cell permissivity. *J. Virol.* **68**, 2398–2408.
55. Nandi, S., and McGrath, C. M. (1973). Mammary neoplasia in mice. *Adv. Cancer Res.* **17**, 353–414.
56. Tsubura, A., Inaba, M., Imai, S., Murakami, A., Oyaizu, N., Yasumizu, R., Ohnishi, Y., Tanaka, H., Morii, S., and Ikehara, S. (1988). Intervention of T-cells in transportation of mouse mammary tumor virus (milk factor) to mammary gland cells *in vivo. Cancer Res.* **48**, 6555–6559.
57. Ponta, H., Gunzburg, W. H., Salmons, B., Groner, B., and Herrlich, P. (1985). Mouse mammary tumour virus: A proviral gene contributes to the understanding of eukaryotic gene expression and mammary tumorigenesis. *J. Gen. Virol.* **66**, 931–943.
58. Marshall, C. J. (1991). Tumor suppressor genes. *Cell* **64**, 313–326.
59. Weinberg, R. A. (1991). Tumor suppressor genes. *Science* **254**, 1138–1146.

60. Bryant, P. J. (1993). Towards the cellular functions of tumour suppresors: An introduction. *Trends Cell Biol.* **3**, 31–35.
61. Knudson, A. G. (1993). Antioncogenes and human cancer. *Proc. Natl. Acad. Sci. U.S.A.* **90**, 10914–10921.
62. Levine, A. J., and Momand, J. (1990). Tumor suppressor genes: The p53 and retinoblastoma sensitivity genes and gene products. *Biochim. Biophys. Acta* **1032**, 119–136.
63. Wiman, K. G. (1993). The retinoblastoma gene: role in cell cycle control and cell differentiation. *FASEB J.* **7**, 841–845.
64. Welch, P. J., and Wang, J. Y. J. (1993). A C-terminal protein-binding domain in the retinoblastoma protein regulates nuclear c-Ab1 tyrosine kinase in the cell cycle. *Cell* **75**, 779–790.
65. Rustgi, A. K., Dyson, N., and Bernards, R. (1991). Amino-terminal domains of c-*myc* and N-*myc* proteins mediate binding to the retinoblastoma gene product. *Nature (London)* **352**, 541–544.
66. Zamanian, M., and La Thangue, N. B. (1992). Adenovirus E1a prevents the retinoblastoma gene product from repressing the activity of a cellular transcription factor. *EMBO J.* **11**, 2603–2610.
67. Wang, C. Y., Petryniak, B., Thompson, C. B., Kaelin, W. G., and Leiden, J. M. (1993). Regulation of the Ets-related transcription factor Elf-1 by binding to the retinoblastoma protein. *Science* **260**, 1330–1335.
68. Ray, S. K., Arroyo, M., Bagchi, S., and Raychaudhuri, P. (1992). Identification of a 60-kilodalton Rb-binding protein, RBP60, that allows the Rb-E2F complex to bind DNA. *J. Biol. Chem.* **267**, 4327–4333.
69. Weintraub, S. J., Prater, C. A., and Dean, D. C. (1992). Retinoblastoma protein switches the E2F site from positive to negative element. *Nature (London)* **358**, 259–261.
70. Gu, W., Schneider, J. W., Condorelli, G., Kaushal, S., Mahdavi, V., and Nadal-Ginard, B. (1993). Interaction of myogenic factors and the retinoblastoma protein mediates muscle cell commitment and differentiation. *Cell* **72**, 309–324.
71. Stirdivant, S. M., Huber, H. E., Patrick, D. R., Defeo-Jones, D., McAvoy, E. M., Garsky, V. M., Oliff, A., and Heimbrook, D. C. (1992). Human papillomavirus type 16 E7 protein inhibits DNA binding by the retinoblastoma gene product. *Mol. Cell. Biol.* **12**, 1905–1914.
72. Dowdy, S. F., Hinds, P. W., Louie, K., Reed, S. I., Arnold, A., and Weinberg, R. A. (1993). Physical interaction of the retinoblastoma protein with human D cyclins. *Cell* **73**, 499–511.
73. Lees, J. A., Buchkovich, K. J., Marshak, D. R., Anderson, C. W., and Harlow, E. (1991). The retinoblastoma protein is phosphorylated on multiple sites by human cdc2. *EMBO J.* **10**, 4279–4290.
74. Hu, Q., Lees, J. A., Buchkovich, K. J., and Harlow, E. (1992). The retinoblastoma protein physically associates with the human cdc2 kinase. *Mol. Cell. Biol.* **12**, 971–980.
75. Templeton, D. J. (1992). Nuclear binding of purified retinoblastoma gene product is determined by cell cycle-regulated phosphorylation. *Mol. Cell. Biol.* **12**, 435–443.
76. Laiho, M., DeCaprio, J. A., Ludlow, J. W., Livingston, D. M., and Massagué, J. (1990). Growth inhibition by TGF-β linked to suppression of retinoblastoma protein phosphorylation. *Cell* **62**, 175–185.

77. Resnitzky, D., Tiefenbrun, N., Berissi, H., and Kimchi, A. (1992). Interferons and interleukin 6 suppress phosphorylation of the retinoblastoma protein in growth-sensitive hematopoietic cells. *Proc. Natl. Acad. Sci. U.S.A.* **89**, 402–406.
78. Bagchi, S., Weinmann, R., and Raychaudhuri, P. (1991). The retinoblastoma protein copurifies with E2F-I, an E1A-regulated inhibitor of the transcription factor E2F. *Cell* **65**, 1063–1072.
79. Chellappan, S. P., Hiebert, S., Mudryj, M., Horowitz, J. M., and Nevins, J. R. (1991). The E2F transcription factor is a cellular target for the RB protein. *Cell* **65**, 1053–1061.
80. Chittenden, T., Livingston, D. M., and Kaelin, W. G. (1991). The T/E1A-binding domain of the retinoblastoma product can interact selectively with a sequence-specific DNA-binding protein. *Cell* **65**, 1073–1082.
81. Szekely, L., Selivanova, G., Magnusson, K. P., Klein, G., and Wiman, K. G. (1993). EBNA-5, an Epstein–Barr virus-encoded nuclear antigen, binds to the retinoblastoma and p53 proteins. *Proc. Natl. Acad. Sci. U.S.A.* **90**, 5455–5459.
82. Levine, A. J. (1990). The p53 protein and its interactions with the oncogene products of the small DNA tumor viruses. *Virology* **177**, 419–426.
83. Donehower, L. A., and Bradley, A. (1993). The tumor suppressor p53. *Biochim. Biophys. Acta* **1155**, 181–205.
84. Zambetti, G. P., and Levine, A. J. (1993). A comparison of the biological activities of wild-type and mutant p53. *FASEB J.* **7**, 855–865.
85. Foord, O. S., Bhattacharya, P., Reich, Z., and Rotter, V. (1991). A DNA binding domain is contained in the C-terminus of *wild type* p53 protein. *Nucleic Acids Res.* **19**, 5191–5198.
86. Li, R., and Botchan, M. R. (1993). The acidic transcriptional activation domains of VP16 and p53 bind the cellular replication protein A and stimulate in vitro BPV-1 DNA replication. *Cell* **73**, 1207–1221.
87. Martin, D. W., Muñoz, R. M., Subler, M. A., and Deb, S. (1993). p53 binds to the TATA-binding protein-TATA complex. *J. Biol. Chem.* **268**, 13062–13067.
88. Ragimov, N., Krauskopf, A., Navot, N., Rotter, V., Oren, M., and Aloni, Y. (1993). Wild-type but not mutant p53 can repress transcription initiation *in vitro* by interfering with the binding of basal transcription factors to the TATA motif. *Oncogene* **8**, 1183–1193.
89. Levine, A. J. (1993). The tumor suppressor genes. *Annu. Rev. Biochem.* **62**, 623–651.
90. Hupp, T. R., Meek, D. W., Midgley, C. A., and Lane, D. P. (1992). Regulation of the specific DNA binding function of p53. *Cell* **71**, 875–886.
91. Milne, D. M., Palmer, R. H., and Meek, D. W. (1992). Mutation of the casein kinase II phosphorylation site abolishes the anti-proliferative activity of p53. *Nucleic Acids Res.* **20**, 5565–5570.
92. Moll, U. M., Riou, G., and Levine, A. J. (1992). Two distinct mechanisms alter p53 in breast cancer: Mutation and nuclear exclusion. *Proc. Natl. Acad. Sci. U.S.A.* **89**, 7262–7266.
93. Frade, R., Gauffre, A., Hermann, J., and Barel, M. (1992). EBV/C3d receptor (CR2) interacts by its intracytoplasmic carboxy-terminal domain and two distinct binding sites with the p53 anti-oncoprotein and the p68 calcium-binding protein. *J. Immunol.* **149**, 3232–3238.
94. Momand, J., Zambetti, G. P., Olson, D. C., George, D., and Levine, A. J. (1992). The *mdm-2* oncogene product forms a complex with the p53 protein and inhibits p53-mediated transactivation. *Cell* **69**, 1237–1245.

95. Feitelson, M. A., Zhu, M., Duan, L. X., and London, W. T. (1993). Hepatitis B X antigen and p53 are associated *in vitro* and in liver tissues from patients with primary hepatocellular carcinoma. *Oncogene* **8**, 1109–1117.

96. Lechner, M. S., Mack, D. H., Finicle, A. B., Crook, T., Vousden, K. H., and Laimins, L. A. (1992). Human papillomavirus E6 proteins bind p53 *in vivo* and abrogate p53-mediated repression of transcription. *EMBO J.* **11**, 3045–3052.

97. Chen, J., Marechal, V., and Levine, A. J. (1993). Mapping of the p53 and mdm-2 interaction domains. *Mol. Cell. Biol.* **13**, 4107–4114.

98. Rauscher, F. J. (1993). The WT1 Wilms tumor gene product: a developmentally regulated transcription factor in the kidney that functions as a tumor suppressor. *FASEB J.* **7**, 896–903.

99. Huff, V., and Saunders, G. F. (1993). Wilms tumor genes. *Biochim. Biophys. Acta* **1155**, 295–306.

100. Wang, Z. Y., Qiu, Q. Q., and Deuel, T. F. (1993). The Wilms' tumor gene product WT1 activates or suppresses transcription through separate functional domains. *J. Biol. Chem.* **268**, 9172–9175.

101. Maheswaran, S., Park, S., Bernard, A., Morris, J. F., Rauscher, F. J., Hill, D. E., and Haber, D. A. (1993). Physical and functional interaction between WT1 and p53 proteins. *Proc. Natl. Acad. Sci. U.S.A.* **90**, 5100–5104.

102. Rauscher, F. J. (1993). The WT1 Wilms tumor gene product: A developmentally regulated transcription factor in the kidney that functions as a tumor suppressor. *FASEB J.* **7**, 896–903.

103. Harrington, M. A., Konicek, B., Song, A., Xia, X., Fredericks, W. J., and Rauscher, F. J. (1993). Inhibition of colony-stimulating factor-1 promoter activity by the product of the Wilms' tumor locus. *J. Biol. Chem.* **268**, 21271–21275.

104. Fischer, E. H., Charbonneau, H., and Tonks, N. K. (1991). Protein tyrosine phosphatases: A diverse family of intracellular and transmembrane enzymes. *Science* **253**, 401–406.

105. Ramponi, G., Ruggiero, M., Raugei, G., Berti, A., Modesti, A., Deglinnocenti, D., Magnelli, L., Pazzagli, C., Chiarugi, V. P., and Camici, G. (1992). Overexpression of a synthetic phosphotyrosine protein phosphatase gene inhibits normal and transformed cell growth. *Int. J. Cancer* **51**, 652–656.

106. Zhai, Y. F., Beittenmiller, H., Wang, B., Gould, M. N., Oakley, C., Esselman, W. J., and Welsch, C. W. (1993). Increased expression of specific protein tyrosine phosphatases in human breast epithelial cells neoplastically transformed by the *neu* oncogene. *Cancer Res.* **53**, 2272–2278.

107. Zander, N. F., Cool, D. E., Diltz, C. D., Rohrschneider, L. R., Krebs, E. G., and Fischer, E. H. (1993). Suppression of v-*fms*-induced transformation by overexpression of a truncated T-cell protein tyrosine phosphatase. *Oncogene* **8**, 1175–1182.

108. Mumby, M. C., and Walter, G. (1991). Protein phosphatases and DNA tumor viruses: Transformation through the back door? *Cell Regul.* **2**, 589–598.

109. Fujiki, H. (1992). Is the inhibition of protein phosphatase 1 and 2A activities a general mechanism of tumor promotion in human cancer development? *Mol. Carcinogen.* **5**, 91–94.

110. Sontag, E., Fedorov, S., Kamibayashi, C., Robbins, D., Cobb, M., and Mumby, M. (1993). The interaction of SV40 small tumor antigen with protein phosphatase 2A stimulates the MAP kinase pathway and induces cell proliferation. *Cell* **75**, 887–897.

111. Cayla, X., Ballmer-Hofer, K., Merlevede, W., and Goris, J. (1993). Phosphatase

2A associated with polyomavirus small-T or middle-T antigen is an okadaic acid-sensitive tyrosyl phosphatase. *Eur. J. Biochem.* **214,** 281–286.

112. Gutmann, D. H., and Collins, F. S. (1993). The neurofibromatosis type 1 gene and its protein product, neurofibromin. *Neuron* **10,** 335–343.
113. Weinberg, R. (1993). Tumor suppressor genes. *Neuron* **11,** 191–196.
114. Rubinfeld, B., Souza, B., Albert, I., Müller, O., Chamberlain, S. H., Masiarz, F. R., Munemitsu, S., and Polakis, P. (1993). Association of the *APC* gene product with β-catenin. *Science* **262,** 1731–1734.
115. Su, L. K., Vogelstein, B., and Kinzler, K. W. (1993). Association of the APC tumor suppressor protein with catenins. *Science* **262,** 1734–1737.
116. Latif, F., Tory, K., Gnarra, J., Yao, M., Duh, F. M., Orcutt, M. L., Stackhouse, T., Kuzmin, I., Modi, W., Geil, L., Schmidt, L., Zhou, F., Li, H., Wei, M. H., Chen, F., Glenn, G., Choyke, P., Walther, M. M., Weng, Y., Duan, D. S. R., Dean, M., Glavać, D., Richards, F. M., Crossey, P. A., Ferguson-Smith, M. A., Le Paslier, D., Chumalov, I., Cohen, D., Chinault, A. C., Maher, E. R., Linehan, W. M., Zbar, B., and Lerman, M. I. (1993). Identification of the von Hippel–Lindau disease tumor suppressor gene. *Science* **260,** 1317–1320.

CHAPTER 17

Molecular Bases of Endocrinopathies

CHAPTER OUTLINE

I. Introduction

Not long ago, clinical endocrinology was very simple: virtually all endocrine diseases involved too much or too little of a certain hormone. If the patient had too little, one administered the appropriate hormone or its agonist; if the patient had too much, one could either partially remove the gland or chemically suppress hormonal synthesis. Technology was not advanced enough to determine why there was too much or too little hormone, but now recombinant DNA techniques have identified the molecular bases for a number of endocrinopathies.

II. Hormones

A. Peptide Hormones

The simplest mechanism for a hypoendocrinopathy is not to have the gene for that hormone. This occurs in *isolated GH deficiency, type IA* (1). There are, in fact two human growth hormone (hGH) genes and both of them, as well as three placental lactogen genes, are clustered along a 48-kb (kilobase) stretch of DNA (Fig. 17–1). hGH-N is expressed in the pituitary gland, whereas hGH-V is expressed in the placenta (2). Human placental lactogen-L (hPL-L) is inactive because an intron mutation blocks proper splicing, but both hPL-A and hPL-B are normal and contribute to serum levels during pregnancy (3).

In isolated GH deficiency, type IA, hGN-N is deleted (1). Although hGH-V remains, it is not secreted from pituitary glands, so patients are short and susceptible to hypoglycemia (see Chapter 2). Several hPL deletions have also been described: isolated hPL-A deletion, hPL-A–hGH-V–hPL-B deletion, and so on. These deletions have no clinical effects in pregnant patients, suggesting that, despite the high levels of hPL found during pregnancy, it serves no essential function. In the triple deletion, growth is normal; this finding confirms the nonfunctional nature of hGH-V in the adult. These multiple deletions occur with relatively high frequency in this region of the genome as a result of recombination among homologous adjacent sequences (4).

Another possible mechanism for a hypoendocrinopathy is to have a defective hormone. These mutations have been suspected for a long time, because certain patients would present with classic signs and symptoms of a hormone deficiency, but hormone levels measured by radioimmunoassay were normal or elevated. There had to be a defective hormone or an end-or-

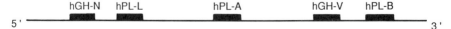

Fig. 17-1. The organization of the hGH–hPL gene cluster.

gan resistance and, since these patients responded normally to exogenous hormone, the latter possibility could be eliminated. Unfortunately, hormones are present in such low concentrations that it is impossible to purify sufficient hormone from a single individual for analysis. In contrast, there are several hundred hemoglobin mutants that have been identified because hemoglobin is present in the blood at a concentration of 15 *grams* per 100 ml. Furthermore, it is neatly packaged in erythrocytes, which in mammals contain little else; purification is quick and simple. Insulin concentrations in serum, however, are only 0.1–0.6 *micrograms* per 100 ml, depending on whether the patient is fasted or fed, respectively. Today, it is easier to purify and clone the gene than to purify the protein; this approach has revealed several mutant hormones.

Insulin deficiency results in *diabetes mellitus* and several mutant insulins have been characterized (5). V3L[1] in the A chain and both F24S and F25L in the B chain have been identified in patients with diabetes. All three residues occur in the receptor-binding domain of insulin. Point mutations have also been described for human GH (6), thyroid-stimulating hormone β (TSHβ) (7), luteinizing hormone β (LHβ) (8), follicle-stimulating hormone β (FSHβ) (9), angiotensinogen (10,11), and the Müllerian inhibiting substance (12) (Table 17–1). The mutant angiotensinogen is of particular interest because of its association with essential hypertension and pre-eclampsia, a form of pregnancy-associated hypertension. Serum levels of angiotensinogen are elevated, suggesting that this mutation may affect the clearance of this hormone. In mice, point mutations and truncations in macrophage colony-stimulating factor (M-CSF) are responsible for the disease mouse osteopetrosis (13,14).

In addition to intrinsic mutations, processing defects have also been described: insulin is synthesized as a single peptide containing a temporary C bridge between the A and B subunits (see Chapter 2). This C peptide is flanked by pairs of basic amino acids that are substrates for a trypsin-like protease. In familial hyperproinsulinemia, the B–C junction is cleaved normally but the A–C junction is not, so the C peptide is retained (5). This latter junction is demarcated by a pair of basic residues at positions 64 and 65; R65H and R65L mutants disrupt this cleavage site. The patients do not have diabetes, because the semi-cleaved proinsulin has 60% of the biological activity of normal insulin and the pancreas makes up the difference by secreting more hormone to elevate the serum levels.

Both antidiuretic hormone (ADH) and its neurophysin are cleaved from a single polyprotein. In *familial neurohypophyseal diabetes insipidus*, the G29V mutation does not alter either ADH, which is located at the amino terminus, or its cleavage site. However, the neurophysin is required for processing and

---

[1] Point mutations are designated by the residue number preceded by the original amino acid and followed by the new substitution. The one letter abbreviation is used for both amino acids.

Table 17-1

Molecular Basis for Some Human Endocrinopathies

Disease	Molecular defect	Comments
Hypothyroidism		
Some hypothyroidism	Mutant TSHβ	Cannot associate with TSHα
Some goiters	Mutant thyroid peroxidase	
	Mutant thyroglobulin	
Generalized resistance to thyroid hormones	Mutant TR	
Idiopathic myxoedema	Antibodies against TSHR	Blocking antibodies
Chronic thyroiditis	Antibodies against thyroglobulin	Inflammatory destruction of thyroid gland
Hyperthyroidism		
Graves' disease	Antibodies against TSHR	Stimulating antibodies
McCune–Albright syndrome	Stimulating mutants of G_α	Somatic mosaic; also ↑ in GH, ACTH, and gonadotropins
GH deficiency		
Isolated GH deficiency, type IA	Deleted or mutant GH	
Familial human dwarfism	Mutant Pit-1	Also PRL and TSH deficiencies
Laron dwarf	Mutant GHR	
GH excess		
Some acromegaly	Antibodies to GHR	Stimulating antibodies
	Stimulating mutants of G_α	Somatic mutations leading to pituitary tumors
Diabetes mellitus		
Some diabetes mellitus	Mutant insulin	Inactive or improper processing depending on mutation
Leprechaunism	Mutant insulin receptor (α subunit)	Severest form; death in early infancy
Rabson–Mendenhall syndrome	Mutant insulin receptor (α subunit)	Severe insulin resistance in children
Type A insulin resistance	Mutant insulin receptor (β subunit or α truncation)	Severe insulin resistance in adult females

Condition	Molecular defect	Comments
Maturity onset diabetes of the young	Mutant glucokinase	
Wolfram syndrome	Mutant tRNA$^{\text{Leu}}_{\text{UUR}}$ and other defects in the respiratory chain	Sensorineural hearing loss
Glucocorticoid deficiency		
Congenital adrenal hyperplasia	Mutant synthetic enzymes	Symptoms depend on defective enzyme
Familial glucocorticoid deficiency	Mutant ACTH receptor	
Isolated, congenital ACTH deficiency	Probable mutant POMC processing protease	
Primary cortisol resistance	Mutant GR	
Addison's disease, adult onset	Antibodies against 21-hydroxylase	
Type 1 polyendocrine autoimmunity syndrome	Antibodies against 17α-hydroxylase	
Hyperaldosterism		
Some hyperaldosterism	Mutant 11β-hydroxysteroid dehydrogenase	Cortisol cannot be inactivated and floods the aldosterone receptor
Glucocorticoid-remediable aldosterism	Mutant CYP11B2	Regulatory mutant; crossover changes 5' end
Hypoaldosteronism		
Type I pseudohypoaldosteronism	Mutant aldosterone receptor	
Bone metabolism		
Vitamin D-resistant rickets	Mutant VDR	
Osteoporosis	Defective VDR regulation	
Hypogonadism		
Kallman syndrome	Mutant adhesion molecule	Defect in migration of GnRH-secreting neurons
Some hypogonadism	Mutant LHβ	Normal ♀ phenotype (♀); no Leydig cells (♂)
	Mutant FSHβ	Normal ♂ phenotype (♂); small breasts, amenorrhea, and infertility (♀)
Testicular feminization	Mutant AR	Completely inactive AR
Male pseudohermaphroditism	Mutant AR	Partially inactive AR
	Mutant 5α-reductase 2	
	Mutant Müllerian inhibiting substance	Also called persistent Müllerian duct syndrome

continues

continued

Disease	Molecular defect	Comments
Kennedy's disease	Mutant AR (polyGln domain)	Also called X-linked spinal and bulbar muscular atrophy
Precocious puberty		
McCune–Albright syndrome	Stimulating mutants of G_α	Elevated gonadotropins
Familial male precocious puberty	Mutant LHR	Constitutively active
Diabetes insipidus		
Familial neurohypophyseal diabetes insipidus	Mutant ADH precursor	ADH precursor cannot be processed or defective neurophysin
Hereditary nephrogenic diabetes insipidus	Mutant ADH receptor (V_2 receptor)	
Hypoparathyroidism		
Familial isolated hypoparathyroidism	Mutant preproparathormone	PTH precursor cannot be processed
Pseudohypoparathyroidism, type IA	Inhibiting mutants of G_α	Also called Albright's heredity osteodystrophy
Hyperparathyroidism		
Familial hypocalciuric hypercalcemia	Defective calcium sensor	Heterozygous
Neonatal severe hyperparathyroidism	Defective calcium sensor	Homozygous

Disorder	Molecular defect	Consequence
Cytokine deficiencies		
Myelodysplasia	CSF-1R deletion	Refractory anemia and abnormal megakaryocytes
X-linked severe combined immunodeficiency	Mutant IL-2Rγ	
Agammaglobulinemia	Mutant Bpk	Soluble tyrosine kinase
Piebaldism	Mutant or deleted SCF receptor (Kit)	Defect in melanocyte migration
Neuromuscular disorders		
Some congenital myasthenia	Possible mutant nAChR	
Myasthenia gravis	Antibodies to nAChR	Usually the α subunit; ↑ receptor degradation
Malignant hyperthermia	Mutant ryanodine receptor (skeletal muscle)	Hypersensitive gating
Central core disease	Mutant ryanodine receptor (skeletal muscle)	Slow calcium leakage
Hereditary hyperekplexia	Mutant $\alpha1$ of GlyR	Muscle rigidity and exaggerated startle response
Miscellaneous disorders		
Some essential hypertension and preeclampsia	Mutant angiotensinogen	Elevated levels of angiotensinogen
Some retinitis pigmentosa	Mutant rhodopsin	
	Mutant cGMP-specific phosphodiesterase	
Angelman syndrome	Deleted GABA$_A$ subunits	Hypopigmentation, craniofacial anomalies, and neurological deficits

packaging, and the mutation impairs this activity (15). A similar defect occurs in the Brattleboro rat (16). A second mutation found in some cases of diabetes insipidus occurs just prior to the signal peptide cleavage site and blocks the removal of the signal peptide (17). A functionally related mutation in para-thormone (PTH) produces *familial isolated hypoparathyroidism* (18).

One final example is the *hpg* mouse, which has hereditary hypogonad-ism secondary to a deficiency of gonadotropin-releasing hormone (GnRH). GnRH also forms the amino terminus of a polyprotein (see Chapter 2); in the *hpg* mouse, a large deletion removes all but the first 11 amino acids of the second peptide (19). GnRH and its cleavage site are intact, but no GnRH is detectable. Either the mRNA is not translated or processing of the truncated polyprotein is impaired and the abnormal polyprotein is rapidly degraded.

Occasionally, a processing defect can be traced to the processing enzyme rather than the hormone. In *isolated congenital adrenocorticotropic hormone (ACTH) deficiency,* there is no detectable ACTH, although the precursor and some of the other products of proopiomelanocortin (POMC) are present in normal concentrations and the POMC gene has a normal sequence (20). It is strongly suspected that one of the proteases responsible for processing POMC is defective or absent.

Defects in regulation are more difficult to detect because the genomic sequence is required to examine the 5' noncoding region of the gene. In African Americans or other persons of African descent with *non-insulin-de-pendent diabetes mellitus* (NIDDM), the insulin gene has a variant promoter that contains an 8-bp repeat and has only 38–49% of the activity of the normal promoter (21). However, this reduced activity appears to be more a contributing factor than a sole determinant of the development of NIDDM. Another regulatory defect would be a mutant transcription factor; because most transcription factors are widely distributed and affect an enormous number of vital genes, few natural mutations have been found. In contrast, Pit-1 is a highly specific factor that induces the transcription of the GH, prolactin (PRL), and thyroid-stimulating hormone (TSH) genes. Mutations in both DNA-binding domains (DBDs) and the transcriptional activation do-main (TAD) of Pit-1 have been reported in humans and mice (22–26). GH deficiency can also arise as a result of inadequate tropic stimulation. Al-though no mutant growth hormone-releasing factor (GHRF) is known, the *little* mouse has a defective growth hormone-releasing factor (GHRF) recep-tor (27).

A second regulatory defect involves the inability of the hormone-secret-ing cell to detect secretagogues or feedback inhibitors. For example, low serum calcium stimulates the parathyroid gland to secrete parathormone (PTH) which then dissolves bone and recovers the cation from urine (see Chapter 1). Rising calcium levels eventually inhibit PTH secretion. However, in *neonatal severe hyperparathyroidism,* the calcium sensor is mutated, the gland cannot detect this feedback inhibitor, and PTH is secreted constitu-tively (28). The heterozygous state produces a milder disease known as *familial hypocalciuric hypercalcemia* or *familial benign hypercalcemia.*

Finally, developmental anomalies can result in hormone deficiencies. Kallman syndrome is characterized by anosmia and hypogonadotropic hypogonadism; it is due to a partial deletion in an adhesion molecule that is required for the proper migration of olfactory and gonadotropin-secreting neurons during embryogenesis (29).

B. Nonpeptide Hormones

1. Steroids

Genes do not encode steroids; they encode the enzymes that synthesize steroids. Therefore, steroid hormone deficiencies are really enzyme deficiencies. The most thoroughly studied system is in the adrenal cortex, and impaired steroid synthesis produces a clinical and biochemical spectrum of diseases known collectively as *congenital adrenal hyperplasia* (30,31). The adrenal cortex becomes hyperplastic because no glucocorticoids are produced to inhibit the pituitary secretion of ACTH.

Any enzyme in the steroid biosynthetic pathway may be missing or defective (Table 17–2); however, the key to understanding the clinical picture of these patients is to determine (i) if androgen synthesis is impaired, (ii) if aldosterone synthesis is impaired, and (iii) what precursors are accumulating. It is also important to remember that the basic embryonic phenotype is female; the presence of androgens is required to masculinize the genitalia of males.

Both the 20,22-desmolase (P450scc) and the 3β-hydroxysteroid dehydrogenase/5-ene-4-ene isomerase act very early in the pathway (see Fig.

Table 17-2
Molecular Defects in Steroid Synthesis or Metabolism

Deficient enzyme activity	Genitalia	Sodium loss	Hypertension
20,22-Desmolase	Female (in ♂)	+	0
3β-Hydroxysteroid dehydrogenase/5-ene-4-ene isomerase	Hypomasculine (♂)	+	0
P450c17			
17α-Dehydrogenase	Female or hypomasculine (♂)	0	+
17,20-Desmolase	Female or hypomasculine (♂)	0	0
21-Hydroxylase	Virilization (♀)	+	0
P450c11			
11β-Hydroxylase	Virilization (♀)	0	+
18-Hydroxylase	Normal	+	0
18-ol-Dehydrogenase	Normal	+	0
11β-Hydroxysteroid dehydrogenase	Normal	0	+
Aromatase	Pseudohermaphroditism (♀)	0	0
5α-Reductase 2	Hypomasculine (♂)	0	0

2–4); therefore, their absence results in a deficiency of aldosterone, gluco-corticoids, and androgens. Without aldosterone, the patients lose sodium (salt wasting); without androgens, male infants have a female (desmolase deficiency) or hypomasculine (dehydrogenase/isomerase deficiency) pheno-type. The difference is due to the formation of dehydroepiandrosterone in the latter patients; although this steroid is only a weak androgen, the hyper-plastic gland produces enough of it to masculinize the fetus partially. Note that the degree of salt wasting in the dehydrogenase/isomerase deficiency is variable, because it is dependent on the severity of the mutation; as little as 10% of normal enzymatic activity is sufficient to prevent salt wasting (32). Like many enzymes in this pathway, the dehydrogenase/isomerase has dual activities. In all these enzymes, the active sites appear to be functionally, if not structurally, distinct since clinically patient can have symptoms related to impairment of only one of the enzymatic activities. In addition, compounds can be synthesized to inhibit one activity, while leaving the other activity intact (33,34). Although nonsense mutations have been reported for the dehydrogenase/isomerase gene, the defect in the desmolase step is still controversial. Even though there is no desmolase activity, some investigators claim that the gene is normal (35), whereas others have shown that the gene is deleted in a rabbit model of this disease (36).

Deficiency of P450c17 also eliminates the androgens, resulting in female or hypomasculine phenotypes in males. Deficiency of the 17,20-desmolase component of P450c17 exclusively affects the androgens, but the absence of the 17α-dehydrogenase component also eliminates cortisol. Its precursor, 11-deoxycortisol, is a weak mineralocorticoid but, again, its accumulation compensates for its low activity. In fact, sodium is retained and hypertension develops. As noted earlier, mutations can selectively affect one or the other activity (37).

There are two P450c11 genes. CYB11B1 has 11β- and 18-hydroxylase activities and is present in the zonae fasciculata and reticularis. Deficiencies of either CYB11B1 or 21-hydroxylase affect both aldosterone and the gluco-corticoids. Because the gland is hyperstimulated, precursors accumulate and are eventually shunted into the androgen pathway. Males appear normal, but females become virilized; for example, the clitoris enlarges to resemble a penis and the labia fuse, creating the appearance of an empty scrotum. The 21-hydroxylase deficiency also leads to sodium loss, but the CYB11B1 defi-ciency still allows the synthesis of 11-deoxycortisol and 11-deoxycorticoster-one. As noted already, these steroids are weak mineralocorticoids whose accumulation is sufficient to overcome the loss of aldosterone; sodium is retained and hypertension results.

The second P450c11 gene is CYB11B2. It has 18-ol-dehydrogenase as well as 11β- and 18-hydroxylase activities and is restricted to the zona glomerulosa. For this reason, it is often called the aldosterone synthase. Deficiency in CYB11B2 selectively eliminates aldosterone, so sexual develop-ment is normal and the only clinical problem is salt wasting. Because this enzyme is 93% identical to CYB11B1, its gene is subject to nonreciprocal crossing over with that encoding CYB11B1 (38). This usually occurs near the 5' end of the gene and results in the CYB11B2 gene having the 5' regulatory region of the CYB11B1 gene, that is, aldosterone synthase is now induced by ACTH. The subsequent elevation of aldosterone leads to sodium retention and hypertension, and can be corrected by glucocorticoids, which suppress ACTH and CYB11B2 gene expression. For this reason, the disease is known as *glucocorticoid-remediable aldosterism.* Hyperaldosterism can also occur with a deficiency of 11β-hydroxysteroid dehydrogenase (39). This enzyme occurs in aldosterone target tissues and rapidly metabolizes cortisol so that it cannot bind and activate the aldosterone receptor, which cannot distinguish between the two steroids. The absence of this enzyme allows cortisol, whose serum levels greatly exceed those of aldosterone, to flood the aldosterone receptor and activate it.

However, the gene for the 21-hydroxylase is most subject to mutations (40,41). Near the normal 21-hydroxylase gene is a second nonfunctional copy; such copies are called *pseudogenes.* Since pseudogenes are never expressed, they are not under any selective pressure to maintain their sequences and many mutations accumulate. As noted earlier, homologous adjacent genes are subject to nonreciprocal crossing over, which can introduce some of the mutations of the pseudogene into the real gene. Such an event is called *gene conversion;* most of the mutations in the 21-hydroxylase gene appear to have arisen in this manner.

The most active androgen for most tissues is dihydrotestosterone, a product of 5α-reductase. The type 2 enzyme is the predominant form in genital tissue and its deficiency produces male pseudohermaphroditism (42,43). Finally, the female sex steroids are generated by an aromatase. Point mutations in this enzyme produce pseudohermaphroditism in female infants (44).

2. Thyroid Hormones

Like steroids, thyroid hormones are enzymatically synthesized. The major enzyme is thyroid peroxidase and several mutations in this enzyme have been reported (45). However, the synthetic enzymes for thyroid hormones differ from those for steroids because the former act on another gene product, thyroglobulin, which is also subject to mutations (46). All known defects of this substrate are truncations that remove the major iodination site. The low triiodothyronine (T_3) and thyroxine (T_4) levels resulting from both the peroxidase and the thyroglobulin mutations lead to elevated TSH concentrations, which induce thyroid growth or *goiter.*

3. Serum Binding Proteins

Although hydrophobic hormones bind serum proteins, these carriers are not essential for hormone function since only the free hormone is active. Mutations in these proteins are often detected by assays that measure total hormone, which is low, even though free hormone is normal and the patient has no symptoms (47). However, such abnormal proteins can cause other problems; for example, mutant transthyretin, also called thyronine-binding prealbumin, can polymerize to form long insoluble fibrils that can precipitate in tissues and disrupt function (48). Such a disease is called *amyloidosis* and the fibrils can arise from many sources. When transthyretin is the culprit, the nervous and cardiac tissue are primarily affected and the maladies are known as *familial amyloid polyneuropathy* and *familial cardiac amyloidosis*.

III. Receptors

A. Nuclear Receptors

1. Genomic Mutations

Before discussing individual receptors and their mutations, several general points should noted. Like hormones, hormone receptors are present in concentrations that are too low for conventional analytical techniques. One of the most sensitive methods of detection is radioligand binding, but this technique would only pick up mutations that affect receptor affinity. This problem explains why most of the mutations identified in nuclear receptors have been restricted to the ligand-binding domain (LBD). In both the androgen (AR) and T_3 (TR) receptors, these sites are further clustered into two major regions (see Fig. 5-4) that are presumably critical for ligand binding (49,50). Another major problem in clinical practice is that there appears to be no correlation between the molecular defect and the phenotype of the patient. For example, the identical mutation in the AR can produce different patient phenotypes ranging from male pseudohermaphroditism to complete testicular feminization (50,51; similar disparities have also been noted in mutant TRs (52) and glucocorticoid receptors (GRs) (53). In the latter case, the effects of the defect may be ameliorated by a higher ratio of normal to mutant TRs (54). Other compensatory mechanisms may also influence the severity of the symptoms of any given mutation.

More mutations have been identified in the AR than in any other hormone receptor (51,55). This is most certainly due to the fact that androgens only affect sexual differentiation and reproduction and have no major impact on the survival of the organism. Furthermore, our society often seems obsessed with sexual characteristics, so anatomical anomalies of the sexual organs are quickly identified for possible treatment. Mutations in the AR span the entire molecule, and their location frequently predicts their physiochemical effects. For example, those in the LBD inhibit steroid binding and others in the DBD reduce binding to the hormone response element (HRE). If there is complete androgen insensitivity, the fetus will develop the female phenotype, although the uterus and oviducts will be missing (see Chapter 2); this condition is known as *testicular feminization*. Less severe insensitivity will result in various degrees of male pseudohermaphroditism; females are unaffected except for their carrier status.

The most interesting mutations involve the polyglutamine stretch in the amino terminus. This tract is produced by a CAG repeat that is unstable and can lengthen (56); normally the track is 21 glutamines long (range 17–26). If the length should double, a disease called *Kennedy's disease* or *X-linked spinal and bulbar muscular atrophy* results (57). This syndrome is characterized by progressive muscular weakness and atrophy, a normal male phenotype, although there is frequently delayed adolescence, and relative signs of androgen insensitivity, such as gynecomastia and reduced fertility. Since complete inactivation of AR does not produce these muscular symptoms, it is thought that the polyglutamine region interacts with some muscle-specific factor and that increasing the length of this tract has some deleterious effect on this interaction; for example, it may bind the factor more tightly and sequester it. Another hypothesis proposes that polyglutamine stretches longer than 33 residues have an increased probability of being substrates for tranglutaminase (58). This enzyme forms cross-links between proteins via isopeptide bonds (see Chapter 10); such cross-links would gradually lead to protein aggregation and cell death. This mechanism would explain the delayed onset of symptoms and the propensity to affect nervous and muscular tissue which cannot regenerate. The length of the tract has been correlated with the onset and severity of the symptoms (59,60). Shortening of the tract has not been reported as an isolated defect but does occur associated with other mutations (61). Halving the tract length does not seem to affect AR function but does accentuate the effect of the other mutations.

Strangely, a similar complement of mutations has not been reported for the estrogen receptor (ER). Gene inactivation experiments in mice do not produce any external anatomical abnormalities in females but they are infertile and have hypoplastic uteri (62). Only one such mutation has been reported: the A86V change is associated with an increased incidence of spontaneous abortions in patients with ER-positive breast cancer but not in normal women (63). As such, its actual role in spontaneous abortions is still unclear.

Molecular defects in the TR are also interesting in that those unable to bind T_3 have dominant phenotypes (64,65). TR can bind its HRE in the absence of T_3 but still requires its ligand for transcription activation; essentially, unoccupied TR acts as an inhibitor by blocking the HRE (see Chapter 12). Mutant TRs that cannot bind T_3 would be permanent inhibitors and would compete with normal TRs for the HRE. Deletions large enough to completely inactivate the TR would be recessive.

Defects in other nuclear receptors have also been reported but they are much less common than those in the AR or TR. Several mutations in the vitamin D receptor (VDR) produce *vitamin D-resistant rickets* (66–71), defects in the aldosterone receptor give rise to *type I pseudohypoaldosteronism* (72), and variants of the GR are responsible for *familial glucocorticoid resistance* (73–75). In addition, a possible regulatory defect in the VDR has been reported in *osteoporosis* (76). This disease of bone-thinning is associated with a VDR allele whose coding sequence is normal. However, regulatory sequences in the flanking region are different and VDR levels are below normal. In addition, when these flanking sequences are used to induce a reporter gene, gene expression is reduced. A second possible regulatory mutation in the GR gene has also been reported: a patient with signs of glucocorticoid excess had normal serum cortisol levels, but her lymphocytes had a 7-fold increase in GR. Since the kinetic and physiochemical characteristics of the receptor appeared to be normal, a regulatory defect was postulated (77). Confirmation of this hypothesis will have to await the sequencing of the 5' end of her GR gene.

2. Somatic Mutations

The previously described mutations occurred in the germ line; however, there has been an increasing interest in somatic mutations and their possible relationship to cancer. For example, breast cancer is one of the leading causes of cancer death in women; in several animal models, it can be induced by estrogens and, in humans, anti-estrogen therapy can cause regression. Unfortunately, many tumors will eventually become unresponsive to endocrine therapy. Since the ER links estradiol to its effects, several groups have sought to explain these phenomena in terms of alterations in the ER.

The T47D breast cancer cell line is estrogen resistant and its ER has been shown to have several mutations that could explain this insensitivity (78). The MCF-7 breast cancer cell line is estrogen dependent, but a subclone is unresponsive to anti-estrogens. These cells have a G400V mutation that binds the antagonist in such a way that it can activate the ER, that is, antagonists are converted to agonists (79).

In actual breast tumors, aberrant processing resulting in deleted exons is much more common than mutation (80,81); in general, there appears to be a deregulation of splicing in tumors. Of the many variant ERs that have been reported in breast cancer, three are of considerable note: deletions of exon 3 containing the second zinc finger or exon 7 in the LBD are dominant negative mutants. These ERs are not only defective but would inhibit the function of normal ERs, therefore, only some mRNAs would have to be affected. The third variant lacks exon 5 and is constitutively active; although this activity is only 10–15% that of the normal ER, it may be enough to remove the tumor from any dependence on exogenous estrogens.

Other tumors closely linked to the endocrine system are the lymphomas and leukemias. Glucocorticoids are toxic to lymphocytes and are very effective drugs in the initial treatment of these cancers. However, many of these malignant cells will eventually develop resistance to these steroids. This resistance is generally a result of defects in the glucocorticoid receptor; several such mutants have been characterized (82). The *nuclear transfer-deficient* mutants have point mutations in the DBD resulting in a decreased affinity for DNA. The *increased nuclear transfer* type has a truncated receptor lacking the amino-terminal modulatory domain. Although it actually has an increased affinity for DNA, it is incapable of triggering transcription. The r^0 mutant does not produce any receptor at all, despite the absence of any obvious deletions or rearrangements; a regulatory defect is suspected. Finally, the *activation-labile* receptor is extremely unstable after activation and quickly loses hormone-binding activity. The molecular basis for this mutant is unknown. Although these mutations occurred in human cell lines, similar defects can occur *in vivo*. For example, the deletion of all or part of the GR has been documented in patients with leukemia or multiple myeloma following therapy (83,84). As in the ER, these deletions in the GR are often the result of abberrant splicing.

Somatic mutations in other receptors have not been as thoroughly studied. Prostate cancer is usually androgen responsive and can contain mutated ARs. Several mutations in the LBD have been reported to have lax binding specificity: androgens, estrogens, progestins, and anti-androgens can all bind this variant AR and activate transcription (85,86). Finally, in addition to point mutations, deletions, and processing defects, nuclear receptors can also be disabled by translocations. Acute promyelocytic leukemia is commonly associated with a t(15;17) chromosomal translocation, which creates a RAR/*myl* fusion gene (87). The function of Myl is unknown, but its replacement of the amino terminus of the retinoic acid receptor (RAR) converts RAR into a dominant negative mutant (88). Since retinoids are often associated with differentiation, the inactivation of one of their receptors might favor growth over differentiation. A deletion of the amino terminus of RAR has also been reported in P19 embryonal cancer cells; this variant is a dominant negative mutant as well (89).

B. Membrane Receptors

1. Receptor Tyrosine Kinases

One of the most heavily studied membrane receptors is the insulin receptor and numerous mutation have been reported (90–92). These mutations can have many effects, depending on their locations: truncations often affect synthesis, mutations in the α subunit frequently impair insulin binding, and defects in the catalytic site reduce kinase activity. In addition, some variants display processing defects. For example, the R735S mutation occurs at the α–β interface and prevents cleavage. Other mutations interfere with transport to the plasma membrane.

Most of these defects produce severe insulin resistance. The severest form is *leprechaunism*; the name is derived from the small size and elfin features of these infants. They also have lipoatrophy and acanthosis nigrans; the latter is a skin condition in which the epidermis is hypertrophied and darkened. It is believed to result from the activation of insulin-like growth factor–insulin receptors (IGF-IRs) by insulin, which is quite elevated in these patients. Insulin receptors are virtually unmeasurable and affected individuals die in early infancy. Growth retardation is less severe and life expectancy is longer for patients with the *Rabson–Mendenhall syndrome*. This syndrome is also characterized by precocious puberty and dystrophic nails and teeth. Most known mutations for both of these diseases are in the α subunit. *Type A insulin resistance* occurs most commonly in adult women, who also have hirsutism and scanty menses. Mutations in either the α or the β subunit have been found in the tissues from these patients. As noted for mutations in the nuclear receptors, the phenotype does not always correspond to the genotype: the W1193L[2] change has been reported for several members of a family (93). Although all are heterozygotes, one had type A insulin resistance, another had minimum symptoms, while a third had no overt disease. It is possible that individual factors may affect whether or not an insulin receptor mutation is dominant. Alternatively, since a tryptophan-to-leucine substitution would normally be considered a conservative one, the receptor may have a quasi-stable structure. Other compensatory factors may then determine the functionality of this protein.

These syndromes are exceedingly rare, whereas NIDDM is very common. It would be far more clinically relevant if insulin receptor defects could be found in NIDDM. Although no such mutations have been proven to be associated with NIDDM, two have been proposed based on their frequency in diabetic patients. The R1152Q mutation displays normal autophosphorylation but impaired phosphorylation of a synthetic substrate (94). The V985M mutation is found in both diabetic and normal individuals, but carriers do have higher serum glucose levels following a glucose load (95). As such, this mutation may be a contributing rather than a causative factor in developing NIDDM. Another candidate is S992P; the rhesus monkey is diabetes prone and has an insulin receptor identical to that for humans except for 12 amino acids (96). All but the S992P substitution are conservative changes; this same alteration occurs in other diabetes-prone species.

Another interesting human disease caused by a defective receptor tyrosine kinase (RTK) is *piebaldism* (97–99) and its murine counterpart *white spotting* (100). Stem cell factor (SCF) is a tropic hormone for stem cells in the blood, pigmentary, and reproductive systems (see Chapter 3). In humans, mutations in the SCF receptor result in depigmented patches on the skin. Since the patches are most commonly located on the ventral surface, this phenotype appears to be a result of a defect in the migration of the melanocytes from the neural crest, where they arise, to the ventral surface. This migration may depend on a gradient of the SCF receptor; if receptor activity is compromised, the entire gradient may be reduced and the lower end may drop below the threshold for melanocyte migration. In addition to depigmentation, rats also show reductions in erythrocytes and mast cells.

An alteration in the gene for at least one other human RTK has been reported: the CSF-1 receptor gene is deleted in *myelodysplasia* (101). CSF-1 is a hematopoietic factor (see Chapter 3) and its loss is associated with refractory anemia and abnormal megakaryocytes.

---

[2] Although the mature insulin receptor is cleaved; mutants are designated by their position in the uncleaved precursor.

2. Serpentine Receptors

The first mutant serpentine receptor to be described was rhodopsin, the light receptor. These defects are responsible for the disease *retinitis pigmentosa*. Reports of mutations in the ADH (V_2) receptor (102,103) and ACTH receptor (104) followed; these variants produce *hereditary nephrogenic diabetes insipidus* and *familial glucocorticoid deficiency*, respectively. In the case of the ADH receptor, the mutations are clustered in the third transmembrane helix, third extracellular domain, and third cytosolic domain. The first two sites are probably involved with ligand binding, whereas the cytoplasmic domain couples to the G protein.

Recently, mutant receptors that are constitutively active have been isolated. Several mutations in the carboxy terminus of the third cytoplasmic loop of the TSHR have been found in hyperfunctioning thyroid adenomas (105). This alteration in receptor structure may mimic the active conformation that stimulates G_s. Another constitutively active receptor, LHR, has been documented in *familial male precocious puberty* (106,107). All these receptors have mutations in the sixth transmembrane helix; these changes may mimic ligand binding. Although males show precocious sexual development, females are normal. Androgen production only requires LH but estrogen synthesis requires LH and FSH; therefore, a hyperactive LHR alone will not elevate estrogen levels in females.

In mice, defects have also been found in the GHRF and melanocyte-stimulating hormone (MSH) receptors (27,108). The former results in dwarf mice whereas the latter alters pigmentation. Three MSH receptor alleles are known. The *e* allele in C57BL mice is characterized by a yellow phenotype, which arises from an inactive receptor truncated just after the fourth transmembrane helix. The other two alleles actually encode hyperactive receptors. E^{50} produces a totally black mouse; the receptor which it encodes has a point mutation in the second transmembrane helix and is constitutively active. E^{tob} produces a black dorsum and encodes a receptor with another point mutation in the first cytoplasmic loop. The basal activity and MSH affinity of the receptor are unchanged, but the receptor couples more efficiently to the G protein.

3. Cytokine Receptors

The best studied cytokine receptor is the GH receptor, whose inactive mutants are responsible for *Laron dwarfism* (109). Both truncations, which lead to defects in synthesis, and point mutations, which result in processing errors, have been reported. IL-2 is a critical hormone in the immune system (see Chapter 3) and the truncation of its receptor dramatically compromises this system (110). The resulting disease is known as *X-linked severe combined immunodeficiency disease*. Cytokine receptors act, in part, by coupling to soluble tyrosine kinases; such a kinase may be Bpk (111). Bpk belongs to the Itk family (see Table 6-3) and its inactive mutants prevent the maturation of B cells and the production of all antibodies: this disease is called *agammaglobulinemia*.

4. Ion Channel Receptors

Several deletions and mutations in the γ-aminobutyric acid receptor A (GABA$_A$) have been described. The *pink-eyed, cleft-palate* mutation in mice is characterized by hypopigmentation, craniofacial anomalies, and neurological deficits and results from the deletion of several GABA$_A$ subunits (112). *Angelman's syndrome* is a very similar human disease that is also associated with deletions of GABA$_A$ subunits (113). Finally, a point mutation in the α6 subunit of the rat GABA$_A$ receptor produces an *alcohol-nontolerant rat* (114). Diazepine cannot bind this variant, nor can it potentiate the inhibition elicited by GABA.

Mutants in the α1 subunit of the glycine receptor (GlyR) produce *hereditary hyperekplexia,* also called *familial startle disease* (115). Glycine is an inhibitory neurotransmitter in the spinal cord. Impairment of its receptor reduces this inhibition and results in overstimulation. Patients exhibit muscle rigidity and an exaggerated startle response.

No documented case of a disease-producing mutant nicotinic acetylcholine receptor (nAChR) has been reported in humans, but one form of congenital myasthenia is a likely candidate. Congenital myasthenia is actually a heterogeneous group of diseases that all affect neuromuscular transmission. In one form, a mutation in the ϵ subunit of the nAChR appears to be either causative or contributory (116).

C. Receptor Antibodies

Another group of endocrinopathies is related to autoimmune diseases. These diseases are characterized by the inability of the immune system to recognize certain endogenous antigens as "self" and the subsequent development of antibodies against them. When these antigens are hormone receptors, several interesting possibilities arise. For example, antibody binding to a receptor may prevent hormone binding and may lead to a hormone-deficient-like state. However, occasionally antibody binding can actually activate the receptor and can lead to a hormone-excess-like state.

The latter is called a *stimulating antibody*; the classic disease of this type is *Graves' disease,* a form of hyperthyroidism (117). These patients have in their serum "long-acting thyroid stimulators," that are in fact IgG antibodies directed against the thyroid plasma membrane. These antibodies are heterogeneous, but some clearly bind to the TSH receptor and all stimulate the adenylate cyclase. In some forms of *acromegaly,* stimulating antibodies against the GH receptor have also been identified (118). Acromegaly is a disease normally produced by an excess of GH in the adult. Since the epiphyses have fused, linear growth is no longer possible; instead, the bones become thicker and the facial features coarser.

The other type of antibody is called a *blocking antibody*; the classic disease of this type is *myasthenia gravis,* a neuromuscular disease (119,120). Clinically, patients have weak and easily fatigued skeletal muscles. Biochemically, these patients have antibodies directed primarily against the α subunit of the nAChR, although epitopes in the γ and δ subunits have also been reported. Interestingly, these antibodies do not prevent ACh binding but do accelerate receptor degradation. Blocking antibodies can also be directed against the TSH receptor; this form of hypothyroidism is called *idiopathic myxoedema* (121).

Because receptors are on the surfaces of cells, they are exposed to the immune system. However, other components of the endocrine system can also be the target of autoimmune diseases. In *adult onset Addison's disease,* antibodies are directed against the 21-hydroxylase (122); in *type 1 polyendocrine autoimmunity syndrome,* against the 17α-hydroxylase (123); and in *chronic thyroiditis,* against thyroglobulin. In all these diseases, the antibodies are neither stimulating nor blocking; rather, they induce a severe inflammatory response that eventually leads to the destruction of the gland and hormone deficiency.

Finally, many insulin-dependent diabetics have antibodies against glutamate decarboxylase, an enzyme involved in the synthesis of GABA (124–126). GABA is an inhibitory neurotransmitter that the β cells use to suppress the secretion of hormones that oppose insulin action. Again, inflammation gradually destroys the gland.

IV. Transduction

A. G and GAP-Like Proteins

The best example in this group of disorders is *pseudohypoparathyroidism, type IA,* or *Albright's heredity osteodystrophy* (127,128). Clinically, the patients appear to have hypoparathyroidism; that is, they have skeletal abnormalities and hypocalcemia, with resulting tetany and seizures (see Chapter 1). However, parathormone (PTH) levels are elevated and hormone receptors appear normal. The adenylate cyclase is also normal, since it can be stimulated by forskolin. However, fluoride and the nonhydrolyzable analogs of GTP do not activate the adenylate cyclase; unlike forskolin, which acts directly on the cyclase, fluoride and the GTP analogs act through the α subunit of G_s (see Chapter 8). There is also a decreased incorporation of labeled ADP–ribose into α_s by cholera toxin. This α_s deficiency was eventually shown to be due to the replacement of the initial methionine by valine (127). Normal initiation is blocked but does occur at an internal site; however, the truncated protein is rapidly degraded. Other truncations and point mutations have also been reported (128,129).

A major question remains: If G_s resides in a common pool for all cAMP-dependent hormones, why is only PTH action affected? In truth, this defect is not just limited to PTH; the deficiency is found in all tissues and affects every cAMP-dependent hormone studied including thyrotropin-releasing hormone (TRH), TSH, gonadotropins, ADH, glucagon, and prostaglandin E_1

(PGE$_1$) (130). However, these effects are usually subclinical; that is, they are not severe enough to produce symptoms and have only been discovered by sophisticated testing. There are several possible explanations for this discrepancy between PTH and the other cAMP-dependent hormones. First, there is actually a family of α_s genes and some hormones may preferentially use one α_s over another. Second, the other hormones may have multiple transducers; for example, in the liver glucagon activates both the adenylate cyclase and the polyphosphoinositide (PPI) pathway. Therefore, the loss of one transducer would not be as devastating to glucagon as it would be to another hormone that acted exclusively through α_s.

There are also mutations that can activate α_s. All known mutations occur at either residue 201 or 227; the former is the mono(ADP–ribosyl)ating site for cholera toxin and the latter occurs in a GAP-like sequence. These mutations impair the GTPase activity of α_s, thereby prolonging its action. It would appear that widespread activation of α_s is not compatible with life, since only somatic mutations have been identified. Two types of somatic mutations have been reported. Those that occur in single cells of an adult generally produce adenomas because cAMP is often mitogenic. In secretory cells, these tumors can also overproduce hormones. For example, these mutants have been found in some GH-secreting pituitary adenomas and thyroid-secreting thyroid adenomas (131); in fact, it has been estimated that as much as 40% of acromegaly may be due to activating mutations in α_s.

The other somatic mutation occurs early in embryogenesis, before the three germ layers form. The mature individual is composed of a mixture of normal and affected tissues; such a person is said to be a *genetic mosaic*. The result is that certain tissues are hyperactive, particularly with respect to hormone secretion or activity. The clinical picture includes bone lesions, café au lait spots (MSH), sexual precocity (gonadotropins), hyperthyroidism (TSH), pituitary adenomas, and adrenal hyperplasia (ACTH). This disease is known as the *McCune–Albright syndrome* (132,133).

Mutations in α_{i2} have also been identified (134). These activate α_{i2} and constitutively inhibit adenylate cyclase. These mutations are somatic and have been found in some adrenocortical and ovarian tumors.

Spontaneous mutations in Ras are similar to those found in oncogenic viruses (see Chapter 16); most interfere with the ability of Ras to interact with RasGAP. Another way to elevate Ras activity would be to inactivate GAP. No such mutations have been reported for RasGAP, but they have been identified in a GAP-like protein in patients with *neurofibromatosis type 1* (135). The physiological role for this protein is unknown, but it has a GAP-like domain and can enhance the GTPase activity of Ras. Therefore, it may keep Ras in check. Most mutations are located in the GAP-like region. The clinical picture reflects growth and hyperactivity: neurofibromas, café au lait spots, and an increased risk of malignancies. Somatic mutations in this gene have also been reported in colon adenocarcinomas, anaplastic astrocytomas, and basal cell carcinomas.

B. cAMP Pathway

Because the transduction systems serve many hormones, defects at this level can have widespread and devastating effects. For that reason, very few have been documented in higher animals; such defects are probably not compatible with life. Therefore, most of the examples given here will be from invertebrates or cell lines.

Several protein kinase A (PKA) mutants have been characterized in cell lines from an adrenocortical tumor (136) and a lymphoma (137). All of these have been in the cAMP-binding sites of RI. Another interesting mutation has been found in a papillary thyroid carcinoma (138); it consists of a fusion protein between RI and Ret, a tyrosine kinase. Tyrosine kinases are activated by dimerization, a process usually induced by ligands (see Chapter 6). In this mutant, RI provides a constitutive dimerization motif for the kinase.

There are only four major serine–threonine phosphatases (see Chapter 11). Because of their broad functions, defects would have a major impact on the viability of the animal. However, there are many more protein tyrosine phosphatases (PTPs), several of which appear to be highly specialized. Point mutations or truncations in the SH2-containing PTP associated with hematopoietic cells is responsible for the *motheaten* mutation in mice (139,140). These mutations lead to developmental and functional defects in immune cells with eventual progression to autoimmune disorders.

Several mutations in the PDE have also been described. The *dunce*+ mutant in *Drosophila* has a defective cAMP-specific PDE and is characterized by impaired memory and female sterility (141). The cGMP-specific PDE is restricted to the retina and its inactivation results in *retinal degeneration* in mice (142), *rod-cone dysplasia 1* in dogs (143), and some forms of retinitis pigmentosa in humans (144). In all three species, the mutations are located in the β subunit.

C. Polyphosphoinositide Pathway

The PPI pathway is also involved in vision in *Drosophila*; because these components are specific for the eye, their loss is still compatible with a viable organism. Phospholipase Cβ (PLCβ) is essential for phototransduction and its inactivation by an insertional mutation renders the flies blind (145). PKC2 deactivates the photoresponse in flies; its variants lead to hyperadaptation to light (146). Finally, retinal degeneration A and B in *Drosophila* are results of a defective diacylglyceride kinase (147) and a mutant membrane-bound PI transfer protein (148), respectively; these proteins are necessary to maintain the supply of PI for the PI cycle (see Chapter 9).

There is one example of a mutant component of the calcium transduction system in humans: the skeletal ryanodine receptor, which gates an intracellular calcium store. Mutations in this protein produce a variety of phenotypes. In *malignant hyperthermia*, the mutant receptor is hypersensitive to several molecules, especially certain anesthetics and skeletal muscle relaxants, which trigger the release of calcium and muscle contraction (149). The resulting hypermetabolism elevates the body temperature to dangerous levels. In *central core disease,* the mutant receptor continuously leaks calcium (150). The periphery of the myofibril is spared any damage because plasma membrane pumps can remove the calcium. However, the additional calcium load in the interior can only be removed by the mitochondria that are eventually destroyed. The result is muscle weakness due to a loss of oxidative metabolism in the center of the myofibrils.

D. Metabolic Pathways

Insulin regulates glucose metabolism; mutations in insulin or its receptor interfere with glucose metabolism and result in diabetes mellitus. However, diabetes can also be produced by mutations affecting the central glucose pathways. For example, *maturity onset diabetes mellitus of the young* is characterized by glucokinase mutants (151,152); in addition to its role in glucose metabolism, glucokinase acts as a glucose sensor for the pancreatic islets. Therefore, a defective glucokinase would impair insulin secretion. *Wolfram syndrome* results from defects in the respiratory chain; a mutant $tRNA^{Leu}_{UUR}$ is associated with diabetes and deafness (153). More extensive mutations will produce more severe neural defects (154). Considering the importance of the glucose transporter in insulin action, it is surprising that no study has been able to document any mutations in these molecules from diabetic patients (155).

V. Transcription Factors

Like transducers, transcription factors are central to many cellular processes and their inactivation would lead to severe cellular dysfunction. However, if the factors were specific enough, their loss would produce more limited disruption. An example would be the nuclear receptors for the sex steroids (see preceding discussion); nuclear receptors are simply ligand-activated transcription factors. Pit-1 is another relatively specific factor; it is predominantly expressed in the pituitary, where it is required for the transcription of the GH, PRL, and TSH genes. In addition, it is essential for the development of the somato-, lacto-, and thyrotropes, at least in the mouse; the Snell dwarf mouse has a point mutation in the recognition helix of POU_H and its pituitary is hypoplastic (22). This phenomenon is not seen in humans, but the defects in humans are located in other parts of the molecule (23–26). In general, the induction of GH is most sensitive to mutations in Pit-1 and homozygotes have more severe symptoms than heterozygotes. The possible exceptions are mutations that do not disrupt DNA binding; such variants behave as dominant repressors, presumably by competing with intact Pit-1 for DNA-binding sites. Constitutively active mutants of several transcription factors are carried by some retroviruses (see Chapter 16).

VI. Summary

The human body obeys Murphy's Law: whatever can go wrong, will go wrong, that is, almost every possible defect in hormone action has, in fact, been observed in patients. Peptide hormone deficiencies include gene deletions, point mutations, and improper processing, whereas steroid hormone deficiencies are results of defective synthetic enzymes. Mutations have also been documented in every class of membrane and nuclear receptor. Examples of mutations in transducers and transcription factors, other than nuclear receptors, are not as common, presumably because they serve many systems and their disruption could have serious effects. However, variant G proteins have been found, especially in tumors in which their effects are more restricted.

Mutations do not always result in deficiencies or inactivation: a nonreciprocal crossover puts the aldosterone synthase gene under the control of another, more active gene, whereas a defective cortisol-metabolizing enzyme allows cortisol to flood and activate the aldosterone receptor. Both of these conditions produce hyperaldosteronism. In addition, mutations in the GTPase site of G proteins can generate a G protein that cannot turn itself off by hydrolyzing GTP. Finally, some mutant serpertine receptors are constitutively active.

Autoimmune diseases can produce other endocrinopathies. Antibodies against membrane receptors can either stimulate the receptor and lead to a hyperactive endocrine state or block or destroy the receptor and result in an endocrine deficiency state. Finally, antibodies against steroid synthetic enzymes or thyroglobulin can initiate an inflammatory reaction that will eventually destroy the affected gland.

References

General References

Fuqua, S. A. W., Chamness, G. C., and McGuire, W. L. (1993). Estrogen receptor mutations in breast cancer. *J. Cell. Biochem.* **51**, 135–139.
Parks, J. S., Kinoshita, E. I., and Pfäffle, R. W. (1993). Pit-1 and hypopituitarism. *Trends Endocrinol. Metab.* **4**, 81–85.
Spiegel, A. M., Weinstein, L. S., and Shenker, A. (1993). Abnormalities in G protein-coupled signal transduction pathways in human disease. *J. Clin. Invest.* **92**, 1119–1125.
See also Refs. 1, 40, 41, 43, 64, 65, 80–82, 90–92, 109, 119, 120, 124–126, 130, 135, 151, and 155.

Cited References

1. Phillips, J. A., and Cogan, J. D. (1994). Molecular basis of familial human growth hormone deficiency. *J. Clin. Endocrinol. Metab.* **78**, 11–16.

2. Frankenne, F., Rentier-Delrue, F., Scippo, M. L., Martial, J., and Hennen, G. (1987). Expression of the growth hormone variant gene in human placenta. *J. Clin. Endocrinol. Metab.* **64,** 635–637.
3. Parks, J. S., Nielsen, P. V., Sexton, L. A., and Jorgensen, E. H. (1985). An effect of gene dosage on production of human chorionic somatomammotropin. *J. Clin. Endocrinol. Metab.* **60,** 993–997.
4. Vnencak-Jones, C. L., and Phillips, J. A. (1990). Hot spots for growth hormone gene deletions in homologous regions outside of Alu repeats. *Science* **250,** 1745–1748.
5. Yano, H., Kitano, N., Morimoto, M., Polonsky, K. S., Imura, H., and Seino, Y. (1992). A novel point mutation in the human insulin gene giving rise to hyper-proinsulinemia (proinsulin Kyoto). *J. Clin. Invest.* **89,** 1902–1907.
6. Cogan, J. D., Phillips, J. A., Sakati, N., Frisch, H., Schober, E., and Milner, R. D. G. (1993). Heterogeneous growth hormone (GH) gene mutations in familial GH deficiency. *J. Clin. Endocrinol. Metabol.* **76,** 1224–1228.
7. Hayashizaki, Y., Hiraoka, Y., Endo, Y., Miyai, K., and Matsubara, K. (1989). Thyroid-stimulating hormone (TSH) deficiency caused by a single base substitution in the CAGYC region of the β-subunit. *EMBO J.* **8,** 2291–2296.
8. Weiss, J., Axelrod, L., Whitcomb, R. W., Harris, P. E., Crowley, W. F., and Jameson, J. L. (1992). Hypogonadism caused by a single amino acid substitution in the β subunit of luteinizing hormone. *N. Engl. J. Med.* **326,** 179–183.
9. Matthews, C. H., Borgato, S., Beck-Peccoz, P., Adams, M., Tone, Y., Gambino, G., Casagrande, S., Tedeschini, G., Benedetti, A., and Chatterjee, V. K. K. (1993). Primary amenorrhoea and infertility due to a mutation in the β-subunit of follicle-stimulating hormone. *Nature Genet.* **5,** 83–86.
10. Jeunemaitre, X., Soubrier, F., Kotelevtsev, Y. V., Lifton, R. P., Williams, C. S., Charru, A., Hunt, S. C., Hopkins, P. N., Williams, R. R., Lalouel, J. M., and Corvol, P. (1992). Molecular basis of human hypertension: Role of angiotensinogen. *Cell* **71,** 169–180.
11. Ward, K., Hata, A., Jeunemaitre, X., Helin, C., Nelson, L., Namikawa, C., Farrington, P. F., Ogasawara, M., Suzumori, K., Tomoda, S., Berrebi, S., Sasaki, M., Corvol, P., Lifton, R. P., and Lalouel, J. M. (1993). A molecular variant of angiotensinogen associated with preeclampsia. *Nature Genet.* **4,** 59–61.
12. Knebelmann, B., Boussin, L., Guerrier, D., Legeai, L., Kahn, A., Josso, N., and Picard, J. Y. (1991). Anti-Müllerian hormone Bruxelles: A nonsense mutation associated with the persistent Müllerian duct syndrome. *Proc. Natl. Acad. Sci. U.S.A.* **88,** 3767–3771.
13. Yoshida, H., Hayashi, S. I., Kunisada, T., Ogawa, M., Nishikawa, S., Okamura, H., Sudo, T., Shultz, L. D., and Nishikawa, S. I. (1990). The murine mutation osteopetrosis is in the coding region of the macrophage colony stimulating factor gene. *Nature (London)* **345,** 442–444.
14. Wiktor-Jedrzejczak, W., Bartocci, A., Ferrante, A. W., Ahmed-Ansari, A., Sell, K. W., Pollard, J. W., and Stanley, E. R. (1990). Total absence of colony-stimulating factor 1 in the macrophage-deficient osteopetrotic (*op/op*) mouse. *Proc. Natl. Acad. Sci. U.S.A.* **87,** 4828–4832.
15. Bahnsen, U., Oosting, P., Swaab, D. F., Nahke, P., Richter, D., and Schmale, H. (1992). A missense mutation in the vasopressin-neurophysin precursor gene cosegregates with human autosomal dominant neurohypophyseal diabetes insipidus. *EMBO J.* **11,** 19–23.
16. Schmale, H., and Richter, D. (1984). Single base deletion in the vasopressin

gene is the cause of diabetes insipidus in Brattleboro rats. *Nature (London)* **308**, 705–709.

17. Ito, M., Oiso, Y., Murase, T., Kondo, K., Saito, H., Chinzei, T., Racchi, M., and Lively, M. O. (1993). Possible involvement of inefficient cleavage of preprovasopressin by signal peptidase as a cause for familial central diabetes insipidus. *J. Clin. Invest.* **91**, 2565–2571.

18. Arnold, A., Horst, S. A., Gardella, T. J., Baba, H., Levine, M. A., and Kronenberg, H. M. (1990). Mutation of the signal peptide-encoding region of the preproparathyroid hormone gene in familial isolated hypoparathyroidism. *J. Clin. Invest.* **86**, 1084–1087.

19. Mason, A. J., Hayflick, J. S., Zoeller, R. T., Young, W. S., Phillips, H. S., Nikolics, K., and Seeburg, P. H. (1986). A deletion truncating the gonadotropin-releasing hormone gene is responsible for hypogonadism in the *hpg* mouse. *Science* **234**, 1366–1371.

20. Nussey, S. S., Soo, S. C., Gibson, S., Gout, I., White, A., Bain, M., and Johnstone, A. P. (1993). Isolated congenital ACTH deficiency: A cleavage enzyme defect? *Clin. Endocrinol. (Oxford)* **39**, 381–385.

21. Olansky, L., Welling, C., Giddings, S., Adler, S., Bourey, R., Dowse, G., Serjeantson, S., Zimmet, P., and Permutt, M. A. (1992). A variant insulin promoter in non-insulin-dependent diabetes mellitus. *J. Clin. Invest.* **89**, 1596–1602.

22. Li, S., Crenshaw, E. B., Rawson, E. J., Simmons, D. M., Swanson, L. W., and Rosenfeld, M. G. (1990). Dwarf locus mutants lacking three pituitary cell types result from mutations in the POU-domain gene *pit-1*. *Nature (London)* **347**, 528–533.

23. Ohta, K., Nobukuni, Y., Mitsubuchi, H., Fujimoto, S., Matsuo, N., Inagaki, H., Endo, F., and Matsuda, I. (1992). Mutations in the Pit-1 gene in children with combined pituitary hormone deficiency. *Biochem. Biophys. Res. Commun.* **189**, 851–855.

24. Pfäffle, R. W., DiMattia, G. E., Parks, J. S., Brown, M. R., Wit, J. M., Jansen, M., Van der Nat, H., and Van den Brande, J. L. (1992). Mutation of the POU-specific domain of Pit-1 and hypopituitarism without pituitary hypoplasia. *Science* **257**, 1118–1121.

25. Radovick, S., Nations, M., Du, Y., Berg, L. A., Weintraub, B. D., and Wondisford, F. E. (1992). A mutation in the POU-homeodomain of Pit-1 responsible for combined pituitary hormone deficiency. *Science* **257**, 1115–1118.

26. Tatsumi, K., Miyai, K., Notomi, T., Kaibe, K., Amino, N., Mizuno, Y., and Kohno, H. (1992). Cretinism with combined hormone deficiency caused by a mutation in the *PIT1* gene. *Nature Genet.* **1**, 56–58.

27. Lin, S. C., Lin, C. R., Gukovsky, I., Lusis, A. J., Sawchenko, P. E., and Rosenfeld, M. G. (1993). Molecular basis of the *little* mouse phenotype and implications for cell type-specific growth. *Nature (London)* **364**, 208–213.

28. Pollak, M. R., Brown, E. M., Chou, Y. H. W., Herbert, S. C., Marx, S. J., Steinmann, B., Levi, T., Seidman, C. E., and Siedman, J. G. (1993). Mutations in the human Ca^{2+}-sensing receptor gene cause familial hypocalciuric and neonatal severe hyperparathyroidism. *Cell* **75**, 1297–1303.

29. Legouis, R., Hardelin, J. P., Levilliers, J., Claverie, J. M., Compain, S., Wunderle, V., Millasseau, P., Le Paslier, D., Cohen, D., Caterina, D., Bougueleret, L., Delemarre-Van de Waal, H., Lutfalla, G., Weissenbach, J., and Petit, C. (1991). The candidate gene for the X-linked Kallmann syndrome encodes a protein related to adhesion molecules. *Cell* **67**, 423–435.

30. White, P. C., and New, M. I. (1988). Molecular genetics of congenital adrenal hyperplasia. *Clin. Endocrinol. Metab.* **2**, 941–965.

31. Strachan, T. (1989). Molecular genetics of congenital adrenal hyperplasia. *Trends Endocrinol. Metab.* **1**, 68–72.

32. Simard, J., Rhéaume, E., Sanchez, R., Laflamme, N., de Launoit, Y., Luu-The, V., van Seters, A. P., Gordon, R. D., Bettendorf, M., Heinrich, U., Moshang, T., New, M. I., and Labrie, F. (1993). Molecular basis of congenital adrenal hyperplasia due to 3β-hydroxysteroid dehydrogenase deficiency. *Mol. Endocrinol.* **7**, 716–728.

33. Luu-The, V., Takahashi, M., de Launoit, Y., Dumont, M., Lachance, Y., and Labrie, F. (1991). Evidence for distinct dehydrogenase and isomerase sites within a single 3β-hydroxysteroid dehydrogenase/5-ene-4-ene isomerase protein. *Biochemistry* **30**, 8861–8865.

34. Luu-The, V., Takahashi, M., and Labrie, F. (1991). Differential inhibition of dehydrogenase and 5-ene→4-ene isomerase activities of purified 3β-hydroxysteroid dehydrogenase. Evidence for two distinct sites. *J. Steroid Biochem. Mol. Biol.* **40**, 545–548.

35. Lin, D., Gitelman, S. E., Saenger, P., and Miller, W. L. (1991). Normal genes for the cholesterol side chain cleavage enzyme, P450scc, in congenital lipoid adrenal hyperplasia. *J. Clin. Invest.* **88**, 1955–1962.

36. Yang, X., Iwamoto, K., Wang, M., Artwohl, J., Mason, J. I., and Pang, S. (1993). Inherited congenital adrenal hyperplasia in the rabbit is caused by a deletion in the gene encoding cytochrome P450 cholesterol side-chain cleavage enzyme. *Endocrinol. (Baltimore)* **132**, 1977–1982.

37. Kitamura, M., Buczko, E., and Dufau, M. L. (1991). Dissociation of hydroxylase and lyase activities by site-directed mutagenesis of the rat P450$_{17\alpha}$. *Mol. Endocrinol.* **5**, 1373–1380.

38. Lifton, R. P., Dluhy, R. G., Powers, M., Rich, G. M., Cook, S., Ulick, S., and Lalouel, J. M. (1992). A chimaeric 11β-hydroxylase/aldosterone synthase gene causes glucocorticoid-remediable aldosteronism and human hypertension. *Nature (London)* **355**, 262–265.

39. Ulick, S., Levine, L. S., Gunczler, P., Zanconato, G., Ramirez, L. C., Rauh, W., Rösler, A., Bradlow, H. L., and New, M. I. (1979). A syndrome of apparent mineralocorticoid excess associated with defects in the peripheral metabolism of cortisol. *J. Clin. Endocrinol. Metab.* **49**, 757–764.

40. Miller, W. L. (1994). Genetics, diagnosis, and management of 21-hydroxylase deficiency. *J. Clin. Endocrinol. Metab.* **78**, 241–246.

41. New, M. I. (1994). 21-Hydroxylase deficiency congenital adrenal hyperplasia. *J. Steroid Biochem. Mol. Biol.* **48**, 15–22.

42. Andersson, S., Berman, D. M., Jenkins, E. P., and Russell, D. W. (1991). Deletion of steroid 5α-reductase 2 gene in male pseudohermaphroditism. *Nature (London)* **354**, 159–161.

43. Wilson, J. D., Griffin, J. E., and Russell, D. W. (1993). Steroid 5α-reductase deficiency. *Endocr. Rev.* **14**, 577–593.

44. Ito, Y., Fisher, C. R., Conte, F. A., Grumbach, M. M., and Simpson, E. R. (1993). Molecular basis of aromatase deficiency in an adult female with sexual infantilism and polycystic ovaries. *Proc. Natl. Acad. Sci. U.S.A.* **90**, 11673–11677.

45. Abramowicz, M. J., Targovnik, H. M., Varela, V., Cochaux, P., Krawiec, L., Pisarev, M. A., Propato, F. V. E., Juvenal, G., Chester, H. A., and Vassart, G.

(1992). Identification of a mutation in the coding sequence of the human thyroid peroxidase gene causing congenital goiter. *J. Clin. Invest.* **90,** 1200–1204.

46. Medeiros-Neto, G., Targovnik, H. M., and Vassart, G. (1993). Defective thyroglobulin synthesis and secretion causing goiter and hypothyroidism. *Endocr. Rev.* **14,** 165–183.

47. Bertenshaw, R., Sarne, D., Tornari, J., Weinberg, M., and Refetoff, S. (1992). Sequencing of the variant thyroxine-binding globulin (TBG)-San Diego reveals two nucleotide substitutions. *Biochim. Biophys. Acta* **1139,** 307–310.

48. Terry, C. J., Damas, A. M., Oliveira, P., Saraiva, M. J. M., Alves, I. L., Costa, P. P., Matias, P. M., Sakaki, Y., and Blake, C. C. F. (1993). Structure of Met30 variant of transthyretin and its amyloidogenic implications. *EMBO J.* **12,** 735–741.

49. Mixson, A. J., Parrilla, R., Ransom, S. C., Wiggs, E. A., McClaskey, J. H., Hauser, P., and Weintraub, B. D. (1992). Correlations of language abnormalities with localization of mutations in the β-thyroid hormone receptor in 13 kindreds with generalized resistance to thyroid hormone: Identification of four new mutations. *J. Clin. Endocrinol. Metab.* **75,** 1039–1045.

50. McPhaul, M. J., Marcelli, M., Zoppi, S., Wilson, C. M., Griffin, J. E., and Wilson, J. D. (1992). Mutations in the ligand-binding domain of the androgen receptor gene cluster in two regions of the gene. *J. Clin. Invest.* **90,** 2097–2101.

51. McPhaul, M. J., Marcelli, M., Zoppi, S., Griffin, J. E., and Wilson, J. D. (1993). The spectrum of mutations in the androgen receptor gene that causes androgen resistance. *J. Clin. Endocrinol. Metab.* **76,** 17–23.

52. Hayashi, Y., Janssen, O. E., Weiss, R. E., Murata, Y., Seo, H., and Refetoff, S. (1993). The relative expression of mutant and normal thyroid hormone receptor genes in patients with generalized resistance to thyroid hormone determined by estimation of their specific messenger ribonucleic acid products. *J. Clin. Endocrinol. Metab.* **76,** 64–69.

53. Ashraf, J., and Thompson, E. B. (1993). Identification of the activation-labile gene: A single point mutation in the human glucocorticoid receptor presents as two distinct receptor phenotypes. *Mol. Endocrinol.* **7,** 631–642.

54. Mixson, A. J., Hauser, P., Tennyson, G., Renault, J. C., Bodenner, D. L., and Weintraub, B. D. (1993). Differential expression of mutant and normal beta T3 receptor alleles in kindreds with generalized resistance to thyroid hormone. *J. Clin. Invest.* **91,** 2296–2300.

55. Sultan, C., Lumbroso, S., Poujol, N., Belon, C., Boudon, C., and Lobaccaro, J. M. (1993). Mutations of androgen receptor gene in androgen insensitivity syndromes. *J. Steroid Biochem. Mol. Biol.* **46,** 519–530.

56. Richards, R. I., and Sutherland, G. R. (1992). Dynamic mutations: A new class of mutations causing human disease. *Cell* **70,** 709–712.

57. La Spada, A., Wilson, E. M., Lubahn, D. B., Harding, A. E., and Fischbeck, K. H. (1991). Androgen receptor gene mutations in X-linked spinal and bulbar muscular atrophy. *Nature (London)* **352,** 77–79.

58. Green, H. (1993). Human genetic diseases due to codon reiteration: Relationship to an evolutionary mechanism. *Cell* **74,** 955–956.

59. Doyu, M., Sobue, G., Mukai, E., Kachi, T., Yasuda, T., Mitsuma, T., and Takahashi, A. (1992). Severity of X-linked recessive bulbospinal neuronopathy correlates with size of the tandem CAG repeat in androgen receptor gene. *Ann. Neurol.* **32,** 707–710.

60. Igarashi, S., Tanno, Y., Onodera, O., Yamazaki, M., Sato, S., Ishikawa, A., Miyatani, N., Nagashima, M., Ishikawa, Y., Sahashi, K., Ibi, T., Miyatake, T., and Tsuji, S. (1992). Strong correlation between the number of CAG repeats in androgen receptor genes and the clinical onset of features of spinal and bulbar muscular atrophy. *Neurology* **42,** 2300–2302.

61. McPhaul, M. J., Marcelli, M., Tilley, W. D., Griffin, J. E., Isidro-Gutierrez, R. F., and Wilson, J. D. (1991). Molecular basis of androgen resistance in a family with a qualitative abnormality of the androgen receptor and responsive to high-dose androgen therapy. *J. Clin. Invest.* **87,** 1413–1421.

62. Lubahn, D. B., Moyer, J. S., Golding, T. S., Couse, J. F., Korach, K. S., and Smithies, O. (1993). Alteration of reproductive function but not prenatal sexual development after insertional disruption of the mouse estrogen receptor gene. *Proc. Natl. Acad. Sci. U.S.A.* **90,** 11162–11166.

63. Lehrer, S. P., Schmutzler, R. K., Rabin, J. M., and Schachter, B. S. (1993). An estrogen receptor genetic polymorphism and a history of spontaneous abortion: Correlation in women with estrogen receptor positive breast cancer but not in women estrogen receptor negative breast cancer or in women without cancer. *Breast Cancer Res. Treat.* **26,** 175–180.

64. Franklyn, J. A. (1991). Syndromes of thyroid hormone resistance. *Clin. Endocrinol. (Oxford)* **34,** 237–245.

65. Refetoff, S., Weiss, R. E., and Usala, S. J. (1993). The syndromes of resistance to thyroid hormone. *Endocr. Rev.* **14,** 348–399.

66. Hughes, M. R., Malloy, P. J., Kieback, D. G., Kesterson, R. A., Pike, J. W., Feldman, D., and O'Malley, B. W. (1988). Point mutation in the human vitamin D receptor gene associated with hypocalcemic rickets. *Science* **242,** 1702–1705.

67. Ritchie, H. H., Hughes, M. R., Thompson, E. T., Malloy, P. J., Hochberg, Z., Feldman, D., Pike, J. W., and O'Malley, B. W. (1989). An ochre mutation in the vitamin D receptor gene causes hereditary 1,25-dihydroxyvitamin D_3-resistant rickets in three families. *Proc. Natl. Acad. Sci. U.S.A.* **86,** 9783–9787.

68. Sone, T., Marx, S. J., Liberman, U. A., and Pike, J. W. (1990). A unique point mutation in the human vitamin D receptor chromosomal gene confers hereditary resistance to 1,25-dihydroxyvitamin D_3. *Mol. Endocrinol.* **4,** 623–631.

69. Saijo, T., Ito, M., Takeda, E., Huq, A. H. M. M., Naito, E., Yokota, I., Sone, T., Pike, J. W., and Kuroda, Y. (1991). A unique mutation in the vitamin D receptor gene in three Japanese patients with vitamin D-dependent rickets type II: Utility of single-strand conformation polymorphism analysis for heterozygous carrier detection. *Am. J. Hum. Genet.* **49,** 668–673.

70. Wiese, R. J., Goto, H., Prahl, J. M., Marx, S. J., Thomas, M., Al-Aqeel, A., and DeLuca, H. F. (1993). Vitamin D-dependency rickets type II: Truncated vitamin D receptor in three kindreds. *Mol. Cell. Endocrinol.* **90,** 197–201.

71. Yagi, H., Ozono, K., Miyake, H., Nagashima, K., Kuroume, T., and Pike, J. W. (1993). A new point mutation in the deoxyribonucleic acid-binding domain of the vitamin D receptor in a kindred with hereditary 1,25-dihydroxyvitamin D-resistant rickets. *J. Clin. Endocrinol. Metab.* **76,** 509–512.

72. Arai, K., Karl, M., Irony, I., Suzuki, Y., and Chrousos, G. P. (1993). The mineralocorticoid receptor cDNA in type I pseudohypoaldosteronism (aldosterone resistance). *Progr. Abstr. 75th Annu. Meet. Endocr. Soc.,* 285.

73. Hurley, D. M., Accili, D., Stratakis, C. A., Karl, M., Vamvakopoulos, N., Rorer, E., Constantine, K., Taylor, S. I., and Chrousos, G. P. (1991). Point mutation causing a single amino acid substitution in the hormone binding domain of the

glucocorticoid receptor in familial glucocorticoid resistance. *J. Clin. Invest.* **87**, 680–686.

74. Karl, M., Lamberts, S. W. J., Detera-Wadleigh, S. D., Encio, I. J., Stratakis, C. A., Hurley, D. M., Accili, D., and Chrousos, G. P. (1993). Familial glucocorticoid resistance caused by a splice site deletion in the human glucocorticoid receptor gene. *J. Clin. Endocrinol. Metab.* **76**, 683–689.

75. Malchoff, D. M., Brufsky, A., Reardon, G., McDermott, P., Javier, E. C., Bergh, C. H., Rowe, D., and Malchoff, C. D. (1993). A mutation of the glucocorticoid receptor in primary cortisol resistance. *J. Clin. Invest.* **91**, 1918–1925.

76. Morrison, N. A., Qi, J. C., Tokita, A., Kelly, P. J., Crofts, L., Nguyen, T. V., Sambrook, P. N., and Eisman, J. A. (1994). Prediction of bone density from vitamin D receptor alleles. *Nature (London)* **367**, 284–287.

77. New, M. I., Gertner, J., Chilton, D., and Thompson, E. B. (1992). A new endocrinopathy: Cushingoid features owing to increased number of glucocorticoid receptors rather than increased cortisol secretion. *Progr. Abstr. 74th Annu. Meet. Endocr. Soc.*, 436.

78. Graham, M. L., Krett, N. L., Miller, L. A., Leslie, K. K., Gordon, D. F., Wood, W. M., Wei, L. L., and Horwitz, K. B. (1990). T47D$_{CO}$ cells, genetically unstable and containing estrogen receptor mutations, are a model for the progression of breast cancers to hormone resistance. *Cancer Res.* **50**, 6208–6217.

79. Jiang, S. Y., Langan-Fahey, S. M., Stella, A. L., McCague, R., and Jordan, V. C. (1992). Point mutation of estrogen receptor (ER) in the ligand-binding domain changes the pharmacology of antiestrogens in ER-negative breast cancer cells stably expressing complementary DNAs for ER. *Mol. Endocrinol.* **6**, 2167–2174.

80. McGuire, W. L., Chamness, G. C., and Fuqua, S. A. W. (1992). Abnormal estrogen receptor in clinical breast cancer. *J. Steroid Biochem. Mol. Biol.* **43**, 243–247.

81. Sluyser, M. (1992). Role of estrogen receptor variants in the development of hormone resistance in breast cancer. *Clin. Biochem.* **25**, 407–414.

82. Gehring, U. (1986). Genetics of glucocorticoid receptors. *Mol. Cell. Endocrinol.* **48**, 89–96.

83. Palmer, L. A., Hukku, B., and Harmon, J. M. (1992). Human glucocorticoid receptor gene deletion following exposure to cancer chemotherapeutic drugs and chemical mutagens. *Cancer Res.* **52**, 6612–6618.

84. Moalli, P. A., Pillay, S., Krett, N. L., and Rosen, S. T. (1993). Alternately spliced glucocorticoid receptor messenger RNAs in glucocorticoid-resistant human multiple myeloma cells. *Cancer Res.* **53**, 3877–3879.

85. Veldscholte, J., Ris-Stalpers, C., Kuiper, G. G. J. M., Jenster, G., Berrevoets, C., Claassen, E., van Rooij, H. C. J., Trapman, J., Brinkman, A. O., and Mulder, E. (1990). A mutation in the ligand binding domain of the androgen receptor of human LNCaP cells affects steroid binding characteristics and response to antiandrogens. *Biochem. Biophys. Res. Commun.* **173**, 534–540.

86. Culig, Z., Hobisch, A., Cronauer, M. V., Cato, A. C. B., Hittmair, A., Radmayr, C., Eberle, J., Bartsch, G., and Klocker, H. (1993). Mutant androgen receptor detected in an advanced-stage prostatic carcinoma is activated by adrenal androgens and progesterone. *Mol. Endocrinol.* **7**, 1541–1550.

87. Chang, K. S., Stass, S. A., Chu, D. T., Deaven, L. L., Trujillo, J. M., and Freireich, E. J. (1992). Characterization of a fusion cDNA (RARA/*myl*) transcribed from the t(15;17) translocation breakpoint in acute promyelocytic leukemia. *Mol. Cell. Biol.* **12**, 800–810.

88. Kastner, P., Perez, A., Lutz, Y., Rochette-Egly, C., Gaub, M. P., Durand, B., Lanotte, M., Berger, R., and Chambon, P. (1992). Structure, localization and transcriptional properties of two classes of retinoic acid receptor α fusion proteins in acute promyelocytic leukemia (APL): Structural similarities with a new family of oncoproteins. *EMBO J.* **11**, 629–642.

89. Kruyt, F. A. E., van der Veer, L. J., Mader, S., van den Brink, C. E., Feijen, A., Jonk, L. J. C., Kruijer, W., and van der Saag, P. T. (1992). Retinoic acid resistance of the variant embryonal carcinoma cell line RAC65 is caused by expression of a truncated RARα. *Differentiation* **49**, 27–37.

90. Makino, H., Taira, M., Shimada, F., Hashimoto, N., Suzuki, Y., Nozaki, O., Hatanaka, Y., and Yoshida, S. (1992). Insulin receptor gene mutation: A molecular genetical and functional analysis. *Cell. Signal.* **4**, 351–363.

91. O'Rahilly, S., and Moller, D. E. (1992). Mutant insulin receptors in syndromes of insulin resistance. *Clin. Endocrinol. (Oxford)* **36**, 121–132.

92. Taylor, S. I., Cama, A., Accili, D., Barbetti, F., Quon, M. J., de la Luz Sierra, M., Suzuki, Y., Koller, E., Levy-Toledano, R., Wertheimer, E., Moncada, V. Y., Kadowaki, H., and Kadawaki, T. (1992). Mutations in the insulin receptor gene. *Endocr. Rev.* **13**, 566–595.

93. Iwanishi, M., Haruta, T., Takata, Y., Ishibashi, O., Sasaoka, T., Egawa, K., Imamura, T., Naitou, K., Itazu, T., and Kobayashi, M. (1993). A mutation (Trp 1193→Leu 1193) in the tyrosine kinase domain of the insulin receptor associated with type A syndrome of insulin resistance. *Diabetologia* **36**, 414–422.

94. Cocozza, S., Porcellini, A., Riccardi, G., Monticelli, A., Condorelli, G., Ferrara, A., Pianese, L., Miele, C., Capaldo, B., Beguinot, F., and Varrone, S. (1992). NIDDM associated with mutation in tyrosine kinase domain of insulin receptor gene. *Diabetes* **41**, 521–526.

95. Elbein, S. C., Sorensen, L. K., and Schumacher, M. C. (1993). Methionine for valine substitution in exon 17 of the insulin receptor gene in a pedigree with familial NIDDM. *Diabetes* **42**, 429–434.

96. Huang, Z., Bodkin, N. L., Ortmeyer, H. K., Hansen, B. C., and Shuldiner, A. R. (1993). The rhesus insulin receptor gene: A thrifty gene in a diabetes-prone species? *Progr. Abstr. 75th Annu. Meet. Endocr. Soc.*, 426.

97. Stephenson, D. A., Mercola, M., Anderson, E., Wang, C., Stiles, C. D., Bowen-Pope, D. F., and Chapman, V. M. (1991). Platelet-derived growth factor receptor α-subunit gene (*Pdgfra*) is deleted in the mouse patch (*Ph*) mutation. *Proc. Natl. Acad. Sci. U.S.A.* **88**, 6–10.

98. Sprintz, R. A., Holmes, S. A., Ramesar, R., Greenberg, J., Curtis, D., and Beighton, P. (1992). Mutations of the *KIT* (mast/stem cell growth factor receptor) proto-oncogene account for a continuous range of phenotypes in human piebaldism. *Am. J. Hum. Genet.* **51**, 1058–1065.

99. Fleischman, R. A. (1993). From white spots to stem cells: The role of the Kit receptor in mammalian development. *Trends Genet.* **9**, 285–290.

100. Tsujimura, T., Hirota, S., Nomura, S., Niwa, Y., Yamazaki, M., Tono, T., Morii, E., Kim, H. M., Kondo, K., Nishimune, Y., and Kitamura, Y. (1991). Characterization of *Ws* mutant allele of rats: A 12-base deletion in tyrosine kinase domain of c-*kit* gene. *Blood* **78**, 1942–1946.

101. Boultwood, J., Rack, K., Kelly, S., Madden, J., Sakaguchi, A. Y., Wang, L. M., Oscier, D. G., Buckle, V. J., and Wainscoat, J. S. (1991). Loss of both *CSF1R* (*FMS*) alleles in patients with myelodysplasia and a chromosome 5 deletion. *Proc. Natl. Acad. Sci. U.S.A.* **88**, 6176–6180.

102. Pan, Y., Metzenberg, A., Das, S., Jing, B., and Gitschier, J. (1992). Mutations in the V2 vasopressin receptor gene are associated with X-linked nephrogenic diabetes insipidus. *Nature Genet.* **2,** 103–106.

103. Rosenthal, W., Seibold, A., Antaramian, A., Lonergan, M., Arthus, M. F., Hendy, G. N., Birnbaumer, M., and Bichet, D. G. (1992). Molecular identification of the gene responsible for congenital nephrogenic diabetes insipidus. *Nature (London)* **359,** 233–235.

104. Clark, A. J. L., McLoughlin, L., and Grossman, A. (1993). Familial glucocorticoid deficiency associated with point mutation in the adrenocorticotropin receptor. *Lancet* **341,** 461–462.

105. Parma, J., Duprez, L., Van Sande, J., Cochaux, P., Gervy, C., Mockel, J., Dumont, J., and Vassart, G. (1993). Somatic mutations in the thyrotropin receptor gene cause hyperfunctioning thyroid adenomas. *Nature (London)* **365,** 649–651.

106. Shenker, A., Laue, L., Kosugi, S., Merendino, J. J., Minegishi, T., and Cutler, G. B. (1993). A constitutively activating mutation of the luteinizing hormone receptor in familial male precocious puberty. *Nature (London)* **365,** 652–654.

107. Kremer, H., Mariman, E., Otten, B. J., Moll, G. W., Stoelinga, G. B. A., Wit, J. M., Jansen, M., Drop, S. L., Faas, B., Ropers, H. H., and Brunner, H. G. (1993). Cosegregation of missense mutations of the luteinizing hormone receptor gene with familial male-limited precocious puberty. *Hum. Mol. Genet.* **2,** 1779–1783.

108. Robbins, L. S., Nadeau, J. H., Johnson, K. R., Kelly, M. A., Roselli-Rehfuss, L., Baack, E., Mountjoy, K. G., and Cone, R. D. (1993). Pigmentation phenotypes of variant extension locus alleles result from point mutations that alter MSH receptor function. *Cell* **72,** 827–834.

109. Phillips, J. A. (1992). Molecular biology of growth hormone receptor dysfunction. *Acta Pædiatr.* **383 (Suppl.)** 127–131.

110. Noguchi, M., Yi, H., Rosenblatt, H. M., Filipovich, A. H., Adelstein, S., Modi, W. S., McBride, O. W., and Leonard, W. J. (1993). Interleukin-2 receptor γ chain mutation results in X-linked severe combined immunodeficiency in humans. *Cell* **73,** 147–157.

111. Vetrie, D., Vorechovsky, I., Sideras, P., Holland, J., Davies, A., Flinter, F., Hammarström, L., Kinnon, D. R., Levinsky, R., Bobrow, M., Smith, C. I. E., and Bentley, D. R. (1993). The gene involved in X-linked agammaglobulinaemia is a member of the *src* family of protein-tyrosine kinases. *Nature (London)* **361,** 226–233.

112. Nakatsu, Y., Tyndale, R. F., DeLorey, T. M., Durham-Pierre, D., Gardner, J. M., McDaniel, H. J., Nguyen, Q., Wagstaff, J., Lalande, M., Sikela, J. M., Olsen, R. W., Tobin, A. J., and Brilliant, M. H. (1993). A cluster of three GABA$_A$ receptor subunit genes is deleted in a neurological mutant of the mouse *p* locus. *Nature (London)* **364,** 448–450.

113. Sinnett, D., Wagstaff, J., Glatt, K., Woolf, E., Kirkness, E. J., and Lalande, M. (1993). High-resolution mapping of the γ-aminobutyric acid receptor subunit β3 and α5 gene cluster on chromosome 15q11-q13, and localization of breakpoints in two Angelman syndrome patients. *Am. J. Hum. Genet.* **52,** 1216–1229.

114. Korpi, E. R., Kleingoor, C., Kettenmann, H., and Seeburg, P. H. (1993). Benzodiazepine-induced motor impairment linked to point mutation in cerebellar GABA$_A$ receptor. *Nature (London)* **361,** 356–359.

115. Shiang, R., Ryan, S. G., Zhu, Y. Z., Hahn, A. F., O'Connell, P., and Wasmuth, J. J. (1993). Mutations in the α1 subunit of the inhibitory glycine receptor cause the dominant neurologic disorder, hyperekplexia. *Nature Genet.* **5,** 351–358.

116. Engel, A. G., Hutchinson, D. O., Nakano, S., Murphy, L., Griggs, R. C., Gu, Y., Hall, Z. W., and Lindstrom, J. (1993). Myasthenic syndromes attributed to mutations affecting the epsilon subunit of the acetylcholine receptor. *Ann. N.Y. Acad. Sci.* **681**, 496–508.

117. Carayon, P., Adler, G., Roulier, R., and Lissitzky, S. (1983). Heterogeneity of the Graves' immunoglobulins directed toward the thyrotropin-adenylate cyclase system. *J. Clin. Endocrinol. Metab.* **56**, 1202–1208.

118. Campino, C., Szecowka, J., Lopez, J. M., Mulchahey, J., and Serón-Ferré, M. (1992). Growth hormone (GH) receptor antibodies with GH-like activity occur spontaneously in acromegaly. *J. Clin. Endocrinol. Metab.* **74**, 751–756.

119. Protti, M. P., Manfredi, A. A., Horton, R. M., Bellone, M., and Conti-Tronconi, B. M. (1993). Myasthenia gravis: Recognition of a human autoantigen at the molecular level. *Immunol. Today* **14**, 363–368.

120. Graus, Y. M. F., and De Baets, M. H. (1993). Myasthenia gravis: An autoimmune response against the acetylcholine receptor. *Immunol. Res.* **12**, 78–100.

121. Libert, F., Lefort, A., Gerard, C., Parmentier, M., Perret, J., Ludgate, M., Dumont, J. E., and Vassart, G. (1989). Cloning, sequencing and expression of the human thyrotropin (TSH) receptor: Evidence for binding of autoantibodies. *Biochem. Biophys. Res. Commun.* **165**, 1250–1255.

122. Bednarek, J., Furmaniak, J., Wedlock, N., Kiso, Y., Baumann-Antczak, A., Fowler, S., Krishnan, H., Craft, J. A., and Smith, B. R. (1992). Steroid 21-hydroxylase is a major autoantigen involved in adult onset autoimmune Addison's disease. *FEBS Lett.* **309**, 51–55.

123. Krohn, K., Uibo, R., Aavik, E., Peterson, P., and Savilahti, K. (1992). Identification by molecular cloning of an autoantigen associated with Addison's disease as steroid 17α-hydroxylase. *Lancet* **339**, 770–773.

124. Atkinson, M. A., and Maclaren, N. K. (1993). Islet cell autoantigens in insulin-dependent diabetes. *J. Clin. Invest.* **92**, 1608–1616.

125. Kaufman, D. L., Clare-Salzler, M., Tian, J., Forsthuber, T., Ting, G. S. P., Robinson, P., Atkinson, M. A., Sercarz, E. E., Tobin, A. J., and Lehmann, P. V. (1993). Spontaneous loss of T-cell tolerance and glutamic acid decarboxylase in murine insulin-dependent diabetes. *Nature (London)* **366**, 69–72.

126. Tisch, R., Yang, X. D., Singer, S. M., Liblau, R. S., Fugger, L., and McDevitt, H. O. (1993). Immune response to glutamic acid decarboxylase correlates with insulitis in non-obese diabetic mice. *Nature (London)* **366**, 72–75.

127. Patten, J. L., Johns, D. R., Valle, D., Eil, C., Gruppuso, P. A., Steele, G., Smallwood, P. M., and Levine, M. A. (1990). Mutation in the gene encoding the stimulatory G protein of adenylate cyclase in Albright's hereditary osteodystrophy. *N. Engl. J. Med.* **322**, 1412–1419.

128. Weinstein, L. S., Gejman, P. V., Friedman, E., Kadowaki, T., Collins, R. M., Gershon, E. S., and Spiegel, A. M. (1990). Mutations of the G_s α-subunit gene in Albright hereditary osteodystrophy detected by denaturing gradient gel electrophoresis. *Proc. Natl. Acad. Sci. U.S.A.* **87**, 8287–8290.

129. Miric, A., Vechio, J. D., and Levine, M. A. (1993). Heterogeneous mutations in the gene encoding the α-subunit of the stimulatory G protein of adenylyl cyclase in Albright hereditary osteodystrophy. *J. Clin. Endocrinol. Metabol.* **76**, 1560–1568.

130. Van Dop, C., and Bourne, H. R. (1983). Pseudohypoparathyroidism. *Annu. Rev. Med.* **34**, 259–266.

131. O'Sullivan, C., Barton, C. M., Staddon, S. L., Brown, C. L., and Lemoine, N. R. (1991). Activating point mutations of the *gsp* oncogene in human thyroid adenomas. *Mol. Carcinog.* **4**, 345–349.

132. Weinstein, L. S., Shenker, A., Gejman, P. V., Merino, M. J., Friedman, E., and Spiegel, A. M. (1991). Activating mutations of the stimulatory G protein in the McCune–Albright syndrome. *N. Engl. J. Med.* **325**, 1688–1695.

133. Schwindinger, W. F., Francomano, C. A., and Levine, M. A. (1992). Identification of a mutation in the gene encoding the α subunit of the stimulatory G protein of adenylyl cyclase in McCune-Albright syndrome. *Proc. Natl. Acad. Sci. U.S.A.* **89**, 5152–5156.

134. Lyons, J., Landis, C. A., Harsh, G., Vallar, L., Grünewald, K., Feichtinger, H., Duh, Q. Y., Clark, O. H., Kawasaki, E., Bourne, H. R., and McCormick, F. (1990). Two G protein oncogenes in human endocrine tumors. *Science* **249**, 655–659.

135. Gutmann, D. H., and Collins, F. S. (1993). The neurofibromatosis type 1 gene and its protein product, neurofibromin. *Neuron* **10**, 335–343.

136. Olson, M. F., Krolczyk, A. J., Gorman, K. B., Steinberg, R. A., and Schimmer, B. P. (1993). Molecular basis for the 3′,5′-cyclic adenosine monophosphate resistance of Kin mutant Y1 adrenocortical tumor cells. *Mol. Endocrinol.* **7**, 477–487.

137. Steinberg, R. A., and Gorman, K. B. (1992). Linked spontaneous CGTTA mutations at CpG sites in the gene for protein kinase regulatory subunit. *Mol. Cell. Biol.* **12**, 767–772.

138. Bongarzone, I., Monzini, N., Borrello, M. G., Carcano, C., Ferraresi, G., Arighi, E., Mondellini, P., Porta, G. D., and Pierotti, M. A. (1993). Molecular characterization of a thyroid tumor-specific transforming sequence formed by the fusion of *ret* tyrosine kinase and the regulatory subunit RIα of cyclic AMP-dependent protein kinase A. *Mol. Cell. Biol.* **13**, 358–366.

139. Shultz, L. D., Schweitzer, P. A., Rajan, T. V., Yi, T., Ihle, J. N., Matthews, R. J., Thomas, M. L., and Beier, D. R. (1993). Mutations at the murine motheaten locus are within the hematopoietic cell protein-tyrosine phosphatase (*Hcph*) gene. *Cell* **73**, 1445–1454.

140. Tsui, H. W., Siminovitch, K. A., de Souza, L., and Tsui, F. W. L. (1993). Motheaten and viable motheaten mice have mutations in the haematopoietic cell phosphatase gene. *Nature Genet.* **4**, 124–129.

141. Chen, C. N., Denome, S., and Davis, R. L. (1986). Molecular analysis of cDNA clones and the corresponding genomic coding sequences of the *Drosophila* dunce⁺ gene, the structural gene for cAMP phosphodiesterase. *Proc. Natl. Acad. Sci. U.S.A.* **83**, 9313–9317.

142. Pittler, S. J., and Baehr, W. (1991). Identification of a nonsense mutation in the rod photoreceptor cGMP phosphodiesterase β-subunit gene of the *rd* mouse. *Proc. Natl. Acad. Sci. U.S.A.* **88**, 8322–8326.

143. Suber, M. L., Pittler, S. J., Qin, N., Wright, G. C., Holcombe, V., Lee, R. H., Craft, C. M., Lolley, R. N., Baehr, W., and Hurwitz, R. L. (1993). Irish setter dogs affected with rod/cone dysplasia contain a nonsense mutation in the rod cGMP phosphodiesterase β-subunit gene. *Proc. Natl. Acad. Sci. U.S.A.* **90**, 3968–3972.

144. McLaughlin, M. E., Sandberg, M. A., Berson, E. L., and Dryja, T. P. (1993). Recessive mutations in the gene encoding the β-subunit of rod phosphodiesterase in patients with retinitis pigmentosa. *Nature Genet.* **4**, 130–134.

145. Bloomquist, B. T., Shortridge, R. D., Schneuwly, S., Perdew, M., Montell, C.,

Steller, H., Rubin, G., and Pak, W. L. (1988). Isolation of a putative phospholipase C gene of Drosophila, *norpA*, and its role in phosphotransduction. *Cell* **54,** 723–733.

146. Smith, D. P., Ranganathan, R., Hardy, R. W., Marx, J., Tsuchida, T., and Zuker, C. S. (1991). Photoreceptor deactivation and retinal degeneration mediated by a photoreceptor-specific protein kinase C. *Science* **254,** 1478–1484.

147. Hay, J. C., and Martin, T. F. J. (1993). Phosphatidylinositol transfer protein required for ATP-dependent priming of Ca^{2+}-activated secretion. *Nature (London)* **366,** 572–576.

148. Vihtelic, T. S., Goebl, M., Milligan, S., O'Tousa, J. E., and Hyde, D. R. (1993). Localization of *Drosophila retinal degeneration B*, a membrane-associated phosphatidylinositol transfer protein. *J. Cell Biol.* **122,** 1013–1022.

149. Fujii, J., Otsu, K., Zorzato, F., de Leon, S., Khanna, V. K., Weiler, J. E., O'Brien, P. J., and MacLennan, D. H. (1991). Identification of a mutation in porcine ryanodine receptor associated with malignant hyperthermia. *Science* **253,** 448–451.

150. Zhang, Y., Chen, H. S., Khanna, V. K., De Leon, S., Phillips, M. S., Schappert, K., Britt, B. A., Brownell, A. K. W., and MacLennan, D. H. (1993). A mutation in the human ryanodine receptor gene associated with central core disease. *Nature Genet.* **5,** 46–50.

151. Bell, G. I., Froguel, P., Nishi, S., Pilkis, S. J., Stoffel, M., Takeda, J., Vionnet, N., and Yasuda, K. (1993). Mutations of the human glucokinase gene and diabetes mellitus. *Trends Endocrinol. Metab.* **4,** 86–90.

152. Froguel, P., Zouali, H., Vionnet, N., Velho, G., Vaxillaire, M., Sun, F., Lesage, S., Stoffel, M., Takeda, J., Passa, P., Permutt, M. A., Beckmann, J. S., Bell, G. I., and Cohen, D. (1993). Familial hyperglycemia due to mutations in glucokinase: Definition of a subtype of diabetes mellitus. *N. Engl. J. Med.* **328,** 697–702.

153. van den Ouweland, J. M. W., Lemkes, H. H. P. J., Ruitenbeek, W., Sandkuijl, L. A., de Vijlder, M. F., Struyvenberg, P. A. A., van de Kamp, J. J. P., and Maassen, J. A. (1992). Mutation in mitochondrial tRNA$^{Leu(UUR)}$ gene in a large pedigree with maternally transmitted type II diabetes mellitus and deafness. *Nature Genet.* **1,** 368–371.

154. Rötig, A., Cormier, V., Chatelain, P., Francois, R., Saudubray, J. M., Rustin, P., and Munnich, A. (1993). Deletion of mitochondrial DNA in a case of early-onset diabetes mellitus, optic atrophy, and deafness (Wolfram syndrome, MIM 222300). *J. Clin. Invest.* **91,** 1095–1098.

155. Leahy, J. L., and Boyd, A. E. (1993). Diabetes genes in non-insulin-dependent diabetes mellitus. *N. Engl. J. Med.* **328,** 56–57.

List of Abbreviations

A	Adenosine receptor
AA	Arachidonic acid
αAR	α-Adrenergic receptor
ACh	Acetylcholine
ACTH	Adrenocorticotropic hormone
ADH	Antidiuretic hormone; also called vasopressin (VP)
AH	Androgenic hormone
Ah	Aromatic hydrocarbon
AKH	Adipokinetic hormone
AMF	Autocrine motility factor
AMPA	α-Amino-3-hydroxy-5-methyl-4-isoxazole propionic acid
ANF(R)	Atrial natriuretic factor (receptor)
ANS	Autonomic nervous system
ARF	ADP-ribosylation factor
Arnt	Aromatic hydrocarbon (Ah) receptor nuclear translocator
Asn	Asparagine (N)
AT	Angiotensin II
ATF	Activating transcription factor
ATP	Adenosine 5'-triphosphate
B	Bradykinin receptor
βAR	β-Adrenergic receptor
βARK	β-Adrenergic receptor kinase
BDNF	Brain-derived neurotrophic factor
bHLH	Basic helix–loop–helix transcription factor
bHLH-ZIP	Basic helix–loop–helix zipper transcription factor
bp	Base pairs of nucleotides
BPCH	Black pigment-concentration hormone
bya	Billion years ago
bZIP	Basic zipper transcription factor

C	Catalytic subunit of PKA
CaM	Calmodulin
CaMK	CaM-dependent protein kinase
cAMP	3′,5′-Cyclic AMP
CBG	Corticosteroid-binding globulin
CCAP	Crustacean cardioactive peptide
CCK	Cholecystokinin
cCMP	3′,5′-Cyclic CMP
Cdc2	Cell division cycle kinase 2; also called MPF
cDNA	DNA synthesized from (and therefore complementary to) mRNA
C/EBP	CCAAT/enhancer-binding protein
cGMP	3′,5′-Cyclic GMP
CGRP	Calcitonin gene-related peptide
CHH	Crustacean hyperglycemic hormone
CK	Casein kinase
CNTF(R)	Ciliary neurotropic factor (receptor)
CO	Carbon monoxide
COUP	Chicken ovalbumin upstream promotor
CRABP	Cellular retinoic acid binding protein
CRBP	Cellular retinal binding protein
CREB	cAMP response element binding protein
CREM	cAMP response element modulator
CRF	Corticotropin (ACTH)-releasing factor
CSF-1(R)	Colony-stimulating factor-1 (receptor): also called macrophage colony stimulating factor (M-CSF)
CT	Calcitonin
CTP	Cytidine 5′-triphosphate
CTSH	Chloride transport-stimulating hormone
CURL	Compartment for uncoupling receptor and ligand
D	Dopamine receptor
DBD	DNA-binding domain
DBI	Diazepam-binding inhibitor
DCC	(Anti-oncogene) deleted in colon carcinoma
DFMO	α-Difluoromethylornithine
DG	Diacylglycerol
DH	Diapause hormone
DHCC	Dihydroxycholecalciferol
DHEA	Dihydroepiandosterone
DHP	Dihydropyridine

DHT	Dihydrotestosterone
DNA-PK	DNA-activated protein kinase
DOPA	Dihydroxyphenylalanine
dsDNA	Double-stranded DNA
E	Epinephrine
E_2	Estradiol
EBV	Epstein–Barr virus
EcR	Ecdysone receptor
EDNH	Egg development neurosecretory hormone
EGF(R)	Epidermal growth factor (receptor)
EGTA	Ethylene glycol-*bis*(β-aminoethyl ether)-N,N,N',N'-tetraacetic acid
EH	Eclosion hormone
eIF-2α	Eukaryotic initiation factor-2α
EPO(R)	Erythropoietin (receptor)
ER	Estrogen receptor
ERE	Estrogen hormone response element
ERK	Extracellular-signal regulated kinase; also called MAP kinase (MAPK)
ERR	Estrogen receptor-related receptor
ET	Endothelin
ETYA	5,8,11,14-Eicosatetraynoic acid
FAK	Focal adhesion kinase
FCTH	Follicle cell tropic hormone
FGF(R)	Fibroblast growth factor (receptor)
FKBP	FK506 binding protein
fMLP	Formylmethionylleucylphenylalanine
FMRFamide	Phenylalanylmethionylarginylphenylalaninamide (a neuroactive tetrapeptide)
FNIII	Fibronectin type III domain
FSH(R)	Follicle-stimulating hormone (receptor)
G	GTP-binding protein (usually followed by a subscript designating the transduction system to which it is associated)
GABA	γ-Aminobutryic acid
GAF	Interferonγ- activated factor
GAP	GTPase-activating protein
GAS	Interferonγ- activated site
GC	Guanylate cyclase
G-CSF(R)	Granulocyte–colony stimulating factor (receptor)
GDI	GDP dissociation inhibitor

GDS	GDP dissociation stimulator
GH(R)	Growth hormone (receptor)
GHRF	Growth hormone-releasing factor
GI	Gastrointestinal
GIH	Gonad-inhibiting hormone
GIP	Gastric inhibitory peptide; GTPase inhibiting protein
GLP	Glucagon-like peptide
Glu(R)	Glutamate (receptor)
Gly	Glycine (G)
GM-CSF(R)	Granulocyte–macrophage colony-stimulating factor (receptor)
GnRH	Gonadotropin-releasing hormone; also called LH-releasing hormone (LHRH)
GR	Glucocorticoid receptor
Grb2	Growth factor receptor-bound protein 2
GRE	Glucocorticoid response element
GRP	Gastrin-releasing peptide
GSK-3	Glycogen synthase kinase-3
GTP	Guanosine 5′-triphosphate
H	Histamine receptor
HAVA	α-Hydrazino-δ-aminovaleric acid
hCG	Human chorionic gonadotropin
HER	Human EGF receptor homolog
HETE	Hydroxy-6,8,11,14-eicosatetraenoic acid
HGF(R)	Hepatocyte growth factor (receptor)
hGH	Human growth hormone
HIV	Human immunodeficiency virus
HMG	High-mobility-group nuclear protein
HMG CoA	Hydroxymethylglutaryl coenzyme A
HPETE	5-Hydroxyperoxy-6,8,11,14-eicosatetraenoic acid
hPL	Human placental lactogen (human chorionic somatomammotropin)
HRE	Hormone response element
hsp	Heat shock protein (usually followed by a number designating its molecular weight)
5-HT	5-Hydroxytryptamine; also called serotonin
HTH	Helix–turn–helix transcription factor
IFN	Interferon
Ig	Immunoglobulin
IGFBP	Insulin-like growth factor binding protein

IGF(R)	Insulin-like growth factor (receptor)
IL	Interleukin
IP_2	Inositol 1,4-bisphosphate
IP_3(R)	Inositol 1,4,5-trisphosphate (receptor)
IP_4	Inositol 1,3,4,5-tetrakisphosphate
IRE	Iron response element
IRF	Iron response factor
IRS-1	Insulin receptor substrate-1
ISGF	IFN-stimulated gene factor
JH	Juvenile hormones
kb	Kilobases of nucleotides
kDa	Kilodalton
KGF	Keratinocyte growth factor
KL	Kit ligand; also called MGF, SCF, and SLF
LBD	Ligand-binding domain
LBS	Ligand-binding subunit
LH(R)	Luteinizing hormone (receptor)
LHRH	Luteinizing hormone-releasing hormone; also called gonado-tropin-releasing hormone (GnRH)
LIF(R)	Leukemia inhibitory factor (receptor)
LNGFR	Low-affinity (or low-molecular-weight) NGF receptor
LTR	Long terminal repeat
LX	Lipoxin
MAPK	Mitogen-activated protein kinase; also called extracellular-signal regulated kinase (ERK)
M-CSF	Macrophage colony-stimulating factor; also called CSF-1
MEK	MAPK-ERK-activating kinase; also called MAPK kinase (MAPKK)
MGBG	Methylglyoxal *bis*(guanylhydrazone)
MGF	Mast cell growth factor; also called KL, SCF, and SLF
mGluR	Metabotropic glutamate receptor
MGSA	Melanocyte growth stimulatory activity
MHC	Major histocompatibility complex
MIH	Molt-inhibiting hormone
MIP	Macrophage inflammatory protein
MIS	Müllerian inhibiting substance
MLCK	Myosin light chain kinase
MMTV	Mouse mammary tumor virus
MPF	Maturation (or M phase) promoting factor; also called Cdc2
MR	Mineralocorticoid receptor

MRCH	Melanization and reddish coloration hormone
mRNA	Messenger RNA
MGBG	Methylglyoxal *bis*(guanylhydrazone)
MSH	Melanocyte-stimulating hormone
Multi-CSF	Multi-colony stimulating factor; also called IL-3
mya	Million years ago
N	Asparagine
nAChR	Nicotinic acetycholine receptor
NAD	Nicotinamide adenine dinucleotide
NDGA	Nordihydroguaiaretic acid
NE	Norepinephrine
NGF	Nerve growth factor
NHE	Sodium (Na)-hydrogen exchanger
NIDDM	Non-insulin-dependent diabetes mellitus
NK(R)	Neurokinin (receptor)
NKSF(R)	Natural killer cell stimulatory factor (receptor); also called IL-12
NLS	Nuclear location signal
NMDA	*N*-Methyl-D-aspartate
NO	Nitric oxide
NSC-CC	Neurosecretory cells-corpus cardiacum
NT	Neurotropin
ODC	Ornithine decarboxylase
ORF	Open reading frame
OT	Oxytocin
p85	Regulatory subunit of PI3K
p110	Catalytic subunit of PI3K
PA	Phosphatidic acid
PACAP	Pituitary adenylate cyclase-activating polypeptide
PAF	Platelet-activating factor
PAK	p21-activated kinase
PBAN	Pheromone biosynthesis-activating neuropeptide
PC	Phosphatidylcholine
PC-PLA$_2$	PC-specific phospholipase A$_2$
PC-PLC	PC-specific phospholipase C
PC-PLD	PC-specific phospholipase D
PDE	Phosphodiesterase
PD-ECGF	Platelet-derived endothelial cell growth factor
PDGF(R)	Platelet-derived growth factor (receptor)
PDH	Pigment dispersing hormone

PDI	Protein disulfide isomerase
PDK	Proline-directed kinase
PDS	Pigment-dispersing factor
PE	Phosphatidylethanolamine
PEP	Phosphoenolpyruvate
PG	Prostaglandin (usually followed by a third letter designating the head group)
pGlu	Pyroglutamic acid
PgR	Progesterone receptor
PH	Pleckstrin homology domain
PI	Phosphoinositide (phosphatidylinositol)
PI3,5-P_2	Phosphatidylinositol 3,5-bisphosphate
PI3K	Phosphatidylinositol-3 kinase
PI-glycan	Phosphatidylinositol-glycan
PIP_2	Phosphatidylinositol 4,5-bisphosphate
PKA	Protein kinase A (cAMP-dependent protein kinase)
PKC	Protein kinase C (calcium-activated, phospholipid-dependent protein kinase)
PKG	Protein kinase G (cGMP-dependent protein kinase)
PKI	Protein kinase inhibitor
PL	Phospholipase
PLC	Phospholipase C
POH	Permanent ovarian hormone
POMC	Proopiomelanocortin
PP	Protein phosphatase
PPAR	Peroxisome proliferator-activated receptor
PPI	Polyphosphoinositide
PRL(R)	Prolactin (receptor)
PTH	Parathormone
PTP	Protein tyrosine phosphatase
PTTH	Prothoracicotropic hormone
R	Regulatory subunit of PKA
RACK	Receptor for activated C kinase
RAR	Retinoic acid receptor
Rb	(Anti-oncogene deleted in) retinoblastoma
RIA	Radioimmunoassay
RNP	Ribonucleoprotein
RPCH	Red pigment-concentration hormone
rRNA	Ribosomal RNA
RSK	Ribosomal S6 kinase; also called S6 kinase (S6K)

RTK	Receptor tyrosine kinase
RXR	Retinoic acid X receptor
S	Serine
S6K	S6 kinase; also called ribosomal S6 kinase (RSK)
SAH	*S*-Adenosylhomocysteine
SAM	*S*-Adenosylmethionine
SCF	Stem cell growth factor; also called KL, MGF, and SLF
Ser	Serine (S)
Serpin	Serine protease inhibitor
SH	Src homology domain
Shc	Src homology 2-containing protein
SIE	*sis*-Inducible element
SIF	*sis*-Inducible factor
SLF	Steel factor; also called KL, MGF, and SCF
SRF	Serum response factor
SRIF	Somatotropin (GH) release-inhibiting factor (somatostatin)
T	Testosterone; threonine
T_3	Triiodothyronine
T_4	Thyroxine
TAD	Transcriptional activation domain
TBG	Thyronine-binding protein
TBPA	Thyronine-binding prealbumin
TCF	Ternary complex factor
TeBG	Testosterone – estrogen-binding globulin
TGF(R)	Transforming growth factor (receptor)
Thr	Threonine (T)
7-TMS	Seven-transmembrane-segment
TNF(R)	Tumor necrosis factor (receptor)
TPA	12-*O*-Tetradecanoylphorbol-13-acetate
TR	Thyroid receptor
TRH	Thyrotropin (TSH)-releasing hormone
tRNA	Transfer RNA
TSH	Thyroid-stimulating hormone (thyrotropin)
TX	Thromboxane
Tyr	Tyrosine (Y)
VDR	Vitamin D receptor
VEGF	Vascular endothelial growth factor
VIP	Vasoactive intestinal peptide
VP	Vasopressin; also called antidiuretic hormone (ADH)

VPF	Vascular permeability factor
VSOH	Vitellogenin-stimulating ovarian hormone
WT1	(Anti-oncogene deleted in) Wilms' tumor
Y	Tyrosine

Index[1]

[1]T refers to table numbers and F to figure numbers.